Study Guide for

Medical-Surgical Nursing: Assessment and Management of Clinical Problems

Ninth Edition

Prepared by:

Susan A. Sandstrom, RN, MSN, BC, CNE
Associate Professor in Nursing, Retired
College of Saint Mary
Omaha, Nebraska

Sharon L. Lewis, RN, PhD, FAAN
Shannon Ruff Dirksen, RN, PhD, FAAN
Margaret McLean Heitkemper, RN, PhD, FAAN
Linda Bucher, RN, PhD, CEN, CNE

Reviewed by:

Charles D. Rogers, RN, MSN
Advanced Cardiac Life Support Provider
Assistant Professor of Nursing
Morehead State University
Morehead, Kentucky

Collin Bowman-Woodall, RN, MS
Assistant Professor
Samuel Merritt University
San Francisco Peninsula Campus
San Mateo, California

ELSEVIER
MOSBY

3251 Riverport Lane
St. Louis, Missouri 63043

STUDY GUIDE FOR MEDICAL-SURGICAL NURSING:
ASSESSMENT AND MANAGEMENT OF CLINICAL PROBLEMS

ISBN: 978-0-323-09147-3

Although for mechanical reasons all pages of this publication are perforated, only those pages imprinted with an Elsevier Inc. copyright notice are intended for removal.

NANDA International Nursing Diagnoses: Definitions and Classifications 2012-2014; Herdman T.H. (ED); copyright © 2012, 1994-2012 NANDA International; published by John Wiley & Sons, Limited.

ISBN: 9780323091473

Executive Content Strategist: Kristin Geen
Content Manager: Jamie Randall
Associate Content Development Specialist: Melissa Rawe
Publishing Services Manager: Jeff Patterson
Project Manager: Megan Isenberg
Design Direction: Maggie Reid
Cover Designer: Maggie Reid

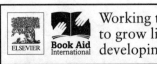
Printed in the United States of America

Last digit is the print number: 9 8 7 6 5 4 3 2 1

Contents

Professional Nursing Practice

1. Using the American Nurses Association's definition of nursing, which activities are within the domain of nursing (*select all that apply*)?

   _____ a. Implementing intake and output for a patient who is vomiting

   _____ b. Establishing and implementing a stress management program for family caregivers of patients with Alzheimer's disease

   _____ c. Explaining the risks associated with the planned surgical procedure when a preoperative patient inquires about risks

   _____ d. Developing and performing a study to compare the health status of older patients who live alone with the status of older patients who live with family members

   _____ e. Identifying the effect of an investigational drug on patients' hemoglobin levels

   _____ f. Using a biofeedback machine to teach a patient with cancer how to manage chronic pain

   _____ g. Preventing pneumonia in an immobile patient by implementing frequent turning, coughing, and deep breathing

   _____ h. Determining and administering fluid replacement therapy needed for a patient with serious burns

   _____ i. Testifying to legislative bodies regarding the effect of health policies on culturally, socially, and economically diverse populations

2. A nurse who has worked on an orthopedic unit for several years is encouraged by the nurse manager to become certified in orthopedic nursing. What will certification in nursing require and/or provide (*select all that apply*)?

   a. A certain amount of clinical experience

   b. Successful completion of an examination

   c. Membership in specialty nursing organizations

   d. Professional recognition of expertise in a specialty area

   e. An advanced practice role that requires graduate education

3. What accurately describes the health care system in which future nurses will be employed?

   a. With improvements in medicine there will be fewer patients with chronic illnesses.

   b. Rapidly changing technology and expanding knowledge will simplify the health care environment.

   c. The Quality and Safety Education for Nurses (QSEN) project measures the ability of nursing graduates to be prepared for the reality of practice.

   d. The Joint Commission establishes National Patient Safety Goals and evidence-based solutions for nurses to promote meeting these goals by all caring for the patient.

4. What are the six competencies from Quality and Safety Education for Nurses (QSEN) that are expected of new nursing graduates?

   a.

   b.

   c.

   d.

   e.

   f.

5. Place the steps of the evidence-based practice (EBP) process in order (0 being the first step; 6 being the last step).
   _____ Make recommendations for practice or generate data
   _____ Ask a clinical question
   _____ Critically analyze the evidence
   _____ Find and collect the evidence
   _____ Evaluate the outcomes in the clinical setting
   _____ Create a spirit of inquiry
   _____ Use evidence, clinical expertise, and patient preferences to determine care

6. The following is an example of an evidence-based practice (EBP) clinical question. "In adult seizure patients, is restraint or medication more effective in protecting them from injury during a seizure?" Which word(s) in the question identify(ies) the C part of the PICOT format?
   a. Restraint
   b. Or medication
   c. During a seizure
   d. Adult seizure patients
   e. Protecting them from injury

7. Two nurses are establishing a smoking cessation program to assist patients with chronic lung disease to stop smoking. To offer the most effective program with the best outcomes, the nurses should initially
   a. search for an article that describes nursing interventions that are effective for smoking cessation.
   b. develop a clinical question that will allow them to compare different cessation methods during the program.
   c. keep comprehensive records that detail each patient's progress and ultimate outcomes from participation in the program.
   d. use evidence-based clinical practice guidelines developed from randomized controlled trials of smoking cessation methods.

8. Which standardized nursing terminologies specifically relate to the steps of the nursing process (select all that apply)?
   a. Omaha System
   b. Nursing Minimum Data Set (NMDS)
   c. Perioperative Nursing Data Set (PNDS)
   d. Nursing Outcomes Classification (NOC)
   e. Nursing Interventions Classification (NIC)
   f. NANDA International: Nursing Diagnoses

9. The nurse working in a health care facility where uniform electronic health records are used explains to the patient that the primary purpose of such a record is to
   a. reduce the cost of health care by eliminating paper records.
   b. prevent medical errors associated with traditional paper records and handwritten orders and prescriptions.
   c. force the use of standardized medical vocabularies and nursing terminologies so that outcomes of patient care can be measured.
   d. provide a single record in which all aspects of a patient's medical information are readily available to any health care provider involved in the patient's care.

10. Which actions are done primarily by an informatics nurse (select all that apply)?
   a. Designs and builds computer systems
   b. Studies the validity of nursing information
   c. Trains health care providers to provide nursing care
   d. Communicates and accesses information for nursing staff
   e. Builds systems that support the processing of nursing information

11. Match the phases of the nursing process with the descriptions (phases may be used more than once).

    _____ a. Analysis of data   1. Assessment
    _____ b. Priority setting   2. Diagnosis
    _____ c. Nursing interventions   3. Planning
    _____ d. Data collection   4. Implementation
    _____ e. Identifying patient strengths   5. Evaluation
    _____ f. Measuring patient achievement of goals
    _____ g. Setting goals
    _____ h. Identifying health problems
    _____ i. Modifying the plan of care
    _____ j. Documenting care provided

12. During the diagnosis phase of the nursing process, both nursing diagnoses and collaborative problems are identified. Which are collaborative problem statements (*select all that apply*)?

    a. Fatigue related to sleep deprivation
    b. Infection related to immunosuppression
    c. Excess fluid volume related to high sodium intake
    d. Constipation related to irregular defecation habits
    e. Hypoxia related to chronic obstructive pulmonary disease
    f. Risk for cardiac dysrhythmias related to potassium deficiency

13. For the nursing diagnoses and written patient outcomes listed below, use the Nursing Interventions Classification (NIC) to identify a specific nursing intervention to help the patient reach the outcome.

    a. Nursing diagnosis: Risk for impaired skin integrity *related to* immobility
       Patient outcome: Patient will demonstrate skin integrity free of pressure ulcers.

    b. Nursing diagnosis: Constipation *related to* inadequate fluid and fiber intake
       Patient outcome: Patient will have daily soft bowel movements in 1 week.

14. A patient with a seizure disorder is admitted to the hospital after a sustained seizure. When she tells the nurse that she has not taken her medication regularly, the nurse makes a nursing diagnosis of ineffective self-health management related to lack of knowledge regarding medication regimen and identifies the Nursing Outcomes Classification (NOC) outcome of *Compliance behavior*, with the indicator *Performs treatment regimen as prescribed, at a target rate of 3 (sometimes demonstrated)*. When the nurse tries to teach the patient about the medication regimen, the patient tells the nurse that she knows about the medication but she does not always have the money to refill the prescription. Where was the mistake made in the nursing process with this patient?

    a. Planning
    b. Diagnosis
    c. Evaluation
    d. Assessment
    e. Implementation

15. Identify the five rights of delegating nursing care (*select all that apply*).

    a. Right time
    b. Right task
    c. Right patient
    d. Right person
    e. Right dosage
    f. Right circumstance
    g. Right supervision and evaluation
    h. Right direction and communication

16. Delegation is a process used by the RN to provide safe and effective care in an efficient manner. Which nursing interventions should not be delegated to unlicensed assistive personnel (UAP) but should be performed by the RN (*select all that apply*)?
    a. Administering patient medications
    b. Ambulating stable patients
    c. Performing patient assessment
    d. Evaluating the effectiveness of patient care
    e. Feeding patients at mealtime
    f. Performing sterile procedures
    g. Providing patient teaching
    h. Obtaining vital signs on a stable patient
    i. Assisting with patient bathing

17. Match the following care planning tools to the description statement(s). There may be more than one statement per tool and some statements may be used more than once.

    Tools
    1. Nursing Care Plan
    2. Concept Maps
    3. Clinical Pathway

    Statements
    _____ A plan that directs an entire health care team
    _____ Used as guides for routine nursing care
    _____ Used in nursing education to teach the nursing process and care planning
    _____ A description of patient care required at specific times during treatment
    _____ Should be personalized and specific to each patient
    _____ A visual diagram representing relationships between patient problems, interventions, and data
    _____ Used for high-volume and highly predictable case types

18. Which nursing actions are in response to the National Patient Safety Goals (*select all that apply*)?
    a. Use restraints to prevent patient falls.
    b. Administer all medications ordered by physicians.
    c. Wash hands before and after every patient contact.
    d. Conduct a "time-out" when too tired to provide care.
    e. Use SBAR for communicating with health professionals.
    f. Evaluate the initial existence of pressure ulcers before patient dismissal.

19. Which quality of care measures influence the payment for health care services by third-party payers (*select all that apply*)?
    a. Clinical outcomes
    b. Regulatory agencies
    c. Use of evidence-based practice
    d. Adoption of information technology
    e. Occurrence of preventable conditions

Health Disparities and Culturally Competent Care

1. A 62-year-old African American man has been diagnosed with lung cancer and has been scheduled for surgery. The nurse recognizes what as the most likely major determinant of this patient's health?
   a. He is African American.
   b. He chose to smoke all of his adult life.
   c. His father died of lung cancer at about the same age.
   d. He has a limited ability to understand and act on health information.

2. A 73-year-old white woman is brought to the emergency department by a neighbor who found the woman experiencing severe abdominal and lower back pain for 2 days and nausea and vomiting for the last 24 hours. She has always refused medical care of any kind and lives by herself "up the mountain" off a dirt road in rural West Virginia. She had two children with the help of a midwife but they both left for the West Coast years ago and she rarely sees them. She was not married to the father of her children and she has not seen him in years. She has barely made a living by sewing for a doll company and receives a small amount of public assistance. As ill as she is, she is insisting that she will return home after she sees the doctor.

   List at least four factors in this situation that contribute to health disparities.
   a.

   b.

   c.

   d.

3. Limited health literacy may be associated with which conditions that lead to health disparities (*select all that apply*)?
   a. Age
   b. Place
   c. Gender
   d. Race/ethnicity
   e. Language barrier
   f. Income/education

4. Cultural safety describes care that prevents cultural imposition. The nurse must be aware of and include the knowledge of which factors in providing safe cultural care for the patient (*select all that apply*)?
   a. Values
   b. Culture
   c. Ethnicity
   d. Stereotyping
   e. Acculturation
   f. Ethnocentricity

5. What are four basic characteristics of culture?
   a. Ever-present, shared by all members, expected by all members, adapted to individuals
   b. Dynamic, shared values, provides a baseline for judging other cultures, learned from parents
   c. Ever-present, not always shared by all members, not accepted by the group, learned at school
   d. Dynamic, not always shared by all members, adapted to specific conditions, learned by communication and imitation

6. Identify the specific component of acquiring cultural competence that is reflected in creating a safe environment in which collection of relevant cultural data can be obtained during the health history and physical examination.
   a. Cultural skill
   b. Cultural encounter
   c. Cultural awareness
   d. Cultural knowledge

7. Identify one example of how each of the following cultural factors may affect the nursing care of a patient of a different culture and one example of the functioning of a health care team made up of individuals from different cultures.

Cultural Factor	Effect on Nursing Care	Health Care Team
Time orientation		
Economic factors		
Nutrition		
Personal space		
Beliefs and practices		

8. When admitting a woman experiencing a spontaneous abortion at the ambulatory care center, the nurse notes that the admission form identifies the patient's religion as Islam. What should the nurse understand about this patient?
   a. She should not receive any pork-derived products.
   b. She probably will not have purchased health insurance.
   c. Artificial contraception and abortion are prohibited.
   d. She will not be able to receive blood or blood products if an emergency develops.

9. A hospitalized Native American patient tells the nurse that later in the day a medicine man from his tribe is coming to perform a healing ceremony to return his world to balance. What should the nurse recognize about this situation?
   a. The patient does not adhere to an organized, formal religion.
   b. The patient's spiritual needs may be met by traditional rituals.
   c. The patient may be putting his health in jeopardy by relying on rituals.
   d. Native American medicine cannot alter the progression of the patient's physical illness.

10. In a Hispanic patient who claims to have empacho, what assessment findings would the nurse expect?
    a. Abdominal pain and cramping
    b. Anxiety, insomnia, anorexia, and social isolation
    c. Nightmares, weakness, and a sense of suffocation
    d. Headaches, stomach problems, and loss of consciousness

11. When the nurse takes a surgical consent form to an Asian woman for a signature after the surgeon has provided the information about the recommended surgery, the patient refuses to sign the consent form. What is the best response by the nurse?
    a. "Didn't you understand what the doctor told you about the surgery?"
    b. "Are there others with whom you want to talk before making this decision?"
    c. "Why won't you sign this form? Do you want to do what the doctor recommended?"
    d. "I'll have to call the surgeon and have your surgery cancelled until you can make a decision."

12. A male nurse would be providing culturally competent care by requesting that a female nurse provide the care for which patient?
    a. Arab male
    b. Latino male
    c. Arab female
    d. African American female

13. Identify the drug classes that have a different response in African Americans when compared with the usual response of whites of European descent (*select all that apply*).
    a. Analgesics
    b. Antipsychotics
    c. Benzodiazepines
    d. Tricyclic antidepressants
    e. Antihypertensive agents

14. Several cultural groups avoid direct eye contact and consider it disrespectful or aggressive. Which cultural group may not return a direct gaze?
    a. Arab
    b. Asian
    c. Hispanic
    d. Native American

15. To communicate with a patient who does not speak the dominant language, the nurse should (*select all that apply*)
    a. speak slowly and enunciate clearly in a slightly louder voice.
    b. use gestures and pantomime words while verbalizing specific words.
    c. use family members rather than strangers as interpreters to increase the patient's feeling of comfort.
    d. use a dictionary or phrase books that translate from both the nurse's language and the patient's language.
    e. avoid the use of any words known in the patient's language because the grammar and pronunciation may be incorrect.

16. Identify measures that the nurse should use to reduce health care disparities (*select all that apply*).
    a. Use cultural competency guidelines
    b. Use a family member as the interpreter
    c. Use standardized, evidence-based care guidelines
    d. Complete the health history as rapidly as possible
    e. Include racial cultural differences in planning care

CHAPTER 3

Health History and Physical Examination

1. During the day, while being admitted to the nursing unit from the emergency department, a patient tells the nurse that she is short of breath and has pain in her chest when she breathes. Her respiratory rate is 28 and she is coughing up yellow sputum. Her skin is hot and moist, and her temperature is 102.2°F (39°C). The laboratory results show white blood cell count elevation and the sputum result is pending. The patient says that coughing makes her head hurt and she aches all over. Identify the subjective and objective assessment findings for this patient.

Subjective	Objective

2. For the patient described in Question 1, the data will lead the night shift nurse to complete a focused nursing assessment of which body part(s)?
   a. Abdomen
   b. Arms and legs
   c. Head and neck
   d. Anterior and posterior chest

3. Give an example of a sensitive way to ask a patient each of the following questions.
   a. Is the patient on antihypertensive medication having a side effect of impotence?

   b. Has the patient with a history of alcoholism had recent alcohol intake?

   c. Who are the sexual contacts of a patient with gonorrhea?

   d. Does the patient skip taking medications because they cost too much?

4. *Priority Decision:* The nurse prepares to interview a patient for a nursing history but finds the patient in obvious pain. Which action by the nurse is the best at this time?
   a. Delay the interview until the patient is free of pain.
   b. Administer pain medication before initiating the interview.
   c. Gather as much information as quickly as possible by using closed questions that require brief answers.
   d. Ask only those questions pertinent to the specific problem and complete the interview when the patient is more comfortable.

5. *Priority Decision:* While the nurse is obtaining a health history the patient tells the nurse, "I am so tired I can hardly function." What is the nurse's best action at this time?
   a. Stop the interview and leave the patient alone to be able to rest.
   b. Arrange another time with the patient to complete the interview.
   c. Question the patient further about the characteristics of the symptoms.
   d. Reassure the patient that the symptoms will improve when treatment has had time to be effective.

6. Rewrite each of the following questions asked by the nurse so that it is an open-ended question designed to gather information about the patient's functional health patterns.
   a. Are you having any pain?

   b. Do you have a good relationship with your spouse?

   c. How long have you been ill?

   d. Do you exercise regularly?

7. A patient has come to the health clinic with diarrhea of 3 days' duration. He says the stools occur five or six times per day and are very watery. Every time he eats or drinks something, he has an urgent diarrhea stool. He denies being out of the country but did attend a large family reunion held at a campground in the mountains about a week ago. Identify the areas of symptom investigation using PQRST that still need to be addressed to provide additional important information (*select all that apply*).
   a. Timing
   b. Quality
   c. Severity
   d. Palliative
   e. Radiation
   f. Precipitating

8. The following data are obtained from a patient during a nursing history. Organize these data according to Gordon's functional health patterns. Patterns may be used more than once and some data may apply to more than one pattern.

   _____ a. 78-year-old woman
   _____ b. Married, three grown children who all live out of town
   _____ c. Cares for invalid husband in home with help of daily homemaker
   _____ d. Vision corrected with glasses; hearing normal
   _____ e. Height 5 ft, 10 in; weight 172 lb
   _____ f. Vital signs: T 99.2°F (37.3°C); HR 82 bpm; RR 32; BP 142/88
   _____ g. 5-year history of adult-onset asthma; smokes two or three cigarettes a day
   _____ h. Coughing, wheezing, with stated shortness of breath
   _____ i. Moderate light-yellow sputum
   _____ j. Says she now has no energy to care for husband
   _____ k. Awakens three or four times per night and has to use a bronchodilator inhaler
   _____ l. Uses a laxative twice a week for bowel function; no urinary problems
   _____ m. Feels her health is good for her age
   _____ n. Allergic to codeine and aspirin
   _____ o. Has esophageal reflux and eats bland foods
   _____ p. Can usually handle the stress of caring for her husband but if she becomes overwhelmed, asthma worsens
   _____ q. Has been menopausal for 26 years; no sexual activity
   _____ r. Takes medications for asthma, hypertension, and hypothyroidism and uses diazepam (Valium) PRN for anxiety
   _____ s. Goes out to lunch with friends weekly
   _____ t. Says she misses going to church with her husband but watches religious services with him on TV

   1. Demographic data
   2. Important health information
   3. Health-perception–health-management pattern
   4. Nutrition-metabolic pattern
   5. Elimination pattern
   6. Activity-exercise pattern
   7. Sleep-rest pattern
   8. Cognitive-perceptual pattern
   9. Self-perception–self-concept pattern
   10. Role-relationship pattern
   11. Sexuality-reproductive pattern
   12. Coping–stress tolerance pattern
   13. Value-belief pattern

9. What is an example of a pertinent negative finding during a physical examination?
   a. Chest pain that does not radiate to the arm
   b. Elevated blood pressure in a patient with hypertension
   c. Pupils that are equal and react to light and accommodation
   d. Clear and full lung sounds in a patient with chronic bronchitis

10. Match the following data with the assessment technique used to obtain the information.

    _____ a. Normal blood flow through arteries   1. Inspection
    _____ b. Abnormal blood flow in carotid artery   2. Palpation
    _____ c. Tympany of the abdomen   3. Percussion
    _____ d. Pitting edema   4. Auscultation
    _____ e. Cyanosis of the lips
    _____ f. Hyperactive peristalsis
    _____ g. Bruising of the lateral left thigh
    _____ h. Cool, clammy skin

11. What is the correct sequence of examination techniques that should be used when assessing the patient's abdomen?
    a. Inspection, palpation, auscultation, percussion   c. Palpation, percussion, auscultation, inspection
    b. Auscultation, inspection, percussion, palpation   d. Inspection, auscultation, percussion, palpation

12. When performing a physical examination, what approach is most important for the nurse to use?
    a. A head-to-toe approach to avoid missing an important area
    b. The same systematic, efficient sequence for all examinations
    c. A sequence that is least revealing and embarrassing for the patient
    d. An approach that allows time to collect the nursing history data while performing the examination

13. The nurse is performing a physical examination on a 90-year-old male patient who has been bedridden for the past year. Which adaptations for performing the examination would be appropriate for the patient (*select all that apply*)?
    a. Make sure that a family member is with him.
    b. Handle the skin with care because of potential fragility.
    c. Keep the patient warm and comfortable during the assessment.
    d. Allow the patient to watch TV to distract him from any painful assessments.
    e. Place the patient in a position of comfort and avoid unnecessary changes in position.

14. In what patient situations would a comprehensive assessment be performed (*select all that apply*)?
    a. Complaints of chest pain
    b. On initial admission to the telemetry unit
    c. On initial evaluation by the home health nurse
    d. The patient is found lying on the floor and is unresponsive
    e. On arrival in the surgery holding area of the operating room

15. Which assessment tools can be used to assess the cardiac system (*select all that apply*)?
    a. Watch   d. Percussion hammer
    b. Stethoscope   e. Blood pressure cuff
    c. Ophthalmoscope

16. What is the term used for assessment data that the patient tells you about?
    a. Focused   c. Subjective
    b. Objective   d. Comprehensive

17. On the first encounter with the patient, the nurse will complete a general survey. Which features are included (*select all that apply*)?
    a. Mental state and behavior   d. Speech and body movements
    b. Lung sounds and bowel tones   e. Body features and obvious physical signs
    c. Body temperature and pulses   f. Abnormal heart murmur and limited mobility

Patient and Caregiver Teaching

1. In each of the nursing situations described below, identify the goal of the patient and caregiver teaching.

Nursing Situation	Goal
Teaching a new mother about the recommended infant immunization schedule	a.
Discussing recommended lifestyle changes with a patient with newly diagnosed heart disease	b.
Counseling a patient with a breast biopsy that is positive for cancer	c.
Demonstrating the proper condom application to sexually active teenagers	d.

2. What is meant by this statement? "Every interaction with a patient or caregiver is potentially a teachable moment."

3. Which statements characterize the teaching-learning process (*select all that apply*)?
   a. Learning can occur without teaching.
   b. Teaching may make learning more efficient.
   c. Teaching must be well planned to be effective.
   d. Learning has not occurred when there is no change in behavior.
   e. Teaching uses a variety of methods to influence knowledge and behavior.

4. From the list of principles of adult learning below, identify which one(s) is (are) used in the following examples of patient teaching. Principles may be used more than once and more than one principle may be used for each example of patient teaching.

   _____ a. The nurse explains why it is important for a patient with Parkinson's disease to walk with wide placement of the feet.

   _____ b. The nurse asks a patient what is most important to her to learn about managing a new colostomy.

   _____ c. The nurse teaches a patient how to reduce the risks for stroke after the patient has had a transient ischemic attack.

   _____ d. The nurse provides a variety of printed materials and Internet resources for a patient with impaired kidney function to use to learn about the disorder.

   _____ e. When caring for a patient with newly diagnosed asthma, the nurse explains that asthma is a disorder the patient can control and allows the patient to decide when teaching should be done and who else should be included.

   _____ f. The patient diagnosed with diabetes mellitus requests to try performing self-monitoring of blood glucose and insulin administration while being taught by the nurse.

   _____ g. During preoperative teaching of a patient scheduled for a total hip replacement, the nurse compares the postoperative care with that of the patient's prior back surgery.

   1. Learner's need to know
   2. Learner's readiness to learn
   3. Learner's prior experiences
   4. Learner's motivation to learn
   5. Learner's orientation to learning
   6. Learner's self-concept

5. When a patient with diabetes tells the nurse that he cannot see any reason to change his eating habits because he is not overweight, what action does the nurse determine as the most appropriate at this stage of the Transtheoretical Model of behavior change?
   a. Help the patient set priorities for managing his diabetes.
   b. Arrange for the dietitian to describe what dietary changes are needed.
   c. Explain that dietary changes can help prevent long-term complications of diabetes.
   d. Emphasize that he must change behaviors if he is going to control his blood glucose levels.

6. Put the following medical terms into phrases that a patient with limited health literacy would be able to understand.
   a. Acute myocardial infarction

   b. Intravenous pyelogram

   c. Diabetic retinopathy

7. What demonstrates an empathetic approach to patient teaching by the nurse?
   a. Assesses the patient's needs before developing the teaching plan.
   b. Provides positive nonverbal messages that promote communication.
   c. Reads and reviews educational materials before distributing them to patients and families.
   d. Overcomes personal frustration when patients are discharged before teaching is complete.

8. Describe one strategy that could be used to overcome the common barriers to teaching patients and caregivers.

Barrier	Strategy
Lack of time	
Your feeling as a teacher	
Patient circumstances	

9. The nurse assesses a 48-year-old male patient and his family for learning needs related to the myocardial infarction the patient experienced 2 days ago. While doing her assessment, she finds out that the patient's father died at age 52 from a myocardial infarction. Which assessment area will influence the teaching plan for this patient and family?
   a. Learner characteristics
   b. Physical characteristics
   c. Psychologic characteristics
   d. Sociocultural characteristics

10. To promote the patient's self-efficacy during the teaching-learning process, the nurse should use which strategy?
    a. Emphasize the relevancy of the teaching to the patient's life.
    b. Begin with concepts and tasks that are easily learned to promote success.
    c. Provide stimulating learning activities that encourage motivation to learn.
    d. Encourage the patient to learn independently without instruction from others.

11. Identify the teaching interventions that are indicated when the following patient characteristics are found.

Patient Characteristic	Teaching Intervention
Impaired hearing	
Patient refuses to see a need for a change in health behaviors	
Drowsiness caused by use of sedatives	
Presence of pain	
Uncertain of reading ability	
Visual learning style	
Primary language is not English	

12. On assessment of a patient's learning needs, the nurse determines that a patient taking potassium-wasting diuretics does not know what foods are high in potassium. What is an appropriate nursing diagnosis for this patient?
    a. Risk for cardiac dysrhythmias related to low potassium intake
    b. Deficient knowledge related to not knowing what foods are high in potassium
    c. Imbalanced nutrition: less than body requirements related to lack of intake of potassium-rich foods
    d. Deficient knowledge related to lack of interest regarding dietary requirements when taking diuretics

13. Write a learning goal for the patient taking potassium-wasting diuretics who does not know what foods are high in potassium.

14. Which teaching strategies should be used when it is difficult to reach the desired goals of the session (*select all that apply*)?
    a. DVD
    b. Role play
    c. Discussion
    d. Printed material
    e. Lecture-discussion

15. When is role playing best used as a teaching strategy (*select all that apply*)?
    a. To rehearse behaviors or feelings
    b. With mature and confident participants
    c. To teach motor skills or procedures to patients
    d. To provide patients and caregivers basic information
    e. In combination with almost any other teaching strategy

16. When selecting audiovisual and written materials as teaching strategies, what is important for the nurse to do?
    a. Provide the patient with these materials before the planned learning experience.
    b. Ensure that the materials include all the information the patient will need to learn.
    c. Review the materials before use for accuracy and appropriateness to learning needs and goals.
    d. Assess the patient's auditory and visual ability because these functions are necessary for these strategies to be effective.

17. A patient with a breast biopsy positive for cancer tells the nurse that she has been using information from the Internet to try to make a decision about her treatment choices. In counseling the patient, the nurse knows that (*select all that apply*)
    a. the patient should be taught how to identify reliable and accurate information available online.
    b. all sites used by the patient should be evaluated by the nurse for accuracy and appropriateness of the information.
    c. most information from the Internet is incomplete and inaccurate and should not be used to make important decisions regarding treatment.
    d. the Internet is an excellent source of health information, and online education programs can provide patients with better instruction than is available at clinics.
    e. the patient should be encouraged to use sites established by universities, the government, or reputable health organizations, such as the American Cancer Society, to access reliable information.

18. Identify what short-term evaluation technique is appropriate to assess whether the patient has met the following learning goals.

Learning Goal	Evaluation Technique
The patient will demonstrate to the nurse the preparation and administration of a subcutaneous insulin injection to himself with correct technique before discharge.	
Before discharge, the patient will identify five serious side effects of Coumadin that should be reported to the doctor.	
The patient's wife will select the foods highest in potassium for each meal from the hospital menu with 80% accuracy.	
The patient will verbalize "no shortness of breath" when ambulating unassisted with the walker each of three times a day.	
The patient's caregiver will state that they are ready to change the patient's dressing today.	

19. What is the best example of documentation of patient teaching regarding wound care?
    a. "The patient was instructed about care of wound and dressing changes."
    b. "The patient demonstrated correct technique of wound care following instruction."
    c. "The patient and caregiver verbalize that they understand the purposes of wound care."
    d. "Written instructions regarding wound care and dressing changes were given to the patient."

20. Which teaching strategies should the nurse plan to use for a baby boomer patient (*select all that apply*)?
    a. Podcast
    b. Role playing
    c. Group teaching
    d. Lecture-discussion
    e. A game or game system
    f. Patient education TV channels

21. An 88-year-old male patient with dementia and a fractured hip is admitted to the clinical unit accompanied by his daughter who is his caregiver. She looks tired and disheveled. She states that she moved in with her father about 6 months ago when he started wandering away from his house. She is concerned about what will happen to her father after this hospitalization. Her brother calls on the phone to tell her what to do but does not help out. What stressors is she experiencing (*select all that apply*)?
    a. Change in role within the family
    b. Lack of respite from caregiving responsibilities
    c. Conflict in the family related to decisions about caregiving
    d. Financial depletion of resources as a result of her inability to work
    e. Social isolation and loss of friends from an inability to have time for herself

22. A 68-year-old female patient was admitted with a stroke 3 days ago. She has weakness on her right side. She states, "I will never be able to take care of myself. I don't want to go to therapy this afternoon." After listening to her, which statement would be included as part of a motivational interview?
    a. "Why not?"
    b. "If you go to therapy, I'll give you a back rub when you get back."
    c. "I know you are tired but look how much easier walking was today than it was last week."
    d. "Well, with that attitude, you will have trouble. The doctor ordered therapy because he thought it would help."

CHAPTER

5

Chronic Illness and Older Adults

1. A 78-year-old female patient is admitted with nausea, vomiting, anorexia, diarrhea, and dehydration. She has a history of diabetes mellitus and 2 years ago had a stroke with residual right-sided weakness. Identify which characteristics of chronic illness the nurse will probably find in this patient (*select all that apply*).
   a. Self-limiting
   b. Residual disability
   c. Permanent impairments
   d. Infrequent complications
   e. Need for long-term management
   f. Nonreversible pathologic changes

2. Seven tasks required for daily living with chronic illness have been identified. From Table 5-4, select at least one of these tasks that would specifically apply to the following common chronic conditions in older adults.

Chronic Condition	Task
Diabetes mellitus	
Visual impairment	prevent social isolation, attempt to normalize interactions w/others
Heart disease	
Hearing impairment	
Alzheimer's disease	
Arthritis	
Orthopedic impairment	

3. Consider the differences between primary and secondary prevention. Fill in the blanks.
   a. Actions aimed at early detection of disease and interventions to prevent progression of disease are

   considered _secondary_ prevention.
   b. Following a proper diet, getting appropriate exercise, and receiving immunizations against specific diseases

   is considered _primary_ prevention.

4. What is the leading cause of death in the United States?
   a. Cancer
   b. Diabetes mellitus
   c. Coronary artery disease
   d. Cerebrovascular accident
   e. Chronic obstructive pulmonary disease

5. According to the Corbin and Strauss chronic illness trajectory, which statement describes a patient with an unstable condition?
   a. Life-threatening situation
   b. Increasing disability and symptoms
   c. Gradual return to acceptable way of life
   d. Loss of control over symptoms and disease course

6. Which statement(s) about older people are only myths and illustrate the concept of ageism (*select all that apply*)?
   a. Can't teach an old dog new tricks.
   b. Old people are not sexually active.
   c. Most old people live independently.
   d. Most older adults can no longer synthesize new information.
   e. Most older people lose interest in life and wish they would die.

7. For each of the nursing diagnoses listed, identify at least two normal expected physiologic changes related to aging that could be etiologic factors of the diagnosis. Changes related to aging are found in the chapters identified in Table 5-6.
   a. Imbalanced nutrition: less than body requirements (see Table 39-5, p. 871.)
      Change:

      Change:

   b. Activity intolerance (see Table 62-1, p. 1494.)
      Change:

      Change:

   c. Risk for injury (see Table 56-4, p. 1344; Table 21-1, p. 371.)
      Change:

      Change:

   d. Urge urinary incontinence (see Table 45-2, p. 1051.)
      Change:

      Change:

   e. Ineffective airway clearance (see Table 26-4, p. 481.)
      Change:

      Change:

   f. Risk for impaired skin integrity (see Table 23-1, p. 417.)
      Change:

      Change:

   g. Ineffective peripheral tissue perfusion (see Table 32-1, p. 691.)
      Change:

      Change:

   h. Constipation (see Table 39-5, p. 871.)
      Change:

      Change:

8. The nurse identifies the presence of age-associated memory impairment in the older adult who states
   a. "I just can't seem to remember the name of my granddaughter."
   b. "I make out lists to help me remember what I need to do but I can't seem to use them."
   c. "I forgot that I went to the grocery store this morning and didn't realize it until I went again this afternoon."
   d. "I forget movie stars' names more often now but I can remember them later after the conversation is over."

9. Indicate what the acronym SCALES stands for in assessment of nutrition indicators in frail older adults.

S	Sadness (mood)
C	cholesterol (high)
A	albumin (low)
L	Loss (or gain) of weight
E	eating problems
S	shopping (& food prep problems)

10. When working with older patients who identify with a specific ethnic group, the nurse recognizes that health care problems may occur in these patients because they
    a. live with extended families who isolate the patient.
    b. live in rural areas where services are not readily available.
    c. eat ethnic foods that do not provide all essential nutrients.
    d. have less income to spend for medications and health care services.

11. An 83-year-old woman is being discharged from the hospital following stabilization of her international normalized ratio (INR) levels (used to assess effectiveness of warfarin therapy). She has chronic atrial fibrillation and has been on warfarin (Coumadin) for several years. Discharge instructions include returning to the clinic weekly for INR (2-3) testing. Which statement by the patient indicates that she may be unable to have the testing done?
    a. "When I have the energy, I have taken the bus to get this test done."
    b. "I will need to ask my son to bring me into town every week for the test."
    c. "Should I just keep taking the same pill every day until I can get a ride to town?"
    d. "It is very important to have this test every week. I have several church friends who can bring me."

12. The old-old population (85 years and older) has an increased risk for frailty. However, old age is just one element of frailty. Identify at least three other assessment findings that contribute to frailty.
    a. unplanned weight loss
    b. weakness
    c.

13. An 80-year-old woman is brought to the emergency department by her daughter, who says her mother has refused to eat for 6 days. The mother says she stays in her room all of the time because the family is mean to her when she eats or watches TV with them. She says her daughter brings her only one meal a day and that meal is cold leftovers from the family's meals days before.
    a. What types of elder mistreatment may be present in this situation?
    b. How would the nurse assess the situation to determine whether abuse is present?

    The daughter says her mother is too demanding and she just cannot cope with caring for her 24 hours a day.
    c. What might be an appropriate nursing diagnosis for the daughter?
    d. What resources can the nurse suggest to the daughter?

14. What are three common factors known to precipitate placement in a long-term care facility?
    a.
    b.
    c.

15. An 88-year-old woman is brought to the health clinic for the first time by her 64-year-old daughter. During the initial comprehensive nursing assessment of the patient, what should the nurse do?
    a. Ask the daughter whether the patient has any urgent needs or problems.
    b. Interview the patient and daughter together so that pertinent information can be confirmed. – want to interview seperately
    c. Obtain a health history using a functional health pattern and assess activities of daily living (ADLs) and mental status.
    d. Refer the patient for an interdisciplinary comprehensive geriatric assessment because at her age she will have multiple needs.

16. What is a mental status assessment of the older adult especially important in determining?
    a. Potential for independent living
    b. Eligibility for federal health programs
    c. Service and placement needs of the individual
    d. Whether the person should be classified as frail

17. What is an important nursing measure in the rehabilitation of an older adult to prevent loss of function from inactivity and immobility?
    a. Using assistive devices such as walkers and canes
    b. Teaching good nutrition to prevent loss of muscle mass
    c. Performance of active and passive range-of-motion (ROM) exercises
    d. Performance of risk appraisals and assessments related to immobility

18. In view of the fact that most older adults take at least six prescription drugs, what are four nursing interventions that can specifically help prevent problems caused by multiple drug use in older patients?
    a.

    b.

    c.

    d.

19. Which nursing actions would demonstrate the nurse's understanding of the concept of providing safe care without using restraints (*select all that apply*)?
    a. Placing patients with fall risk in low beds.
    b. Asking simple yes-or-no questions to clarify patient needs.
    c. Making hourly rounds on patients to assess for pain and toileting needs.
    d. Placing a disruptive patient near the nurses' station in a chair with a seat belt.
    e. Applying a jacket vest loosely so the patient can turn but cannot climb out of bed.

20. When teaching a 69-year-old patient about self-care, what will promote health (*select all that apply*)?
    a. Proper diet
    b. Immunizations
    c. Teaching chair yoga
    d. Demonstrating balancing techniques
    e. Participation in health promotion activities

21. The 58-year-old male patient will be transferred from the acute care clinical unit of the hospital to another care area. The patient requires complicated dressing changes for several weeks. To which practice setting should the patient be transitioned?
    a. Acute rehabilitation
    b. Long-term acute care
    c. Intermediate care facility
    d. Transitional subacute care

p.322

Complementary and Alternative Therapies

1. Which National Center for Complementary and Alternative Medicine (NCCAM) category is described by the use of dietary supplements and unrefined plants or plant parts for specific effects?
   a. Natural products
   b. Mind-body medicine
   c. Other CAM therapies
   d. Manipulative and body-based practices

2. What therapies are included in the mind-body medicine National Center for Complementary and Alternative Medicine (NCCAM) category (*select all that apply*)?
   a. Use of hands to realign energy flow
   b. Communication with the Creator or the Sacred
   c. Learned control of physiologic responses of the body
   d. Self-directed practice of focusing, centering, and relaxing
   e. Spinal manipulation and realignment to promote health and well-being
   f. Soft tissue manipulation to relax, stimulate the immune system, and increase flexibility

3. What describes the whole medical system of Ayurveda?
   a. Manipulation of energy channels with fine needles
   b. Uses the principle of "like cures like" with small doses of prepared extracts
   c. Use of finger and hand pressure at energy meridians to improve energy flow
   d. Considers disease as an imbalance of life force and basic metabolic condition

4. What is the focus of the integrative model of health care?
   a. Costs paid by insurance
   b. Treatment of symptoms
   c. Mind-body-spirit connections
   d. Care directed by nurse practitioners

5. Which statement accurately describes the use of complementary and alternative medicine (CAM)?
   a. CAM therapy incorporates only the emotional and spiritual realms of the patient.
   b. The increase in the use of CAM therapies is due to an increase in cost of conventional therapy.
   c. Research and education in CAM therapies are financially supported by the American Holistic Nurses Association.
   d. Practices that are considered complementary and alternative in one culture or time might be considered conventional in another culture or time.

6. What is the rationale behind many nurses advocating complementary and alternative therapies?
   a. They promote self-care and self-determination by patients.
   b. They are congruent with a view of humans as holistic beings.
   c. They are less expensive for patients than conventional therapies.
   d. They cause few adverse effects while achieving positive outcomes.

7. According to Traditional Chinese Medicine, when does disease occur?
   a. Yin and yang become imbalanced, altering the flow of Qi.
   b. Acupoints in Qi channels become obstructed, preventing the release of Qi.
   c. The body's natural healing abilities are impaired by obstruction of fluid channels.
   d. The individual is out of harmony with nature and requires spiritualism and mysticism to reestablish balance.

8. What is acupuncture used for (*select all that apply*)?
   a. Relieve pain by causing counterirritation in another area of the body.
   b. Reestablish the flow of Qi through meridians to simulate the body's self-healing mechanism.
   c. Create an inflammatory response at an acupoint, increasing blood circulation and healing energy.
   d. Relieve nausea and vomiting postoperatively, with pregnancy, or related to chemotherapy.
   e. Stimulate the electrical activity of the central nervous system, promoting movement of vital energy through the body.

9. When the family members of a postoperative patient leave after a visit, the patient tells the nurse that his family gave him a headache by fussing over him so much. What is an appropriate intervention by the nurse?
   a. Administer the PRN analgesic prescribed for his postoperative pain.
   b. Ask the patient's permission to use acupressure to ease his headache.
   c. Reassure the patient that his headache will subside now that his family has gone.
   d. Teach the patient biofeedback methods to relieve his headaches by controlling cerebral blood flow.

10. *Priority Decision:* A bedridden patient tells the nurse she has low back pain and asks if the area could be massaged. What is the best action by the nurse?
    a. Ask the patient if she has ever tried acupuncture for back pain.
    b. Explain to the patient that massage may be done only by a licensed therapist and offer a PRN analgesic instead.
    c. Comfortably position the patient to expose the area and massage the back with effleurage and petrissage strokes.
    d. Call the physical therapy department to request that a physical therapist see the patient to provide a therapeutic massage.

11. A patient who is receiving radiation therapy for breast cancer tells the nurse that she cannot verbalize her fears about her treatment. Which complementary or alternative therapy would be most beneficial for the nurse to teach this patient about at this time?
    a. Journaling
    b. Yoga therapy
    c. Herbal therapy
    d. Chiropractic therapy

12. When discussing herbal therapy with a patient, what should the nurse advise the patient?
    a. Preparations should be purchased only from reputable manufacturers.
    b. Herbs rarely cause harm or side effects because they are natural plants.
    c. Herbs are safe and there are no known contraindications to the use of herbal therapy.
    d. Most herbal preparations have been clinically tested for safety and efficacy before marketing.

13. *Priority Decision:* While the nurse is obtaining a health history for a patient, the patient tells the nurse that he uses a number of herbs to maintain his health. What is the most important thing the nurse can do to address the patient's use of these products?
    a. Ask the patient what effects the various products have.
    b. Have a working knowledge of commonly used herbs and dietary supplements.
    c. Reassure the patient that the products can continue to be used with conventional therapies.
    d. Warn the patient that there is limited research on the therapeutic and harmful effects of herbal products.

14. A patient newly diagnosed with type 2 diabetes has been given a prescription to start on an oral hypoglycemic. The patient tells the nurse she would rather control her blood sugar with herbal therapy. Which action should the nurse take?
    a. Advise the patient to discuss using herbal therapy with her physician.
    b. Advise the patient that herbal therapy is not safe and should not be used.
    c. Advise the patient to give the prescriptive medication time to work before using herbal therapy.
    d. Advise the patient that if she takes herbal therapy, she will have to monitor her blood sugar more often.

15. What is the role of the professional nurse related to the use of complementary and alternative therapies (CAT) (*select all that apply*)?
    a. Seeking further education on CAT
    b. Evaluating the evidence regarding CAT
    c. Collecting data on the use of CAT as part of the nursing assessment
    d. Suggesting specific herbs the patient should take to help with his or her condition
    e. Advising patients to not use these therapies because there are so many side effects
    f. Investigating which of these therapies fall within the nursing practice domain in the nurse's state.

16. Which statement accurately describes the common use of feverfew?
    a. Frequently used for insomnia and anxiety
    b. Most commonly used for prevention of migraine headaches
    c. Frequently used to prevent and treat upper respiratory infections
    d. Often used by perimenopausal women to relieve menopausal symptoms

17. Which spice may be used to treat the nausea and vomiting related to pregnancy?
    a. Aloe
    b. Ginger
    c. Cranberry
    d. Evening primrose

18. Melatonin's use is based on scientific evidence. The patient with which problem would benefit from melatonin?
    a. Sleep problems
    b. Mild depression
    c. High cholesterol
    d. Benign prostatic hyperplasia

19. Which herb may relieve anxiety but can cause hepatotoxicity?
    a. Kava
    b. Ginseng
    c. Milk thistle
    d. Ginkgo biloba

Stress and Stress Management

1. When a patient at the clinic is informed that testing indicates the presence of gonorrhea, the patient sighs and says, "That, I can handle." What does the nurse understand about the patient in this situation?
   a. The patient is in denial about the possible complications of gonorrhea.
   b. The patient does not perceive the gonorrhea infection as a threatening stressor.
   c. The patient does not have other current stressors that require adaptation or coping mechanisms.
   d. The patient knows how to cope with gonorrhea from dealing with previous gonorrhea infections.

2. Number the stages of the general adaptation syndrome (GAS) according to the signs and symptoms the nurse would expect to see (see Table 7-1). Use 1 for the Alarm stage, the first stage; 2 for the Resistance stage, the second stage; and 3 for the Exhaustion stage, the third stage.
   _____ a. Increased agitation
   _____ b. Increased heart rate
   _____ c. Continuous viral infections
   _____ d. Bleeding ulcer
   _____ e. Increased blood glucose levels
   _____ f. No signs or symptoms evident

3. Identify four personal characteristics that promote adaptation to stressors.
   a.

   b.

   c.

   d.

4. Using the word and phrase list below, fill in the boxes below with the numbers of the words or phrases that illustrate the physiologic response to stress.

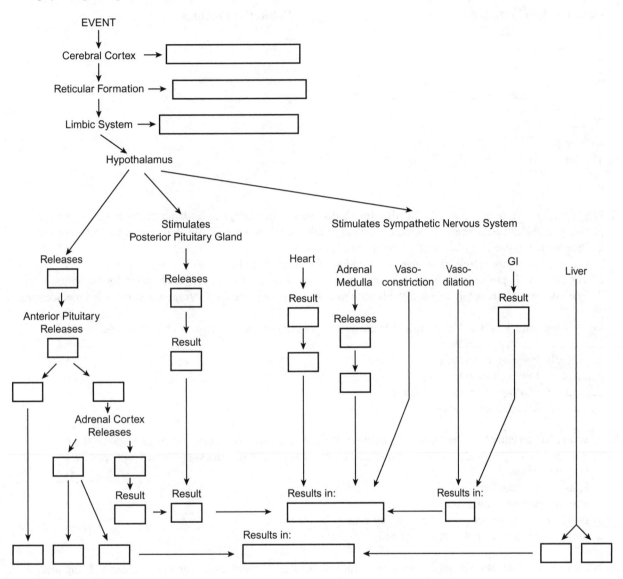

Word and Phrase List

1. Interpretation of event
2. ↑ ADH (antidiuretic hormone)
3. Cortisol
4. ↑ Blood volume
5. ↑ HR and stroke volume
6. ↑ Water retention
7. Wakefulness and alertness
8. ↑ Sympathetic response
9. β-Endorphin
10. Self-preservation behaviors
11. ↑ Cardiac output
12. Corticotropin-releasing hormone
13. Aldosterone
14. ACTH (adrenocorticotropic hormone)
15. Blunted pain perception
16. ↑ Gluconeogenesis
17. ↑ Epinephrine and norepinephrine
18. ↓ Digestion
19. ↑ Pro-opiomelanocortin (POMC)
20. ↑ Systolic blood pressure
21. ↓ Inflammatory response
22. Glycogenolysis
23. ↑ Blood to vital organs and large muscles
24. ↑ Blood glucose
25. ↑ Na and H_2O reabsorption

5. Using the diagram in Question 4 and the physiologic responses that are noted, identify eight objective clinical or laboratory manifestations and four subjective findings that the nurse might expect.

Objective Manifestations	**Subjective Findings**
a.	a.
b.	b.
c.	c.
d.	d.
e.	
f.	
g.	
h.	

6. While caring for a female patient with Alzheimer's disease and her caregiver husband, the nurse finds that the patient's husband is experiencing increased asthma problems. What is a possible explanation for this finding?
   a. Progressive worsening of asthma occurs in people as they age.
   b. Chronic and intense stress can cause exacerbation of immune-based diseases.
   c. The husband is probably smoking more to help him cope with needing to care continually for his wife.
   d. The husband inadequately copes with his wife's condition by unconsciously forgetting to take his medications.

7. Identify the behaviors listed below as either positive coping (P) or negative coping (N) strategies.
   _____ a. Smoking cigarettes
   _____ b. Ignoring a situation
   _____ c. Joining a support group
   _____ d. Starting an exercise program
   _____ e. Increasing time spent with friends

8. A patient has recently had a myocardial infarction. What emotion-focused coping strategies should the nurse encourage him to use to adapt to the physical and emotional stress of his illness (*select all that apply*)?
   a. Use meditation
   b. Plan dietary changes
   c. Start an exercise program
   d. Do favorite escape activities (e.g., playing cards)
   e. Share feelings with spouse or other family members

9. While teaching relaxation therapy to a patient with fibromyalgia, what does the nurse recognize as being most important to incorporate?
   a. Relaxation breathing
   b. Soft background music
   c. Progressive muscle relaxation
   d. Concentration on a single focus

10. *Priority Decision:* After receiving the assigned patients for the day, the nurse determines that stress-relieving interventions are a priority for which patient?
    a. The man with peptic ulcer disease
    b. The newly admitted woman with cholecystitis
    c. The man with a bacterial exacerbation of chronic bronchitis
    d. The woman who is 1 day postoperative for knee replacement

11. A 32-year-old man is admitted to the hospital with an acute exacerbation of Crohn's disease. Coping strategies that might be suggested by the nurse during his hospitalization include (*select all that apply*)
    a. Humor
    b. Exercise
    c. Journaling
    d. A cleansing diet
    e. Relaxation therapy

CASE STUDY
Stress
Patient Profile

M.J., a 26-year-old female single secretary, is admitted to the hospital with right lower quadrant pain rated as 9 on a scale of 0 to 10; 10 to 12 watery, blood-streaked stools in the past 24 hours; and a low-grade fever. She has a 7-year history of inflammatory bowel disease.

Subjective Data

Patient relates the following:
- She has been hospitalized four times in the past year.
- She is not currently working because of the illness and has no income.
- She has no insurance.
- Her boyfriend has lived with her for 2 years.
- She does not want her boyfriend to visit because she thinks he has enough problems of his own.
- She has been in bed for the past week because of weakness, nausea, and malaise and has been crying and depressed.

Objective Data

- Height: 5 ft, 6 in (168 cm)
- Weight: 104 lb (47.3 kg)
- Hemoglobin: 10.5 g/dL (105 g/L)
- Hematocrit: 30%
- Temp: 100°F (37.8°C)

Discussion Questions

Using a separate sheet of paper, answer the following questions:

1. What physiologic and psychologic stressors can be identified or anticipated in M.J.'s situation? Describe the possible effects of these stressors on the course of her illness.
2. What factors identified in the nursing assessment could affect M.J.'s current adaptation to stress?
3. What physiologic changes would be expected in M.J. as she begins to respond to prescribed treatment?
4. Describe an approach that the nurse could use to assess M.J.'s perception of her situation. Include several specific questions to be asked by the nurse.
5. *Priority Decision:* What are the priority nursing interventions that can be implemented for M.J. to enhance her adaptation to stress?
6. *Priority Decision:* Based on the assessment data provided, what are the priority nursing diagnoses? Are there any collaborative problems?
7. *Priority Decision:* What is the priority nursing diagnosis for M.J. on admission?

Sleep and Sleep Disorders

1. Which statement about sleep is accurate?
   a. Lack of sleep causes medical and psychiatric disorders.
   b. Adults generally require at least 5 hours of sleep every 24 hours.
   c. During sleep an individual is not consciously aware of his or her environment.
   d. Less than 10% of adults report at least one sleep problem, such as difficulty falling asleep.

2. What are clinical manifestations of insomnia (*select all that apply*)?
   a. Narcolepsy
   b. Fragmented sleep
   c. Long sleep latency
   d. Morning headache
   e. Daytime sleepiness
   f. Difficulty concentrating

3. What is a typical parasomnia?
   a. Cataplexy
   b. Hypopnea
   c. Sleep apnea
   d. Sleep terrors

4. What controls the cyclic changes between waking and sleep?
   a. Fluctuating levels of melatonin
   b. The environmental light-dark cycles
   c. Key nuclei in the brainstem, hypothalamus, and thalamus
   d. A variety of neuropeptides released from the nervous system

5. Match the descriptions to the stages of sleep. Some descriptions may have more than one stage and some stages may be used more than once.

   _____ a. Brain waves resemble wakefulness
   _____ b. Deepest sleep, lasting 20 to 40 minutes
   _____ c. Associated with specific EEG waveforms
   _____ d. Most vivid dreaming occurs
   _____ e. 20% to 25% of sleep
   _____ f. Person easily awakened
   _____ g. Most of the night of sleep
   _____ h. Slow eye movements
   _____ i. Slowed heart rate, decreased body temperature
   _____ j. Decreased occurrence in older adults

   1. NREM stage 1
   2. NREM stage 2
   3. NREM stage 3
   4. REM

6. List at least three behaviors or practices that can contribute to insomnia.
   a.

   b.

   c.

7. A clinical polysomnography (PSG) may be performed on a patient with signs and symptoms of a sleep disorder. What measures and observations does this study include (*select all that apply*)?
   a. Heart rate monitoring
   b. Noninvasive oxygen saturation (SpO_2)
   c. Surface body temperature fluctuations
   d. Blood pressure monitoring (noninvasive)
   e. Airflow measured at the nose and mouth
   f. Muscle tone measured by electromyogram (EMG)
   g. Respiratory effort around the chest and abdomen
   h. Eye movements recorded by electrooculogram (EOG)
   i. Brain activity recorded by electroencephalogram (EEG)
   j. Actigraph watch worn on the wrist to monitor motor activity
   k. Gross body movements monitored via audio and visual recordings

8. What is first-line therapy for insomnia?
   a. Complementary therapies such as melatonin
   b. Cognitive-behavioral therapies such as relaxation therapy
   c. Benzodiazepine-receptor-like agents (e.g., zolpidem [Ambien])
   d. Over-the-counter medication such as diphenhydramine (Benadryl)

9. The nurse knows that a patient taught sleep hygiene practices needs further instruction when he says
   a. "Once I go to bed, I should get up if I am not asleep after 20 minutes."
   b. "It's okay to have my usual two glasses of wine in the evening before bed."
   c. "A couple of crackers with cheese and a glass of milk may help to relax before bed."
   d. "I should go to the gym earlier in the day so that I'm done at least 6 hours before bedtime."

10. The patient is complaining of insomnia. Which bedtime snack would be the best option for this patient?
    a. Hershey's bar
    b. 8 oz hot chocolate
    c. 8 oz Dannon coffee yogurt
    d. 1 cup Ben & Jerry's nonfat coffee fudge frozen yogurt

11. A nurse caring for a patient in the intensive care unit (ICU) implements strategies to create an environment conducive to sleep. Which strategy would be most effective?
    a. Turning off the lights in the room during the night
    b. Having the television on at all times for background noise
    c. Silencing the alarms on the bedside monitor and infusion pumps
    d. Administering ordered analgesics around the clock, even if the patient denies pain

12. Which medication is a nonamphetamine wake-promotion drug?
    a. Modafinil (Provigil)
    b. Protriptyline (Vavactil)
    c. Desipramine (Norpramin)
    d. Methylphenidate (Concerta)

13. The nurse in a clinic is talking with a patient who will be traveling from the Midwest time zone to Moscow to attend a 4-day conference. The patient asks the nurse how he can minimize the effects of jet lag. What are at least two recommendations that the nurse could give to the patient?

14. Place the events below in the order they occur in the patient with obstructive sleep apnea (beginning with 1).

_____ a. Apnea lasting 10 to 90 seconds

_____ b. Brief arousal and airway opened

_____ c. Generalized startle response, snorting, or gasping

_____ d. Hypoxemia and hypercapnia

_____ e. Narrowing of air passages with muscle relaxation during sleep

_____ f. Risk factors: obesity, large neck circumference, craniofacial abnormalities, acromegaly, smoking

_____ g. Occurs 200 to 400 times during 6 to 8 hours of sleep

_____ h. Tongue and soft palate obstruct pharynx

15. The physician has ordered continuous positive airway pressure (CPAP) for a patient with serious obstructive sleep apnea. How will CPAP help the patient?

a. Prevent airway occlusion by bringing the tongue forward

b. Be easily tolerated by both the patient and the patient's bed partner

c. Provide enough positive pressure in the airway to prevent airway collapse

d. Deliver a high inspiratory pressure and a low expiratory pressure to prevent airway collapse

16. While caring for a patient following an uvulopalatopharyngoplasty (UPPP), the nurse monitors the patient for which complications in the immediate postoperative period?

a. Snoring and foul-smelling breath

b. Infection and electrolyte imbalance

c. Loss of voice and severe sore throat

d. Airway obstruction and hemorrhage

17. An older patient asks the nurse why she has so much trouble sleeping. What is the most appropriate response by the nurse?

a. "Disturbed sleep is a normal result of aging."

b. "Have you tried any over-the-counter medications to help you sleep?"

c. "Don't worry. You don't need as much sleep as you did when you were younger."

d. "Tell me more about the trouble you are having. There may be some things we can do to help."

18. Nurses who rotate shifts or work nights are at risk for developing shift work sleep disorder characterized by insomnia, sleepiness, and fatigue. Identify at least three negative implications for the nurse.

19. What strategies could decrease the distress of rotating shifts for nurses (*select all that apply*)?

a. Take a brief onsite nap

b. Use sleep hygiene practices

c. Sleep just before going to work

d. Maintain consistent sleep/wake schedules even on days off (if possible)

e. Negotiate to control work schedule rather than having someone else impose the schedule

1. Pain has been defined as "whatever the person experiencing the pain says it is, existing whenever the patient says it does." This definition is problematic for the nurse when caring for which type of patient?
   a. A patient placed on a ventilator
   b. A patient with a history of opioid addiction
   c. A patient with decreased cognitive function
   d. A patient with pain resulting from severe trauma

2. On the first postoperative day following a bowel resection, the patient complains of abdominal and incisional pain rated 9 on a scale of 0 to 10. Postoperative orders include morphine, 4 mg IV q2 hr, for pain and may repeat morphine, 4 mg IV, for breakthrough pain. The nurse determines that it has been only 2 hours since the last dose of morphine and wants to wait a little longer. What effect does the nurse's action have on the patient?
   a. Protects the patient from addiction and toxic effects of the drug
   b. Prevents hastening or causing a patient's death from respiratory dysfunction
   c. Contributes to unnecessary suffering and physical and psychosocial dysfunction
   d. Indicates that the nurse understands the adage of "start low and go slow" in administering analgesics

3. List and briefly describe the five dimensions of pain.
   a.
   b.
   c. onset
   d.
   e.

4. Once generated, what may block the transmission of an action potential along a peripheral nerve fiber to the dorsal root of the spinal cord?
   a. The transmission may be interrupted by drugs such as local anesthetics.
   b. Nothing can stop the action potential along an intact nerve until it reaches the spinal cord.
   c. The action potential must cross several synapses, points at which the impulse may be blocked by drugs.
   d. The nerve fiber produces neurotransmitters that may activate nearby nerve fibers to transmit pain impulses.

5. A patient comes to the clinic with a complaint of a dull pain in the anterior and posterior neck. On examination, the nurse notes that the patient has full range of motion (ROM) of the neck and no throat redness or enlarged head or neck lymph nodes. What will be the nurse's next appropriate assessment indicated by these findings?
   a. Palpation of the liver
   b. Auscultation of bowel sounds
   c. Inspection of the patient's ears
   d. Palpation for the presence of left flank pain

   neck pain may be liver issues

6. While caring for an unconscious patient, the nurse discovers a stage 2 pressure ulcer on the patient's heel. During care of the ulcer, what is the nurse's understanding of the patient's perception of pain?
   a. The patient will have a behavioral response if pain is perceived.
   b. The area should be treated as a painful lesion, using gentle cleansing and dressing.
   c. The area can be thoroughly scrubbed because the patient is not able to perceive pain.
   d. All nociceptive stimuli that are transmitted to the brain result in the perception of pain.

7. List in order the nociceptive processes that occur to communicate tissue damage to the CNS. No. 1 is the first process and No. 4 is the last process.

3 a. Perception
4 b. Modulation
2 c. Transmission
1 d. Transduction

8. Match the following types of pain in the left column with a category of pain from the upper right column and an example of the source of the pain from the lower right column.

Types of Pain

_2, 7_ a. Pain from loss of afferent input
_____ b. Pain persisting from sympathetic nervous system (SNS) activity
_____ c. Pain caused by dysfunction in the central nervous system (CNS)
_1, 3_ d. Pain arising from skin and subcutaneous tissue; well localized
_____ e. Pain arising from muscles and bones; localized or diffuse and radiating
_____ f. Pain felt along the distribution of peripheral nerve(s) from nerve damage
_____ g. Pain arising from visceral organs; well or poorly localized; referred cutaneously

Categories of Pain
1. Nociceptive pain
2. Neuropathic pain

Sources of Pain
3. Sunburn
4. Pancreatitis
5. Osteoarthritis
6. Poststroke pain
7. Phantom limb pain
8. Trigeminal neuralgia
9. Postmastectomy pain

9. Amitriptyline (Elavil) is prescribed for a patient with chronic pain from fibromyalgia. When the nurse explains that this drug is an antidepressant, the patient states that she is in pain, not depressed. What is the nurse's best response to the patient?
   a. Antidepressants will improve the patient's attitude and prevent a negative emotional response to the pain.
   b. Chronic pain almost always leads to depression, and the use of this drug will prevent depression from occurring.
   c. Some antidepressant drugs relieve pain by releasing neurotransmitters that prevent pain impulses from reaching the brain.
   d. Certain antidepressant drugs are metabolized in the liver to substances that numb the ends of nerve fibers, preventing the onset of pain.

10. A patient with trigeminal neuralgia has moderate to severe burning and shooting pain. In helping the patient to manage the pain, the nurse recognizes what about this type of pain?
    a. Treatment includes the use of adjuvant analgesics
    b. Will be chronic in nature and require long-term treatment
    c. Responds to small to moderate around-the-clock doses of oral opioids
    d. Can be well controlled with salicylates or nonsteroidal antiinflammatory drugs (NSAIDs)

11. In the following scenario, identify the elements of a pain assessment that are present.

    A 62-year-old male patient is admitted to the medical unit from the emergency department. On arrival he is trembling and nearly doubled over with severe, cramping abdominal pain. He indicates that he has severe right upper quadrant pain that radiates to his back and he is more comfortable walking bent forward than lying in bed. He notes that he has had several similar bouts of abdominal pain in the last month but "not as bad as this. This is the worst pain I can imagine." The other episodes lasted only about 2 hours. Today he experienced an acute onset of pain and nausea after eating fish and chips at a fast-food restaurant about 4 hours ago.

    a.

    b.

    c.

    d.

    e.

    f.

    g.

12. List the 10 basic principles that should guide the treatment of all pain.

    a.

    b.

    c.

    d.

    e.

    f.

    g.

    h.

    i.

    j.

13. A patient with colorectal cancer has continuous, poorly localized abdominal pain at an intensity of 5 on a scale of 0 to 10. How does the nurse teach the patient to use pain medications?
    a. On an around-the-clock schedule
    b. As often as necessary to keep the pain controlled
    c. By alternating two different types of drugs to prevent tolerance
    d. When the pain cannot be controlled with distraction or relaxation

14. A patient who has been taking ibuprofen (Motrin) and imipramine (Tofranil) for control of cancer pain is having increased pain. What would the health care provider recommend as an appropriate change in the medication plan?
    a. Add PO oxycodone (Oxycontin) to the other medications
    b. Substitute PO propoxyphene (Darvon), a mild opioid, for imipramine
    c. Add transdermal fentanyl (Duragesic) to the use of the other medications
    d. Substitute PO hydrocodone with acetaminophen (Lortab, Vicodin) for the other medications

15. A patient with chronic cancer-related pain has started using MS Contin for pain control and has developed common side effects of the drug. The nurse reassures the patient that tolerance will develop to most of these side effects but that continued treatment will most likely be required for what?
    a. Pruritus
    b. Dizziness
    c. Constipation
    d. Nausea and vomiting

16. A postoperative 68-year-old opioid-naive patient is receiving morphine by patient-controlled analgesia (PCA) for postoperative pain. What is the rationale for not initiating the PCA analgesic with a basal dose of analgesic as well?
    a. Opioid overdose
    b. Nausea and itching
    c. Lack of pain control
    d. Adverse respiratory outcomes

17. Which measures or drugs may be effective in controlling pain in the physiologic pain process stage of transduction (*select all that apply*)?
    a. Distraction
    b. Corticosteroids
    c. Epidural opioids
    d. Local anesthetics
    e. Antiseizure medications
    f. Nonsteroidal antiinflammatory drugs (NSAIDs)

18. A patient is receiving a continuous infusion of morphine via an epidural catheter following major abdominal surgery. Which actions should the nurse include in the plan of care (*select all that apply*)?
    a. Label the catheter as an epidural access.
    b. Assess the patient's pain relief frequently.
    c. Use sterile technique when caring for the catheter.
    d. Monitor the patient's level of consciousness (LOC).
    e. Monitor patient vital signs (blood pressure, heart rate, respirations).
    f. Assess the motor and sensory function of the patient's lower extremities.

19. A patient with multiple injuries resulting from an automobile accident tells the nurse that he has "bad" pain but that he can "tough it out" and does not require pain medication. To gain the patient's participation in pain management, what should the nurse explain to the patient?
    a. Patients have a responsibility to keep the nurse informed about their pain.
    b. Unrelieved pain has many harmful effects on the body that can impair recovery.
    c. Using pain medications rarely leads to addiction when they are used for actual pain.
    d. Nonpharmacologic therapies can be used to relieve his pain if he is afraid to use pain medications.

20. The patient has chronic pain that is no longer relieved with oral morphine. Which medication would the nurse expect to be ordered to provide better pain relief for this patient?
    a. Duragesic
    b. Oramorph SR
    c. Hydrocodone
    d. Intranasal butorphanol (Stadol)

CASE STUDY

Pain

Patient Profile

R.D. is a 62-year-old man being evaluated for a change in his pain therapy for chronic malignant pain from metastatic cancer.

Subjective Data

- Patient desires zero pain but will accept pain level of 3 to 4 on a scale of 0 to 10.
- He has been taking two Percocet tablets q4hr while awake but his pain is now usually at 4 to 5 with the medication.
- Patient reports that pain varies over 24 hours from 5 to 10.
- He always awakens in the morning with pain at 10 with nervousness, nausea, and a runny nose.
- When pain becomes severe he stays in bed and concentrates on blocking the pain by emptying his mind.
- He is worried that increased pain means his disease is worsening.
- He is afraid to take additional doses or other opioids because he fears addiction.

Objective Data

- Height: 6 ft, 0 in (183 cm)
- Weight: 150 lb (68 kg)
- Rigid posturing, slow gait

Discussion Questions

Using a separate sheet of paper, answer the following questions:

1. What additional assessment data should the nurse obtain from R.D. before making any decisions about his problem?
2. What data from the nursing assessment are characteristic of the affective, behavioral, and cognitive dimensions of the pain experience?
3. Based on R.D.'s lack of pain control with his current dosage of opioid and his symptoms on arising in the morning, what changes are indicated in his medication regimen?
4. *Priority Decision:* What are the priority teaching needs that should be included in a teaching plan for R.D. to titrate his analgesic dose effectively?
5. How could the nurse best help R.D. overcome his fear of addiction to opioid drugs?
6. What additional pain therapies could the nurse plan to help R.D. manage his pain?
7. *Priority Decision:* Based on the assessment data provided, what are the priority nursing diagnoses? Are there any collaborative problems?

CHAPTER 10

Palliative Care at End of Life

1. According to the World Health Organization, palliative care is an approach that improves quality of life for patients and their families who face problems associated with life-threatening illnesses. From the list below, identify the specific goals of palliative care (*select all that apply*).
   a. Regard dying as a normal process.
   b. Minimize the financial burden on the family.
   c. Provide relief from symptoms, including pain.
   d. Affirm life and neither hasten nor postpone death.
   e. Prolong the patient's life with aggressive new therapies.
   f. Support holistic patient care and enhance quality of life.
   g. Offer support to patients to live as actively as possible until death.
   h. Assist the patient and family to identify and access pastoral care services.
   i. Offer support to the family during the patient's illness and their own bereavement.

2. *Priority Decision:* The husband and daughter of a Hispanic woman dying from pancreatic cancer refuse to consider using hospice care. What is the first thing the nurse should do?
   a. Assess their understanding of what hospice care services are.
   b. Ask them how they will care for the patient without hospice care.
   c. Talk directly to the patient and family to see if she can change their minds.
   d. Accept their decision since they are Hispanic and prefer to care for their own.

3. List the two criteria for admission to a hospice program.
   a.

   b.

4. For each of the following body systems, identify three physical manifestations that the nurse would expect to see in a patient approaching death.

   Respiratory
   a.

   b.

   c.

   Skin
   a.

   b.

   c.

   Gastrointestinal
   a.

   b.

   c.

   Musculoskeletal
   a.

   b.

   c.

5. *Priority Decision:* A terminally ill patient is unresponsive and has cold, clammy skin with mottling on the extremities. The patient's husband and two grown children are arguing at the bedside about where the patient's funeral should be held. What should the nurse do first?
   a. Ask the family members to leave the room if they are going to argue.
   b. Take the family members aside and explain that the patient may be able to hear them.
   c. Tell the family members that this decision is premature because the patient has not yet died.
   d. Remind the family that this should be the patient's decision and to ask her if she regains consciousness.

6. A 20-year-old patient with a massive head injury is on life support, including a ventilator to maintain respirations. What three criteria for brain death are necessary to discontinue life support?
   a.

   b.

   c.

7. A patient with end-stage liver failure tells the nurse, "If I can just live to see my first grandchild who is expected in 5 months, then I can die happy." The nurse recognizes that the patient is demonstrating which of the following stages of grieving?
   a. Prolonged grief disorder
   b. Kübler-Ross's stage of bargaining
   c. Kübler-Ross's stage of depression
   d. The new normal stage of the Grief Wheel

8. A terminally ill man tells the nurse, "I have never believed there is a God or an afterlife, but now it is too terrible to imagine that I will not exist. Why was I here in the first place?" What does this comment help the nurse recognize about the patient's needs?
   a. He is experiencing spiritual distress.
   b. This man most likely will not have a peaceful death.
   c. He needs to be reassured that his feelings are normal.
   d. This patient should be referred to a clergyman for a discussion of his beliefs.

9. In most states, directives to physicians, durable power of attorney for health care, and medical power of attorney are included in which legal documents?
   a. Natural death acts
   b. Allow natural death
   c. Advance care planning
   d. Do Not Resuscitate order

10. A patient is receiving care to manage symptoms of a terminal illness when the disease no longer responds to treatment. What is this type of care known as?
    a. Terminal care
    b. Palliative care
    c. Supportive care
    d. Maintenance care

11. *Priority Decision:* A patient in the last stages of life is experiencing shortness of breath and air hunger. Based on practice guidelines, what is the most appropriate action by the nurse?
    a. Administer oxygen.
    b. Administer bronchodilators.
    c. Administer antianxiety agents.
    d. Use any methods that make the patient more comfortable.

12. End-of-life palliative nursing care involves
    a. constant assessment for changes in physiologic functioning.
    b. administering large doses of analgesics to keep the patient sedated.
    c. providing as little physical care as possible to prevent disturbing the patient.
    d. encouraging the patient and family members to verbalize their feelings of sadness, loss, and forgiveness.

13. The dying patient and family have many interrelated psychosocial and physical care needs. Which ones can the nurse begin to manage with the patient and family (*select all that apply*)?
    a. Anxiety
    b. Fear of pain
    c. The dying process
    d. Care being provided
    e. Anger toward the nurse
    f. Feeling powerless and hopeless

14. A deathly ill patient from a culture different than the nurse's is admitted. Which question is appropriate to help the nurse provide culturally competent care?
    a. "If you die, will you want an autopsy?"
    b. "Are you interested in learning about palliative or hospice care?"
    c. "Do you have any preferences for what happens if you are dying?"
    d. "Tell me about your expectations of care during this hospitalization."

CASE STUDY
End-of-Life Palliative Care
Patient Profile

S.J., a 42-year-old woman, had unsuccessful treatment for breast cancer 1 year ago and now has metastasis to the lung and vertebrae. She lives at home with her husband, a 15-year-old daughter, and a 12-year-old son. She has been referred to hospice because of her deteriorating condition and increasing pain. Her husband is an accountant and tries to do as much of his work at home as possible so that he can help care for his wife. Their children have become withdrawn, choosing to spend as much time as possible at their friends' homes and in outside activities.

Subjective Data

- S.J. reports that she stays in bed most of the time because it is too painful to stand and sit.
- She reports her pain as an 8 on a scale of 0 to 10 while taking oral MS Contin q12hr.
- She reports shortness of breath with almost any activity, such as getting up to go to the bathroom.
- S.J. says she knows she is dying but her greatest suffering results from her children not caring about her.
- She and her husband have not talked with the children about her dying.
- Her husband reports that he does not know how to help his wife anymore and that he feels guilty sometimes when he just wishes it were all over.

Objective Data

- Height: 5 ft, 2 in (157 cm)
- Weight: 97 lb (44 kg)
- Skin intact
- Vital signs: Temp 99°F (37.2°C), HR 92 bpm, RR 30, BP 102/60

Discussion Questions

Using a separate sheet of paper, answer the following questions:

1. What additional assessment data should the nurse obtain from S.J. and her husband before making any decisions about care of the family?
2. What types of grieving appear to be occurring in the family?
3. *Priority Decision*: What physical care should the nurse include in a plan for S.J. at this time?
4. What is the best way to facilitate healthy grieving in this family?
5. What resources of a hospice team are available to assist this patient and her family?
6. *Priority Decision:* Based on the assessment data provided, what are the priority nursing diagnoses?

Substance Abuse

1. What is the definition of substance abuse?
   a. A compulsive need to experience pleasure
   b. Behavior associated with maintaining an addiction
   c. Absence of a substance will cause withdrawal symptoms
   d. Overuse and dependence on a substance that negatively affects functioning

2. What term is used to describe a decreased effect of a substance following repeated exposure?
   a. Relapse
   b. Tolerance
   c. Abstinence
   d. Withdrawal

3. As health care professionals, nurses have a responsibility to help reduce the use of tobacco. List the recommended "five As" as brief clinical interventions.

   a.

   b

   c.

   d.

   e.

4. On admission to the hospital for a knee replacement, a patient who has smoked for 20 years expresses an interest in quitting. What is the best response by the nurse?
   a. "Good for you! You should talk to your doctor about that."
   b. "Why did you ever start in the first place? It's so hard to quit."
   c. "Since you won't be able to smoke while you are in the hospital, just don't start again when you are discharged.
   d. "Great! I'll help you make a plan and work with your doctor to get you what you need to start while you are here."

5. List two major health problems commonly seen in the acute care setting related to the abuse of the following substances.

   Nicotine
   a.

   b.

   Alcohol
   a.

   b.

   Cocaine and amphetamines
   a.

   b.

   Opioids
   a.

   b.

   Cannabis
   a.

   b.

6. What are the physiologic effects associated with cocaine and amphetamines (*select all that apply*)?
   a. Drowsiness
   b. Nasal damage
   c. Sexual arousal
   d. Constricted pupils
   e. Increase in appetite
   f. Tachycardia with hypertension

7. Which substance, when abused, can cause euphoria, drowsiness, decreased respiratory rate, and slurred speech?
   a. Opioids
   b. Alcohol
   c. Cannabis
   d. Depressants

8. Which manifestation(s) is (are) experienced by a patient when withdrawing from sedative-hypnotic addiction (*select all that apply*)?
   a. Seizures
   b. Violence
   c. Suicidal thoughts
   d. Tremors and chills
   e. Sweating, nausea, and cramps

9. When the nurse is encouraging a woman who smokes 1½ packs of cigarettes per day to quit with the use of nicotine replacement therapy, the woman asks how the nicotine in a patch or gum differs from the nicotine she gets from cigarettes. What should the nurse explain about nicotine replacement?
   a. It includes a substance that eventually creates an aversion to nicotine.
   b. It provides a noncarcinogenic nicotine, unlike the nicotine in cigarettes.
   c. It prevents the weight gain that is a concern to women who stop smoking.
   d. It eliminates the thousands of toxic chemicals that are inhaled with smoking.

10. Match the following drugs used for treatment of cocaine toxicity with their specific uses (answers may be used more than once).
    _____ a. Haloperidol (Haldol)   1. Tachycardia
    _____ b. IV lidocaine   2. Hallucinations
    _____ c. IV diazepam (Valium)   3. Dysrhythmias
    _____ d. Propranolol (Inderal)   4. Seizures
    _____ e. Bretylium (Bretylol)
    _____ f. IV lorazepam (Ativan)
    _____ g. Procainamide (Pronestyl)

11. A patient who is a heavy caffeine user has been NPO all day in preparation for a late afternoon surgery. The nurse monitors the patient for effects of caffeine withdrawal that may include
    a. headache.
    b. nervousness.
    c. mild tremors.
    d. shortness of breath.

12. The third day after an alcohol-dependent patient was admitted to the hospital for pancreatitis, the nurse determines that the patient is experiencing alcohol withdrawal. What are the signs of withdrawal on which the nurse bases this judgment (*select all that apply*)?
    a. Apathy
    b. Seizures
    c. Gross tremors
    d. Severe depression
    e. Cardiovascular collapse
    f. Visual and auditory hallucinations

13. Which question is the best approach by the nurse to assess a newly admitted patient's use of addictive drugs?
    a. "How do you relieve your stress?"
    b. "You don't use any illegal drugs, do you?"
    c. "Which alcohol or recreational drugs do you use?"
    d. "Do you have any addictions we should know about to prevent complications?"

14. To stop the behavior that leads to the most preventable cause of death in the United States, the nurse should support programs that
    a. prohibit alcohol use in public places.
    b. prevent tobacco use in children and adolescents.
    c. motivate individuals to enter addiction treatment.
    d. recognize addictions as illnesses rather than crimes.

15. A young woman is brought to the emergency department by police who found her lying on a downtown sidewalk. The initial nursing assessment finds that she is unresponsive and has a weak pulse of 112; shallow respirations of 8 breaths/minute; and cold, clammy skin. Identify the two medications that would most likely be given immediately to this patient and explain why they would be given.
    a.

    b.

16. *Priority Decision:* A patient with a history of alcohol abuse is admitted to the hospital following an automobile accident. What is most important for the nurse to assess to plan care for the patient?
    a. When the patient last had alcohol intake
    b. How much alcohol has recently been used
    c. What type of alcohol has recently been ingested
    d. The patient's current blood alcohol concentration

17. *Priority Decision:* A patient in alcohol withdrawal has a nursing diagnosis of ineffective protection related to sensorimotor deficits, seizure activity, and confusion. Which nursing intervention is most important for the patient?
    a. Provide a darkened, quiet environment free from external stimuli.
    b. Force fluids to assist in diluting the alcohol concentration in the blood.
    c. Monitor vital signs frequently to detect an extreme autonomic nervous system response.
    d. Use restraints as necessary to prevent the patient from reacting violently to hallucinations.

18. What is an important postoperative intervention indicated for the alcoholic patient who is alcohol intoxicated and is undergoing emergency surgery?
    a. Monitor weight because of malnutrition.
    b. Give an emergency dose of IV magnesium.
    c. Decrease pain medication to prevent cross-tolerance to opiates.
    d. Closely monitor for signs of withdrawal and respiratory and cardiac problems.

19. *Priority Decision:* During admission to the emergency department, a patient with chronic alcoholism is intoxicated and very disoriented and confused. Which drug will the nurse administer first?
    a. IV thiamine
    b. IV benzodiazepines
    c. IV haloperidol (Haldol)
    d. IV naloxone (Narcan) in normal saline

20. The nurse is working with a patient at the clinic who does not want to quit smoking even though he is having trouble breathing at times and has a frequent cough. Which clinical practice guideline strategies should the nurse use with this patient?
    a. Cost, cough, cleanliness, Chantix
    b. Ask, advise, assess, assist, arrange
    c. Deduce, describe, decide, deadline
    d. Relevance, risks, rewards, roadblocks, repetition

21. When assessing an older patient for substance abuse, the nurse specifically asks the patient about the use of alcohol and which other types of medications?
    a. Opioids
    b. Sedative-hypnotics
    c. Central nervous system stimulants
    d. Prescription and over-the-counter (OTC) medications

CASE STUDY
Cocaine Toxicity
Patient Profile

N.C. is a 34-year-old man who was admitted to the emergency department with chest pain, tachycardia, dizziness, nausea, and severe migraine-like headache.

Subjective Data

- He thinks he is having a heart attack.
- Admits he was at a party earlier in the evening drinking alcohol, smoking pot, and snorting cocaine.
- States he became irritable and restless.
- States he has experienced an increased need for cocaine in the past few months.

Objective Data

- Appears extremely nervous and irritable
- Appears pale and diaphoretic
- Has tremors
- BP 210/110, HR 100 bpm, RR 30

Discussion Questions

Using a separate sheet of paper, answer the following questions:

1. What other information is needed to assess N.C.'s condition?
2. How should questions related to these areas be addressed?
3. What other clues should the nurse be alert for in assessing N.C.'s drug use?
4. What emergency conditions must be carefully monitored?
5. *Priority Decision:* What are the priority nursing interventions?
6. What is the best way to approach N.C. to engage him in a treatment program?
7. *Priority Decision:* Based on the assessment data presented, what are the priority nursing diagnoses? Are there any collaborative problems?

Inflammation and Wound Healing

1. A patient with an inflammatory disease has the following clinical manifestations. Identify the primary chemical mediators involved in producing the manifestation and the physiologic change that causes the manifestation.

Clinical Manifestation	Chemical Mediators	Physiologic Change
Fever		
Redness		
Edema		
Leukocytosis		

2. In a patient with leukocytosis with a shift to the left, what does the nurse recognize as causing this finding?
   a. The complement system has been activated to enhance phagocytosis.
   b. Monocytes are released into the blood in larger-than-normal amounts.
   c. The response to cellular injury is not adequate to remove damaged tissue and promote healing.
   d. The demand for neutrophils causes the release of immature neutrophils from the bone marrow.

3. What does the mechanism of chemotaxis accomplish?
   a. Causes the transformation of monocytes into macrophages
   b. Involves a pathway of chemical processes resulting in cellular lysis
   c. Attracts the accumulation of neutrophils and monocytes to an area of injury
   d. Slows the blood flow in a damaged area, allowing migration of leukocytes into tissue

4. What effect does the action of the complement system have on inflammation?
   a. Modifies the inflammatory response to prevent stimulation of pain
   b. Increases body temperature, resulting in destruction of microorganisms
   c. Produces prostaglandins and leukotrienes that increase blood flow, edema, and pain
   d. Increases inflammatory responses of vascular permeability, chemotaxis, and phagocytosis

5. *Priority Decision:* Key interventions for treating soft tissue injury and resulting inflammation are remembered using the acronym RICE. What are the most important actions for the emergency department nurse to do for the patient with an ankle injury?
   a. Reduce swelling, shine light on wound, control mobility, and elicit the history of the injury
   b. Rub the wound clean, immobilize the area, cover the area protectively, and exercise that leg
   c. Rest with immobility, apply a cold compress, apply a compress bandage, and elevate the ankle
   d. Rinse the wounded ankle, image the ankle, carry the patient, and extend the ankle with imaging

6. What is characteristic of chronic inflammation?
   a. It may last 2 to 3 weeks.
   b. The injurious agent persists or repeatedly injures tissue.
   c. Infective endocarditis is an example of chronic inflammation.
   d. Neutrophils are the predominant cell type at the site of inflammation.

7. During the healing phase of inflammation, which cells would be mostly likely to regenerate?
   a. Skin
   b. Neurons
   c. Cardiac muscle
   d. Skeletal muscle

8. Place the following events that occur during healing by primary intention in sequential order from 1 (first) to 10 (last).

1 _____ a. Blood clots form

10 _____ b. Avascular, pale, mature scar present

2 _____ c. Accumulation of inflammatory debris

4 _____ d. Enzymes from neutrophils digest fibrin

8 _____ e. Epithelial cells migrate across wound surface

6 _____ f. Fibroblasts migrate to site and secrete collagen

7 _____ g. Budding capillaries result in pink, vascular friable wound

9 _____ h. Contraction of healing area by movement of myofibroblasts

3 _____ i. Macrophages ingest and digest cellular debris and red blood cells

5 _____ j. Fibrin clot that serves as meshwork for capillary growth and epithelial cell migration

9. What is the primary difference between healing by primary intention and healing by secondary intention?
   a. Secondary healing requires surgical debridement for healing to occur.
   b. Primary healing involves suturing two layers of granulation tissue together.
   c. Presence of more granulation tissue in secondary healing results in more scarring.
   d. Healing by secondary intention takes longer because more steps in the healing process are necessary.

10. A patient had abdominal surgery 3 months ago and calls the clinic with complaints of severe abdominal pain and cramping, vomiting, and bloating. What should the nurse most likely suspect as the cause of the patient's problem?
    a. Infection
    b. Adhesion
    c. Contracture
    d. Evisceration

11. A patient had a complicated vaginal hysterectomy. The student nurse provided perineal care after the patient had a bowel movement. The student nurse tells the nurse there was a lot of light brown, smelly drainage seeping from the perianal area. What should the nurse suspect when assessing this patient?
    a. Dehiscence
    b. Hemorrhage
    c. Keloid formation
    d. Fistula formation

12. Which nutrients aid in capillary synthesis and collagen production by the fibroblasts in wound healing?
    a. Fats
    b. Proteins
    c. Vitamin C
    d. Vitamin A

13. What role do the B-complex vitamins play in wound healing?
    a. Decrease metabolism
    b. Protect protein from being used for energy
    c. Provide metabolic energy for the inflammatory process
    d. Coenzymes for fat, protein, and carbohydrate metabolism

14. The patient is admitted from home with a stage II pressure ulcer. This wound is classified as a yellow wound using the red-yellow-black concept of wound care. What is the nurse likely to observe when she does her wound assessment?
    a. Serosanguineous drainage
    b. Adherent gray necrotic tissue
    c. Clean, moist granulating tissue
    d. Creamy ivory to yellow-green exudate

15. What type of dressing will the nurse most likely use for the patient in Question 14?
    a. Dry, sterile dressing — closed wound
    b. Absorptive dressing — yellow
    c. Negative pressure wound therapy — black
    d. Telfa dressing with antibiotic ointment — red wound

16. The patient's wound is not healing, so the health care provider is going to send the patient home with negative pressure wound therapy or a "wound vac" device. What will the caregiver need to understand about the use of this device?
    a. The wound must be cleaned daily. — weekly
    b. The patient will be placed in a hyperbaric chamber.
    c. The occlusive dressing must be sealed tightly to the skin.
    d. The diet will not be as important with this sort of treatment.

17. *Priority Decision:* During care of patients, what is the most important precaution for preventing transmission of infections?
    a. Wearing face and eye protection during routine daily care of the patient
    b. Wearing nonsterile gloves when in contact with body fluids, excretions, and contaminated items
    c. Wearing a gown to protect the skin and clothing during patient care activities likely to soil clothing
    d. Hand washing after touching fluids and secretions and removing gloves, as well as between patient contacts

18. Which patient is at the greatest risk for developing pressure ulcers?
    a. A 42-year-old obese woman with type 2 diabetes
    b. A 78-year-old man who is confused and malnourished
    c. A 30-year-old man who is comatose following a head injury
    d. A 65-year-old woman who has urge and stress incontinence

19. *Priority Decision:* What is the most important nursing intervention for the prevention and treatment of pressure ulcers?
    a. Using pressure-reduction devices
    b. Massaging pressure areas with lotion
    c. Repositioning the patient a minimum of every 2 hours
    d. Using lift sheets and trapeze bars to facilitate patient movement

20. The patient is transferring from another facility with the description of a sore on her sacrum that is deep enough to see the muscle. What stage of pressure ulcer does the nurse expect to see on admission?
    a. Stage I
    b. Stage II
    c. Stage III
    d. Stage IV

21. A patient's documentation indicates he has a stage III pressure ulcer on his right hip. What should the nurse expect to find on assessment of the patient's right hip?
    a. Exposed bone, tendon, or muscle
    b. An abrasion, blister, or shallow crater
    c. Deep crater through subcutaneous tissue to fascia
    d. Persistent redness (or bluish color in darker skin tones)

22. *Delegation Decision*: Which nursing interventions for a patient with a Stage IV sacral pressure ulcer are most appropriate to assign or delegate to a licensed practical nurse (LPN) (*select all that apply*)?
    a. Assess and document wound appearance.
    b. Teach the patient pressure ulcer risk factors.
    c. Choose the type of dressing to apply to the ulcer.
    d. Measure the size (width, length, depth) of the ulcer.
    e. Assist the patient to change positions at frequent intervals.

CASE STUDY
Inflammation
Patient Profile

G.K., a 28-year-old patient who has type 1 diabetes, is admitted to the hospital with cellulitis of her left lower leg. She had been applying heating pads to the leg for the last 48 hours but the leg has become more painful and she has developed chills.

Subjective Data
- States that she has severe pain and heaviness in her leg
- States she cannot bear weight on her leg and has been in bed for 3 days
- Lives alone and has not had anyone to help her with meals

Objective Data
Physical Examination

- Irregular shape, yellow-red, 2-cm diameter, 1-cm deep, open wound above the left medial malleolus with moderate amount of thick, yellow drainage
- Left leg red and swollen from ankle to knee
- Calf measurement on left 3 inches larger than on right
- Temp: 102°F (38.9°C)
- Height: 5 ft, 4 in (160 cm)
- Weight: 184 lb (83.7 kg)

Laboratory Tests

- White blood cell (WBC) count: 18,300/μL (18.3 × 10³/L; 80% neutrophils, 12% bands)
- Wound culture: *Staphylococcus aureus*

Discussion Questions

Using a separate sheet of paper, answer the following questions:

1. What clinical manifestations of inflammation are present in G.K.?
2. What type of exudate is draining from the open wound?
3. What type of ulcer is this likely to be?
4. What is the significance of her WBC count and differential?
5. What factors are present in G.K.'s situation that could delay wound healing?
6. Her health care provider orders acetaminophen to be given PRN for a temperature above 102°F (38.9°C). How does the acetaminophen act to interfere with the fever mechanism? Why is the acetaminophen to be given only if the temperature is above 102°F? To prevent cycling of chills and diaphoresis, how should the nurse administer the acetaminophen?
7. What type of wound dressing would promote healing of the open wound?
8. *Priority Decision*: What are the priority precautions to prevent transmission of infection in the care of G.K.?
9. *Priority Decision*: Based on the assessment data provided, what are the priority nursing diagnoses? Are there any collaborative problems?

Genetics and Genomics

1. Physical traits expressed by an individual is the definition for which term?
   a. Allele
   b. Genomics
   c. Phenotype
   d. Chromosomes

2. Which definition is the best description of the term *genotype*?
   a. Basic unit of heredity; arranged on chromosome
   b. Transmission of a disease from parent to child
   c. Genetic identity of an individual not seen as outward characteristics
   d. Family tree containing genetic characteristics and disorders of that family

3. A 26-year-old man was adopted. What health information related to his biological parents and family will be most useful to him when he gets married (*select all that apply*)?
   a. Cholecystitis occurring in family members
   b. Occurrence of prostate cancer in one uncle
   c. Ages of family members diagnosed with diseases
   d. Kidney stones present in extended family members
   e. Age and cause of death of deceased family members

4. The new parents of an infant born with Down syndrome ask the nurse what happened to cause the chromosomal abnormality. What is the best response by the nurse?
   a. "During cell division of the reproductive cells there is an error causing an abnormal number of chromosomes."
   b. "A mutation in one of the chromosomes created an autosomal recessive gene that is expressed as Down syndrome."
   c. "An abnormal gene on one of the two chromosomes was transferred to the fetus, causing an abnormal chromosome."
   d. "A process of translocation caused the exchange of genetic material between the two chromosomes in the cell, resulting in abnormal chromosomes."

5. When a father has Huntington's disease with a heterozygous genotype, the nurse uses the Punnett square to illustrate the inheritance patterns and the probability of transmission of the autosomal dominant disease. The mother does not carry the Huntington's disease gene. Complete the Punnett square below to illustrate this inheritance pattern, using "H" as the normal gene and "h" as the gene for Huntington's disease.

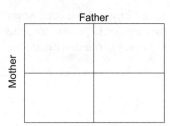

There is a _____ % chance that offspring will be unaffected.

There is a _____ % chance that offspring will be affected.

6. Which of the following statements accurately describe genetic testing (*select all that apply*)?
   a. Results of genetic testing may raise psychologic and emotional issues.
   b. An ethical issue that is raised with genetic testing is protection of privacy to prevent discrimination.
   c. Genetic testing of the mother can be used to determine an unborn child's risk of having genetic conditions.
   d. An example of genetic testing that is required by all states is premarital testing of women for the hemophilia gene.
   e. Genetic testing for *BRCA1* and *BRCA2* mutations can identify women who may choose to have mastectomies to prevent breast cancer.

7. Tay-Sachs disease is an autosomal recessive disease. Both parents have been identified as heterozygous. There is a _____% chance that their offspring will be affected.

8. A couple lost a second baby to miscarriage. They are both considering having genetic testing done before trying to get pregnant again. What should the nurse include when teaching about genetic testing?
   a. A particular genetic test will tell them if there is a specific genetic change.
   b. The test results will identify the diseases their children will inherit from them.
   c. Genetic testing will determine if they are predisposed to developing a genetic disease.
   d. Genetic testing kits that are available on the Internet are just as good and less costly than going to a genetic counselor.

9. The daughter of a man with Huntington's disease is having presymptomatic genetic testing done. What does a positive result mean for her?
   a. She will get the disease.
   b. She is a carrier of Huntington's disease.
   c. She will be at increased risk for developing the disease.
   d. She should change her diet, exercise, and environment to prevent the disease.

10. A 21-year-old patient says no one in his family has type 1 diabetes mellitus but he has had it since childhood. He asks how his diabetes was transmitted to him. The nurse should explain to him that this disease is
    a. a single gene disorder
    b. a chromosome disorder
    c. an acquired genetic disorder
    d. a multifactorial genetic disorder

11. The physician plans to prescribe trastuzumab (Herceptin) for the patient with breast cancer. What testing will the physician order before prescribing this medication?
    a. HER2 protein levels
    b. *BRCA2* gene mutation
    c. *BRCA1* gene mutation
    d. Stage II cancer identification

12. The physician is having difficulty finding the appropriate dose for the patient taking warfarin (Coumadin). What can the nurse suggest that may solve this problem?
    a. Pharmacogenetic testing
    b. Start bivalirudin (Angiomax) IV
    c. Change from warfarin (Coumadin) to clopidogrel (Plavix) and aspirin
    d. Change from warfarin (Coumadin) to enoxaparin (Lovenox) injections

13. A 20-year-old patient has a family history of colon cancer. Genetic testing shows he has the gene for familial adenomatous polyposis. What should the nurse teach the patient to do?
    a. Change his diet
    b. Have annual colonoscopies
    c. Consider a referral for gene therapy
    d. Not to have children so they will not be affected

14. What statement accurately describes gene therapy?
    a. May activate a mutated gene that is functioning improperly.
    b. Is a risky technique under study for genetic diseases with no cure.
    c. Is frequently done by replacing a healthy gene with a mutated gene.
    d. Introduces a new gene into reproductive cells to help fight a genetic disease.

15. The National Marrow Donor Program obtains hematopoietic stem cells from donors for recipients in need. When discussing this donation with the donor, what should the nurse know about these stem cells?
    a. They must come from an embryo or umbilical cord.
    b. These cells will form new blood cells for the recipient.
    c. Taking these cells will cause the donor to become anemic.
    d. These cells must be removed with a bone marrow aspiration.

CASE STUDY

Genetics

Patient Profile

D.L., a 24-year-old woman, is concerned about having children because her younger brother has Duchenne muscular dystrophy (MD). She is seeking genetic testing.

Subjective Data

- She is engaged to be married.
- She has many questions about her risks. (See questions below.)

Objective Data

- Her eyes are darting around the room.
- Her hands and feet are trembling.
- She is chewing her fingernails.

Discussion Questions

Using a separate sheet of paper, answer the following questions:

1. What are the nurse's responsibilities in working with D.L.?
2. What type of genetic disorder is Duchenne MD?
3. D.L. asks, "Will I develop MD?" How should the nurse respond?
4. D.L. wants to know: "What are the chances my children will develop MD?"
5. D.L. is also worried about who will see her genetic testing results and if they will affect her future health insurance. What should the nurse tell her?

Altered Immune Responses and Transplantation

1. Which type of immunity is the result of contact with the antigen through infection and is the longest lasting type of immunity?
   a. Active innate immunity
   b. Passive innate immunity
   c. Active acquired immunity
   d. Passive acquired immunity

2. What accurately describes passive acquired immunity (*select all that apply*)?
   a. Pooled gamma globulin
   b. Immunization with antigen
   c. Temporary for several months
   d. Immediate, lasting several weeks
   e. Maternal immunoglobulins in neonate
   f. Boosters may be needed for extended protection

3. How does an antigen stimulate an immune response?
   a. It is captured, processed, and presented to a lymphocyte by a macrophage.
   b. It circulates in the blood, where it comes in contact with circulating lymphocytes.
   c. It is a foreign protein that has antigenic determinants different from those of the body.
   d. It combines with larger molecules that are capable of stimulating production of antibodies.

4. Which T lymphocytes are involved in direct attack and destruction of foreign pathogens?
   a. Dendritic cells
   b. Natural killer cells
   c. T helper (CD4) cells
   d. T cytotoxic (CD8) cells

5. How does interferon help the body's natural defenses?
   a. Directly attacks and destroys virus-infected cells
   b. Augments the immune response by activating phagocytes
   c. Induces production of antiviral proteins in cells that prevent viral replication
   d. Is produced by viral infected cells and prevents the transmission of the virus to adjacent cells

6. What is included in the humoral immune response?
   a. Surveillance for malignant cell changes
   b. Production of antigen-specific immunoglobulins
   c. Direct attack of antigens by activated B lymphocytes
   d. Releasing cytokines responsible for destruction of antigens

7. Where and into what do activated B lymphocytes differentiate?
   a. Spleen; natural killer cells that destroy infected cells
   b. Bone marrow; plasma cells that secrete immunoglobulins
   c. Thymus; memory B-cells that retain a memory of the antigen
   d. Bursa of Fabricius; helper cells that in turn activate additional B lymphocytes

8. Which immunoglobulin is responsible for the primary immune response and forms antibodies to ABO blood antigens?
   a. IgA
   b. IgD
   c. IgG
   d. IgM

9. Which immunoglobulins will initially protect a newborn baby of a breastfeeding mother (*select all that apply*)?
   a. IgA
   b. IgD
   c. IgE
   d. IgG
   e. IgM

10. Which characteristic describes immunoglobulin E (*select all that apply*)?
    - (a.) Assists in parasitic infections
    - (b.) Responsible for allergic reactions
    - c. Present on the lymphocyte surface
    - d. Assists in B-lymphocyte differentiation
    - e. Predominant in secondary immune response
    - f. Protects body surfaces and mucous membranes

11. What are the important functions of cell-mediated immunity (*select all that apply*)?
    - (a.) Fungal infections
    - b. Transfusion reactions
    - (c.) Rejection of transplanted tissues
    - (d.) Contact hypersensitivity reactions
    - e. Immunity against pathogens that survive outside cells

12. A 69-year-old woman asks the nurse whether it is possible to "catch" cancer because many of her friends of the same age have been diagnosed with different kinds of cancer. In responding to the woman, the nurse understands that what factor increases the incidence of tumors in older adults?
    - a. An increase in autoantibodies
    - b. Decreased activity of the bone marrow
    - c. Decreased differentiation of T lymphocytes
    - (d.) Decreased size and activity of the thymus gland

13. What describes the occurrence of a type IV or delayed hypersensitivity transplant reaction?
    - a. Antigen links with specific IgE antibodies bound to mast cells or basophils releasing chemical mediators
    - b. Cellular lysis or phagocytosis through complement activation following antigen-antibody binding on cell surfaces
    - (c.) Sensitized T lymphocytes attack antigens or release cytokines that attract macrophages that cause tissue damage
    - d. Antigens combined with IgG and IgM too small to be removed by mononuclear phagocytic system deposit in tissue and cause fixation of complement

14. What are examples of type I or IgE-mediated hypersensitivity reactions (*select all that apply*)?
    - a. Asthma
    - b. Urticaria
    - c. Angioedema
    - d. Allergic rhinitis
    - e. Atopic dermatitis
    - f. Contact dermatitis
    - g. Anaphylactic shock
    - h. Transfusion reactions
    - i. Goodpasture syndrome

15. Which type of hypersensitivity reaction occurs with rheumatoid arthritis and acute glomerulonephritis?
    - a. Type I or IgE-mediated hypersensitivity reaction
    - b. Type II or cytotoxic hypersensitivity reaction
    - (c.) Type III or immune-complex mediated hypersensitivity reaction
    - d. Type IV or delayed hypersensitivity reaction

16. For the patient with allergic rhinitis, which therapy should the nurse expect to be ordered first?
    - a. Corticosteroids
    - b. Immunotherapy
    - c. Antipruritic drugs
    - (d.) Sympathomimetic/decongestant drugs

17. A patient was given an IM injection of penicillin in the gluteus maximus and developed dyspnea and weakness within minutes following the injection. Which additional assessment findings indicate that the patient is having an anaphylactoid reaction (*select all that apply*)?
    - a. Wheezing
    - b. Hypertension
    - c. Rash on arms
    - d. Constricted pupils
    - e. Slowed strong pulse
    - f. Feeling of impending doom

18. **Priority Decision:** The patient is admitted from a nearby park with an apparent anaphylactic reaction to a bee sting. He is experiencing dyspnea and hypotension with swelling at the site. Number the following actions in the order of priority that the nurse should implement for this patient.
    - _____ a. Provide oxygen
    - _____ b. Remove the stinger
    - _____ c. Ensure a patent airway
    - _____ d. Prepare to administer epinephrine
    - _____ e. Start IV for fluid and medication access
    - _____ f. Position patient flat with the legs elevated
    - _____ g. Anticipate intubation with severe respiratory distress
    - _____ h. Have diphenhydramine (Benadryl) and nebulized albuterol available

19. Which rationale describes treatment of atopic allergies with immunotherapy?
    a. It decreases the levels of allergen-specific T helper cells.
    b. It decreases the level of IgE so that it does not react as readily with an allergen.
    c. It stimulates increased IgG to bind with allergen-reactive sites, preventing mast cell–bound IgE reactions.
    d. It gradually increases the amount of allergen in the body until it is no longer recognized as foreign and does not elicit an antibody reaction.

20. Which description about a nurse who develops a contact dermatitis from wearing latex gloves is accurate?
    a. This demonstrates a type I allergic reaction to natural latex proteins.
    b. Use powder-free latex gloves to prevent the development of symptoms.
    c. Use an oil-based hand cream when wearing gloves to prevent latex allergy.
    d. This demonstrates a type IV allergic reaction to chemicals used in the manufacture of latex gloves.

21. A 28-year-old male Gulf War veteran tells the nurse he gets a headache, sore throat, shortness of breath, and nausea when his girlfriend wears perfume and when he was painting her apartment. He is afraid he has cancer. What does the nurse suspect may be the patient's problem?
    a. He has posttraumatic stress disorder.
    b. He has multiple chemical sensitivities.
    c. He needs to wear a mask when he paints.
    d. He is looking for an excuse to break up with his girlfriend.

22. Although the cause of autoimmune disorders is unknown, which factors are believed to be present in most conditions (*select all that apply*)?
    a. Younger age
    b. Male gender
    c. Inheritance of susceptibility genes
    d. Initiation of autoreactivity by triggers
    e. Frequent viruses throughout the lifetime

23. Why is plasmapheresis indicated in the treatment of autoimmune disorders?
    a. Obtain plasma for analysis and evaluation of specific autoantibodies
    b. Decrease high lymphocyte levels in the blood to prevent immune responses
    c. Remove autoantibodies, antigen-antibody complexes, and inflammatory mediators of immune reactions
    d. Add monocytes to the blood to promote removal of immune complexes by the mononuclear phagocyte system

24. Before the patient receives a kidney transplant, a crossmatch test is ordered. What does a positive crossmatch indicate?
    a. Matches tissue types for a successful transplantation
    b. Determines paternity and predicts risk for certain diseases
    c. Establishes racial background and predicts risk for certain diseases
    d. Cytotoxic antibodies to the donor contraindicate transplanting this donor's organ

25. What is the most common cause of secondary immunodeficiency disorders?
    a. Chronic stress
    b. T-cell deficiency from HIV
    c. Drug-induced immunosuppression
    d. Common variable hypogammaglobulinemia

26. Which characteristics are seen with acute transplant rejection (*select all that apply*)?
    a. Treatment is supportive
    b. Only occurs with transplanted kidneys
    c. Organ must be removed when it occurs
    d. The recipient's T cytotoxic lymphocytes attack the foreign organ
    e. Long-term use of immunosuppressants necessary to combat the rejection
    f. Usually reversible with additional or increased immunosuppressant therapy

27. The patient is experiencing fibrosis and glomerulopathy a year after a kidney transplant. Which type of rejection is occurring?
    a. Acute
    b. Chronic
    c. Delayed
    d. Hyperacute

28. What are the most common immunosuppressive agents used to prevent rejection of transplanted organs?
    a. Cyclosporine, sirolimus, and muromonab-CD3
    b. Prednisone, polyclonal antibodies, and cyclosporine
    c. Azathioprine, mycophenolate mofetil, and sirolimus
    d. Tacrolimus, prednisone, and mycophenolate mofetil

29. The patient has received a bone marrow transplant. Soon after the transplant there is a rash on the patient's skin. She says her skin is itchy and she has severe abdominal pain. What best summarizes what is happening to the patient and how she will be treated?
    a. Graft rejection occurring; treat with different immunosuppressive agents
    b. Dry skin and nausea are side effects of immunosuppressants; decrease the dose
    c. Transplanted bone marrow is rejecting her tissue; prevent with immunosuppressive agents
    d. Dry skin from the dry air and nausea from the food in the hospital; treat with humidifier and home food

CASE STUDY

Allergy

Patient Profile

M.W., a 54-year-old male patient, has been diagnosed as having chronic allergic rhinitis. His health care provider pre-scribed oral antihistamines for control of his symptoms, which has not been completely effective. He is to undergo skin testing to identify specific allergens.

Subjective Data

- Itching of eyes, nose, and throat
- Stuffy nose, head congestion

Objective Data

- Clear nasal drainage; reddened eyes and lacrimation

Discussion Questions

Using a separate sheet of paper, answer the following questions:

1. What assessments of M.W. should be included by the nurse?
2. What immunoglobulins and chemical mediators are involved in M.W.'s allergic reaction?
3. Describe the procedure the nurse uses to perform the skin testing. What results indicate a positive response?
4. What precautions should be taken by the nurse during skin testing?
5. How do antihistamines act to relieve allergic symptoms? What information should the nurse include in teaching M.W. about using the antihistamines?
6. Skin testing indicates M.W. has an allergy to household dust. What information should the nurse include in teaching M.W. to control his exposure to this allergen?
7. M.W. is to begin immunotherapy. What would be the advantages and disadvantages of using sublingual immunotherapy?
8. What precautions does the nurse use during the subcutaneous administration of the allergen extract?
9. *Priority Decision:* Based on the assessment data provided, what are the priority nursing diagnoses? Are there any collaborative problems?

CHAPTER

15 Infection and Human Immunodeficiency Virus Infection

1. To what is the increase in emerging and untreatable infections attributed (*select all that apply*)?
   - a. The evolution of new infectious agents
   - b. Use of antibiotics to treat viral infections
   - c. Human population encroachment into wilderness areas
   - d. Transmission of infectious agents from humans to animals
   - e. An increased number of immunosuppressed and chronically ill people

2. The three antibiotic-resistant bacteria that are of most current concern in North America are _____, _____, and _____.

3. What are the recommended measures to prevent the transmission of health care–associated infections (HAIs) (*select all that apply*)?
   - a. Empty bedpans as soon as possible
   - b. Limit fresh flowers in patient rooms
   - c. Remove urinals from bedside tables
   - d. Use personal protective equipment
   - e. Hand washing or alcohol-based sanitizing
   - f. Have patients wear sandals in the shower

4. A patient with diarrhea has been diagnosed with *Clostridium difficile*. Along with standard precautions, which kind of transmission-based precautions will be used when the nurse is caring for this patient?
   - a. Droplet precautions
   - b. Contact precautions
   - c. Isolation precautions
   - d. Airborne precautions

5. A 78-year-old patient has developed *Haemophilus influenzae*. In addition to standard precautions, what should the nurse use to protect herself and other patients when working within 3 feet of the patient?
   - a. Mask
   - b. Gown
   - c. Gloves
   - d. Shoe covers

6. An 82-year-old male patient with pneumonia who is in the intensive care unit (ICU) is beginning to have decreased cognitive function. What should the nurse first suspect as a potential cause of this change?
   - a. Fatigue
   - b. Infection
   - c. ICU psychosis
   - d. Medication allergy

7. The nurse realizes that the patient understands the teaching about decreasing the risk for antibiotic-resistant infection when the patient says which of the following?
   - a. "I know I should take the antibiotic for one day after I feel better."
   - b. "I want an antibiotic ordered for my cold so I can feel better sooner."
   - c. "I always save some pills because I get the illness again after I first feel better."
   - d. "I will follow the directions for taking the antibiotic so I will get over this infection."

8. In each of the following situations identify which option has the highest risk for human immunodeficiency virus (HIV) transmission?
   - a. Transmission to women OR to men during sexual intercourse
   - b. Hollow-bore needle used for vascular access OR used for IM injection
   - c. First 2 to 6 months of infection OR 1 year after infection
   - d. Perinatal transmission from HIV-infected mothers taking antiretroviral therapy OR HIV-infected mothers using no therapy
   - e. A splash exposure of HIV-infected blood on skin with an open lesion OR a needle-stick exposure to HIV-infected blood

9. Place the following events of HIV infection of a cell in sequence from 1 (first) to 7 (last).

   _____ a. Viral RNA is converted to single-stranded viral DNA with assistance of reverse transcriptase

   _____ b. Viral DNA is spliced into cell genome using the enzyme integrase

   _____ c. gp 120 proteins on viral envelope combine with CD4 receptors of body cells

   _____ d. Cell replicates infected daughter cells and makes more HIV

   _____ e. Viral RNA and reverse transcriptase enzyme enter host CD4$^+$ T cell

   _____ f. Long strands of viral RNA are cut in the presence of protease

   _____ g. Single-stranded viral DNA replicates into double-stranded DNA

10. Indicate below which event (from Question 9) of HIV infection of a cell is controlled by each drug. This would also be the mechanism of action of the drug.

Drug	Mechanism of Action
Entry inhibitors	
Reverse transcriptase inhibitors	
Integrase inhibitors	
Protease inhibitors	

11. What is a primary reason that the normal immune response fails to contain the HIV infection?
    a. CD4$^+$ T cells become infected with HIV and are destroyed.
    b. The virus inactivates B cells, preventing the production of HIV antibodies.
    c. Natural killer cells are destroyed by the virus before the immune system can be activated.
    d. Monocytes ingest infected cells, differentiate into macrophages, and shed viruses in body tissues.

12. Which characteristic corresponds with the acute stage of HIV infection?
    a. Burkitt's lymphoma   c. Persistent fevers and night sweats
    b. Temporary fall of CD4$^+$ T cells   d. *Pneumocystis jiroveci* pneumonia

13. What finding supports the diagnosis of acquired immunodeficiency syndrome (AIDS) in the individual with HIV?
    a. Flu-like symptoms   c. CD4$^+$ T cells 200–500/μL
    b. Oral hairy leukoplakia   d. Cytomegalovirus retinitis

14. Why do opportunistic diseases develop in an individual with AIDS?
    a. They are side effects of drug treatment of AIDS.
    b. They are sexually transmitted to individuals during exposure to HIV.
    c. They are characteristic in individuals with stimulated B and T lymphocytes.
    d. These infections or tumors occur in a person with an incompetent immune system.

15. Which characteristics describe *Pneumocystis jiroveci* infection, an opportunistic disease that can be associated with HIV?
    a. May cause fungal meningitis
    b. Diagnosed by lymph node biopsy
    c. Pneumonia with dry, nonproductive cough
    d. Viral retinitis, stomatitis, esophagitis, gastritis, or colitis

16. Which opportunistic disease associated with AIDS is characterized by hyperpigmented lesions of skin, lungs, and gastrointestinal (GI) tract?
    a. Kaposi sarcoma   c. Herpes simplex type 1 infection
    b. *Candida albicans*   d. Varicella-zoster virus infection

✳ 17. A patient comes to the clinic and requests testing for HIV infection. Before administering testing, what is most important for the nurse to do?
  a. Ask the patient to identify all sexual partners
  b. Determine when the patient thinks exposure to HIV occurred
  c. Explain that all test results must be repeated at least twice to be valid
  d. Discuss prevention practices to prevent transmission of the HIV to others

18. The "rapid" HIV antibody testing is performed on a patient at high risk for HIV infection. What should the nurse explain about this test?
  a. The test measures the activity of the HIV and reports viral loads as real numbers.
  b. This test is highly reliable, and in 5 minutes the patient will know if HIV infection is present.
  c. If the results are positive, another blood test and a return appointment for results will be necessary.
  d. This test detects drug-resistant viral mutations that are present in viral genes to evaluate resistance to antiretroviral drugs.

19. Treatment with two nucleoside reverse transcriptase inhibitors (NRTIs) and a protease inhibitor (PI) is prescribed for a patient with HIV infection who has a CD4$^+$ T-cell count of <400/µL. The patient asks why so many drugs are necessary for treatment. What should the nurse explain as the primary rationale for combination therapy?
  a. Cross-resistance between specific antiretroviral drugs is reduced when drugs are given in combination.
  b. Combinations of antiretroviral drugs decrease the potential for development of antiretroviral-resistant HIV variants.
  c. Side effects of the drugs are reduced when smaller doses of three different drugs are used rather than large doses of one drug.
  d. When CD4$^+$ T-cell counts are <500/µL, a combination of drugs that have different actions is more effective in slowing HIV growth.

20. What is one of the most significant factors in determining when to start antiretroviral therapy in a patient with HIV infection?
  a. Whether the patient has high levels of HIV antibodies
  b. Confirmation that the patient has contracted HIV infection
  c. The patient's readiness to commit to a complex, lifelong, uncomfortable drug regimen
  d. Whether the patient has a support system to help manage the costs and side effects of the drugs

21. After teaching a patient with HIV infection about using antiretroviral drugs, the nurse recognizes that further teaching is needed when the patient says
  a. "I should never skip doses of my medication, even if I develop side effects."
  b. "If my viral load becomes undetectable, I will no longer be able to transmit HIV to others."
  c. "I should not use any over-the-counter drugs without checking with my health care provider."
  d. "If I develop a constant headache that is not relieved with aspirin or acetaminophen, I should report it within 24 hours."

22. Prophylactic measures that are routinely used as early as possible in HIV infection to prevent opportunistic and debilitating secondary problems include administration of
  a. isoniazid (INH) to prevent tuberculosis
  b. trimethoprim/sulfamethoxazole (TMP/SMX) for toxoplasmosis
  c. vaccines for pneumococcal pneumonia, influenza, and hepatitis A and B
  d. varicella-zoster immune globulin (VZIG) to prevent chickenpox or shingles

23. A patient identified as HIV antibody–positive 1 year ago manifests acute HIV infection but does not want to start antiretroviral therapy at this time. What is an appropriate nursing intervention for the patient at this stage of illness?
  a. Assist with end-of-life issues
  b. Provide care during acute exacerbations
  c. Provide physical care for chronic diseases
  d. Teach the patient about immune enhancement

24. Identify three methods to eliminate or reduce the risk for HIV transmission related to sexual intercourse and drug use and two methods to reduce the risk for perinatal transmission.

Sexual Intercourse	**Drug Use**	**Perinatal Transmission**
a.	a.	a.
b.	b.	b.
c.	c.	

25. A patient with advanced AIDS has a nursing diagnosis of impaired memory related to neurologic changes. In planning care for the patient, what should the nurse set as the highest priority?
    a. Maintain a safe patient environment
    b. Provide a quiet, nonstressful environment to avoid overstimulation
    c. Use memory cues such as calendars and clocks to promote orientation
    d. Provide written instructions of directions to promote understanding and orientation

---

CASE STUDY

HIV Infection

Patient Profile

A.K., a 28-year-old single man, had HIV antibody screening performed 2 weeks ago when he was seen at a health clinic for flu-like symptoms. At that time he revealed that he had a history of multiple sexual partners. He has returned to the clinic for the results of his screening.

Subjective Data

- Vague symptoms of fatigue and headache
- Reports occasional night sweats

Objective Data

- Positive Western blot test for HIV
- Temp: 100°F (37.8°C)
- Enlarged cervical and femoral lymph nodes

Discussion Questions

Using a separate sheet of paper, answer the following questions:

1. *Priority Decision:* What are the priority posttest counseling activities that should be performed by the nurse during A.K.'s visit?
2. A.K.'s $CD4^+$ T-cell count is 650/μL. What stage of HIV infection is he most likely experiencing?
3. What additional diagnostic tests might be performed at this visit?
4. What prophylactic treatments should be used at this time to prevent the development of opportunistic diseases?
5. The health care provider encourages A.K. to consider starting combination antiretroviral therapy. What can the nurse tell A.K. about the expected effect of this therapy?
6. If A.K. does not respond to treatment with an increased $CD4^+$ T-cell count and a decreased viral load, what tests could be used to identify resistance to the antiretroviral agents?
7. *Priority Decision:* Based on the assessment data presented, what are the priority nursing diagnoses? Are there any collaborative problems?

1. The nurse is presenting a community education program related to cancer prevention. Based on current cancer death rates, the nurse emphasizes what as the most important preventive action for both women and men?
   a. Smoking cessation
   b. Routine colonoscopies
   c. Protection from ultraviolet light
   d. Regular examination of reproductive organs

2. What defect in cellular proliferation is involved in the development of cancer?
   a. A rate of cell proliferation that is more rapid than that of normal body cells
   b. Shortened phases of cell life cycles with occasional skipping of G1 or S phases
   c. Rearrangement of stem cell RNA that causes abnormal cellular protein synthesis
   d. Indiscriminate and continuous proliferation of cells with loss of contact inhibition

3. What does the presence of carcinoembryonic antigens (CEAs) and α-fetoprotein (AFP) on cell membranes indicate has happened to the cells?
   a. They have shifted to more immature metabolic pathways and functions.
   b. They have spread from areas of original development to different body tissues.
   c. They produce abnormal toxins or chemicals that indicate abnormal cellular function.
   d. They have become more differentiated as a result of repression of embryonic functions.

4. What factor differentiates a malignant tumor from a benign tumor?
   a. It causes death.
   b. It grows at a faster rate.
   c. It is often encapsulated.
   d. It invades and metastasizes.

5. A patient is admitted with acute myelogenous leukemia and a history of Hodgkin's lymphoma. What is the nurse likely to find in the patient's history?
   a. Work as a radiation chemist
   b. Epstein-Barr virus diagnosed in vitro
   c. Intense tanning throughout the lifetime
   d. Alkylating agents for treating the Hodgkin's lymphoma

6. Which mutated tumor suppressor gene is most likely to contribute to many types of cancer, including bladder, breast, colorectal, and lung?
   a. *p53*
   b. *APC*
   c. *BRCA1*
   d. *BRCA2*

7. Cancer cells go through stages of development. What accurately describes the stage of promotion (*select all that apply*)?
   a. Obesity is an example of a promoting factor.
   b. The stage is characterized by increased growth rate and metastasis.
   c. Withdrawal of promoting factors will reduce the risk of cancer development.
   d. Tobacco smoke is a complete carcinogen that is capable of both initiation and promotion.
   e. Promotion is the stage of cancer development in which there is an irreversible alteration in the cell's DNA.

8. The patient was told she has carcinoma in situ, and the student nurse wonders what that is. How should the nurse explain this to the student nurse?
   a. Evasion of the immune system by cancer cells
   b. Lesion with histologic features of cancer except invasion
   c. Capable of causing cellular alterations associated with cancer
   d. Tumor cell surface antigens that stimulate an immune response

9. Which word identifies a mutation of protooncogenes?
   a. Oncogenes
   b. Retrogenes
   c. Oncofetal antigens
   d. Tumor angiogenesis factor

10. What is the name of a tumor from the embryonal mesoderm tissue of origin located in the anatomic site of the meninges that has malignant behavior?
    a. Meningitis
    b. Meningioma –benign
    c. Meningocele
    d. Meningeal sarcoma

11. A patient's breast tumor originates from embryonal ectoderm. It has moderate dysplasia and moderately differentiated cells. It is a small tumor with minimal lymph node involvement and no metastases. What is the best description of this tumor?
    a. Sarcoma, grade II, $T_3N_4M_0$
    b. Leukemia, grade I, $T_1N_2M_1$
    c. Carcinoma, grade II, $T_1N_1M_0$
    d. Lymphoma, grade III, T_1N_0M

12. The nurse is counseling a group of individuals over the age of 50 with average risk for cancer about screening tests for cancer. Which screening recommendation should be performed to screen for colorectal cancer?
    a. Barium enema every year
    b. Colonoscopy every 10 years
    c. Fecal occult blood every 5 years
    d. Annual prostate-specific antigen (PSA) and digital rectal exam

13. A small lesion is discovered in a patient's lung when an x-ray is performed for cervical spine pain. What is the definitive method of determining if the lesion is malignant?
    a. Lung scan
    b. Tissue biopsy
    c. Oncofetal antigens in the blood
    d. CT or positron emission tomography (PET) scan

14. A patient with a genetic mutation of *BRCA1* and a family history of breast cancer is admitted to the surgical unit where she is scheduled that day for a bilateral simple mastectomy. What is the reason for this procedure?
    a. Prevent breast cancer
    b. Diagnose breast cancer
    c. Cure or control breast cancer
    d. Provide palliative care for untreated breast cancer

15. Match the surgical procedures with their primary purposes in cancer treatment (answers may be used more than once).

_____4_____ a. Mammoplasty
_____1_____ b. Bowel resection
_____3_____ c. Cordotomy for pain control
_____2_____ d. Insertion of feeding tube into stomach
_____3_____ e. Colostomy to bypass bowel obstruction
_____2_____ f. Placement of a central venous catheter
_____1_____ g. Debulking procedure to enhance radiation therapy
_____2_____ h. Surgical fixation of bones at risk for pathologic fracture

1. Cure, control, or both
2. Supportive care
3. Palliation
4. Rehabilitation

16. Which patient would be most likely to be cured with chemotherapy as a treatment measure?
    a. Small cell lung cancer
    b. New neuroblastoma
    c. Small tumor of the bone
    d. Large hepatocellular carcinoma

17. Which classification of chemotherapy drugs is cell cycle phase–nonspecific, breaks the DNA helix which interferes with DNA replication, and crosses the blood-brain barrier?
    a. Nitrosureas
    b. Antimetabolites
    c. Mitotic inhibitors
    d. Antitumor antibiotics

18. The nurse uses many precautions during IV administration of vesicant chemotherapeutic agents, primarily to prevent
    a. septicemia.
    b. extravasation.
    c. catheter occlusion.
    d. anaphylactic shock.

19. For which type of malignancy should the nurse expect the use of the intravesical route of regional chemotherapy delivery?
    a. Bladder
    b. Leukemia
    c. Osteogenic sarcoma
    d. Metastasis to the brain

20. Which delivery system would be used to deliver regional chemotherapy for metastasis from a primary colorectal cancer?
    a. Intrathecal → Spinal theca
    b. Intraarterial → Specific vessel
    c. Intravenous – Systemic
    d. Intraperitoneal

21. When teaching the patient with cancer about chemotherapy, which approach should the nurse take?
    a. Avoid telling the patient about possible side effects of the drugs to prevent anticipatory anxiety.
    b. Explain that antiemetics, antidiarrheals, and analgesics will be provided as needed to control side effects.
    c. Assure the patient that the side effects from chemotherapy are uncomfortable but never life threatening.
    d. Inform the patient that chemotherapy-related alopecia is usually permanent but can be managed with lifelong use of wigs.

22. Which normal tissues manifest early, acute responses to radiation therapy?
    a. Spleen and liver
    b. Kidney and nervous tissue
    c. Bone marrow and gastrointestinal (GI) mucosa
    d. Hollow organs such as the stomach and bladder

23. The patient is learning about skin care related to the external radiation that he is receiving. Which instructions should the nurse include in this teaching?
    a. Moisturize skin with lotion
    b. Keep the area covered if it is sore
    c. Dry the skin thoroughly after cleansing it
    d. Avoid extreme temperatures to the area

24. When a patient is undergoing brachytherapy, what is it important for the nurse to be aware of when caring for this patient?
    a. The patient will undergo simulation to identify and mark the field of treatment.
    b. The patient is a source of radiation and personnel must wear film badges during care.
    c. The goal of this treatment is only palliative and the patient should be aware of the expected outcome.
    d. Computerized dosimetry is used to determine the maximum dose of radiation to the tumor within an acceptable dose to normal tissue.

25. To prevent the debilitating cycle of fatigue-depression-fatigue in patients receiving radiation therapy, what should the nurse encourage the patient to do?
    a. Implement a walking program
    b. Ignore the fatigue as much as possible
    c. Do the most stressful activities when fatigue is tolerable
    d. Schedule rest periods throughout the day whether fatigue is present or not

26. When the patient asks about the late effects of chemotherapy and high-dose radiation, what areas of teaching should the nurse plan to include when describing these effects?
    a. Third space syndrome
    b. Secondary malignancies
    c. Chronic nausea and vomiting
    d. Persistent myelosuppression

27. What describes a primary use of biologic therapy in cancer treatment?
    a. Protect normal, rapidly reproducing cells of the gastrointestinal system from damage during chemotherapy
    b. Prevent the fatigue associated with chemotherapy and high-dose radiation as seen with bone marrow depression
    c. Enhance or supplement the effects of the host's immune responses to tumor cells that produce flu-like symptoms
    d. Depress the immune system and circulating lymphocytes as well as increase a sense of well-being by replacing central nervous system deficits

28. *Priority Decision:* While caring for a patient who is at the nadir of chemotherapy, the nurse establishes the highest priority for nursing actions related to
    a. diarrhea.
    b. grieving.
    c. risk for infection.
    d. inadequate nutritional intake.

29. An allogenic hematopoietic stem cell transplant is considered as treatment for a patient with acute myelogenous leukemia. What information should the nurse include when teaching the patient about this procedure?
    a. There is no risk for graft-versus-host disease because the donated marrow is treated to remove cancer cells.
    b. The patient's bone marrow will be removed, treated, stored, and then reinfused after intensive chemotherapy.
    c. Peripheral stem cells are obtained from a donor who has a human leukocyte antigen (HLA) match with the patient.
    d. There is no need for posttransplant protective isolation because the stem cells are infused directly into the blood.

30. During initial chemotherapy a patient with leukemia develops hyperkalemia and hyperuricemia. The nurse recognizes these symptoms as an oncologic emergency and anticipates that the priority treatment will be to
    a. increase urine output with hydration therapy.
    b. establish electrocardiographic (ECG) monitoring.
    c. administer a bisphosphonate such as pamidronate (Aredia).
    d. restrict fluids and administer hypertonic sodium chloride solution.

31. ***Priority Decision:*** The patient with advanced cancer is having difficulty controlling her pain. She says she is afraid she will become addicted to the opioids. What is the first thing the nurse should do for this patient?
    a. Administer a nonsteroidal antiinflammatory drug.
    b. Assess the patient's vital signs and behavior to determine the medication to use.
    c. Have the patient keep a pain diary to better assess the patient's potential addiction.
    d. Obtain a detailed pain history including quality, location, intensity, duration, and type of pain.

32. Which factors will assist a patient in coping positively with having cancer (*select all that apply*)?
    a. Feeling of control
    b. Strong support system
    c. Internalization of feelings
    d. Possibility of cure or control
    e. A young person will adapt more easily
    f. Not having had to cope with previous stressful events

CASE STUDY

Cancer

Patient Profile

R.M. is a 65-year-old African American man who was recently diagnosed with metastatic lung cancer. He began treatment with chemotherapy through a peripherally inserted central venous catheter 5 days ago.

Subjective Data

- States he has almost continuous nausea, which becomes severe and causes vomiting following his dose of chemotherapy
- States he has no appetite
- Expresses no hope that the chemotherapy will have a positive effect

Objective Data

- Temp: 99.4°F (37.4°C)
- WBC count: 3200/μL (3.2×10^9/L)
- Neutrophils: 500/μL (0.5×10^9/L)
- Skin warm with decreased turgor

Discussion Questions

Using a separate sheet of paper, answer the following questions:

1. What factors may be responsible for R.M.'s decreased WBC and neutrophil count?
2. What assessment data indicate that R.M. may be experiencing an infection?
3. What additional assessment data should be collected from R.M. to determine the presence of an infection?
4. What factors may contribute to his negative attitude toward the chemotherapy?
5. ***Priority Decision:*** What are the priority nursing measures that should be used to help control his anorexia, nausea, and vomiting?
6. His daughter is visiting and wants to know how the cancer metastasized to his lung. What should the nurse teach her about metastasis?
7. During her visit, R.M.'s daughter questions how likely she is to get cancer. What should the nurse explain to her about risk factors and screening tests?
8. ***Priority Decision:*** What are the priority teaching measures that should be included in the teaching plan for R.M. and his family to prevent infection?
9. ***Priority Decision:*** Based on the assessment data presented, what are the priority nursing diagnoses? Are there any collaborative problems?

17

p.341

Fluid, Electrolyte, and Acid-Base Imbalances

1. A patient with consistent dietary intake who loses 1 kg of weight in 1 day has lost ___1000___ mL of fluid.

? 2. A man who weighs 90 kg has a total body water content of approximately $90\ kg \times 60\% = 54$ ___ L.

3. Which statements about fluid in the human body are true (select all that apply)?
   (a.) The primary hypothalamic mechanism of water intake is thirst.
   2nd – b. Third spacing refers to the abnormal movement of fluid into interstitial spaces.
   c. A cell surrounded by hypoosmolar fluid will shrink and die as water moves out of the cell.
   (d.) A cell surrounded by hyperosmolar fluid will shrink and die as water moves out of the cell.
   (e.) Concentrations of Na^+ and K^+ in interstitial and intracellular fluids are maintained by the sodium-potassium pump.

4. Match the following descriptions with the mechanisms of fluid and electrolyte movement.

   ___3___ a. Adenosine triphosphate (ATP) required
   ___6___ b. Uses a carrier molecule
   ___7___ c. Force exerted by a fluid
   ___4___ d. Pressure exerted by proteins
   ___5___ e. Force determined by osmolality of a fluid
   ___1___ f. Flow of water from low-solute concentration to high-solute concentration
   ___2___ g. Passive movement of molecules from a high concentration to lower concentration

   1. Osmosis
   2. Diffusion
   3. Active transport
   4. Oncotic pressure
   5. Osmotic pressure
   6. Facilitated diffusion
   7. Hydrostatic pressure

   oncotic → pulls created by proteins

5. A patient has a serum Na^+ of 147 mEq/L (147 mmol/L) and a blood glucose level of 126 mg/dL (7.0 mmol/L). Osmolality = (2 × Na concentration) + (glucose concentration/18). The patient's effective serum osmolality is

   _____ mOsm/kg. Is the patient's serum osmolality normal, increased, or decreased?

6. As fluid circulates through the capillaries, there is movement of fluid between the capillaries and the interstitium. What describes the fluid movement that would cause edema (select all that apply)?
   a. Plasma hydrostatic pressure is less than plasma oncotic pressure.
   b. Plasma oncotic pressure is higher than interstitial oncotic pressure.
   (c.) Plasma hydrostatic pressure is higher than plasma oncotic pressure.
   d. Plasma hydrostatic pressure is less than interstitial hydrostatic pressure.
   (e.) Interstitial hydrostatic pressure is lower than plasma hydrostatic pressure.

7. Fill in the blanks in the table below to indicate the direction of fluid shift (may use answers more than once) and the mechanism of fluid movement that is involved (may use answers more than once)

Event or Factor	Direction of Fluid Shift	Mechanism of Fluid Movement Involved
Burns		
Dehydration		
Fluid overload		
Hyponatremia		
Low serum albumin		
Administration of 10% glucose		
Application of elastic bandages		

Direction of Fluid Shifts	Mechanism of Fluid Movement Involved
1. From blood vessels to interstitium 2. From extracellular compartment to the cell 3. From cell to extracellular compartment 4. From interstitium to vessels	a. Osmosis b. Plasma hydrostatic pressure c. Interstitial hydrostatic pressure d. Tissue oncotic pressure e. Oncotic pressure

8. A woman has ham with gravy and green beans cooked with salt pork for dinner.
   a. What could happen to the woman's serum osmolality as a result of this meal?

   b. What fluid regulation mechanisms are stimulated by the intake of these foods?

9. What stimulates aldosterone secretion from the adrenal cortex?
   a. Excessive water intake
   b. Increased serum osmolality
   c. Decreased serum potassium
   d. Decreased sodium and water

10. While caring for an 84-year-old patient, the nurse monitors the patient's fluid and electrolyte balance, recognizing what as a normal change of aging?
    a. Hyperkalemia
    b. Hyponatremia
    c. Decreased insensible fluid loss
    d. Increased plasma oncotic pressures

11. The nurse is admitting a patient to the clinical unit from surgery. Being alert to potential fluid volume alterations, what assessment data will be important for the nurse to monitor to identify early changes in the patient's postoperative fluid volume (*select all that apply*)?
    a. Intake and output
    b. Skin turgor
    c. Lung sounds
    d. Respiratory rate
    e. Level of consciousness

12. Which patient is at risk for hypernatremia?
    a. Has a deficiency of aldosterone
    b. Has prolonged vomiting and diarrhea   *lead to hyponatremia*
    c. Receives excessive IV 5% dextrose solution
    d. Has impaired consciousness and decreased thirst sensitivity

13. In a patient with sodium imbalances, the primary clinical manifestations are related to alterations in what body system?
    a. Kidneys
    b. Cardiovascular system
    c. Musculoskeletal system
    d. Central nervous system   *causes shrinking or swelling in the brain*

14. Match the electrolyte imbalances with their associated causes (answers may be used more than once and imbalances may have more than one associated cause).
    ___8___ a. Alcohol withdrawal
    ___4___ b. Metabolic alkalosis
    ___6___ c. Parathyroidectomy
    ___1___ d. Diabetes insipidus
    ___7___ e. Fleet enemas
    ___2___ f. Primary polydipsia
    ___9___ g. Milk of magnesia use in renal failure
    ___3___ h. Early burn stage
    _6,10_ i. Chronic alcoholism
    ___6___ j. Vitamin D deficiency
    ___1___ k. Osmotic diuresis
    ___5___ l. Prolonged immobilization
    _1,4,10_ m. Hyperaldosteronism
    _____ n. Chronic kidney disease
    _____ o. Loop and thiazide diuretics

    1. Hypernatremia
    2. Hyponatremia
    3. Hyperkalemia
    4. Hypokalemia
    5. Hypercalcemia
    6. Hypocalcemia
    7. Hyperphosphatemia
    8. Hypophosphatemia
    9. Hypermagnesemia
    10. Hypomagnesemia

15. A patient is taking diuretic drugs that cause sodium loss from the kidney. Which fluid or electrolyte imbalance is most likely to occur in this patient?
    a. Hyperkalemia
    b. Hyponatremia
    c. Hypocalcemia
    d. Hypotonic fluid loss

16. A common collaborative problem related to both hyperkalemia and hypokalemia is which potential complication?
    a. Seizures
    b. Paralysis
    c. Dysrhythmias
    d. Acute kidney injury

17. What is hyperkalemia frequently associated with?
    a. Hypoglycemia
    b. Metabolic acidosis
    c. Respiratory alkalosis
    d. Decreased urine potassium levels

18. In a patient with a positive Chvostek's sign, the nurse would anticipate the IV administration of which medication?
    a. Calcitonin
    b. Vitamin D
    c. Loop diuretics
    d. Calcium gluconate

19. A patient with chronic kidney disease has hyperphosphatemia. What is a commonly associated electrolyte imbalance?
    a. Hypokalemia
    b. Hyponatremia
    c. Hypocalcemia
    d. Hypomagnesemia

20. What is the normal pH range of the blood and what ratio of base to acid does this reflect?
    a. 7.32 to 7.42; 25 to 2
    b. 7.32 to 7.42; 28 to 2
    c. 7.35 to 7.45; 20 to 1
    d. 7.35 to 7.45; 30 to 1

21. What are the characteristics of the carbonic acid–bicarbonate buffer system (*select all that apply*)?
    a. CO_2 is eliminated by the lung
    b. Neutralizes HCl acid to yield carbonic acid and salt
    c. H_2CO_3 formed by neutralization dissociates into H_2O and CO_2
    d. Shifts H^+ in and out of cell in exchange for other cations such as potassium and sodium
    e. Free basic radicals dissociate into ammonia and OH^- that combines with H^+ to form water

22. What are characteristics of the phosphate buffer system (*select all that apply*)?
    a. Neutralizes a strong base to a weak base and water
    b. Resultant sodium biphosphate is eliminated by kidneys
    c. Free acid radicals dissociate into H^+ and CO_2, buffering excess base
    d. Neutralizes a strong acid to yield sodium biphosphate, a weak acid, and salt
    e. Shifts chloride in and out of red blood cells in exchange for sodium bicarbonate, buffering both acids and bases

23. A patient who has a large amount of carbon dioxide in the blood also has what in the blood?
    a. Large amount of carbonic acid and low hydrogen ion concentration
    b. Small amount of carbonic acid and low hydrogen ion concentration
    c. Large amount of carbonic acid and high hydrogen ion concentration
    d. Small amount of carbonic acid and high hydrogen ion concentration

24. Match the acid-base imbalances with their mechanisms.
    _____ a. Increased carbonic acid (H_2CO_3)
    _____ b. Decreased carbonic acid (H_2CO_3)
    _____ c. Increased base bicarbonate (HCO_3^-)
    _____ d. Decreased base bicarbonate (HCO_3^-)

    1. Metabolic acidosis
    2. Metabolic alkalosis
    3. Respiratory acidosis
    4. Respiratory alkalosis

25. What is a compensatory mechanism for metabolic alkalosis?
    a. Shifting of bicarbonate into cells in exchange for chloride
    b. Kidney conservation of bicarbonate and excretion of hydrogen ions
    c. Deep, rapid respirations (Kussmaul respirations) to increase CO_2 excretion
    d. Decreased respiratory rate and depth to retain CO_2 and kidney excretion of bicarbonate

p. 342

26. Match the acid-base imbalances with their common causes (answers may be used more than once).
    _____ a. Renal failure
    _____ b. Severe shock
    _____ c. Diabetic ketosis
    _____ d. Respiratory failure
    _____ e. Prolonged vomiting
    _____ f. Baking soda used as antacid
    _____ g. Mechanical overventilation
    _____ h. Sedative or opioid overdose
    _____ i. Response to anxiety, fear, and pain

    1. Metabolic acidosis
    2. Metabolic alkalosis
    3. Respiratory acidosis
    4. Respiratory alkalosis

27. A patient with a pH of 7.29 has metabolic acidosis. Which value is useful in determining whether the cause of the acidosis is an acid gain or a bicarbonate loss?
    a. $PaCO_2$
    (b.) Anion gap
    c. Serum Na^+ level
    d. Bicarbonate level

28. Identify the acid-base imbalances represented by the following laboratory values.
    a. pH 7.50 ↑
       $PaCO_2$ 30 mm Hg ↓
       HCO_3^- 24 mEq/L
       Interpretation:
       Respiratory alkalosis;
       no comp

    b. pH 7.20 ↓
       $PaCO_2$ 25 mm Hg ↓
       HCO_3^- 15 mEq/L ↓
       Interpretation:
       Metabolic acidosis
       w/ partical comp.

    c. pH 7.26 ↓
       $PaCO_2$ 56 mm Hg ↑
       HCO_3^- 24 mEq/L —
       Interpretation:
       Respiratory acidosis
       no comp.

    d. pH 7.62 ↑
       $PaCO_2$ 48 mm Hg ↑
       HCO_3^- 45 mEq/L ↑
       Interpretation:
       Metabolic Alkalosis
       w/ partial comp.

    e. pH 7.44
       $PaCO_2$ 54 mm Hg ↑
       HCO_3^- 36 mEq/L ↑
       Interpretation:
       Metabolic alkalosis
       w/ full comp.

    f. pH 7.35
       $PaCO_2$ 60 mm Hg ↑
       HCO_3^- 40 mEq/L ↑
       Interpretation:
       Respiratory acidosis
       w/ full comp.

29. To provide free water and intracellular fluid hydration for a patient with acute gastroenteritis who is NPO, the nurse would expect administration of which infusion?
    (a.) Dextrose 5% in water
    b. Dextrose 10% in water
    c. Lactated Ringer's solution
    d. Dextrose 5% in normal saline (0.9%)

30. What is an example of an IV solution that would be appropriate to treat an extracellular fluid volume deficit?
    a. D_5W
    b. 3% saline
    (c.) Lactated Ringer's solution
    d. D_5W in ½ normal saline (0.45%)

31. *Priority Decision:* On assessment of a central venous access device (CVAD) site, the nurse observes that the transparent dressing is loose along two sides. What should the nurse do immediately?
    a. Wait and change the dressing when it is due.
    b. Tape the two loose sides down and document.
    c. Apply a gauze dressing over the transparent dressing and tape securely.
    (d.) Remove the dressing and apply a new transparent dressing using sterile technique.

32. ***Priority Decision:*** Number the following nursing actions related to care of the patient's central venous access device (CVAD) in the correct order to complete these actions. Number 1 is the first action and number 8 is the last action.

____1____ a. Perform hand hygiene
_____ b. Flush each line with 10 mL of normal saline
_____ c. Use strict sterile technique to change the dressing
_____ d. Clamp unused lines after flushing if not using positive pressure valve caps
_____ e. Assess the CVAD insertion site for redness, edema, warmth, drainage, and pain
_____ f. Use friction to cleanse the CVAD insertion site with chlorhexidine-based preparation
_____ g. Turn the patient's head to the side away from the CVAD insertion site when changing the caps
_____ h. Obtain chest x-ray results to verify placement of the catheter in the distal end of the superior vena cava

central line

33. A patient is scheduled to have a tunneled catheter placed for administration of chemotherapy for breast cancer. When preparing the patient for the catheter insertion, what does the nurse explain about this method of chemotherapy administration?
a. Decreases the risk for extravasation at the infusion site
b. Reduces the incidence of systemic side effects of the drug
c. Does not become occluded as peripherally inserted catheters can
d. Allows continuous infusion of the drug directly to the area of the tumor

34. The nurse is reviewing a patient's morning laboratory results. Which result is of greatest concern?
a. Serum Na$^+$ of 150 mEq/L *135-145*   c. Serum PO$_4^{3-}$ of 4.5 mg/dL *2.5-4.5*
b. Serum Mg^{2+} of 1.1 mEq/L *1.5-2.5*   d. Serum Ca^{2+} (total) of 8.6 mg/dL *8.6-10.2*

CASE STUDY
Fluid and Electrolyte Imbalance
Patient Profile
P.B., a 74-year-old woman who lives alone, is admitted to the hospital because of weakness and confusion. She has a history of chronic heart failure and chronic diuretic use.

Objective Data
Physical Examination
- Neurologic: Confusion, slow to respond to questioning, generalized weakness
- Cardiovascular: BP 90/62, HR 112 bpm and irregular, peripheral pulses weak; ECG indicates sinus tachycardia
- Pulmonary: RR 12 and shallow
- Additional findings: Decreased skin turgor, dry mucous membranes

Laboratory Results
- Serum electrolytes
  - Na$^+$: 141 mEq/L (141 mmol/L) *normal*
  - K$^+$: 2.5 mEq/L (2.5 mmol/L) *Low*
  - Cl$^-$: 85 mEq/L (85 mmol/L) *Low*
  - HCO$_3^-$: 34 mEq/L (34 mmol/L) *High*
- BUN: 42 mg/dL (15 mmol/L)
- Hct: 49%
- Arterial blood gases
  - pH: 7.52 ↑
  - PaCO$_2$: 55 mm Hg ↑
  - PaO$_2$: 88 mm Hg
  - HCO$_3^-$: 34 mEq/L (34 mmol/L) ↑

Metabolic alkalosis w/ partial compensation

Discussion Questions

Using a separate sheet of paper, answer the following questions:

1. Evaluate P.B.'s fluid volume and electrolyte status. Which physical assessment findings support your analysis? Which laboratory results support your analysis? What is the most likely etiology of these imbalances?
2. Explain the reasons for her ECG changes.
3. Analyze the arterial blood gas results. What is the etiology of the primary imbalance? Is the body compensating for this imbalance?
4. Why has P.B.'s advanced age placed her at risk for fluid imbalance?
5. Discuss the role of aldosterone in the regulation of fluid and electrolyte balance. How will changes in aldosterone affect P.B.'s fluid and electrolyte imbalances?
6. *Priority Decision:* Develop a plan of care for P.B. while she is in the hospital. What are the priority daily assessments that should be included in this plan of care?
7. *Priority Decision:* Based on the assessment data presented, what are the priority nursing diagnoses? Are there any collaborative problems?

Normal Na^+ = 135-145 mEq/Liter
Normal Mg^{2+} = 1.5-2.5 mEq/Liter
Normal PO_4^{3-} = 2.4-4.5 mg/dL
Normal Ca^{2+} = 8.5-10.2 mg/dL
Normal K^+ = 3.5-5 mEq/L
~~Normal Cl^- = 96-106 mEq/L~~

Potassium → 3.5-5
Sodium → 135-145
Mg → 1.5-2.5
Phosphorus → 2.4-4.1
Calcium → 8.5-10.2
Chloride → 96-106

CHAPTER

18

Nursing Management: Preoperative Care

1. Which procedures are done for curative purposes (*select all that apply*)?
   a. Gastroscopy
   b. Rhinoplasty
   c. Tracheotomy
   d. Hysterectomy
   e. Herniorrhaphy

2. A patient is scheduled for a hemorrhoidectomy at an ambulatory day-surgery center. An advantage of performing surgery at an ambulatory center is a decreased need for
   a. laboratory tests and perioperative medications.
   b. preoperative and postoperative teaching by the nurse.
   c. psychologic support to alleviate fears of pain and discomfort.
   d. preoperative nursing assessment related to possible risks and complications.

3. A patient who is being admitted to the surgical unit for a hysterectomy paces the floor, repeatedly saying, "I just want this over." What should the nurse do to promote a positive surgical outcome for the patient?
   a. Ask the patient what her specific concerns are about the surgery.
   b. Reassure the patient that the surgery will be over soon and she will be fine.
   c. Redirect the patient's attention to the necessary preoperative preparations.
   d. Tell the patient she should not be so anxious because she is having a common, safe surgery.

4. Many herbal products that are commonly taken cause surgical problems. Which herbs listed below should the nurse teach the patient to avoid before surgery to prevent an increase in bleeding for the surgical patient (*select all that apply*)?
   a. Garlic
   b. Fish oil
   c. Valerian
   d. Vitamin E
   e. Astragalus
   f. Ginkgo biloba

5. *Priority Decision:* When the nurse asks a preoperative patient about allergies, the patient reports a history of seasonal environmental allergies and allergies to a variety of fruits. What should the nurse do next?
   a. Note this information in the patient's record as hay fever and food allergies.
   b. Place an allergy alert wristband that identifies the specific allergies on the patient.
   c. Ask the patient to describe the nature and severity of any allergic responses experienced from these agents.
   d. Notify the anesthesia care provider (ACP) because the patient may have an increased risk for allergies to anesthetics.

6. During a preoperative review of systems, the patient reveals a history of renal disease. This finding suggests the need for which preoperative diagnostic tests?
   a. ECG and chest x-ray
   b. Serum glucose and CBC
   c. ABGs and coagulation tests
   d. BUN, serum creatinine, and electrolytes

66

Copyright © 2014 by Mosby, an imprint of Elsevier Inc. All rights reserved.

7. During a preoperative physical examination, the nurse is alerted to the possibility of compromised respiratory function during or after surgery in a patient with which problem?
   a. Obesity
   b. Dehydration
   c. Enlarged liver
   d. Decreased peripheral pulses

8. What type of procedural information should be given to a patient in preparation for ambulatory surgery (*select all that apply*)?
   a. How pain will be controlled
   b. Any fluid and food restrictions
   c. Characteristics of monitoring equipment
   d. What odors and sensations may be experienced
   e. Technique and practice of coughing and deep breathing, if appropriate

9. The nurse asks a preoperative patient to sign a surgical consent form as specified by the surgeon and then signs the form after the patient does so. By this action, what is the nurse doing?
   a. Witnessing the patient's signature
   b. Obtaining informed consent from the patient for the surgery
   c. Verifying that the consent for surgery is truly voluntary and informed
   d. Ensuring that the patient is mentally competent to sign the consent form

10. When the nurse prepares to administer a preoperative medication to a patient, the patient tells the nurse that she really does not understand what the surgeon plans to do.
    a. What action should be taken by the nurse?

    b. What criterion of informed consent has not been met in this situation?

11. A patient scheduled for hip replacement surgery in the early afternoon is NPO but receives and ingests a breakfast tray with clear liquids on the morning of surgery. What response does the nurse expect when the anesthesia care provider is notified?
    a. Surgery will be done as scheduled.
    b. Surgery will be rescheduled for the following day.
    c. Surgery will be postponed for 8 hours after the fluid intake.
    d. A nasogastric tube will be inserted to remove the fluids from the stomach.

12. What is the rationale for using preoperative checklists on the day of surgery?
    a. The patient is correctly identified.
    b. All preoperative orders and procedures have been carried out and records are complete.
    c. Patients' families have been informed as to where they can accompany and wait for patients.
    d. Preoperative medications are the last procedure before the patient is transported to the operating room.

13. A common reason that a nurse may need extra time when preparing older adults for surgery is their
    a. ineffective coping.
    b. limited adaptation to stress.
    c. diminished vision and hearing.
    d. need to include caregivers in activities.

14. The nurse is reviewing the laboratory results for a preoperative patient. Which test result should be brought to the attention of the surgeon immediately?
    a. Serum K^+ of 3.8 mEq/L
    b. Hemoglobin of 15 g/dL
    c. Blood glucose of 100 mg/dL
    d. White blood cell (WBC) count of 18,500/µL

15. The nurse is preparing a patient for transport to the operating room. The patient is scheduled for a right knee arthroscopy. What actions should the nurse take at this time (*select all that apply*)?
    a. Ensure that the patient has voided.
    b. Verify that the informed consent is signed.
    c. Complete preoperative nursing documentation.
    d. Verify that the right knee is marked with indelible marker.
    e. Ensure that the H&P, diagnostic reports, and vital signs are on the chart.

CASE STUDY

Preoperative Patient

Patient Profile

C.J., a 49-year-old construction worker, is scheduled for a bronchoscopy for biopsy of a right lung lesion. He initially sought medical care for hemoptysis and increasing fatigue. When the nurse asked him to sign the operative permit, he stated that he was not certain if he should go ahead with the procedure because he fears a diagnosis of cancer.

Subjective Data

- Has never been hospitalized
- Has had no medical problems except mild obesity
- Has a cigarette smoking history of 40 pack-years
- Is married with two children, ages 6 and 8; both children have cystic fibrosis
- Is fearful that his wife will not be able to manage without him

Objective Data

- Diagnostic studies: chest x-ray revealed mass in upper lobe of right lung
- Hematocrit: 31%

Discussion Questions

Using a separate sheet of paper, answer the following questions:

1. What factors in C.J.'s background or personal situation might influence his emotional response and physical reactions to this surgery?
2. What should C.J. know if his consent for surgery is to be truly informed?
3. *Priority Decision:* C.J. will be an outpatient for this procedure. What is the priority preoperative teaching that should be done to prepare him for surgery?
4. What risk factors for surgical and anesthetic complications might you anticipate for C.J.? What are the potential interventions that might minimize the risks?
5. *Priority Decision:* Based on the assessment data provided, what are the priority nursing diagnoses? Are there any collaborative problems?

Nursing Management: Intraoperative Care

1. What is the physical environment of a surgery suite primarily designed to promote?
   a. Electrical safety
   b. Medical and surgical asepsis
   c. Comfort and privacy of the patient
   d. Communication among the surgical team

2. When transporting an inpatient to the surgical department, which area is a nurse from another area of the hospital able to access?
   a. Clean core
   b. Holding area
   c. Corridors of surgical suite
   d. Unprepared operating room

3. Which nursing actions are completed by the scrub nurse (*select all that apply*)?
   a. Prepares instrument table
   b. Documents intraoperative care
   c. Remains in the sterile area of the OR
   d. Checks mechanical and electrical equipment
   e. Passes instruments to surgeon and assistants
   f. Monitors blood and other fluid loss and urine output

4. What is the primary goal of the circulating nurse during preparation of the operating room, transferring and positioning the patient, and assisting the anesthesia team?
   a. Avoiding any type of injury to the patient
   b. Maintaining a clean environment for the patient
   c. Providing for patient comfort and sense of well-being
   d. Preventing breaks in aseptic technique by the sterile members of the team

5. Goals for patient safety in the OR include the Universal Protocol. What is included in this protocol?
   a. All surgical centers of any type must submit reports on patient safety infractions to the accreditation agencies.
   b. Members of the surgical team stop whatever they are doing to check that all sterile items have been prepared properly.
   c. Members of the surgical team pause right before surgery to meditate for 1 minute to decrease stress and possible errors.
   d. A surgical timeout is performed just before the procedure is started to verify patient identity, surgical procedure, and surgical site.

6. A break in sterile technique occurs during surgery when the scrub nurse touches
   a. the mask with sterile gloved hands.
   b. sterile gloved hands to the gown at chest level.
   c. the drape at the incision site with sterile gloved hands.
   d. the lower arm to the instruments on the instrument tray.

7. During surgery, a patient has a nursing diagnosis of risk for perioperative positioning injury. What is a common risk factor for this nursing diagnosis?
   a. Skin lesions
   b. Break in sterile technique
   c. Musculoskeletal deformities
   d. Electrical or mechanical equipment failure

8. At the end of the surgical procedure, the perioperative nurse evaluates the patient's response to the nursing care delivered during the perioperative period. What reflects a positive outcome related to the patient's physical status?
   a. The patient's right to privacy is maintained.
   b. The patient's care is consistent with the perioperative plan of care.
   c. The patient receives consistent and comparable care regardless of the setting.
   d. The patient's respiratory function is consistent with or improved from baseline levels established preoperatively.

9. Which short-acting barbiturates are most commonly used for induction of general anesthesia (*select all that apply*)?
   a. Nitrous oxide
   b. Propofol (Diprivan)
   c. Isoflurane (Florane)
   d. Thiopental sodium (Pentothal)
   e. Sodium methohexital (Brevital)

10. Because of the rapid elimination of volatile liquids used for general anesthesia, what should the nurse anticipate the patient will need early in the anesthesia recovery period?
    a. Warm blankets
    b. Analgesic medication
    c. Observation for respiratory depression
    d. Airway protection in anticipation of vomiting

11. What is the primary advantage of the use of midazolam (Versed) as an adjunct to general anesthesia?
    a. Amnestic effect
    b. Analgesic effect
    c. Prolonged action
    d. Antiemetic effect

12. Identify the rationale for the use of each of the following drugs during surgery and one nursing implication indicated in the care of the patient immediately postoperatively related to the drug.

Drug	Use	Nursing Implication
Ketamine (Ketalar)		
Fentanyl (Sublimaze)		
Desflurane (Suprane)		
Succinylcholine (Anectine)		

13. Monitored anesthesia care (MAC) is being considered for a patient undergoing a cervical dilation and endometrial biopsy in the health care clinic. The patient asks the nurse, "What is this MAC?" The nurse's response is based on the knowledge that MAC
    a. can be administered only by anesthesiologists or nurse anesthetists.
    b. should never be used outside of the OR because of the risk of serious complications.
    c. is so safe that it can be administered by nurses with direction from health care providers.
    d. provides maximum flexibility to match the sedation level with the patient and procedure needs.

14. Match the methods of local anesthetic administration with their descriptions.
    _____ a. Injection of agent into subarachnoid space
    _____ b. Injection of anesthetic agent directly into tissues
    _____ c. Injection of a specific nerve with an anesthetic agent
    _____ d. Injection of anesthetic agent into space around the vertebrae
    _____ e. Injection of agent into veins of extremity after limb is exsanguinated

    1. Nerve block
    2. IV nerve block
    3. Spinal block
    4. Epidural block
    5. Local infiltration

15. The patient will be placed under moderate sedation to allow realignment of a fracture in the emergency department. When the family asks about this anesthesia, what should the nurse tell them?
    a. Includes inhalation agents
    b. Induces high levels of sedation
    c. Frequently used for traumatic injuries
    d. Patients remain responsive and breathe without assistance

16. What condition should the nurse anticipate that might occur during epidural and spinal anesthesia?
    a. Spinal headache
    b. Hypotension and bradycardia
    c. Loss of consciousness and seizures
    d. Downward extension of nerve block

17. A preoperative patient reveals that an uncle died during surgery because of a fever and cardiac arrest. Knowing the patient is at risk for malignant hyperthermia, the perioperative nurse alerts the surgical team. What is likely to happen next?
    a. The surgery will have to be cancelled.
    b. Specific precautions can be taken to safely anesthetize the patient.
    c. Dantrolene (Dantrium) must be given to prevent hyperthermia during surgery.
    d. The patient should be placed on a cooling blanket during the surgical procedure.

CASE STUDY

Intraoperative Patient

Patient Profile

T.M., a 76-year-old retired police officer, is admitted to the OR for an inguinal hernia repair. He has a history of severe chronic obstructive pulmonary disease (COPD) and heart failure. Therefore, the anesthesia care provider (ACP) has decided to administer spinal anesthesia. The circulating nurse has verified the baseline data (vital signs, height, weight, age; allergies; level of consciousness; NPO status; and comfort level). A signed informed consent is on the chart. T.M. has no allergies.

Discussion Questions

Using a separate sheet of paper, answer the following questions:

1. *Priority Decision*: What are the priority nursing actions that should be taken when T.M. arrives in the OR?
2. What specific precautions should be taken when positioning T.M. for surgery?
3. What complications of spinal anesthesia should T.M. be monitored for during surgery?
4. T.M. is 76 years old. What gerontologic considerations should be taken?
5. *Priority Decision:* Based on the data presented, what are the priority nursing diagnoses?

CHAPTER

20

Nursing Management: Postoperative Care

1. What does progression of patients through various phases of care in a postanesthesia care unit (PACU) primarily depend on?
   a. Condition of patient
   b. Type of anesthesia used
   c. Preference of surgeon
   d. Type of surgical procedure

2. *Priority Decision*: Upon admission of a patient to the PACU, the nurse's priority assessment is
   a. vital signs.
   b. surgical site.
   c. respiratory adequacy.
   d. level of consciousness.

3. How is the initial information given to the PACU nurses about the surgical patient?
   a. A copy of the written operative report
   b. A verbal report from the circulating nurse
   c. A verbal report from the anesthesia care provider (ACP)
   d. An explanation of the surgical procedure from the surgeon

4. To prevent agitation during the patient's recovery from anesthesia, when should the nurse begin orientation explanations?
   a. When the patient is awake
   b. When the patient first arrives in the PACU
   c. When the patient becomes agitated or frightened
   d. When the patient can be aroused and recognizes where he or she is

5. What is included in the routine assessment of the patient's cardiovascular function on admission to the PACU?
   a. Monitoring arterial blood gases
   b. Electrocardiographic (ECG) monitoring
   c. Determining fluid and electrolyte status
   d. Direct arterial blood pressure monitoring

6. With what are the postoperative respiratory complications of atelectasis and aspiration of gastric contents associated?
   a. Hypoxemia
   b. Hypercapnia
   c. Hypoventilation
   d. Airway obstruction

7. To prevent airway obstruction in the postoperative patient who is unconscious or semiconscious, what will the nurse do?
   a. Encourage deep breathing
   b. Elevate the head of the bed
   c. Administer oxygen per mask
   d. Position the patient in a side-lying position

8. *Priority Decision:* To promote effective coughing, deep breathing, and ambulation in the postoperative patient, what is most important for the nurse to do?
   a. Teach the patient controlled breathing
   b. Explain the rationale for these activities
   c. Provide adequate and regular pain medication
   d. Use an incentive spirometer to motivate the patient

9. While assessing a patient in the PACU, the nurse finds that the patient's blood pressure is below the preoperative baseline. The nurse determines that the patient has residual vasodilating effects of anesthesia when what is assessed?
   a. A urinary output >30 mL/hr
   b. An oxygen saturation of 88%
   c. A normal pulse with warm, dry, pink skin
   d. A narrowing pulse pressure with normal pulse

10. *Priority Decision:* A patient in the PACU has emergence delirium manifested by agitation and thrashing. What should the nurse assess for first in the patient?
    a. Hypoxemia
    b. Neurologic injury
    c. Distended bladder
    d. Cardiac dysrhythmias

11. The PACU nurse applies warm blankets to a postoperative patient who is shivering and has a body temperature of 96.0°F (35.6°C). What treatment also may be used to treat the patient?
    a. Oxygen
    b. Vasodilating drugs
    c. Antidysrhythmic drugs
    d. Analgesics or sedatives

12. Which patient is ready for discharge from Phase I PACU care to the clinical unit?
    a. Arouses easily, pulse is 112 bpm, respiratory rate is 24, dressing is saturated, SaO_2 is 88%
    b. Difficult to arouse, pulse is 52, respiratory rate is 22, dressing is dry and intact, SaO_2 is 91%
    c. Awake, vital signs stable, dressing is dry and intact, no respiratory depression, SaO_2 is 92%
    d. Arouses, blood pressure (BP) higher than preoperative and respiratory rate is 10, no excess bleeding, SaO_2 is 90%

13. For which nursing diagnoses or collaborative problems common in postoperative patients has ambulation been found to be an appropriate intervention (*select all that apply*)?
    a. Impaired skin integrity related to incision
    b. Impaired mobility related to decreased muscle strength
    c. Risk for aspiration related to decreased muscle strength
    d. Ineffective airway clearance related to decreased respiratory excursion
    e. Constipation related to decreased physical activity and impaired gastrointenstinal (GI) motility
    f. Venous thromboembolism related to dehydration, immobility, vascular manipulation, or injury

14. A patient who had major surgery is experiencing emotional stress as well as physiologic stress from the effects of surgery. What can this stress cause?
    a. Diuresis
    b. Hyperkalemia
    c. Fluid retention
    d. Impaired blood coagulation

15. In addition to ambulation, which nursing intervention could be implemented to prevent or treat the postoperative complication of syncope?
    a. Monitor vital signs after ambulation
    b. Do not allow the patient to eat before ambulation
    c. Slowly progress to ambulation with slow changes in position
    d. Have the patient deep breathe and cough before getting out of bed

16. Which tubes drain gastric contents (*select all that apply*)?
    a. T-tube
    b. Hemovac
    c. Nasogastric tube
    d. Indwelling catheter
    e. Gastrointestinal tube

17. Which drainage is drained with a Hemovac?
    a. Bile
    b. Urine
    c. Gastric contents
    d. Wound drainage

18. *Priority Decision:* The nurse notes drainage on the surgical dressing when the patient is transferred from the PACU to the clinical unit. In what order of priority should the nurse do the following actions? Number the options with 1 for the first action and 5 for the last action.
    _____ a. Reinforce the surgical dressing.
    _____ b. Change the dressing and assess the wound as ordered.
    _____ c. Notify the surgeon of excessive drainage type and amount.
    _____ d. Recall the report from PACU for the number and type of drains in use.
    _____ e. Note and record the type, amount, and color and odor of the drainage.

19. Thirty-six hours postoperatively a patient has a temperature of 100°F (37.8°C). What is the most likely cause of this temperature elevation?
    a. Dehydration
    b. Wound infection
    c. Lung congestion and atelectasis
    d. Normal surgical stress response

20. The health care provider has ordered IV morphine q2-4hr PRN for a patient following major abdominal surgery. When should the nurse plan to administer the morphine?
    a. Before all planned painful activities
    b. Every 2 to 4 hours during the first 48 hours
    c. Every 4 hours as the patient requests the medication
    d. After assessing the nature and intensity of the patient's pain

21. What should be included in the instructions given to the postoperative patient before discharge?
    a. Need for follow-up care with home care nurses
    b. Directions for maintaining routine postoperative diet
    c. Written information about self-care during recuperation
    d. Need to restrict all activity until surgical healing is complete

---

CASE STUDY
Postoperative Patient
Patient Profile

S.B., a 28-year-old female school teacher, is admitted to the PACU following a cystoscopy for recurrent bladder infections and hematuria. The procedure was scheduled as outpatient surgery and was performed under IV sedation.

Postoperative Orders

- Vital signs per routine
- Discontinue IV before discharge
- Patient to void before discharge
- Cipro 500 mg PO every 6 hr for 10 days
- Tylenol #3 1–2 tabs every 3–4 hr PRN for pain
- Patient to call office to schedule follow-up appointment

Discussion Questions

Using a separate sheet of paper, answer the following questions:

1. ***Priority Decision:*** What priority nursing actions will be required to progress S.B. toward discharge?
2. What precautions will be required in ambulating S.B. after surgery?
3. What problems might interfere with discharging S.B. home in a timely manner?
4. How will the nurse determine that S.B. is ready to be discharged home?
5. What are the unique needs of discharging a patient home as opposed to a clinical unit?
6. ***Priority Decision:*** Based on the data presented, what are the priority nursing diagnoses? Are there any collaborative problems?

Nursing Assessment: Visual and Auditory Systems

1. Use the following terms to fill in the labels in the illustration below.

Terms

Anterior chamber	Optic nerve
Choroid	Posterior chamber
Ciliary body	Pupil
Cornea	Retina
Iris	Sclera
Lens	Vitreous cavity
Optic disc	

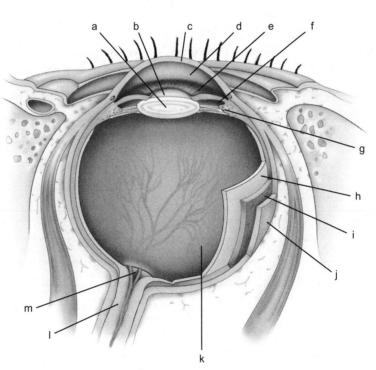

a. _____

b. _____

c. _____

d. _____

e. _____

f. _____

g. _____

h. _____

i. _____

j. _____

k. _____

l. _____

m. _____

2. What is in the posterior cavity of the eye?
   a. Zonules
   b. Cornea
   c. Aqueous humor
   d. Vitreous humor

3. What is the function of the sclera?
   a. Secrete aqueous humor
   b. Focus light rays on the retina
   c. Protective white outer layer of the eyeball
   d. Photoreceptor cells stimulated in dim environments

4. What accurately describes the conjunctiva?
   a. Junction of the upper and lower eyelids
   b. Point where the optic nerve exits the eyeball
   c. Transparent mucous membrane lining the eyelids
   d. Drains tears from the surface of the eye into the lacrimal canals

5. Which tissue nourishes the ciliary body, iris, and part of the retina?
   a. Pupil
   b. Cones
   c. Choroid
   d. Canal of Schlemm

6. Identify the cranial nerves that are responsible for the following eye functions.

Eye Function	Cranial Nerve
Eyelid movement	
Pupil constriction	
Pupil dilation	
Visual acuity	

7. Identify the causes of the following assessment findings of the eye that are associated with aging.

Assessment Finding	Cause
Floaters	
Ectropion	
Pinguecula	
Arcus senilis	
Yellowish sclera	
Dry, irritated eyes	
Decreased pupil size	
Changes in color percept	

8. *Priority Decision:* When obtaining a health history from a patient with cataracts, what is most important for the nurse to ask about the use of?
   a. Corticosteroids
   b. Oral hypoglycemic agents
   c. Antihistamines and decongestants
   d. β-Adrenergic blocking agents

9. Identify a specific finding identified by the nurse during assessment of each of the patient's functional health patterns that indicates either a risk factor for visual problems or the response of the patient to an eye problem.

Functional Health Pattern	Risk Factor or Response to Visual Problem
Health perception–health management	
Nutritional-metabolic	
Elimination	
Activity-exercise	
Sleep-rest	
Cognitive-perceptual	
Self-perception–self-concept	
Role-relationship	
Sexuality-reproductive	
Coping–stress tolerance	
Value-belief	

10. Describe what is meant by the finding that the patient has a visual acuity of OD: 20/40; OS: 20/50.

11. The nurse documents PERRLA following assessment of a patient's eyes. What is one finding that supports this statement?
   a. A slightly oval shape of the pupils
   b. The presence of nystagmus on far lateral gaze
   c. Dilation of the pupil when a light is shined in the opposite eye
   d. Constriction of the pupils when an object is brought closer to the eyes

12. Identify the assessment techniques used to obtain the following assessment data.

Assessment Data	Assessment Technique
Peripheral vision field	
Extraocular muscle functions	
Near visual acuity	
Visual acuity	
Intraocular pressure	

13. In which individuals should the nurse expect to find a yellow cast to the sclera?
   a. Infants
   b. Dark-skinned persons
   c. Persons with brown irises
   d. Patients with eye infections

14. To determine the presence of corneal abrasions or defects in a patient with an eye injury, what would the nurse provide?
   a. A tonometer
   b. Fluorescein dye
   c. Pocket penlight
   d. An ophthalmoscope

15. What are possible abnormal assessment findings when assessing the eyelid (*select all that apply*)?
    a. Ptosis
    b. Strabismus
    c. Blepharitis
    d. Anisocoria
    e. Swelling of the pinna

16. When the patient has a diagnosis of hyperthyroidism, which abnormal assessment of the eye could be found?
    a. Light intolerance
    b. Unequal pupil size
    c. Protrusion of eyeball
    d. Deviation of eye position

17. When examining the patient's eye with an ophthalmoscope, which finding would be of most concern to the nurse?
    a. Depression at the center of the optic disc
    b. Blurring of the nasal margin of the optic disc
    c. A break in the retina at the site of the macula
    d. Pieces of liquefied vitreous in the vitreous chamber

18. To prepare a patient for a fluorescein angiography, what should the nurse explain about the test?
    a. Measures curvature of the cornea
    b. Involves IV dye injection to evaluate blood flow through epithelial and retinal blood vessels
    c. Application of eyedrops containing a dye that will localize arterial abnormalities in the retina
    d. Anesthetizes the eye so that probes can be inserted into the anterior chamber to measure intraocular pressure

19. What is the organ of balance and equilibrium?
    a. Cochlea
    b. Organ of Corti
    c. Ossicular chain
    d. Semicircular canals

20. How does the eustachian tube assist the auditory system?
    a. Transmits sound stimuli to the brain
    b. Sets bones of the middle ear in motion
    c. Allows for equalization of pressure in the middle ear
    d. Transmits stimuli from the semicircular canals to the brain

21. Which changes of aging can impair hearing in the older adult (*select all that apply*)?
    a. Atrophy of eardrum (middle ear)
    b. Increased hair growth (external ear)
    c. Increased production of and dryness of cerumen (external ear)
    d. Increased vestibular apparatus in semicircular canals (inner ear)
    e. Decreased cochlear efficiency from increased blood supply (inner ear)
    f. Neuron degeneration in auditory nerve and central pathways (inner ear)

22. The nurse suspects a patient has presbycusis when she says she has
    a. ringing in the ears.
    b. a sensation of fullness in the ears.
    c. difficulty understanding the meaning of words.
    d. a decrease in the ability to hear high-pitched sounds.

23. Describe the significance of the following questions asked of the patient while obtaining subjective data during assessment of the auditory system.

Question	Significance
Do you have a history of childhood ear infections or ruptured eardrums?	
Do you use any over-the-counter or prescription medications on a regular basis?	
Have you ever been treated for a head injury?	
Is there a history of hearing loss in your parents?	
Have you been exposed to excessive noise levels in your work or recreational activities?	
Has the amount of social activities you are involved in changed?	

24. What accurately describes an assessment of the ear?
    a. Major landmarks of the tympanic membrane include the umbo, handle of malleus, and cone of light.
    b. The presence of a retracted eardrum on otoscopic examination is indicative of positive pressure in the middle ear.
    c. In chronic otitis media, the nurse would expect to find a lack of landmarks and a bulging eardrum on otoscopic examination.
    d. To straighten the ear canal in an adult before insertion of the otoscope, the nurse grasps the auricle and pulls downward and backward.

25. What indicates sensorineural hearing loss (*select all that apply*)?
    a. Positive Rinne test
    b. Negative Rinne test
    c. Weber lateralization to impaired ear
    d. Weber lateralization to good ear
    e. External or middle ear pathology
    f. Inner ear or nerve pathway pathology

26. ***Priority Decision:*** Results of an audiometry indicate that a patient has a 10-dB hearing loss at 8000 Hz. What is the most appropriate action by the nurse?
    a. Encourage the patient to start learning to lip-read
    b. Speak at a normal speed and volume with the patient
    c. Avoid words in conversation that have many high-pitched consonants
    d. Discuss the advantages and disadvantages of various hearing aids with the patient

27. When does caloric testing indicate disease of the vestibular system of the ear?
    a. Hearing is improved with irrigation of the external ear canal
    b. No nystagmus is elicited with application of water in the external ear
    c. The patient experiences intolerable pain with irrigation of the external ear
    d. Irrigation of the external ear with water produces nystagmus opposite the side of instillation

28. Identify a specific finding identified by the nurse during assessment of each of the patient's functional health patterns that indicates either a risk factor for hearing problems or the response of the patient to an ear problem.

Functional Health Pattern	Risk Factor for or Response to Hearing Problem
Health perception–health management	
Nutritional-metabolic	
Elimination	
Activity-exercise	
Sleep-rest	
Cognitive-perceptual	
Self-perception–self-concept	
Role-relationship	
Sexuality-reproductive	
Coping–stress tolerance	
Value-belief	

CHAPTER 22

Nursing Management: Visual and Auditory Problems

1. Myopia is present in 25% of Americans. Which characteristics are associated with myopia (*select all that apply*)?
   a. Excessive light refraction
   b. Abnormally short eyeball
   c. Unequal corneal curvature
   d. Corrected with concave lens
   e. Image focused in front of retina

2. The patient is diagnosed with presbyopia. When he asks the nurse what that is, what is the best explanation the nurse can give to the patient?
   a. Abnormally long eyeballs
   b. Absence of crystalline lens
   c. Correctable with cylinder lens
   d. Loss of accommodation associated with age

3. To determine if an unconscious patient has contact lenses in place, what should be done by the nurse?
   a. Use a penlight to shine a light obliquely over the eyeball.
   b. Apply drops of fluorescein dye to the eye to stain the lenses yellow.
   c. Touch the cornea lightly with a dry cotton ball to see if the patient reacts.
   d. Tense the lateral canthus to cause a lens to be ejected if it is present in the eye.

4. What surgical choices are available for correction of a refractive error (*select all that apply*)?
   a. LASIK
   b. Contact lenses
   c. Corrective lenses
   d. Photorefractive keratectomy (PRK)
   e. Surgical implantation of intraocular lens

5. A patient tells the nurse on admission to the health care facility that he recently has been classified as legally blind. What does the nurse understand about the patient's vision?
   a. Has lost usable vision but has some light perception
   b. Will need time for grieving and adjusting to living with total blindness
   c. Will be dependent on others to ensure a safe environment for functioning
   d. May be able to perform many tasks and activities with vision enhancement techniques

6. Identify five nursing measures that should be implemented to increase a visually impaired patient's safety and comfort.
   a.   d.
   b.   e.
   c.

7. A patient is admitted to the emergency department with a wood splinter imbedded in the right eye. Which intervention by the nurse is most appropriate?
   a. Irrigate the eye with a large amount of sterile saline.
   b. Carefully remove the splinter with a pair of sterile forceps.
   c. Cover the eye with a dry sterile patch and a protective shield.
   d. Apply light pressure on the closed eye to prevent bleeding or loss of aqueous humor.

8. What best describes pinkeye?
   a. Blindness
   b. Acute bacterial conjunctivitis
   c. Epidemic keratoconjunctivitis
   d. Chronic inflammation of sebaceous glands

9. What describes inflammation of the cornea?
   a. Keratitis
   b. Blepharitis
   c. Hordeolum
   d. Conjunctivitis

10. What should the nurse teach all patients with conjunctival infections to use?
    a. Artificial tears to moisten and soothe the eyes
    b. Dark glasses to prevent the discomfort of photophobia
    c. Warm moist compresses to the eyes to promote drainage and healing
    d. Frequent and thorough hand washing to avoid spreading the infection

11. Endophthalmitis can be a complication of intraocular surgery or penetrating ocular injury. What manifestations are expected when the nurse assesses a patient with this disorder (*select all that apply*)?
    a. Ocular pain
    b. Photophobia
    c. Eyelid edema
    d. Reddened sclera
    e. Bleeding conjunctiva
    f. Decreased visual acuity

12. A patient with early cataracts tells the nurse that he is afraid cataract surgery may cause permanent visual damage. What should the nurse teach the patient?
    a. The cataracts will only worsen with time and should be removed as early as possible to prevent blindness.
    b. Cataract surgery is very safe and with the implantation of an intraocular lens, the need for glasses will be eliminated.
    c. Progression of the cataracts can be prevented by avoidance of ultraviolet (UV) light and good dietary management.
    d. Vision enhancement techniques may improve vision until surgery becomes an acceptable option to maintain desired activities.

13. A 60-year-old patient is being prepared for outpatient cataract surgery. When obtaining admission data from the patient, what would the nurse expect to find in the patient's history?
    a. A painless, sudden, severe loss of vision
    b. Blurred vision, colored halos around lights, and eye pain
    c. A gradual loss of vision with abnormal color perception and glare
    d. Light flashes, floaters, and a "cobweb" in the field of vision with loss of central or peripheral vision

14. A patient with bilateral cataracts is scheduled for an extracapsular cataract extraction with an intraocular lens implantation of one eye. What should be done by the nurse preoperatively?
    a. Assess the visual acuity in the unoperated eye to plan the need for postoperative assistance.
    b. Inform the patient that the operative eye will need to be patched for 3 to 4 days postoperatively.
    c. Assure the patient that vision in the operative eye will be improved to near normal on the first postoperative day.
    d. Teach the patient routine coughing and deep-breathing techniques to use postoperatively to prevent respiratory complications.

15. For the patient with a retinal break, what extraocular techniques may be used with sclera buckling to seal the break by creating an inflammatory reaction that causes a chorioretinal adhesion or scar (*select all that apply*)?
    a. Cryopexy
    b. Vitrectomy → intraocular
    c. Pneumatic retinopexy
    d. Laser photocoagulation
    e. Penetrating keratoplasty

16. Following a pneumatic retinopexy, what does the nurse need to know about the postoperative care for the patient?
    a. Specific positioning and activity restrictions are likely to be required for several days.
    b. The patient is frequently hospitalized for 7 to 10 days on bed rest until healing is complete.
    c. Patients experience little or no pain, and development of pain indicates hemorrhage or infection.
    d. Reattachment of the retina commonly fails, and patients can be expected to grieve for loss of vision.

17. *Priority Decision:* What nursing action is most important for the patient with age-related macular degeneration (AMD)?
    a. Teach the patient how to use topical eyedrops for treatment of AMD.
    b. Emphasize the use of vision enhancement techniques to improve what vision is present.
    c. Encourage the patient to undergo laser treatment to slow the deposit of extracellular debris.
    d. Explain that nothing can be done to save the patient's vision because there is no treatment for AMD.

18. A patient with wet AMD is treated with photodynamic therapy. What does the nurse instruct the patient to do after the procedure?
    a. Maintain the head in an upright position for 24 hours.
    b. Avoid blowing the nose or causing jerking movements of the head.
    c. Completely cover all the skin to avoid a thermal burn from sunlight.
    d. Expect to experience blind spots where the laser has caused retinal damage.

19. What is an important health promotion nursing intervention related to glaucoma?
    a. Teaching individuals at risk for glaucoma about early signs and symptoms of the disease
    b. Preparing patients with glaucoma for lifestyle changes necessary to adapt to eventual blindness
    c. Promoting regular measurements of intraocular pressure for early detection and treatment of glaucoma
    d. Informing patients that glaucoma is curable if eye medications are administered before visual impairment has occurred

20. Which characteristics of glaucoma are associated with only primary open-angle glaucoma (POAG) (*select all that apply*)?
    a. Gradual loss of peripheral vision
    b. Treated with iridotomy or iridectomy
    c. Causes loss of central vision with corneal edema
    d. May be caused by increased production of aqueous humor
    e. Treated with cholinergic agents such as pilocarpine (Pilocar)
    f. Resistance to aqueous outflow through trabecular meshwork

21. Which characteristics of glaucoma are associated with only primary angle-closure glaucoma (PACG) (*select all that apply*)?
    a. Caused by lens blocking papillary opening
    b. Treated with trabeculoplasty or trabeculectomy
    c. Causes loss of central vision with corneal edema
    d. Treated with β-adrenergic blockers such as betaxolol (Betoptic)
    e. Causes sudden, severe eye pain associated with nausea and vomiting
    f. Treated with hyperosmotic oral and IV fluids to lower intraocular pressure

22. The health care provider has prescribed optic drops of betaxolol (Betoptic), dipivefrin (Propine), and carbachol (Isopto Carbachol) in addition to oral acetazolamide (Diamox) for treatment of a patient with chronic open-angle glaucoma. What is the rationale for the use of each of these drugs in the treatment of glaucoma? *IOP*

Drug	Rationale for Use
Betaxolol	*decreases aqueous humor production*
Dipivefrin	*decreases aqueous humor production + increases outflow activity*
Carbachol	*increase outflow*
Acetazolamide	

23. What is one of the nurse's roles in preservation of hearing?
    a. Advise patients to keep the ears clear of wax with cotton-tipped applicators.
    b. Monitor patients at risk for drug-induced ototoxicity for tinnitus and vertigo.
    c. Promote the use of ear protection in work and recreational activity with noise levels above 120 dB.
    d. Advocate for MMR (measles, mumps, rubella) immunization in susceptible women as soon as pregnancy is confirmed.

24. Number the following high-noise environments from 1 for the highest risk for ear injury to 6 for the lowest risk for ear injury.
    _____ a. Noisy restaurant for 12 hours
    _____ b. Heavy factory noise for 8 hours
    _____ c. Using a chainsaw continuously for 2 hours
    _____ d. Working in a quiet home office for 8 hours
    _____ e. Guiding jet planes to and from airport gates
    _____ f. Sitting in front of amplifiers at a rock concert

25. A 74-year-old man has moderate presbycusis and heart disease. He takes one aspirin a day as an antiplatelet agent and uses quinidine, furosemide (Lasix), and enalapril (Vasotec) for his heart condition. What risk factors are present for ototoxicity in this situation?

26. Which nursing action should be included in the management of the patient with external otitis?
    a. Irrigate the ear canal with body temperature saline several hours after instilling lubricating eardrops.
    b. Insert an ear wick into the external canal before each application of eardrops to disperse the medication.
    c. Teach the patient to prevent further infections by instilling antibiotic drops into the ear canal before swimming.
    d. Administer eardrops without touching the dropper to the auricle and position the ear upward for 2 minutes afterward.

27. What characteristics describe the care of a patient with chronic otitis media (*select all that apply*)?
    a. It is most commonly treated with antibiotics.
    b. It is an infection in the inner ear that may lead to headaches.
    c. Impairment of the eustachian tube is most commonly associated with effusion.
    d. Formation of an acoustic neuroma may destroy the structures of the middle ear or invade the dura of the brain.
    e. The patient who has had a myringotomy with placement of a tympanostomy tube should be instructed to avoid getting water in the ear.

28. While caring for a patient with otosclerosis, which finding would the nurse expect in the patient's history and physical?
    a. A strong family history of the disease
    b. Symptoms of sensorineural hearing loss
    c. A positive Rinne test and lateralization to the good or better ear on Weber testing
    d. An immediate and consistent improvement in hearing at the time of surgical treatment

29. The nurse identifies a nursing diagnosis of risk for injury for a patient following a stapedectomy based on what knowledge about this surgery?
    a. Nystagmus may result from perilymph disturbances caused by surgery.
    b. Stimulation of the labyrinth during surgery may cause vertigo and loss of balance.
    c. Blowing the nose or coughing may precipitate dislodgement of the tympanic graft.
    d. Postoperative tinnitus may decrease the patient's awareness of environmental hazards.

30. What makes up the triad of symptoms that occur with inner ear problems (*select all that apply*)?
    a. Vertigo
    b. Nausea
    c. Tinnitus
    d. Sensorineural hearing loss
    e. Inflammation of the ear canal

31. An appropriate nursing intervention for the patient during an acute attack of Meniere disease includes providing
    a. frequent repositioning.
    b. a quiet, darkened room.
    c. a television for diversion.
    d. padded side rails on the bed.

32. What knowledge guides the nurse in providing care for a patient with an acoustic neuroma?
    a. Widespread metastasis usually occurs before symptoms of the tumor are noticed.
    b. Facial nerve function will be sacrificed during surgical treatment to preserve hearing.
    c. Early diagnosis and treatment of the tumor can preserve hearing and vestibular function.
    d. Treatment is usually delayed until hearing loss is significant because a neuroma is a benign tumor.

33. What characteristics of hearing loss are associated with conductive loss (*select all that apply*)?
    a. Presbycusis
    b. Speaks softly
    c. Related to otitis media
    d. Result of ototoxic drugs
    e. Hears best in noisy environment
    f. May be caused by impacted cerumen

34. What characteristics of hearing loss are associated with sensorineural loss (*select all that apply*)?
    a. Hearing aid is helpful
    b. Related to otitis media
    c. Caused by noise trauma
    d. Linked with otosclerosis
    e. Associated with Meniere disease

35. When teaching a patient to use a hearing aid, where does the nurse encourage the patient to initially use the aid?
    a. Outdoors, where sounds are distinct
    b. At social functions, where simultaneous conversations take place
    c. In a quiet, controlled environment to experiment with tone and volume
    d. In public areas such as malls or stores, where others will not notice its use

---

CASE STUDY
Chronic Open-Angle Glaucoma
Patient Profile

A.G., a 58-year-old African American woman, was seen in her ophthalmologist's office for a routine eye examination. Her last examination was 5 years ago.

Subjective Data

- Has no current ocular complaints
- Has not kept annually scheduled examinations because her eyes have not bothered her
- Takes metoprolol tartrate (Lopressor) for hypertension
- Has a family history of glaucoma
- Uses over-the-counter diphenhydramine (Benadryl) for her seasonal allergies

Objective Data

- BP: 130/78
- HR: 72 bpm

Ophthalmic Examination

- Visual acuity: OD 20/20, OS 20/20
- Intraocular pressure: OD 25, OS 28; by Tono-Pen tonometry
- Direct and indirect ophthalmoscopy: small, scattered retinal hemorrhages; optic discs appear normal with no cupping
- Visual field perimetry: early glaucomatous changes, OU

Collaborative Care

The health care provider prescribes betaxolol (Betoptic) gtt 1 OU. The nurse instructs A.G. on the reasons for the drug and how to do punctal occlusion.

Discussion Questions

Using a separate sheet of paper, answer the following questions:

1. Why should A.G. have been seeing an ophthalmologist on a yearly basis even though she had no ocular complaints?
2. What should the nurse teach A.G. about administering the eyedrops?
3. Why is it permissible for A.G. to use her antihistamine? What would the nurse have told her if gonioscopy had revealed angle-closure glaucoma?
4. Will A.G. be able to discontinue her eyedrops once her intraocular pressures are within the normal range? Explain your answer.
5. If topical therapy does not control A.G.'s intraocular pressures, what should she be told about alternative therapies?
6. Describe the probable appearance of A.G.'s optic discs in the future if her glaucoma is left untreated. What would her visual complaints be?
7. ***Priority Decision:*** Based on the assessment data presented, what are the priority nursing diagnoses? Are there any collaborative problems?

1. Use the following terms to fill in the labels in the illustration below.

Terms

adipose tissue   connective tissue   hair shaft   stratum germinativum
apocrine sweat gland   hair follicle   stratum corneum   epidermis
arrector pili muscle   sebaceous gland   eccrine sweat gland   nerves
blood vessels   dermis   melanocyte   subcutaneous tissue

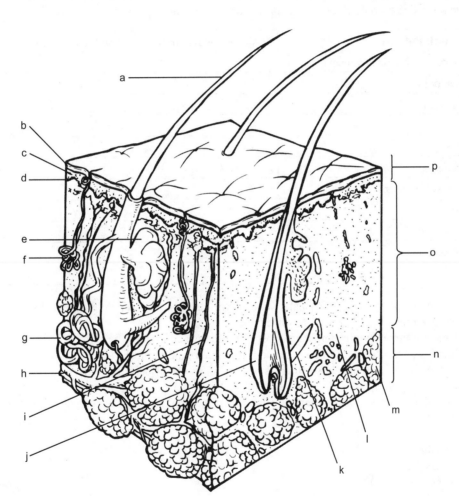

a. _____   g. _____   m. _____

b. _____   h. _____   n. _____

c. _____   i. _____   o. _____

d. _____   j. _____   p. _____

e. _____   k. _____

f. _____   l. _____

2. When the nurse is assessing the skin of an older adult, which factor is likely to contribute to dry skin?
   a. Increased bruising
   b. Excess perspiration
   c. Decreased extracellular fluid
   d. Decreased peripheral blood supply

3. When obtaining important health information from a patient during assessment of the skin, it is important for the nurse to ask about
   a. a history of freckles as a child.
   b. patterns of weight gain and loss.
   c. communicable childhood illnesses.
   d. skin problems related to the use of medications.

4. Identify one specific finding identified by the nurse during assessment of each of the patient's functional health patterns that would indicate a risk factor for skin problems or a patient response to a skin problem.

Functional Health Pattern	Risk Factor for or Response to Skin Problem
Health perception–health management	
Nutritional-metabolic	
Elimination	
Activity-exercise	
Sleep-rest	
Cognitive-perceptual	
Self-perception–self-concept	
Role-relationship	
Sexuality-reproductive	
Coping–stress tolerance	
Value-belief	

5. *Priority Decision:* When performing a physical assessment of the skin, what should the nurse do first?
   a. Palpate the temperature of the skin with the fingertips.
   b. Assess the degree of turgor by pinching the skin on the forearm.
   c. Inspect specific lesions before performing a general examination of the skin.
   d. Ask the patient to undress completely so all areas of the skin can be inspected.

6. The nurse observes that redness remains after palpation of a discolored lesion on the patient's leg. This finding is characteristic of
   a. varicosities.
   b. intradermal bleeding.
   c. dilated blood vessels.
   d. erythematous lesions.

7. A woman calls the health clinic and describes a rash that she has over the abdomen and chest. She tells the nurse it has raised, fluid-filled, small blisters that are distinct.
   a. Identify the type of primary skin lesion described by this patient.
   b. What is the distribution terminology for these lesions?
   c. What additional information does the nurse need to document the critical components of these lesions?

8. What is the primary difference between an excoriation and an ulcer?
   a. Ulcers do not penetrate below the epidermal junction.
   b. Excoriations involve only thinning of the epidermis and dermis.
   c. Excoriations will form crusts or scabs whereas ulcers remain open.
   d. An excoriation heals without scarring because the dermis is not involved.

9. A patient has a plaque lesion on the dorsal forearm. Which type of biopsy is most likely to be used for diagnosis of the lesion?
   a. Punch biopsy
   b. Shave biopsy
   c. Incisional biopsy
   d. Excisional biopsy

10. What is the most common diagnostic test used to determine a causative agent of skin infections?
    a. Culture
    b. Tzanck test
    c. Immunofluorescent studies
    d. Potassium hydroxide (KOH) slides

11. The patient asks the nurse what telangiectasia looks like. Which is the best description for the nurse to give the patient?
    a. A circumscribed, flat discoloration
    b. Small, superficial, dilated blood vessels
    c. Benign tumor of blood or lymph vessels
    d. Tiny purple spots resulting from tiny hemorrhages

12. An active athletic person calls the clinic and describes her feet as having linear breaks through the skin. What is the most likely diagnosis of this problem?
    a. Scales
    b. Fissure
    c. Pustule
    d. Comedo

13. A home health nurse is visiting an older obese woman who has recently had hip surgery. She tells the patient's caregiver that the patient has intertrigo. When the caregiver asks what that is, the nurse should tell the caregiver that it is
    a. thickening of the skin.
    b. dermatitis in the folds of her skin.
    c. loss of color in diffuse areas of her skin.
    d. a firm plaque caused by fluid in the dermis.

Nursing Management: Integumentary Problems

1. Which statements are true about skin and skin care (*select all that apply*)?
   a. One of the detrimental effects of obesity on the skin is increased sweating.
   b. The nutrient that is critical in maintaining and repairing the structure of epithelial cells is vitamin C.
   c. Exposure to UVA rays is believed to be the most important factor in the development of skin cancer.
   d. The photosensitivity caused by various drugs can be blocked by the use of topical hydrocortisone.
   e. Photosensitivity results when certain chemicals in body cells and tissues absorb light from the sun and release energy that harms the tissues and cells.
   f. When teaching a patient about the use of sunscreens that protect against exposure to both UVA and UVB rays, the nurse advises the patient to look for the inclusion of benzophenones.

2. Which statements characterize malignant melanomas (*select all that apply*)?
   a. Lesion is keratotic and firm
   b. Neoplastic growth of melanocytes
   c. Skin cancer with highest mortality rate
   d. Irregular color and asymmetric shape
   e. Frequently occurs on previously damaged skin

3. What is the most common skin cancer and has pearly borders?
   a. Actinic keratosis
   b. Basal cell carcinoma
   c. Malignant melanoma
   d. Squamous cell carcinoma

4. What skin condition has keratotic and firm lesions, is a precursor of squamous cell carcinoma, and is treated with topical fluorouracil (5-FU)?
   a. Actinic keratosis
   b. Basal cell carcinoma
   c. Malignant melanoma
   d. Squamous cell carcinoma

5. What characteristic is commonly seen with dysplastic nevus syndrome?
   a. Associated with sun exposure
   b. Precursor of squamous cell carcinoma
   c. Slow-growing tumor with rare metastasis
   d. Lesion has irregular color and asymmetric shape

6. Describe what is indicated by the ABCDEs of malignant melanoma.
   A
   B
   C
   D
   E

7. ***Priority Decision:*** A 46-year-old African American patient is scheduled to have a basal cell carcinoma on his cheek excised in the health care provider's office. What factor is most important for the nurse to obtain in the patient's history?
   a. Protected sun exposure
   b. Radiation treatment for acne
   c. Prior treatments for the lesion
   d. Exposure to harsh irritants such as ammonia

8. The nurse plans care for a patient with a newly diagnosed malignant melanoma based on the knowledge that initial treatment may involve (*select all that apply*)
   a. shave biopsy.
   b. Mohs' surgery.
   c. surgical excision.
   e. localized radiation.
   f. fluorouracil (5-FU).
   g. topical nitrogen mustard.

9. A patient is a 78-year-old woman who has had chronic respiratory disease for 30 years. She weighs 212 lb (96.4 kg) and is 5 ft, 1 in (152.5 cm) tall. She has recently completed corticosteroid and antibiotic treatment for an exacerbation of her respiratory disease. Identify four specific predisposing factors for bacterial skin infection in this patient.
   a.   c.
   b.   d.

10. What is the name for papillomavirus infection seen on the skin?
    a. Furuncle   c. Erysipelas
    b. Carbuncle   d. Plantar wart

11. Which description characterizes seborrheic keratosis?
    a. White patchy yeast infection   c. Excessive turnover of epithelial cells
    b. Warty, irregular papules or plaques   d. Deep inflammation of subcutaneous tissue

12. Which skin condition occurs as an allergic reaction to mite eggs?
    a. Scabies   c. Folliculitis
    b. Impetigo   d. Pediculosis

13. Which skin conditions are more common in immunosuppressed patients (*select all that apply*)?
    a. Acne   d. Herpes zoster
    b. Lentigo   e. Herpes simplex 1
    c. Candidiasis   f. Kaposi sarcoma

14. What should the nurse include in the instructions for a patient with urticaria?
    a. Apply topical benzene hexachloride.
    b. Avoid contact with the causative agent.
    c. Gradually expose the area to increasing amounts of sunlight.
    d. Use over-the-counter antihistamines routinely to prevent the condition.

15. A nurse caring for a disheveled patient with poor hygiene observes that the patient has small red lesions flush with the skin on the head and body. The patient complains of severe itching at the sites. For what should the nurse further assess the patient?
    a. Nits on the shafts of his head hair
    b. A history of sexually transmitted diseases
    c. The presence of ticks attached to the scalp
    d. The presence of burrows in the interdigital webs

16. A patient with a contact dermatitis is treated with calamine lotion. What is the rationale for using this base for a topical preparation?
    a. A suspension of oil and water to lubricate and prevent drying
    b. An emulsion of oil and water used for lubrication and protection
    c. Insoluble powders suspended in water that leave a residual powder on the skin
    d. A mixture of a powder and ointment that causes drying when moisture is absorbed

17. A patient with psoriasis is being treated with psoralen plus UVA light (PUVA) phototherapy. During the course of therapy, for what duration should the nurse teach the patient to wear protective eyewear that blocks all UV rays?
    a. Continuously for 6 hours after taking the medication
    b. Until the pupils are able to constrict on exposure to light
    c. For 12 hours following treatment to prevent retinal damage
    d. For 24 hours following treatment when outdoors or when indoors near a bright window

18. Identify one instruction the nurse should provide to a patient receiving the following medications for dermatologic problems.

Medication	Nursing Instruction
Topical antibiotics	
Topical corticosteroids	
Systemic antihistamines	
Topical fluorouracil	

19. Match the surgical interventions with conditions that they are used to treat (interventions may be used for more than one condition).

_____ a. Electrodessication or electrocoagulation

_____ b. Excision

_____ c. Mohs' surgery

_____ d. Curettage

_____ e. Cryosurgery

1. Malignant melanoma
2. Common and genital warts
3. Basal and squamous cell carcinomas
4. Telangiectasia
5. Lesions involving the dermis
6. Seborrheic keratoses

20. What are the most appropriate dressings to use to promote comfort for a patient with an inflamed, pruritic dermatitis?
   a. Cool tap water dressings
   b. Cool acetic acid dressings
   c. Warm sterile saline dressings
   d. Warm potassium permanganate dressings

21. What is an appropriate intervention to promote debridement and removal of scales and crusts of skin lesions?
   a. Warm oatmeal baths
   b. Warm saline dressings
   c. Cool sodium bicarbonate baths
   d. Cool magnesium sulfate dressings

22. Identify the rationale for using the following interventions to control pruritus.

Intervention	Rationale
Cool environment	
Topical menthol, camphor, or phenol	
Soaks and baths	

23. A female patient with chronic skin lesions of the face and arms tells the nurse that she cannot stand to look at herself in the mirror anymore because of her appearance. Based on this information, the nurse identifies which nursing diagnosis?
   a. Anxiety *related to* personal appearance
   b. Disturbed body image *related to* perception of unsightly lesions
   c. Social isolation *related to* decreased activities as a result of poor self-image
   d. Ineffective self-health management *related to* lack of knowledge of cover-up techniques

24. To prevent lichenification related to chronic skin problems, what does the nurse encourage the patient to do?
   a. Use measures to control itching.
   b. Wear sterile gloves when touching the lesions.
   c. Use careful hand washing and safe disposal of soiled dressings.
   d. Use topical antibiotics with wet-to-dry dressings over the lesions.

25. What is the most common reason elective cosmetic surgery is requested by patients?
    a. Improve self-image
    b. Remove deep acne scars
    c. Lighten the skin in pigmentation problems
    d. Prevent skin changes associated with aging

26. Which skin condition would be treated with laser surgery?
    a. Preauricular lesion
    b. Redundant soft tissue conditions
    c. Obesity with subcutaneous fat accumulation
    d. Fine wrinkle reduction or facial lesion removal

27. What is a skin graft that is used to transfer skin and subcutaneous tissue to large areas of deep tissue destruction called?
    a. Skin flap
    b. Free graft
    c. Soft tissue extension
    d. Free graft with vascular anastomoses

28. *Priority Decision:* A patient is receiving chemotherapy. She calls the physician's office and says she is experiencing itching in her groin and under her breasts. What is the first nursing assessment that would be done before the nurse makes an appointment for the patient with the physician to determine the treatment?
    a. Her height and weight
    b. What the areas look like
    c. If chemotherapy was completed
    d. Culture and sensitivity of the areas

29. The patient has diabetes mellitus and chronic obstructive pulmonary disease that has been treated with high-dose corticosteroids for the past several years. Which dermatologic manifestations could be related to these systemic problems (*select all that apply*)?
    a. Acne
    b. Increased sweating
    c. Dry, coarse, brittle hair
    d. Impaired wound healing
    e. Erythematous plaques of the shins
    f. Decreased subcutaneous fat over extremities

CASE STUDY
Cellulitis
Patient Profile

W.B., a 72-year-old man, cut his lower arm on a kitchen knife. At the time of the injury he did not seek medical attention. On the third day following the injury he began to be concerned about the condition of the wound and the way he was feeling.

Subjective Data

- States he has a fever and has had a general feeling of malaise
- Has pain in the area of the cut and the entire lower arm

Objective Data

- 4-cm area around cut is hot, erythematous, and edematous with redness extending both up and down his arm
- Temp: 100.8°F (38.2°C)

Discussion Questions

Using a separate sheet of paper, answer the following questions:

1. What other assessment data are needed before treatment begins?
2. What care of the wound should W.B. have taken to prevent the occurrence of cellulitis?
3. What are the usual etiologies of this type of infection?
4. What would you tell W.B. about the usual treatment of cellulitis?
5. What could result if treatment is not initiated and maintained?
6. *Priority Decision:* Based on the assessment data presented, what are the priority nursing diagnoses? Are there any collaborative problems?

25

Nursing Management: Burns

1. Which type of burn injury would cause myoglobinuria, long bone fractures, and cardiac dysrhythmias and/or cardiac arrest?
   a. Thermal
   b. Electrical
   c. Chemical
   d. Smoke and inhalation

2. Which characteristics are true about chemical burns (*select all that apply*)?
   a. Metabolic asphyxiation may occur.
   b. Metabolic acidosis occurs immediately following the burn.
   c. The visible skin injury often does not represent the full extent of tissue damage.
   d. Lavaging with large amounts of water is important to stop the burning process with these injuries.
   e. Alkaline substances that cause these burns continue to cause tissue damage even after being neutralized.

3. When assessing a patient's full-thickness burn injury during the emergent phase, what would the nurse expect to find?
   a. Leathery, dry, hard skin
   b. Red, fluid-filled vesicles
   c. Massive edema at the injury site
   d. Serous exudate on a shiny, dark brown wound

4. A patient has the following mixed deep partial-thickness and full-thickness burn injuries: face, anterior neck, right anterior trunk, and anterior surfaces of the right arm and lower leg.
   a. According to the Lund-Browder chart, what is the extent of the patient's burns?
      _____% total body surface area (TBSA)
   b. According to the rule of nines chart, what is the extent of the patient's burns?
      _____% TBSA
   c. Is it possible to determine the actual extent and depth of burn injury during the emergent phase of the burn? Why or why not?

5. *Priority Decision:* Number the following actions in the order they should be done in the emergency management of a burn of any type, beginning with number 1 for the first action.
   _____a. Establish and maintain an airway.
   _____b. Assess for other associated injuries.
   _____c. Establish an IV line with a large-gauge needle.
   _____d. Remove the patient from the burn source and stop the burning process.

6. The patient was admitted to the burn center with a full-thickness burn 42 hours after the thermal burn occurred. The nurse will apply actions related to which phase of burn management for this patient's care?
   a. Acute
   b. Emergent
   c. Postacute
   d. Rehabilitative

7. During the early emergent phase of burn injury, the patient's laboratory results would most likely include
   a. ↑ Hct, ↓ serum albumin, ↓ serum Na, ↑ serum K.
   b. ↓ Hct, ↓ serum albumin, ↓ serum Na, ↓ serum K.
   c. ↓ Hct, ↑ serum albumin, ↑ serum Na, ↑ serum K.
   d. ↑ Hct, ↑ serum albumin, ↓ serum Na, ↓ serum K.

8. What is the initial cause of hypovolemia during the emergent phase of burn injury?
   a. Increased capillary permeability
   b. Loss of sodium to the interstitium
   c. Decreased vascular oncotic pressure
   d. Fluid loss from denuded skin surfaces

9. How is the immune system altered in a burn injury?
   a. Bone marrow stimulation
   b. Increase in immunoglobulin levels
   c. Impaired function of white blood cells (WBCs)
   d. Overwhelmed by microorganisms entering denuded tissue

10. What is one clinical manifestation the nurse would expect to find during the emergent phase in a patient with a full-thickness burn over the lower half of the body?
    a. Fever
    b. Shivering
    c. Severe pain
    d. Unconsciousness

11. A patient has a 20% TBSA deep partial-thickness and full-thickness burn to the right anterior chest and entire right arm. What is important for a nurse to assess in this patient?
    a. Presence of pain
    b. Swelling of the arm
    c. Formation of eschar
    d. Presence of pulses in the arms

12. Which burn patient should have nasotracheal or endotracheal intubation?
    a. Carbon monoxide poisoning
    b. Electrical burns causing cardiac dysrhythmias
    c. Thermal burn injuries to the face, neck, or airway
    d. Respiratory distress from eschar formation around the chest

13. A patient is admitted to the emergency department at 10:15 PM following a flame burn at 9:30 PM. The patient has 40% TBSA deep partial-thickness and full-thickness burns and weighs 132 lb.
    a. According to the Parkland formula, the type of fluid prescribed for the patient would be _____ and the total amount to be administered during the first 24 hours would be _____ mL.
    b. The schedule for the fluid administration would be _____ mL between _____ and _____(time), _____mL between _____ and _____, and _____ mL between _____ and _____.
    c. Colloidal solutions are given in the second 24 hours. Based on the patient's body weight, what amount of these solutions will be given during this time?
    d. The adequacy of the patient's fluid replacement is determined by _____ and _____.

14. A patient's deep partial-thickness burns are treated with the open method. What should the nurse do when caring for the patient?
    a. Ensure that sterile water is used in the debridement tank.
    b. Wear a cap, mask, gown, and gloves during patient contact.
    c. Use sterile gloves to remove the dressings and wash the wounds.
    d. Apply topical antimicrobial ointment with clean gloves to prevent wound trauma.

15. A patient with deep partial-thickness burns over 45% of his trunk and legs is going for debridement in the cart shower 48 hours post burn. What is the drug of choice to control the patient's pain during this activity?
    a. IV morphine
    b. Midazolam (Versed)
    c. IM meperidine (Demerol)
    d. Long-acting oral morphine

16. The nurse assesses that bowel sounds are absent and abdominal distention is present in a patient 12 hours post burn. The nurse notifies the health care provider and anticipates doing what action?
    a. Withhold all oral intake except water
    b. Insert a nasogastric tube for decompression
    c. Administer a H_2-histamine blocker such as cimetidine (Tagamet)
    d. Administer nutritional supplements through a feeding tube placed in the duodenum

17. How should the nurse position the patient with ear, face, and neck burns?
    a. Prone
    b. On the side
    c. Without pillows
    d. With extra padding around the head

18. Identify the factors that increase nutritional needs of the patient during the emergent and acute phases of burn injury (*select all that apply*).
    a. Electrolyte imbalance
    b. Core temperature elevation
    c. Calories and protein are used for tissue repair
    d. Hypometabolic state secondary to decreased gastrointestinal (GI) function
    e. Massive catabolism characterized by protein breakdown and increased gluconeogenesis

19. At the end of the emergent phase and the initial acute phase of burn injury, a patient has a serum sodium level of 152 mEq/L (152 mmol/L) and a serum potassium level of 2.8 mEq/L (2.8 mmol/L). What could have caused these imbalances?
    a. Free oral water intake
    b. Prolonged hydrotherapy
    c. Mobilization of fluid and electrolytes in the acute phase
    d. Excessive fluid replacement with dextrose in water without potassium supplementation

20. A burn patient has a nursing diagnosis of impaired physical mobility related to a limited range of motion (ROM) resulting from pain. What is an appropriate nursing intervention for this patient?
    a. Have the patient perform ROM exercises when pain is not present.
    b. Provide analgesic medications before physical activity and exercise.
    c. Teach the patient the importance of exercise to prevent contractures.
    d. Arrange for the physical therapist to encourage exercise during hydrotherapy.

21. The nurse initially suspects the possibility of sepsis in the burn patient based on what changes?
    a. Vital signs
    b. Urinary output
    c. Gastrointestinal function
    d. Burn wound appearance

22. Identify one major complication of burns that is believed to be stress-related that may occur in each of the following systems during the acute burn phase.

Body System	Complication
Neurologic	
Gastrointestinal	
Endocrine	

23. Complete the following sentences.
    a. A permanent skin graft that may be available for the patient with large body surface area burns who has limited skin for donor harvesting is _____.
    b. Early excision and grafting of burn wounds involve excising _____ down to clean viable tissue and applying an _____ whenever possible.
    c. Blebs can be removed from skin grafts by _____.

24. The burn patient has developed an increasing dread of painful dressing changes. What would be the most appropriate treatment to ask the health care provider to prescribe?
    a. Midazolam (Versed) to be used with morphine before dressing changes
    b. Morphine in a dosage range so that more may be given before dressing changes
    c. Buprenorphine (Buprenex) to be administered with morphine before dressing changes
    d. Patient-controlled analgesia so that the patient may have control of analgesic administration

25. During the rehabilitation phase of a burn injury, what can control the contour of the scarring?
    a. Pressure garments
    b. Avoidance of sunlight
    c. Splinting joints in extension
    d. Application of emollient lotions

26. A 24-year-old female patient does not want the wound cleansing and dressing change to take place. She states, "What difference will it make anyway?" What will the nurse encourage the patient to do?
    a. Have the wound cleaned and the dressing changed
    b. Have a snack before having the treatments completed
    c. Talk about what is troubling her with the nurse and/or her family
    d. Call the chaplain to come and talk to her and convince her to have the care

27. **Priority Decision:** The nurse has received the change-of-shift report on his group of patients. Indicate the priority order in which the nurse should see these patients.
    _____a. A 40-year-old female who is returning from the postanesthesia care unit (PACU) following surgical debridement of her back and legs
    _____b. A 76-year-old male with partial-thickness burns of his arms and abdomen who is complaining of severe pain
    _____c. A 62-year-old female who was just admitted following partial-thickness burns to her anterior chest, face, and neck
    _____d. An 18-year-old male with full-thickness burns of his lower extremities who is refusing to go for his scheduled dressing change

CASE STUDY

Burn Patient in Rehabilitation Phase

Patient Profile

D.K. is a 30-year-old woman who has been in the burn center for 3 weeks. She sustained partial- and full-thickness burns to both hands and forearms while cooking. She has undergone three surgeries for escharotomy and split-thickness skin grafting. She is married and has three young children at home. Her health care providers feel she is nearly ready for discharge but she has been tearful and noncompliant with therapy. D.K. and her husband refuse to look at her hand grafts, which continue to require light dressings. She has not seen her children since admission.

Discussion Questions

Using a separate sheet of paper, answer the following questions:

1. When should discharge planning be initiated with D.K.? Who should be involved in the planning and implementation of the educational process before discharge?
2. Describe the nutritional needs D.K. will have after discharge and interventions to meet those needs.
3. D.K. has been wearing hand and elbow splints at night while in the burn center. What instructions will D.K. need regarding her splinting and exercise routine at home?
4. D.K. complains of tightness in her hands, which restricts her motion. She uses this excuse to avoid exercise and independent performance of her activities of daily living. What activities and teaching would be beneficial to address this issue?
5. *Priority Decision:* D.K. and her husband have been extremely upset and anxious regarding D.K.'s discharge. They are not actively participating in the discharge planning process. What priority interventions should the staff implement to assist the couple?
6. What are some of the feelings D.K. and her family may experience following her return home? What can the nurse do to prepare the family?
7. *Priority Decision:* What are the priority needs that must be addressed with D.K. and her husband regarding dressing changes and graft care before discharge from the burn center? Discuss how this should be managed.
8. *Priority Decision:* Based on the assessment data presented, what are the priority nursing diagnoses? Are there any collaborative problems?

Nursing Assessment: Respiratory System

1. Number the following organs in the order of the pathway of inspired air. Number 1 is the first organ after the environment and number 13 is the last organ before the alveoli.
   _____a. Carina
   _____b. Larynx
   _____c. Glottis
   _____d. Trachea
   _____e. Epiglottis
   _____f. Nasal cavity
   _____g. Bronchioles
   _____h. Oropharynx
   _____i. Nasopharynx
   _____j. Alveolar duct
   _____k. Laryngopharynx
   _____l. Mainstem bronchi
   _____m. Segmental bronchi

2. A 92-year-old female patient is being admitted to the emergency department with severe shortness of breath. Being aware of the patient's condition, what approach should the nurse use to assess the patient's lungs (*select all that apply*)?
   a. Apex to base
   b. Base to apex
   c. Lateral sequence
   d. Anterior then posterior
   e. Posterior then anterior

3. What keeps alveoli from collapsing?
   a. Carina
   b. Surfactant
   c. Empyema
   d. Thoracic cage

4. What accurately describes the alveolar sacs?
   a. Line the lung pleura
   b. Warm and moisturize inhaled air
   c. Terminal structures of the respiratory tract
   d. Contain dead air that is not available for gas exchange

5. What covers the larynx during swallowing?
   a. Trachea
   b. Epiglottis
   c. Turbinates
   d. Parietal pleura

6. *Priority Decision:* A 75-year-old patient who is breathing room air has the following arterial blood gas (ABG) results: pH 7.40, PaO_2 74 mm Hg, SaO_2 92%, $PaCO_2$ 40 mm Hg. What is the most appropriate action by the nurse?
   a. Document the results in the patient's record.
   b. Repeat the ABGs within an hour to validate the findings.
   c. Encourage deep breathing and coughing to open the alveoli.
   d. Initiate pulse oximetry for continuous monitoring of the patient's oxygen status.

7. A patient's ABGs include a PaO_2 of 88 mm Hg and a $PaCO_2$ of 38 mm Hg, and mixed venous blood gases include a PvO_2 of 40 mm Hg and $PvCO_2$ of 46 mm Hg. What do these findings indicate?
   a. Impaired cardiac output
   b. Unstable hemodynamics
   c. Inadequate delivery of oxygen to the tissues
   d. Normal capillary oxygen–carbon dioxide exchange

8. *Priority Decision:* A pulse oximetry monitor indicates that the patient has a drop in SpO_2 from 95% to 85% over several hours. What is the first action the nurse should take?
   a. Order stat ABGs to confirm the SpO_2 with a SaO_2.
   b. Start oxygen administration by nasal cannula at 2 L/min.
   c. Check the position of the probe on the finger or earlobe.
   d. Notify the health care provider of the change in baseline PaO_2.

9. Pulse oximetry may not be a reliable indicator of oxygen saturation in which patient?
   a. Patient with a fever
   b. Patient who is anesthetized
   c. Patient in hypovolemic shock
   d. Patient receiving oxygen therapy

10. A 73-year-old patient has an SpO_2 of 70%. What other assessment should the nurse consider before making a judgment about the adequacy of the patient's oxygenation?
    a. What the oxygenation status is with a stress test
    b. Trend and rate of development of the hyperkalemia
    c. Comparison of patient's SpO_2 values with the normal values
    d. Comparison of patient's current vital signs with normal vital signs

11. Which values are indicators of the criteria needed for the use of continuous oxygen therapy?
    a. SpO_2 of 92%; PaO_2 of 65 mm Hg
    b. SpO_2 of 95%; PaO_2 of 70 mm Hg
    c. SpO_2 of 90%; PaO_2 of 60 mm Hg
    d. SpO_2 of 88%; PaO_2 of 55 mm Hg

12. Why does a patient's respiratory rate increase when there is an excess of carbon dioxide in the blood?
    a. CO_2 displaces oxygen on hemoglobin, leading to a decreased PaO_2.
    b. CO_2 causes an increase in the amount of hydrogen ions available in the body.
    c. CO_2 combines with water to form carbonic acid, which lowers the pH of cerebrospinal fluid.
    d. CO_2 directly stimulates chemoreceptors in the medulla to increase respiratory rate and volume.

13. Which respiratory defense mechanism is most impaired by smoking?
    a. Cough reflex
    b. Filtration of air
    c. Mucociliary clearance
    d. Reflex bronchoconstriction

14. Which age-related changes in the respiratory system cause decreased secretion clearance (*select all that apply*)?
    a. Decreased functional cilia
    b. Decreased force of cough
    c. Decreased chest wall compliance
    d. Small airway closure earlier in expiration
    e. Decreased functional immunoglobulin A (IgA)

15. Identify one specific finding identified by the nurse during assessment of each of the patient's functional health patterns that indicates a risk factor for respiratory problems or a patient response to an actual respiratory problem.

Functional Health Pattern	Risk Factor for or Response to Respiratory Problem
Health perception–health management	
Nutritional-metabolic	
Elimination	
Activity-exercise	
Sleep-rest	
Cognitive-perceptual	
Self-perception–self-concept	
Role-relationship	
Sexuality-reproductive	
Coping–stress tolerance	
Value-belief	

16. The abnormal assessment findings of dullness and hyperresonance are found with which assessment technique?
    a. Inspection
    b. Palpation
    c. Percussion
    d. Auscultation

17. Palpation is the assessment technique used to find which abnormal assessment findings (*select all that apply*)?
    a. Stridor
    b. Finger clubbing
    c. Tracheal deviation
    d. Limited chest expansion
    e. Increased tactile fremitus
    f. Use of accessory muscles

18. How does the nurse assess the patient's chest expansion?
    a. Put the palms of the hands against the chest wall.
    b. Put the index fingers on either side of the trachea.
    c. Place the thumbs at the midline of the lower chest.
    d. Place one hand on the lower anterior chest and one hand on the upper abdomen.

19. When does the nurse record the presence of an increased anteroposterior (AP) diameter of the chest?
    a. There is a prominent protrusion of the sternum.
    b. The width of the chest is equal to the depth of the chest.
    c. There is equal but diminished movement of the two sides of the chest.
    d. The patient cannot fully expand the lungs because of kyphosis of the spine.

20. How is the presence of bronchovesicular breath sounds in the peripheral lung fields described?
    a. Rhonchi
    b. Crackles
    c. Adventitious sounds
    d. Abnormal lung sounds

21. Match the descriptions or possible etiologies with the appropriate abnormal assessment findings.
    _____ a. Finger clubbing
    _____ b. Stridor
    _____ c. Wheezes
    _____ d. Pleural friction rub
    _____ e. Increased tactile fremitus
    _____ f. Hyperresonance
    _____ g. Fine crackles
    _____ h. Absent breath sounds

    1. Lung consolidation with fluid or exudate
    2. Air trapping
    3. Atelectasis
    4. Interstitial filling with fluid
    5. Bronchoconstriction
    6. Partial obstruction of trachea or larynx
    7. Chronic hypoxemia
    8. Pleurisy

22. A nurse has been exposed to tuberculosis (TB) during care of a patient with TB and has a TB skin test performed. When is the nurse considered infected?
    a. There is no redness or induration at the injection site.
    b. There is an induration of only 5 mm at the injection site.
    c. A negative skin test is followed by a negative chest x-ray.
    d. Testing causes a 10-mm red, indurated area at the injection site.

23. What is a primary nursing responsibility after obtaining a blood specimen for ABGs?
    a. Adding heparin to the blood specimen
    b. Applying pressure to the puncture site for 2 full minutes
    c. Taking the specimen immediately to the laboratory in an iced container
    d. Avoiding any changes in oxygen intervention for 20 minutes following the procedure

24. What should the nurse do when preparing a patient for a pulmonary angiogram scan?
    a. Assess the patient for iodine allergy.
    b. Implement NPO orders for 6 to 12 hours before the test.
    c. Explain the test before the patient signs the informed consent form.
    d. Inform the patient that radiation isolation for 24 hours after the test is necessary.

25. The nurse is preparing the patient for and will assist the physician with a thoracentesis in the patient's room. Number the following actions in the order the nurse should complete them. Use 1 for the first action and 7 for the last action.

_____ a. Verify breath sounds in all fields.

_____ b. Obtain the supplies that will be used.

_____ c. Send labeled specimen containers to the lab.

_____ d. Direct the family members to the waiting room.

_____ e. Observe for signs of hypoxia during the procedure.

_____ f. Instruct the patient not to talk during the procedure.

_____ g. Position the patient sitting upright with the elbows on an over-the-bed table.

26. After which test should the nurse observe the patient for symptoms of a pneumothorax?

a. Thoracentesis

b. Pulmonary function test

c. Ventilation-perfusion scan

d. Positron emission tomography (PET) scan

27. The health care provider orders a pulmonary angiogram for a patient admitted with dyspnea and hemoptysis. For which problem is this test most commonly used as a diagnostic measure?

a. Tuberculosis (TB)

b. Cancer of the lung

c. Airway obstruction

d. Pulmonary embolism

28. Match the following pulmonary capacities and function tests with their descriptions.

_____ a. Vt

_____ b. RV

_____ c. TLC

_____ d. VC

_____ e. FVC

_____ f. PEFR

_____ g. FEV_1

_____ h. FRC

1. Amount of air exhaled in first second of forced vital capacity
2. Maximum amount of air lungs can contain
3. Volume of air inhaled and exhaled with each breath
4. Maximum amount of air that can be exhaled after maximum inhalation
5. Amount of air that can be quickly and forcefully exhaled after maximum inspiration
6. Maximum rate of airflow during forced expiration
7. Amount of air remaining in lungs after forced expiration
8. Volume of air in lungs after normal exhalation

Nursing Management:
Upper Respiratory Problems

1. A patient develops epistaxis upon removal of a nasogastric tube. What action should the nurse take?
   a. Pinch the soft part of the nose.
   b. Position the patient on the side.
   c. Have the patient hyperextend the neck.
   d. Apply an ice pack to the back of the neck.

2. *Priority Decision:* The nurse receives an evening report on a patient who underwent posterior nasal packing for epistaxis earlier in the day. What is the first patient assessment the nurse should make?
   a. Patient's temperature
   b. Level of the patient's pain
   c. Drainage on the nasal dressing
   d. Oxygen saturation by pulse oximetry

3. What does the nurse teach the patient with intermittent allergic rhinitis is the most effective way to decrease allergic symptoms?
   a. Undergo weekly immunotherapy.
   b. Identify and avoid triggers of the allergic reaction.
   c. Use cromolyn nasal spray prophylactically year-round.
   d. Use over-the-counter antihistamines and decongestants during an acute attack.

4. During assessment of the patient with a viral upper respiratory infection, the nurse recognizes that antibiotics may be indicated based on what finding?
   a. Cough and sore throat
   b. Copious nasal discharge
   c. Temperature of 100°F (38°C)
   d. Dyspnea and severe sinus pain

5. A 36-year-old patient with type 1 diabetes mellitus asks the nurse whether an influenza vaccine is necessary every year. What is the best response by the nurse?
   a. "You should get the trivalent inactivated influenza vaccine that is injected every year."
   b. "Only health care workers in contact with high-risk patients should be immunized each year."
   c. "An annual vaccination is not necessary because previous immunity will protect you for several years."
   d. "Antiviral drugs, such as zanamivir (Relenza), eliminate the need for vaccine except in the older adult."

6. A patient with an acute pharyngitis is seen at the clinic with fever and severe throat pain that affects swallowing. On inspection, the throat is reddened and edematous with patchy yellow exudates. The nurse anticipates that collaborative management will include
   a. treatment with antibiotics.
   b. treatment with antifungal agents.
   c. a throat culture or rapid strep antigen test.
   d. treatment with medication only if the pharyngitis does not resolve in 3 to 4 days.

7. While the nurse is feeding a patient, the patient appears to choke on the food. Which symptoms indicate to the nurse that the patient has a partial airway obstruction (*select all that apply*)?
   a. Stridor
   b. Cyanosis
   c. Wheezing
   d. Bradycardia
   e. Rapid respiratory rate

8. What is an advantage of a tracheostomy over an endotracheal (ET) tube for long-term management of an upper airway obstruction?
    a. A tracheostomy is safer to perform in an emergency.
    b. An ET tube has a higher risk of tracheal pressure necrosis.
    c. A tracheostomy tube allows for more comfort and mobility.
    d. An ET tube is more likely to lead to lower respiratory tract infection.

9. What are the characteristics of a fenestrated tracheostomy tube (*select all that apply*)?
    a. The cuff passively fills with air.
    b. Cuff pressure monitoring is not required.
    c. It has two tubings with one opening just above the cuff.
    d. Patient can speak with an attached air source with the cuff inflated.
    e. Airway obstruction is likely if the exact steps are not followed to produce speech.
    f. Airflow around the tube and through the window allows speech when the cuff is deflated and the plug is inserted.

10. During care of a patient with a cuffed tracheostomy, the nurse notes that the tracheostomy tube has an inner cannula. To care for the tracheostomy appropriately, what should the nurse do?
    a. Deflate the cuff, then remove and suction the inner cannula.
    b. Remove the inner cannula and replace it per institutional guidelines.
    c. Remove the inner cannula if the patient shows signs of airway obstruction.
    d. Keep the inner cannula in place at all times to prevent dislodging the tracheostomy tube.

11. Which actions prevent the dislodgement of a tracheostomy tube in the first 3 days after its placement (*select all that apply*)?
    a. Provide tracheostomy care every 24 hours.
    b. Keep the patient in the semi-Fowler position at all times.
    c. Keep a same size or larger replacement tube at the bedside.
    d. Tracheostomy ties are not changed for 24 hours after tracheostomy procedure.
    e. Suction the tracheostomy tube when there is a moist cough or a decreased SpO_2.
    f. A physician performs the first tube change, no sooner than 7 days after the tracheostomy.

12. ***Delegation Decision:*** In planning the care for a patient with a tracheostomy who has been stable and is to be discharged later in the day, the RN may delegate which interventions to the licensed practical nurse (LPN) (*select all that apply*)?
    a. Suction the tracheostomy.
    b. Provide tracheostomy care.
    c. Determine the need for suctioning.
    d. Assess the patient's swallowing ability.
    e. Teach the patient about home tracheostomy care.

13. What is included in the nursing care of the patient with a cuffed tracheostomy tube?
    a. Change the tube every 3 days.
    b. Monitor cuff pressure every 8 hours.
    c. Perform mouth care every 12 hours.
    d. Assess arterial blood gases every 8 hours.

14. ***Priority Decision:*** A patient's tracheostomy tube becomes dislodged with vigorous coughing. What should be the nurse's first action?
    a. Attempt to replace the tube.
    b. Notify the health care provider.
    c. Place the patient in high Fowler position.
    d. Ventilate the patient with a manual resuscitation bag until the health care provider arrives.

15. When obtaining a health history from a patient with possible cancer of the mouth, what would the nurse expect the patient to report?
    a. Long-term denture use
    b. Heavy tobacco and/or alcohol use
    c. Persistent swelling of the neck and face
    d. Chronic herpes simplex infections of the mouth and lips

16. The patient has been diagnosed with an early vocal cord malignancy. The nurse explains that usual treatment includes
    a. radiation therapy that preserves the quality of the voice.
    b. a hemilaryngectomy that prevents the need for a tracheostomy.
    c. a radical neck dissection that removes possible sites of metastasis.
    d. a total laryngectomy to prevent development of second primary cancers.

17. During preoperative teaching for the patient scheduled for a total laryngectomy, what should the nurse include?
    a. The postoperative use of nonverbal communication techniques
    b. Techniques that will be used to alleviate a dry mouth and prevent stomatitis
    c. The need for frequent, vigorous coughing in the first 24 hours postoperatively
    d. Self-help groups and community resources for patients with cancer of the larynx

18. When assessing the patient on return to the surgical unit following a total laryngectomy and radical neck dissection, what would the nurse expect to find?
    a. A closed-wound drainage system
    b. A nasal endotracheal tube in place
    c. A nasogastric tube with orders for tube feedings
    d. A tracheostomy tube and mechanical ventilation

19. Following a supraglottic laryngectomy, the patient is taught how to use the supraglottic swallow to minimize the risk of aspiration. In teaching the patient about this technique, what should the nurse instruct the patient to do?
    a. Perform Valsalva maneuver immediately after swallowing.
    b. Breathe between each Valsalva maneuver and cough sequence.
    c. Cough after swallowing to remove food from the top of the vocal cords.
    d. Practice swallowing thin, watery fluids before attempting to swallow solid foods.

20. What should the nurse include in discharge teaching for the patient with a total laryngectomy?
    a. How to use esophageal speech to communicate
    b. How to use a mirror to suction the tracheostomy
    c. The necessity of never covering the laryngectomy stoma
    d. The need to use baths instead of showers for personal hygiene

21. What is the most normal functioning method of speech restoration in the patient with a total laryngectomy?
    a. Esophageal speech
    b. A transesophageal puncture
    c. An electrolarynx held to the neck
    d. An electrolarynx placed in the mouth

CASE STUDY
Rhinoplasty
Patient Profile

F.N. is a 28-year-old male patient who sustained bilateral fractures of the nose, three rib fractures, and a comminuted fracture of the tibia in an automobile crash 5 days ago. An open reduction and internal fixation of the tibia were performed the day of the trauma. F.N. is now scheduled for a rhinoplasty to reestablish an adequate airway and improve cosmetic appearance.

Subjective Data

- Reports facial pain at a level of 6 on a 10-point scale
- Expresses concern about his facial appearance
- Complains of dry mouth

Objective Data

- RR 24
- HR 68 bpm
- Bilateral ecchymosis of eyes (raccoon eyes)
- Periorbital edema and edema of face reduced by about half since second hospital day
- Has been NPO since midnight in preparation for surgery

Discussion Questions

Using a separate sheet of paper, answer the following questions:

1. When F.N. was admitted, examination of his nose revealed clear drainage. What is the significance of the drainage? What testing is indicated?
2. What is the reason for delaying repair of F.N.'s nose for several days after the trauma?
3. What measures should be taken to maintain F.N.'s airway before and after surgery?
4. *Priority Decision:* When F.N. arrives in the postanesthesia care unit (PACU) following surgery, what priority assessments should the nurse make in the immediate postoperative period?
5. *Priority Decision:* F.N.'s nasal packing is removed in 24 hours and he is to be discharged. What priority predischarge teaching should the nurse provide?
6. *Priority Decision:* Based on the assessment data presented, what are the priority nursing diagnoses? Are there any collaborative problems?

1. How do microorganisms reach the lungs and cause pneumonia (*select all that apply*)?
   a. Aspiration
   b. Lymphatic spread
   c. Inhalation of microbes in the air
   d. Touch contact with the infectious microbes
   e. Hematogenous spread from infections elsewhere in the body

2. Why is the classification of pneumonia as community-acquired pneumonia (CAP) or medical care-associated pneumonia (MCAP) clinically useful?
   a. Atypical pneumonia syndrome is more likely to occur in MCAP.
   b. Diagnostic testing does not have to be used to identify causative agents.
   c. Causative agents can be predicted and empiric treatment is often effective.
   d. IV antibiotic therapy is necessary for MCAP but oral therapy is adequate for CAP.

3. The microorganisms *Pneumocystis jiroveci* (PCP) and cytomegalovirus (CMV) are associated with which type of pneumonia?
   a. Bronchial pneumonia
   b. Opportunistic pneumonia
   c. Hospital-associated pneumonia
   d. Community-acquired pneumonia

4. Which of the following microorganisms are associated with both CAP and MCAP (*select all that apply*)?
   a. *Klebsiella*
   b. *Staphylococcus aureus*
   c. *Haemophilus influenzae*
   d. *Mycoplasma pneumonia*
   e. *Pseudomonas aeruginosa*
   f. *Streptococcus pneumonia*

5. Place the most common pathophysiologic stages of pneumonia in order. Number the first stage with 1 and the last stage with 4.
   _____ a. Macrophages lyse the debris and normal lung tissue and function is restored.
   _____ b. Mucus production increases and can obstruct airflow and further decrease gas exchange.
   _____ c. Inflammatory response in the lungs with neutrophils is activated to engulf and kill the offending organism.
   _____ d. Increased capillary permeability contributes to alveolar filling with organisms and neutrophils interrupt normal oxygen transportation.

6. When obtaining a health history from a 76-year-old patient with suspected CAP, what does the nurse expect the patient or caregiver to report?
   a. Confusion
   b. A recent loss of consciousness
   c. An abrupt onset of fever and chills
   d. A gradual onset of headache and sore throat

7. What is the initial antibiotic treatment for pneumonia based on?
   a. The severity of symptoms
   b. The presence of characteristic leukocytes
   c. Gram stains and cultures of sputum specimens
   d. History and physical examination and characteristic chest x-ray findings

8. ***Priority Decision:*** After the health care provider sees a patient hospitalized with a stroke who developed a fever and adventitious lung sounds, the following orders are written. Which order should the nurse implement first?
   a. Anterior/posterior and lateral chest x-rays
   b. Start IV levofloxacin (Levaquin) 500 mg every 24 hr
   c. Sputum specimen for Gram stain and culture and sensitivity
   d. Complete blood count (CBC) with white blood cell (WBC) count and differential

9. Identify four clinical situations in which hospitalized patients are at risk for aspiration pneumonia and one nursing intervention for each situation that is indicated to prevent pneumonia.

Clinical Situation	Nursing Intervention

10. Following assessment of a patient with pneumonia, the nurse identifies a nursing diagnosis of impaired gas exchange based on which finding?
    a. SpO_2 of 86%
    b. Crackles in both lower lobes
    c. Temperature of 101.4°F (38.6°C)
    d. Production of greenish purulent sputum

11. A patient with pneumonia has a nursing diagnosis of ineffective airway clearance related to pain, fatigue, and thick secretions. What is an expected outcome for this patient?
    a. SpO_2 is 90%
    b. Lungs clear to auscultation
    c. Patient tolerates walking in hallway
    d. Patient takes three or four shallow breaths before coughing to minimize pain

12. During an annual health assessment of a 65-year-old patient at the clinic, the patient tells the nurse he had the pneumonia vaccine when he was age 58. What should the nurse advise him about the best way for him to prevent pneumonia?
    a. Seek medical care and antibiotic therapy for all upper respiratory infections
    b. Obtain the pneumococcal vaccine this year with an annual influenza vaccine
    c. Obtain the pneumococcal vaccine if he is exposed to individuals with pneumonia
    d. Obtain only the influenza vaccine every year because he has immunity to the pneumococcus

13. What was the resurgence in tuberculosis (TB) resulting from the emergence of multidrug-resistant strains of *Mycobacterium tuberculosis* related to?
    a. A lack of effective means to diagnose TB
    b. Poor compliance with drug therapy in patients with TB
    c. Indiscriminate use of antitubercular drugs in treatment of other infections
    d. Increased population of immunosuppressed individuals with acquired immunodeficiency syndrome (AIDS)

14. *Priority Decision:* A patient diagnosed with class 3 TB 1 week ago is admitted to the hospital with symptoms of chest pain and coughing. What nursing action has the highest priority?
    a. Administering the patient's antitubercular drugs
    b. Admitting the patient to an airborne infection isolation room
    c. Preparing the patient's room with suction equipment and extra linens
    d. Placing the patient in an intensive care unit where he can be closely monitored

15. When obtaining a health history from a patient suspected of having early TB, what manifestations should the nurse ask the patient about?
    a. Chest pain, hemoptysis, and weight loss
    b. Fatigue, low-grade fever, and night sweats
    c. Cough with purulent mucus and fever with chills
    d. Pleuritic pain, nonproductive cough, and temperature elevation at night

16. Which medications would be used in four-drug treatment for the initial phase of TB (*select all that apply*)?
    a. Isoniazid (INH)
    b. Rifampin (Rifadin)
    c. Pyrazinamide (PZA)
    d. Rifabutin (Mycobutin)
    e. Levofloxacin (Levaquin)
    f. Ethambutol (Myambutol)

17. A patient with active TB continues to have positive sputum cultures after 6 months of treatment. She says she cannot remember to take the medication all the time. What is the best action for the nurse to take?
    a. Schedule the patient to come to the clinic every day to take the medication.
    b. Have a patient who has recovered from TB tell the patient about his successful treatment.
    c. Schedule more teaching sessions so the patient will understand the risks of noncompliance.
    d. Arrange for directly observed therapy by a responsible family member or a public health nurse.

18. *Priority Decision:* To reduce the risk for most occupational lung diseases, what is the most important measure the occupational nurse should promote?
    a. Maintaining smoke-free work environments for all employees.
    b. Using masks and effective ventilation systems to reduce exposure to irritants.
    c. Inspection and monitoring of workplaces by national occupational safety agencies.
    d. Requiring periodic chest x-rays and pulmonary function tests for exposed employees.

19. During a health promotion program, why should the nurse plan to target women in a discussion of lung cancer prevention (*select all that apply*)?
    a. Women develop lung cancer at a younger age than men.
    b. More women die of lung cancer than die from breast cancer.
    c. Women have a worse prognosis from lung cancer than do men.
    d. Women are more likely to develop small cell carcinoma than men.
    e. Nonsmoking women are at greater risk for developing lung cancer than men.

20. A patient with a 40 pack-year smoking history has recently stopped smoking because of the fear of developing lung cancer. The patient asks the nurse what he can do to learn about whether he develops lung cancer. What is the best response from the nurse?
    a. "You should get a chest x-ray every 6 months to screen for any new growths."
    b. "It would be very rare for you to develop lung cancer now that you have stopped smoking."
    c. "You should monitor for any persistent cough, wheezing, or difficulty breathing, which could indicate tumor growth."
    d. "Screening measures for lung cancers are controversial, but we can discuss the advantages and disadvantages of various measures."

21. A patient with a lung mass found on chest x-ray is undergoing further testing. The nurse explains that a diagnosis of lung cancer can be confirmed using which diagnostic test?
    a. Lung tomograms
    b. Pulmonary angiography
    c. Biopsy done via bronchoscopy
    d. Computed tomography (CT) scans

22. Match the following treatments for lung cancer with their descriptions.
    _____ a. Considered primary treatment for small cell lung cancer (SCLC)
    _____ b. Drug activated by laser light that destroys cancer cells
    _____ c. Electric current heats and destroys tumor cells
    _____ d. Palliative treatment for airway collapse or external compression
    _____ e. Best procedure for cure of lung cancer
    _____ f. Medications that block molecules involved in tumor growth
    _____ g. Palliative treatment by bronchoscope to remove obstructing bronchial tumors
    _____ h. Used to treat both non–small cell lung cancer (NSCLC) and SCLC
    _____ i. Used to prevent metastasis to the brain

    1. Surgical therapy
    2. Radiation therapy
    3. Chemotherapy
    4. Prophylactic cranial radiation
    5. Bronchoscopic laser
    6. Photodynamic therapy
    7. Airway stenting
    8. Radiofrequency ablation
    9. Biologic and targeted therapy

23. A patient with advanced lung cancer refuses pain medication, saying, "I deserve everything this cancer can give me." What is the nurse's best response to this patient?
    a. "Would talking to a counselor help you?"
    b. "Can you tell me what the pain means to you?"
    c. "Are you using the pain as a punishment for your smoking?"
    d. "Pain control will help you to deal more effectively with your feelings."

24. A male patient has chronic obstructive pulmonary disease (COPD) and is a smoker. The nurse notices respiratory distress and no breath sounds over the left chest. Which type of pneumothorax should the nurse suspect is occurring?
    a. Tension pneumothorax
    b. Iatrogenic pneumothorax
    c. Traumatic pneumothorax
    d. Spontaneous pneumothorax

25. To determine whether a tension pneumothorax is developing in a patient with chest trauma, for what does the nurse assess the patient?
    a. Dull percussion sounds on the injured side
    b. Severe respiratory distress and tracheal deviation
    c. Muffled and distant heart sounds with decreasing blood pressure
    d. Decreased movement and diminished breath sounds on the affected side

26. Following a motor vehicle accident, the nurse assesses the driver for which distinctive sign of flail chest?
    a. Severe hypotension
    b. Chest pain over ribs
    c. Absence of breath sounds
    d. Paradoxical chest movement

27. Identify the A, B, C, D, and E labels on the chest drainage devices pictured below (note that only figure 2 has an E label).

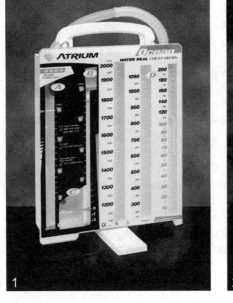 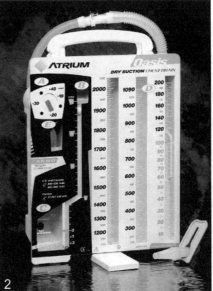

    A. _____   D. _____
    B. _____   E. _____
    C. _____

28. Describe the function of each chamber.

Chamber	Function
Water-seal	
Suction control	
Collection	
Suction monitor bellows	

29. When should the nurse check for leaks in the chest tube and pleural drainage system?
    a. There is continuous bubbling in the water-seal chamber.
    b. There is constant bubbling of water in the suction control chamber.
    c. Fluid in the water-seal chamber fluctuates with the patient's breathing.
    d. The water levels in the water-seal and suction control chambers are decreased.

30. An unlicensed assistive personnel (UAP) is taking care of a patient with a chest tube. The nurse should intervene when she observes the UAP
    a. looping the drainage tubing on the bed.
    b. securing the drainage container in an upright position.
    c. stripping or milking the chest tube to promote drainage.
    d. reminding the patient to cough and deep breathe every 2 hours.

31. Which chest surgery is used for the stripping of a fibrous membrane?
    a. Lobectomy
    b. Decortication
    c. Thoracotomy
    d. Wedge resection

32. What is the purpose of video-assisted thoracic surgery (VATS)?
    a. Removal of a lung
    b. Removal of one or more lung segments
    c. Removal of lung tissue by multiple wedge excisions
    d. Used to inspect, diagnose, and manage intrathoracic injuries

33. Following a thoracotomy, the patient has a nursing diagnosis of ineffective airway clearance related to inability to cough as a result of pain and positioning. What is the best nursing intervention for this patient?
    a. Have the patient drink 16 oz of water before attempting to deep breathe.
    b. Auscultate the lungs before and after deep-breathing and coughing regimens.
    c. Place the patient in the Trendelenburg position for 30 minutes before the coughing exercises.
    d. Medicate the patient with analgesics 20 to 30 minutes before assisting to cough and deep breathe.

34. Match the following restrictive lung conditions with the mechanisms that cause decreased vital capacity (VC) and decreased total lung capacity (TLC).
    _____ a. Pleurisy
    _____ b. Empyema
    _____ c. Atelectasis
    _____ d. Kyphoscoliosis
    _____ e. Pleural effusion
    _____ f. Muscular dystrophy
    _____ g. Pickwickian syndrome
    _____ h. Opioid and sedative overdose
    _____ i. Idiopathic pulmonary fibrosis

    1. Paralysis of respiratory muscles
    2. Presence of collapsed, airless alveoli
    3. Spinal angulation restricting ventilation
    4. Central depression of respiratory rate and depth
    5. Excessive scar tissue in connective tissue in lungs
    6. Lung expansion restricted by fluid in pleural space
    7. Lung expansion restricted by pus in intrapleural space
    8. Inflammation of the pleura restricting lung movement
    9. Excess fat restricts chest wall and diaphragmatic excursion

35. *Priority Decision:* Two days after undergoing pelvic surgery, a patient develops marked dyspnea and anxiety. What is the first action that the nurse should take?
    a. Raise the head of the bed.
    b. Notify the health care provider.
    c. Take the patient's pulse and blood pressure.
    d. Determine the patient's SpO_2 with an oximeter.

36. A pulmonary embolus is suspected in a patient with a deep vein thrombosis who develops hemoptysis, tachycardia, and chest pain. Diagnostic testing is scheduled. Which test should the nurse plan to teach the patient about?
    a. Chest x-rays
    b. Spiral (helical) CT scan
    c. Take the patient's pulse and blood pressure.
    d. Ventilation-perfusion lung scan

37. Which condition contributes to secondary pulmonary arterial hypertension by causing pulmonary capillary and alveolar damage?
    a. COPD
    b. Sarcoidosis
    c. Pulmonary fibrosis
    d. Pulmonary embolism

38. While caring for a patient with idiopathic pulmonary arterial hypertension (IPAH), the nurse observes that the patient has exertional dyspnea and chest pain in addition to fatigue. What are these symptoms related to?
    a. Decreased left ventricular output
    b. Right ventricular hypertrophy and dilation
    c. Increased systemic arterial blood pressure
    d. Development of alveolar interstitial edema

39. What is a primary treatment goal for cor pulmonale?
    a. Controlling dysrhythmias
    b. Dilating the pulmonary arteries
    c. Strengthening the cardiac muscle
    d. Treating the underlying pulmonary condition

40. Six days after a heart-lung transplant, the patient develops a low-grade fever, dyspnea, and decreased SpO_2. What should the nurse recognize that this may indicate?
    a. A normal response to extensive surgery
    b. A frequently fatal cytomegalovirus infection
    c. Acute rejection that may be treated with corticosteroids
    d. Obliterative bronchiolitis that plugs terminal bronchioles

---

CASE STUDY

Pulmonary Hypertension

Patient Profile

T.S. is a 46-year-old female patient who was diagnosed with idiopathic pulmonary arterial hypertension at the age of 42. At that time she presented to her primary care health care provider with a history of increasing fatigue and recent onset of swelling in her feet and ankles. A chest x-ray revealed severe cardiomegaly with pulmonary congestion. She underwent a right-sided cardiac catheterization, which showed very high pulmonary artery pressures. Since then, she has been treated with several drugs but her pulmonary hypertension has never been controlled and her peripheral edema has progressively worsened.

Subjective Data

- Short of breath at rest and exercise intolerant to the extent that she had to quit her job
- Recently divorced from her husband
- Has two children: a girl, 10 years old, and a boy, 4 years old

Objective Data

- 3+ pitting edema from her feet to her knees
- RR: 28 at rest
- HR: 92 bpm and bounding

Discussion Questions

Using a separate sheet of paper, answer the following questions:

1. What drugs might T.S. have been given to treat her pulmonary hypertension?
2. Is T.S. a candidate for heart-lung or lung transplantation? Why or why not?
3. What transplant procedure would be considered for T.S.? What is the rationale?
4. *Priority Decision:* What priority preoperative teaching is necessary for T.S. to prepare for a transplant procedure?
5. *Priority Decision:* Based on the assessment data presented, what are the priority nursing interventions?

29

Nursing Management: Obstructive Pulmonary Diseases

1. While assisting a patient with intermittent asthma to identify specific triggers of asthma, what should the nurse explain?
   a. Food and drug allergies do not manifest in respiratory symptoms.
   b. Exercise-induced asthma is seen only in individuals with sensitivity to cold air.
   c. Asthma attacks are psychogenic in origin and can be controlled with relaxation techniques.
   d. Viral upper respiratory infections are a common precipitating factor in acute asthma attacks.

2. *Priority Decision:* A patient is admitted to the emergency department with an acute asthma attack. Which patient assessment is of greatest concern to the nurse?
   a. The presence of a pulsus paradoxus
   b. Markedly diminished breath sounds with no wheezing
   c. Use of accessory muscles of respiration and a feeling of suffocation
   d. A respiratory rate of 34 and increased pulse and blood pressure

3. A patient with asthma has the following arterial blood gas (ABG) results early in an acute asthma attack: pH 7.48, $PaCO_2$ 30 mm Hg, PaO_2 78 mm Hg. What is the most appropriate action by the nurse?
   a. Prepare the patient for mechanical ventilation.
   b. Have the patient breathe in a paper bag to raise the $PaCO_2$.
   c. Document the findings and monitor the ABGs for a trend toward alkalosis.
   d. Reduce the patient's oxygen flow rate to keep the PaO_2 at the current level.

4. Indicate the role or relationship of the following agents to asthma.

Agent	Role or Relationship to Asthma
Salicylates	
α-Adrenergic blockers	
Beer and wine	

5. What is an indication of marked bronchoconstriction with air trapping and hyperinflation of the lungs in a patient with asthma?
   a. SaO_2 of 85%
   b. PEF rate of <150 L/min
   c. FEV_1 of 85% of predicted
   d. Chest x-ray showing a flattened diaphragm

6. *Priority Decision:* Which medication should the nurse anticipate being used first in the emergency department for relief of severe respiratory distress related to asthma?
   a. Prednisone orally
   b. Ipratopium inhaler
   c. Fluticasone inhaler
   d. Albuterol nebulizer

7. Which medications are the most effective in improving asthma control by reducing bronchial hyperresponsiveness, blocking the late-phase reaction, and inhibiting migration of inflammatory cells (*select all that apply*)?
   a. Zileuton (Zyflo CR)
   b. Omalizumab (Xolair)
   c. Fluticasone (Flovent)
   d. Salmeterol (Serevent)
   e. Montelukast (Singulair)
   f. Budesonide (Pulmicort)
   g. Beclomethasone (Qvar)
   h. Methylxanthine (theophylline)
   i. Mometasone (Asmanex Twisthaler)

8. When teaching the patient about going from a metered-dose inhaler (MDI) to a dry powder inhaler (DPI), which statement by the patient shows the nurse that the patient needs more teaching?
   a. "I do not need to use the spacer like I used to."
   b. "I will hold my breath for 10 seconds or longer if I can."
   c. "I will not shake this inhaler like I did with my old inhaler."
   d. "I will store it in the bathroom so I will be able to clean it when I need to."

9. Which statements by a patient with moderate asthma inform the nurse that the patient needs more teaching about medications (*select all that apply*)?
   a. "If I can't afford all of my medicines, I will only use the salmeterol (Serevent)."
   b. "I will stay inside if there is a high pollen count to prevent having an asthma attack."
   c. "I will rinse my mouth after using fluticasone (Flovent HFA) to prevent oral candidiasis."
   d. "I must have omalizumab (Xolair) injected every 2 to 4 weeks because inhalers don't help my asthma."
   e. "I can use my inhaler three times, every 20 minutes, before going to the hospital if my peak flow has not improved."
   f. "My gastroesophageal reflux disease (GERD) medications will help my asthma and my asthma medications will help my GERD."

10. *Priority Decision:* To decrease the patient's sense of panic during an acute asthma attack, what is the best action for the nurse to do?
    a. Leave the patient alone to rest in a quiet, calm environment.
    b. Stay with the patient and encourage slow, pursed lip breathing.
    c. Reassure the patient that the attack can be controlled with treatment.
    d. Let the patient know that frequent monitoring is being done using measurement of vital signs and SpO_2.

11. When teaching the patient with mild asthma about the use of the peak flow meter, what should the nurse instruct the patient to do?
    a. Carry the flow meter with the patient at all times in case an asthma attack occurs
    b. Use the flow meter to check the status of the patient's asthma every time the patient takes quick-relief medication
    c. Follow the written asthma action plan (e.g., take quick-relief medication) if the expiratory flow rate is in the yellow zone
    d. Use the flow meter by emptying the lungs, closing the mouth around the mouthpiece, and inhaling through the meter as quickly as possible

12. The nurse recognizes that additional teaching is needed when the patient with asthma says
    a. "I should exercise every day if my symptoms are controlled."
    b. "I may use over-the-counter bronchodilator drugs occasionally if I develop chest tightness."
    c. "I should inform my spouse about my medications and how to get help if I have a severe asthma attack."
    d. "A diary to record my medication use, symptoms, peak expiratory flow rates, and activity levels will help in adjusting my therapy."

13. Tobacco smoke causes defects in multiple areas of the respiratory system. What is a long-term effect of smoking?
    a. Bronchospasm and hoarseness
    b. Decreased mucus secretions and cough
    c. Increased function of alveolar macrophages
    (d.) Increased risk of infection and hyperplasia of mucous glands

14. Indicate whether the following clinical manifestations are most characteristic of asthma (A), chronic obstructive pulmonary disease (COPD) (C), or both (B).
    __A__ a. Wheezing
    C __B__ b. Weight loss
    __C__ c. Barrel chest
    C __B__ d. Polycythemia
    __C__ e. Cor pulmonale
    __B__ f. Persistent cough
    __C__ g. Flattened diaphragm
    __B__ h. Decreased breath sounds
    __B__ i. Increased total lung capacity
    __C__ j. Frequent sputum production
    __A__ k. Increased fractional exhaled nitric oxide (FENO)

15. What causes the pulmonary vasoconstriction leading to the development of cor pulmonale in the patient with COPD?
    a. Increased viscosity of the blood
    (b.) Alveolar hypoxia and hypercapnia
    c. Long-term low-flow oxygen therapy
    d. Administration of high concentrations of oxygen

16. In addition to smoking cessation, what treatment is included for COPD to slow the progression of the disease?
    a. Use of bronchodilator drugs
    b. Use of inhaled corticosteroids
    c. Lung volume–reduction surgery
    (d.) Prevention of respiratory tract infections

17. Which method of oxygen administration is the safest system to use for a patient with COPD?
    (a.) Venturi mask
    b. Nasal cannula
    c. Simple face mask
    d. Non-rebreathing mask

18. What is characteristic of a partial rebreathing mask?
    a. Used for long-term O_2 therapy
    (b.) Reservoir bag conserves oxygen
    c. Provides highest oxygen concentrations
    d. Most comfortable and causes the least restriction on activities

19. A patient is being discharged with plans for home O_2 therapy provided by an O_2 concentrator with an O_2-conserving portable unit. In preparing the patient to use the equipment, what should the nurse teach the patient?
    a. The portable unit will last about 6 to 8 hours.
    b. The unit is strictly for portable and emergency use.
    (c.) The unit concentrates O_2 from the air, providing a continuous O_2 supply.
    d. Weekly delivery of one large cylinder of O_2 will be necessary for a 7- to 10-day supply of O_2.

20. Which breathing technique should the nurse teach the patient with moderate COPD to promote exhalation?
    a. Huff coughing
    b. Thoracic breathing
    (c.) Pursed lip breathing
    d. Diaphragmatic breathing

21. What does the nurse include when planning for postural drainage for the patient with COPD?
    a. Schedules the procedure 1 hour before and after meals
    b. Has the patient cough before positioning to clear the lungs
    c. Assesses the patient's tolerance for dependent (head-down) positions
    d. Ensures that percussion and vibration are performed before positioning the patient

22. Which dietary modification helps to meet the nutritional needs of patients with COPD?
    a. Eating a high-carbohydrate, low-fat diet
    b. Avoiding foods that require a lot of chewing
    c. Preparing most foods of the diet to be eaten hot
    d. Drinking fluids with meals to promote digestion

23. *Delegation Decision:* The nurse is caring for a patient with COPD. Which intervention could be delegated to unlicensed assistive personnel (UAP)?
    a. Assist the patient to get out of bed.
    b. Auscultate breath sounds every 4 hours.
    c. Plan patient activities to minimize exertion.
    d. Teach the patient pursed lip breathing technique.

24. Which medication is a dry powder inhaler (DPI) that is used only for COPD?
    a. Roflumilast (Daliresp)
    b. Salmeterol (Serevent)
    c. Ipratropium (Atrovent HFA)
    d. Indacterol (Arcapta Neohaler)

25. *Priority Decision:* During an acute exacerbation of mild COPD, the patient is severely short of breath and the nurse identifies a nursing diagnosis of ineffective breathing pattern related to obstruction of airflow and anxiety. What is the best action by the nurse?
    a. Prepare and administer routine bronchodilator medications.
    b. Perform chest physiotherapy to promote removal of secretions.
    c. Administer oxygen at 5 L/min until the shortness of breath is relieved.
    d. Position the patient upright with the elbows resting on the over-the-bed table.

26. The husband of a patient with severe COPD tells the nurse that he and his wife have not had any sexual activity since she was diagnosed with COPD because she becomes too short of breath. What is the nurse's best response?
    a. "You need to discuss your feelings and needs with your wife so she knows what you expect of her."
    b. "There are other ways to maintain intimacy besides sexual intercourse that will not make her short of breath."
    c. "You should explore other ways to meet your sexual needs since your wife is no longer capable of sexual activity."
    d. "Would you like for me to talk to you and your wife about some modifications that can be made to maintain sexual activity?"

27. What should the nurse include when teaching the patient with COPD about the need for physical exercise?
    a. All patients with COPD should be able to increase walking gradually up to 20 minutes per day.
    b. A bronchodilator inhaler should be used to relieve exercise-induced dyspnea immediately after exercise.
    c. Shortness of breath is expected during exercise but should return to baseline within 5 minutes after the exercise.
    d. Monitoring the heart rate before and after exercise is the best way to determine how much exercise can be tolerated.

28. The patient has had COPD for years and his ABGs usually show hypoxia (PaO_2 <60 mm Hg or SaO_2 <88%) and hypercapnia ($PaCO_2$ >45 mm Hg). Which ABG results show movement toward respiratory acidosis and further hypoxia indicating respiratory failure?
    a. pH 7.35, PaO_2 62 mm Hg, $PaCO_2$ 45 mm Hg
    b. pH 7.34, PaO_2 45 mm Hg, $PaCO_2$ 65 mm Hg
    c. pH 7.42, PaO_2 90 mm Hg, $PaCO_2$ 43 mm Hg
    d. pH 7.46, PaO_2 92 mm Hg, $PaCO_2$ 32 mm Hg

29. Pulmonary rehabilitation (PR) is designed to reduce symptoms and improve the patient's quality of life. Along with improving exercise capacity, what are the anticipated results of PR (*select all that apply*)?
    a. Decreased FEV_1
    b. Decreased anxiety
    c. Decreased depression
    d. Increased oxygen need
    e. Decreased hospitalizations

30. What is the pathophysiologic mechanism of cystic fibrosis leading to obstructive lung disease?
    a. Fibrosis of mucous glands and destruction of bronchial walls
    b. Destruction of lung parenchyma from inflammation and scarring
    c. Production of secretions low in sodium chloride and therefore thickened mucus
    d. Increased serum levels of pancreatic enzymes that are deposited in the bronchial mucosa

31. What is the most effective treatment for cystic fibrosis?
    a. Heart-lung transplant
    b. Administration of prophylactic antibiotics
    c. Administration of nebulized bronchodilators
    d. Vigorous and consistent chest physiotherapy

32. Meeting the developmental tasks of young adults with cystic fibrosis becomes a major problem primarily because
    a. they eventually need a lung transplant.
    b. they must also adapt to a chronic disease.
    c. any children they have will develop cystic fibrosis.
    d. their illness keeps them from becoming financially independent.

33. In an adult patient with bronchiectasis, what is a nursing assessment likely to reveal?
    a. Chest trauma
    b. Childhood asthma
    c. Smoking or oral tobacco use
    d. Recurrent lower respiratory tract infections

34. In planning care for the patient with bronchiectasis, which nursing intervention should the nurse include?
    a. Relieve or reduce pain
    b. Prevent paroxysmal coughing
    c. Prevent spread of the disease to others
    d. Promote drainage and removal of mucus

35. Which obstructive pulmonary disease would a 30-year-old white female patient with a parent with the disease be most likely to be diagnosed with?
    a. COPD
    b. Asthma
    c. Cystic fibrosis
    d. α_1-Antitrypsin (AAT) deficiency

36. What is the primary principle involved in the various airway clearance devices used for mobilizing secretions?
    a. Vibration
    b. Inhalation therapy
    c. Chest physiotherapy
    d. Positive expiratory pressure

CASE STUDY

Asthma

Patient Profile

E.S. is a 35-year-old mother of two school-age boys who arrives via ambulance in the emergency department (ED) with severe wheezing, dyspnea, and anxiety. She was in the ED 6 hours earlier with an asthma attack.

Subjective Data

- Treated during previous ED visit with nebulized albuterol and responded quickly
- Allergic to cigarette smoke
- Began to experience increasing tightness in her chest and shortness of breath when she returned home following her previous ED visit
- Used the albuterol several times after she returned home with no relief
- Diagnosed with asthma 2 years ago
- Does not have a health care provider and is not on any medications

Objective Data

Physical Examination
- Sitting upright and using accessory muscles to breathe
- Talks in one- to three-word sentences
- RR: 34 and shallow
- Audible wheezing
- Auscultation of lung fields reveals no air movement in lower lobes
- HR: 126 bpm
- Noted to be extremely anxious and restless

Diagnostic Studies
- ABGs: pH 7.46, $PaCO_2$ 36 mm Hg, PaO_2 76 mm Hg, O_2 saturation 88%
- Chest x-ray: bilateral lung hyperinflation with lower lobe atelectasis
- CBC with differential and electrolytes: within normal limits

An IV is started in her left forearm with normal saline infusing at 100 mL/hr.

Discussion Questions

Using a separate sheet of paper, answer the following questions:

1. What other assessment information should be obtained from E.S.?
2. *Priority Decision:* What is the priority collaborative intervention for E.S.?
3. What data obtained from the brief history, physical examination, and diagnostic studies indicate that E.S. is experiencing a severe or life-threatening asthma attack?
4. Identify two classifications of medications the nurse should expect to be administered to this patient. What effect is expected with these medications?
5. In addition to medication administration and close monitoring of the patient, what other key role can the nurse take in helping the patient through this episode?
6. What value would peak expiratory flow rate (PEFR) measures have during the care of E.S.?
7. What health care teaching should be included for this patient related to her asthma?
8. *Priority Decision:* Based on the assessment data presented, what are the priority nursing diagnoses? What are the collaborative problems?

CHAPTER

30

Nursing Assessment: Hematologic System

1. What are the characteristics of neutrophils (*select all that apply*)?
   a. Also known as "segs"
   b. Band is immature cell
   c. First WBC at injury site
   d. Arises from megakaryocyte
   e. Increased in individuals with allergies
   f. 50% to 70% of white blood cells (WBCs)

2. An increase in which blood cell indicates an increased rate of erythropoiesis?
   a. Basophil
   b. Monocyte
   c. Reticulocyte
   d. Lymphocyte

3. Which cells are classified as granulocytes (*select all that apply*)?
   a. Basophil
   b. Monocyte
   c. Eosinophil
   d. Neutrophil
   e. Lymphocyte

4. After a woman had a right breast mastectomy, her right arm became severely swollen. What hematologic problem caused this?
   a. Lymphedema
   b. Right-sided heart failure
   c. Wound on her right hand
   d. Refusal to use her right arm

5. Which nutrients are essential for red blood cell production (*select all that apply*)?
   a. Iron
   b. Folic acid
   c. Vitamin C
   d. Vitamin D
   e. Vitamin B$_{12}$
   f. Carbohydrates

6. Number the components of normal hemostasis in the order of occurrence, beginning with 1 for the first component and ending with 4 for the last component.
   ___4___ a. Lysis of clot
   ___1___ b. Vascular response
   ___3___ c. Plasma clotting factors
   ___2___ d. Platelet plug formation

7. Which component of normal hemostasis involves the processes of protein C and protein S and plasminogen?
   a. Lysis of clot
   b. Vascular response
   c. Plasma clotting factors
   d. Platelet plug formation

8. A patient who was in a car accident had abdominal trauma. Which organs may be damaged and contribute to altered function of the hematologic system (*select all that apply*)?
   a. Liver
   b. Spleen
   c. Stomach
   d. Gallbladder
   e. Lymph nodes

9. Laboratory test results indicate increased fibrin split products (FSPs). An appropriate nursing action is to monitor the patient for
   a. fever.
   b. bleeding.
   c. faintness.
   d. thrombotic episodes.

10. When reviewing the results of an 83-year-old patient's blood tests, which finding would be of most concern to the nurse?
    a. Platelets 150,000/μL
    b. Serum iron 50 mcg/dL
    c. Partial thromboplastin time (PTT) 60 seconds *(45-70)*
    d. Erythrocyte sedimentation rate (ESR) 35 mm in 1 hour

11. A patient with a bone marrow disorder has an overproduction of myeloblasts. The nurse would expect the results of a complete blood count (CBC) to include an increase in which cell types (*select all that apply*)?
    a. Basophils
    b. Eosinophils
    c. Monocytes
    d. Neutrophils
    e. Lymphocytes

12. During the nursing assessment of a patient with anemia, what specific information should the nurse ask the patient about?
    a. Stomach surgery
    b. Recurring infections
    c. Corticosteroid therapy
    d. Oral contraceptive use

13. Identify one specific finding identified by the nurse during assessment of each of the patient's functional health patterns that indicates a risk factor for hematologic problems or a patient response to an actual hematologic problem.

Functional Health Pattern	Risk Factor for or Response to Hematologic Problem
Health perception–health management	
Nutritional-metabolic	
Elimination	
Activity-exercise	
Sleep-rest	
Cognitive-perceptual	
Self-perception–self-concept	
Role-relationship	
Sexuality-reproductive	
Coping–stress tolerance	
Value-belief	

14. Using light pressure with the index and middle fingers, the nurse cannot palpate any of the patient's superficial lymph nodes. How should the nurse respond to this assessment?
    a. Record this finding as normal.
    b. Reassess the lymph nodes using deeper pressure.
    c. Ask the patient about any history of radiation therapy.
    d. Notify the health care provider that x-rays of the nodes will be necessary.

15. During physical assessment of a patient with thrombocytopenia, what would the nurse expect to find?
    a. Sternal tenderness
    b. Petechiae and purpura
    c. Jaundiced sclera and skin
    d. Tender, enlarged lymph nodes

16. A patient with a hematologic disorder has a smooth, shiny, red tongue. Which laboratory result would the nurse expect to see?
    a. Neutrophils 45%
    b. Hgb 9.6 g/dL (96 g/L)
    c. WBC count 13,500/μL
    d. Red blood cell (RBC) count 6.4 × 10⁶/μL

17. A patient is being treated with chemotherapy. The nurse revises the patient's care plan based on which result?
    a. WBC count 4000/μL
    b. RBC count 3.8 × 10⁶/μL
    c. Platelets 50,000/μL
    d. Hematocrit (Hct) 39%

18. Identify a possible etiology for the abnormal laboratory study results.

Laboratory Finding	Possible Etiology
Serum iron 40 mcg/dL (7 μmol/L)	
ESR 30 mm/hr	
Increased band neutrophils	
Activated partial thromboplastin time 60 sec	
Indirect bilirubin 2.0 mg/dL (34 μmol/L)	
Bence Jones protein in urine	

19. If a patient with blood type O Rh⁺ is given AB Rh⁻ blood, what would the nurse expect to happen?
    a. The patient's Rh factor will react with the RBCs of the donor blood.
    b. The anti-A and anti-B antibodies in the patient's blood will hemolyze the donor blood.
    c. The anti-A and anti-B antibodies in the donor blood will hemolyze the patient's blood.
    d. No adverse reaction is expected because the patient has no antibodies against the donor blood.

20. *Priority Decision:* A patient is undergoing a contrast computed tomography (CT) of the spleen. What is most important for the nurse to ask the patient about before the test?
    a. Iodine sensitivity
    b. Prior blood transfusions
    c. Phobia of confined spaces
    d. Internal metal implants or appliances

21. When teaching a patient about a bone marrow examination, what should the nurse explain?
    a. The procedure will be done under general anesthesia because it is so painful.
    b. The patient will not have any pain after the area at the puncture site is anesthetized.
    c. The patient will experience a brief, very sharp pain during aspiration of the bone marrow.
    d. There will be no pain during the procedure, but an ache will be present several days afterward.

22. A lymph node biopsy is most often performed to diagnose
    a. leukemia.
    b. cause of lymphedema.
    c. hemorrhagic tendencies.
    d. neoplastic cells in lymph nodes.

23. The patient's laboratory results show a marked decrease in RBCs, WBCs, and platelets. What term should the nurse use when reporting the results to the physician?
    a. Hemolysis
    b. Leukopenia
    c. Pancytopenia
    d. Thrombocytosis

24. Molecular cytogenetics and gene analysis may be done to diagnose, stage, and help to determine treatment options for various hematologic disorders. Which sites are preferred to obtain the sample for this testing (*select all that apply*)?
    a. Skin sample
    b. Lymph node
    c. Bone marrow
    d. Arterial blood
    e. Inner cheek mucosa

1. Match each of the anemic states with both the etiologic and morphologic classifications (answers may be used more than once).

Type or Cause of Anemia	Etiology	Morphology
Malaria		
Thalassemia		
Acute trauma		
Aplastic anemia		
Pernicious anemia		
Sickle cell anemia		
Anemia of gastritis		
Anemia of leukemia		
Iron-deficiency anemia		
Anemia of renal failure		
Glucose-6-phosphate dehydrogenase (G6PD)		
Anemia associated with prosthetic heart valve		

Etiologic
1. Decreased RBC production
2. Blood loss
3. Increased RBC destruction

Morphologic
4. Normocytic, normochromic
5. Macrocytic, normochromic
6. Microcytic, hypochromic

2. A patient with a hemoglobin (Hgb) level of 7.8 g/dL (78 g/L) has cardiac palpitations, a heart rate of 102 bpm, and an increased reticulocyte count. At this severity of anemia, what other manifestation would the nurse expect the patient to exhibit?
   a. Pallor
   b. Dyspnea
   c. A smooth tongue
   d. Sensitivity to cold

3. *Priority Decision:* A 76-year-old woman has an Hgb of 7.3 g/dL (73 g/L) and is experiencing ataxia and confusion on admission to the hospital. What is a priority nursing intervention for this patient?
   a. Provide a darkened, quiet room.
   b. Have the family stay with the patient.
   c. Keep top bedside rails up and call bell in close reach
   d. Question the patient about possible causes of anemia

4. During the physical assessment of the patient with severe anemia, which finding is of the most concern to the nurse?
   a. Anorexia
   b. Bone pain
   c. Hepatomegaly
   d. Dyspnea at rest

5. Which anemia is manifested with pancytopenia?
   a. Thalassemia
   b. Aplastic anemia
   c. Megaloblastic anemia
   d. Anemia of chronic disease

6. Which descriptions are characteristic of iron-deficiency anemia (*select all that apply*)?
   a. Lack of intrinsic factor
   b. Autoimmune-related disease
   c. Most common type of anemia
   d. Associated with chronic blood loss
   e. May occur with removal of the stomach
   f. May occur with removal of the duodenum

7. A 20-year-old female patient is in the emergency department for anorexia and fatigue. She takes phenytoin (Dilantin) for a seizure disorder and oral contraceptives. Which type of anemia is this patient most at risk for?
   a. Aplastic anemia
   b. Hemolytic anemia
   c. Iron-deficiency anemia
   d. Folic acid deficiency anemia

8. Explain the following laboratory findings in anemia.

Finding	Explanation
Reticulocyte counts are increased in chronic blood loss but decreased in cobalamin (vitamin B$_{12}$) deficiency.	
Bilirubin levels are increased in sickle cell anemia but are normal in acute blood loss.	
Mean corpuscular volume (MCV) is increased in folic acid deficiency but decreased in iron-deficiency anemia.	

9. When teaching the patient about a new prescription for oral iron supplements, what does the nurse instruct the patient to do?
   a. Increase fluid and dietary fiber intake
   b. Take the iron preparations with meals
   c. Use enteric-coated preparations taken with orange juice
   d. Report the presence of black stools to the health care provider

10. In teaching the patient with pernicious anemia about the disease, the nurse explains that it results from a lack of
    a. folic acid.
    b. intrinsic factor.
    c. extrinsic factor.
    d. cobalamin intake.

11. During the assessment of a patient with cobalamin deficiency, what manifestation would the nurse expect to find in the patient?
    a. Icteric sclera
    b. Hepatomegaly
    c. Paresthesia of the hands and feet
    d. Intermittent heartburn with acid reflux

12. The nurse determines that teaching about pernicious anemia has been effective when the patient says
    a. "This condition can kill me unless I take injections of the vitamin for the rest of my life."
    b. "My symptoms can be completely reversed if I take cobalamin (vitamin B$_{12}$) supplements."
    c. "If my anemia does not respond to cobalamin therapy, my only other alternative is a bone marrow transplant."
    d. "The least expensive and most convenient treatment of pernicious anemia is to use a diet with foods high in cobalamin."

13. The strict vegetarian is at highest risk for the development of which anemia?
    a. Thalassemia
    b. Iron-deficiency anemia
    c. Folic acid deficiency anemia
    d. Cobalamin deficiency anemia

14. A patient with aplastic anemia has a nursing diagnosis of impaired oral mucous membrane. The etiology of this diagnosis can be related to the effects of what deficiencies (*select all that apply*)?
    a. RBCs
    b. Ferritin
    c. Platelets
    d. Coagulation factor VIII
    e. White blood cells (WBCs)

15. Nursing interventions for the patient with aplastic anemia are directed toward the prevention of which complications?
    a. Fatigue and dyspnea
    b. Hemorrhage and infection
    c. Thromboemboli and gangrene
    d. Cardiac dysrhythmias and heart failure

16. Which statements describe anemia related to blood loss (*select all that apply*)?
    a. A major concern is prevention of shock.
    b. This anemia is most frequently treated with increased dietary iron intake.
    c. In addition to the general symptoms of anemia, this patient also manifests jaundice.
    d. Clinical symptoms are the most reliable way to evaluate the effect and degree of blood loss.
    e. A patient who has acute blood loss may have postural hypotension and increased heart rate.

17. What causes the anemia of sickle cell disease?
    a. Intracellular hemolysis of sickled RBCs
    b. Accelerated breakdown of abnormal RBCs
    c. Autoimmune antibody destruction of RBCs
    d. Isoimmune antibody-antigen reactions with RBCs

18. A patient with sickle cell anemia asks the nurse why the sickling crisis does not stop when oxygen therapy is started. Which explanation should the nurse give to the patient?
    a. Sickling occurs in response to decreased blood viscosity, which is not affected by oxygen therapy.
    b. When RBCs sickle, they occlude small vessels, which causes more local hypoxia and more sickling.
    c. The primary problem during a sickle cell crisis is destruction of the abnormal cells, resulting in fewer RBCs to carry oxygen.
    d. Oxygen therapy does not alter the shape of the abnormal erythrocytes but only allows for increased oxygen concentration in hemoglobin.

19. What is a nursing intervention that is indicated for the patient during a sickle cell crisis?
    a. Frequent ambulation
    b. Application of antiembolism hose
    c. Restriction of sodium and oral fluids
    d. Administration of large doses of continuous opioid analgesics

20. During discharge teaching of a patient with newly diagnosed sickle cell disease, what should the nurse teach the patient to do?
    a. Limit fluid intake
    b. Avoid humid weather
    c. Eliminate exercise from the lifestyle
    d. Seek early medical intervention for upper respiratory infections

21. Which statements accurately describe thrombocytopenia (*select all that apply*)?
    a. Patients with platelet deficiencies can have internal or external hemorrhage.
    b. The most common acquired thrombocytopenia is thrombotic thrombocytopenic purpura (TTP).
    c. Immune thrombocytopenic purpura (ITP) is characterized by increased platelet destruction by the spleen.
    d. TTP is characterized by decreased platelets, decreased RBCs, and enhanced aggregation of platelets.
    e. A classic clinical manifestation of thrombocytopenia that the nurse would expect to find on physical examination of the patient is ecchymosis.

22. A 45-year-old patient has symptoms including arthralgia, impotence, weight loss, and liver enlargement. His laboratory results include an elevated serum iron, total iron binding capacity (TIBC), and serum ferritin levels. Which disorder does this describe and which treatment will be used?
    a. Thalassemia; combination chemotherapy
    b. Hemochromatosis; deferoxamine (Desferal)
    c. Myelodysplastic syndrome; filgrastim (Neupogen)
    d. Delayed transfusion reaction; deferasirox (Exjade)

23. In providing care for a patient hospitalized with an acute exacerbation of polycythemia vera, the nurse gives priority to which activity?
    a. Maintaining protective isolation
    b. Promoting leg exercises and ambulation
    c. Protecting the patient from injury or falls
    d. Promoting hydration with a large oral fluid intake

24. A patient has a platelet count of 50,000/μL and is diagnosed with ITP. What does the nurse anticipate that initial treatment will include?
    a. Splenectomy
    b. Corticosteroids
    c. Administration of platelets
    d. Immunosuppressive therapy

25. *Priority Decision:* A patient is admitted to the hospital for evaluation and treatment of thrombocytopenia. Which action is most important for the nurse to implement?
    a. Taking the temperature every 4 hours to assess for fever
    b. Maintaining the patient on strict bed rest to prevent injury
    c. Monitoring the patient for headaches, vertigo, or confusion
    d. Removing the oral crusting and scabs with a soft brush four times a day

26. The nurse caring for a patient with heparin-induced thrombocytopenia (HIT) identifies risk for bleeding as the priority nursing diagnosis. Identify at least five nursing interventions that should be implemented.
    a.
    b.
    c.
    d.
    e.

27. In reviewing the laboratory results of a patient with hemophilia A, what would the nurse expect to find?
    a. An absence of factor IX
    b. A decreased platelet count
    c. A prolonged bleeding time
    d. A prolonged partial thromboplastin time (PTT)

28. A patient with hemophilia comes to the clinic for treatment. What should the nurse anticipate that he or she will need to administer?
    a. Whole blood
    b. Thromboplastin
    c. Factor concentrates
    d. Fresh frozen plasma

29. A patient with hemophilia is hospitalized with acute knee pain and swelling. What is an appropriate nursing intervention for the patient?
    a. Wrapping the knee with an elastic bandage
    b. Placing the patient on bed rest and applying ice to the joint
    c. Administering nonsteroidal antiinflammatory drugs (NSAIDs) as needed for pain
    d. Gently performing range-of-motion (ROM) exercises to the knee to prevent adhesions

30. Which bleeding disorder affects both genders, is autosomal dominant, and will have laboratory results showing prolonged bleeding time?
    a. Hemophilia A
    b. Hemophilia B
    c. Thrombocytopenia
    d. von Willebrand disease

31. Number in sequence the events that occur in disseminated intravascular coagulation (DIC).
    _____ a. Activation of fibrinolytic system
    _____ b. Uncompensated hemorrhage
    _____ c. Widespread fibrin and platelet deposition in capillaries and arterioles
    _____ d. Release of fibrin-split products
    _____ e. Fibrinogen converted to fibrin
    _____ f. Inhibition of normal blood clotting
    _____ g. Production of intravascular thrombin
    _____ h. Depletion of platelets and coagulation factors

32. A patient has a WBC count of 2300/µL and a neutrophil percentage of 40%.
    a. Does the patient have leukopenia?
    b. What is the patient's neutrophil count?
    c. Does the patient have neutropenia?
    d. Is the patient at risk for developing a bacterial infection? If so, why?

33. What is the most important method for identifying the presence of infection in a neutropenic patient?
    a. Frequent temperature monitoring
    b. Routine blood and sputum cultures
    c. Assessing for redness and swelling
    d. Monitoring white blood cell (WBC) count

34. What is a major method of preventing infection in the patient with neutropenia?
    a. Prophylactic antibiotics
    b. A diet that eliminates fresh fruits and vegetables
    c. High-efficiency particulate air (HEPA) filtration rooms
    d. Strict hand washing by all persons in contact with the patient

35. How does myelodysplastic syndrome (MDS) differ from acute leukemias?
    a. MDS has a slower disease progression.
    b. MDS does not result in bone marrow failure.
    c. MDS is a clonal disorder of hematopoietic cells.
    d. MDS affects only the production and function of platelets and WBCs.

36. Which leukemia is seen in 80% of adults with acute leukemia and exhibits proliferation of precursors of granulocytes?
    a. Acute lymphocytic leukemia (ALL)   c. Acute myelogenous leukemia (AML)
    b. Chronic lymphocytic leukemia (CLL)   d. Chronic myelogenous leukemia (CML)

37. Which statements accurately describe chronic lymphocytic leukemia (*select all that apply*)?
    a. Most common leukemia of adults   d. Increased incidence in survivors of atomic bombs
    b. Only cure is bone marrow transplant   e. Philadelphia chromosome is a diagnostic hallmark
    c. Neoplasm of activated B lymphocytes   f. Mature-appearing but functionally inactive lymphocytes

38. What is the underlying cause of lymphadenopathy, splenomegaly, and hepatomegaly in leukemia?
    a. The development of infection at these sites
    b. Increased compensatory production of blood cells by these organs
    c. Infiltration of the organs by increased numbers of WBCs in the blood
    d. Normal hypertrophy of the organs in an attempt to destroy abnormal cells

39. A patient with acute myelogenous leukemia is considering a hematopoietic stem cell transplant and asks the nurse what is involved. What is the best response the nurse can give the patient?
    a. "Your bone marrow is destroyed by radiation and new bone marrow cells from a matched donor are injected into your bones."
    b. "A specimen of your bone marrow may be aspirated and treated to destroy any leukemic cells and then reinfused when your disease becomes worse."
    c. "Leukemic cells and bone marrow stem cells are eliminated with chemotherapy and/or total-body radiation and new bone marrow cells from a donor are infused."
    d. "During chemotherapy and/or total-body irradiation to destroy all of your blood cells, you may be given transfusions of red blood cells and platelets to prevent complications."

40. Indicate whether the following characteristics are associated with Hodgkin's lymphoma (HL), non-Hodgkin's lymphoma (NHL), or both (B).
    _____ a. Affects all ages
    _____ b. Presence of Reed-Sternberg cells
    _____ c. Associated with Epstein-Barr virus
    _____ d. Multiple histopathologic classifications
    _____ e. Treated with radiation and chemotherapy
    _____ f. Originates in lymph nodes in most patients
    _____ g. Greater than 85% cure rate in stage I disease
    _____ h. Often widely disseminated at time of diagnosis
    _____ i. Ingested alcohol-induced pain at the site of disease
    _____ j. Primary initial clinical manifestation is painless lymph node enlargement

41. What characteristics should the nurse be aware of in planning care for the patient with Hodgkin's lymphoma?
    a. Staging of Hodgkin's lymphoma is not important to predict prognosis.
    b. Nursing management of the patient undergoing treatment for Hodgkin's lymphoma includes measures to prevent infection.
    c. Hodgkin's lymphoma is characterized by proliferation of malignant activated B cells that destroy the kidneys.
    d. An important nursing intervention in the care of patients with Hodgkin's lymphoma is increasing fluids to manage hypercalcemia.

42. Following a splenectomy for the treatment of ITP, the nurse would expect the patient's laboratory test results to reveal which of the following?
    a. Decreased RBCs
    b. Decreased WBCs
    c. Increased platelets
    d. Increased immunoglobulins

43. *Priority Decision:* While receiving a unit of packed RBCs, the patient develops chills and a temperature of 102.2°F (39°C). What is the priority action for the nurse to take?
    a. Stop the transfusion and instill normal saline.
    b. Notify the health care provider and the blood bank.
    c. Add a leukocyte reduction filter to the blood administration set.
    d. Recognize this as a mild allergic transfusion reaction and slow the transfusion.

44. A patient with thrombocytopenia with active bleeding is to receive two units of platelets. To administer the platelets, what should the nurse do?
    a. Check for ABO compatibility.
    b. Agitate the bag periodically during the transfusion.
    c. Take vital signs every 15 minutes during the procedure.
    d. Refrigerate the second unit until the first unit has transfused.

45. Which type of transfusion reaction occurs with leukocyte or plasma protein incompatibility and may be avoided with leukocyte reduction filters?
    a. Febrile reaction
    b. Allergic reaction
    c. Acute hemolytic reaction
    d. Massive blood transfusion reaction

46. Which characteristics are related to an acute hemolytic transfusion reaction (*select all that apply*)?
    a. ABO incompatibility
    b. Hypothermia common
    c. Destruction of donor RBCs
    d. Acute kidney injury occurs
    e. Hypocalcemia and hyperkalemia
    f. Epinephrine used for severe reaction

47. *Delegation Decision:* While administering an infusion of packed RBCs, which actions can the RN delegate to unlicensed assistive personnel (UAP) (*select all that apply*)?
    a. Verify that the IV is patent.
    b. Obtain the blood products from the blood bank.
    c. Obtain vital signs before and after the first 15 minutes.
    d. Monitor the blood transfusion rate and adjust as needed.
    e. Assist the RN with checking patient identification and blood product identification data.

48. *Priority Decision:* The nurse is preparing to administer a blood transfusion. Number the actions in order of priority (1 is first priority action; 10 is last priority action).
    _____ a. Verify the order for the transfusion.
    _____ b. Ensure that the patient has a patent 18-gauge IV.
    _____ c. Prime the transfusion tubing and filter with normal saline.
    _____ d. Verify that the physician has discussed risks, benefits, and alternatives with the patient.
    _____ e. Obtain the blood product from the blood bank.
    _____ f. Ask another licensed person (nurse or MD) to assist in verifying the product identification and the patient identification.
    _____ g. Document outcomes in the patient record. Document vital signs, names of personnel, and starting and ending times.
    _____ h. Adjust the infusion rate and continue to monitor the patient every 30 minutes for up to an hour after the product is infused.
    _____ i. Infuse the first 50 mL over 15 minutes, staying with the patient.
    _____ j. Obtain the patient's vital signs before starting the transfusion.

CASE STUDY

Disseminated Intravascular Coagulation

Patient Profile

N.T., a 35-year-old mother of two, is admitted in active labor to the labor and delivery department for delivery of her third child. She delivers a 9-lb boy following an unusually difficult and prolonged labor.

Objective Data

- During her recovery period, N.T. continues to have heavy uterine bleeding and a boggy fundus
- Her skin is pale and diaphoretic
- BP: 70/40
- HR: 150 bpm
- Although the placenta appeared intact on examination, she is suspected of having retained placental fragments, causing DIC

Discussion Questions

Using a separate sheet of paper, answer the following questions:

1. What is the pathologic mechanism that triggers DIC in N.T.?
2. What additional clinical findings would indicate the presence of DIC?
3. Describe the common laboratory findings that are indicative of DIC.
4. What therapeutic modalities are most appropriate for N.T. and why?
5. *Priority Decision:* Based on the assessment data presented, what are the priority nursing diagnoses? Are there any collaborative problems?

1. Using the list of terms below, identify the structures in the following illustration.

   Terms

   Chordae tendineae
   Mitral valve
   Pulmonic (semilunar) valve
   Papillary muscle

   Tricuspid valve
   Interventricular septum
   Aortic (semilunar) valve

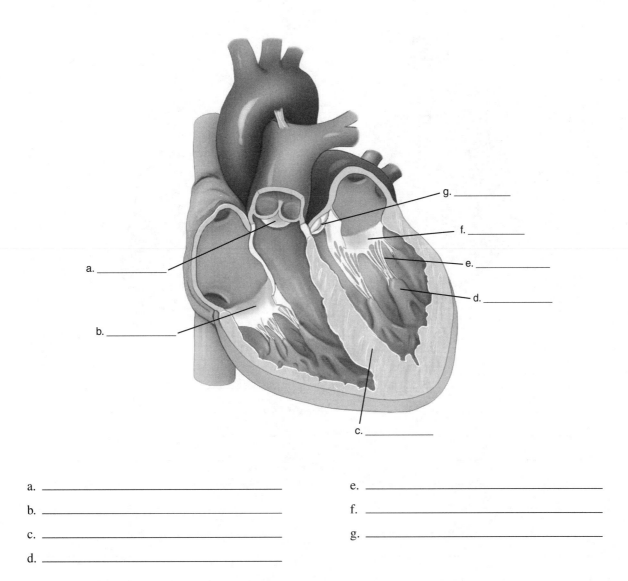

g. _____

f. _____

e. _____

d. _____

a. _____

b. _____

c. _____

a. _____

b. _____

c. _____

d. _____

e. _____

f. _____

g. _____

2. Identify the structures in the following illustrations by placing the correct term from the list below in the corresponding answer blank at the bottom of the page (some terms will be used more than once).

Terms

Left anterior descending artery
Aorta
Circumflex artery
Coronary sinus
Great cardiac vein
Left atrium
Left coronary artery
Left marginal artery
Left ventricle
Middle cardiac vein

Posterior descending artery
Posterior vein
Pulmonary trunk
Right atrium
Right coronary artery
Right marginal artery
Right ventricle
Small cardiac vein
Superior vena cava

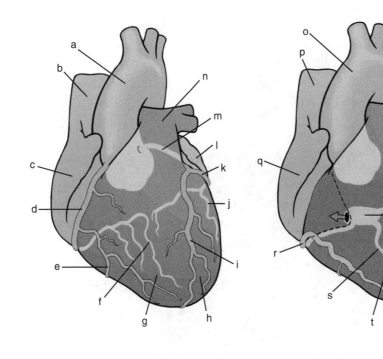

a. _____   n. _____

b. _____   o. _____

c. _____   p. _____

d. _____   q. _____

e. _____   r. _____

f. _____   s. _____

g. _____   t. _____

h. _____   u. _____

i. _____   v. _____

j. _____   w. _____

k. _____   x. _____

l. _____   y. _____

m. _____   z. _____

3. Which arteries are the major providers of coronary circulation (*select all that apply*)?
   a. Left marginal artery
   b. Right marginal artery
   c. Left circumflex artery
   d. Right coronary artery
   e. Posterior descending artery
   f. Left anterior descending artery

4. Number in sequence the path of the action potential along the conduction system of the heart.
   _____ a. Atrioventricular (AV) node
   _____ b. Purkinje fibers
   _____ c. Internodal pathways
   _____ d. Bundle of His
   _____ e. Ventricular cells
   _____ f. Sinoatrial (SA) node
   _____ g. Right and left atrial cells
   _____ h. Right and left bundle branches

5. On the following illustration, locate and letter the following normal electrocardiographic (ECG) pattern deflections and indicate where to locate and measure the intervals. (Use Table 36-2 to assist with this exercise.)
   P
   PR interval
   Q
   QRS interval
   QT interval
   R
   S
   T
   U

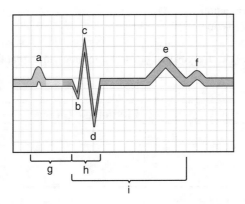

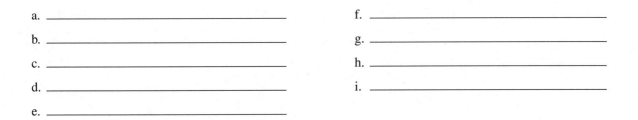

a. _____   f. _____

b. _____   g. _____

c. _____   h. _____

d. _____   i. _____

e. _____

6. Match the cardiac activity and time frames characteristic of the waveforms of the electrocardiogram (answers may be used more than once).

    _____ a. Measured from beginning of P wave to beginning of QRS complex

    _____ b. Repolarization of the ventricles

    _____ c. 0.12 to 0.20 sec

    _____ d. 0.16 sec

    _____ e. Time of depolarization and repolarization of ventricles

    _____ f. <0.12 sec

    _____ g. Depolarization from the AV node throughout ventricles

    _____ h. 0.06 to 0.12 sec

1. P wave
2. PR interval
3. QRS interval
4. T wave
5. QT interval

7. Indicate what factor of stroke volume (i.e., preload, afterload, or contractility) is primarily affected (i.e., increased or decreased) by the following situations and whether cardiac output (CO) is increased or decreased by the factor.

Situation	Stroke Volume Factor	Cardiac Output
Valsalva maneuver		
Venous dilation		
Hypertension		
Administration of epinephrine		
Obstruction of pulmonary artery		
Hemorrhage		

8. Which effects result from sympathetic nervous system stimulation of β-adrenergic receptors (*select all that apply*)?

a. Vasoconstriction

b. Increased heart rate

c. Decreased heart rate

d. Increased rate of impulse conduction

e. Decreased rate of impulse conduction

f. Increased force of cardiac contraction

9. What are the age-related physiologic changes that occur in the older adult that result in the following cardiovascular problems?

Cardiovascular Problem	Physiologic Change
Widened pulse pressure	
Decreased cardiac reserve	
Increased cardiac dysrhythmias	
Decreased response to sympathetic stimulation	
Aortic or mitral valve murmurs	

10. What is a significant finding in the health history of a patient during an assessment of the cardiovascular system?
    a. Metastatic cancer
    b. Frequent viral pharyngitis
    c. Calcium supplementation
    d. Frequent use of recreational drugs

11. Identify one specific finding identified by the nurse during assessment of each of the patient's functional health patterns that indicates a risk factor for cardiovascular disease or a patient response to an actual cardiovascular problem.

Functional Health Pattern	Risk Factor for or Response to Cardiovascular Problem
Health perception–health management	
Nutritional-metabolic	
Elimination	
Activity-exercise	
Sleep-rest	
Cognitive-perceptual	
Self-perception–self-concept	
Role-relationship	
Sexuality-reproductive	
Coping–stress tolerance	
Value-belief	

12. When palpating the patient's popliteal pulse, the nurse feels a vibration at the site. How should the nurse record this finding?
    a. Thready, weak pulse
    b. Bruit at the artery site
    c. Bounding pulse volume
    d. Thrill of the popliteal artery

13. Locate the following points or locations that are inspected and palpated on the chest wall.

Angle of Louis   Mitral area (apex) and point of maximal impulse (PMI)
Aortic area   Pulmonic area
Erb's point   Tricuspid area

a. _____   d. _____

b. _____   e. _____

c. _____   f. _____

14. Indicate whether the following are characteristic of the first heart sound (S_1) or the second heart sound (S_2).
    _____ a. Soft lub sound
    _____ b. Sharp dup sound
    _____ c. Indicates beginning of systole
    _____ d. Indicates the onset of diastole
    _____ e. Loudest at pulmonic and aortic areas
    _____ f. Loudest at tricuspid and mitral areas

15. What can be auscultated in a patient with cardiac valve problems (*select all that apply*)?
    a. Arterial bruit
    b. Pulsus alternans
    c. Cardiac murmurs
    d. Third heart sound (S_3)
    e. Pericardial friction rub
    f. Fourth heart sound (S_4)

16. The nursing student is seeking assistance in hearing the patient's abnormal heart sounds. What should the nurse tell the student to do for a more effective assessment?
    a. Use the diaphragm of the stethoscope with the patient prone
    b. Use the diaphragm of the stethoscope with the patient supine
    c. Use the bell of the stethoscope with the patient leaning forward
    d. Use the bell of the stethoscope with the patient on the right side

17. Which finding is associated with a blue tinge around the lips and conjunctiva?
    a. Finger clubbing
    b. Central cyanosis
    c. Peripheral cyanosis
    d. Delayed capillary filling time

18. A patient is scheduled for exercise nuclear imaging stress testing. The nurse explains to the patient that this test involves
    a. IV administration of a radioisotope at the maximum heart rate during exercise to identify the heart's response to physical stress.
    b. placement of electrodes inside the right-sided heart chambers through a vein to record the electrical activity of the heart directly.
    c. exercising on a treadmill or stationary bicycle with continuous ECG monitoring to detect ischemic changes during exercise.
    d. placement of a small transducer in four positions on the chest to record the direction and flow of blood through the heart by the reflection of sound waves.

19. *Priority Decision:* The nurse caring for a patient immediately following a transesophageal echocardiogram (TEE) should consider which action the highest priority?
    a. Monitor the ECG
    b. Monitor pulse oximetry
    c. Assess vital signs (BP, HR, RR, temperature)
    d. Maintain NPO status until gag reflex has returned

20. Which method is used to evaluate the ECG responses to normal activity over a period of 1 or 2 days?
    a. Serial ECGs
    b. Holter monitoring
    c. 6-minute walk test
    d. Event monitor or loop recorder

21. When caring for a patient after a cardiac catheterization with coronary angiography, which finding would be of most concern to the nurse?
    a. Swelling at the catheter insertion site
    b. Development of raised wheals on the patient's trunk
    c. Absence of pulses distal to the catheter insertion site
    d. Patient pain at the insertion site as 4 on a scale of 0 to 10

22. A female patient has a total cholesterol level of 232 mg/dL (6.0 mmol/L) and a high-density lipoprotein (HDL) of 65 mg/dL (1.68 mmol/L). A male patient has a total cholesterol level of 200 mg/dL and an HDL of 32 mg/dL. Based on these findings, which patient has the highest cardiac risk?
    a. The man, because his HDL is lower
    b. The woman, because her HDL is higher
    c. The woman, because her cholesterol is higher
    d. The man, because his cholesterol-to-HDL ratio is higher

23. Increases in which factors are predictors of an increased risk for coronary artery disease or evidence of myocardial injury (*select all that apply*)?
    a. Creatine kinase (CK)-MM
    b. Cardiac troponin T (cTnT)
    c. B-type natriuretic peptide (BNP)
    d. High-sensitivity C-reactive protein
    e. Lipoprotein-associated phospholipase A_2

1. In the regulation of normal blood pressure (BP), indicate whether the following mechanisms elevate BP by increasing cardiac output (CO), increasing systemic vascular resistance (SVR), or increasing both, and identify how these mechanisms cause the increases indicated.

	Increasing Cardiac Output	Increasing Systemic Vascular Resistance	Mechanisms Causing Increases
β_1-Adrenergic stimulation			
α_1-Adrenergic stimulation			
α_2-Adrenergic stimulation			
Endothelin release			
Angiotensin II			
Aldosterone release			
Antidiuretic hormone (ADH) release			

2. A patient is given an α_1-adrenergic agonist and experiences a reflex bradycardia. What normal mechanism of BP control is stimulated in this situation?

3. A patient uses a mixed β-adrenergic blocking drug for treatment of migraine headaches. What effect might this drug have on BP and why?

4. What are nonmodifiable risk factors for primary hypertension (*select all that apply*)?
   a. Age
   b. Obesity
   c. Gender
   d. Ethnicity
   e. Genetic link

5. How is secondary hypertension differentiated from primary hypertension?
   a. Has a more gradual onset than primary hypertension
   b. Does not cause the target organ damage that occurs with primary hypertension
   c. Has a specific cause, such as renal disease, that often can be treated by medicine or surgery
   d. Is caused by age-related changes in BP regulatory mechanisms in people over 65 years of age

6. What is the patient with primary hypertension likely to report?
   a. No symptoms
   b. Cardiac palpitations
   c. Dyspnea on exertion
   d. Dizziness and vertigo

7. What is most organ damage in hypertension related to?
   a. Increased fluid pressure exerted against organ tissue
   b. Atherosclerotic changes in vessels that supply the organs
   c. Erosion and thinning of blood vessels from constant pressure
   d. Increased hydrostatic pressure causing leakage of plasma into organ interstitial spaces

8. The patient who is being admitted has had a history of uncontrolled hypertension. High SVR is most likely to cause damage to which organ?
   a. Brain
   b. Heart
   c. Retina
   d. Kidney

9. Identify the significance of the following laboratory test results when found in patients with hypertension.

Laboratory Test Result	Significance
Blood urea nitrogen (BUN): 48 mg/dL (17.1 mmol/L) Creatinine: 4.3 mg/dL (380 mmol/L)	
Serum K$^+$: 3.1 mEq/L (3.1 mmol/L)	
Serum uric acid: 9.2 mg/dL (547 mmol/L)	
Fasting blood glucose: 183 mg/dL (10.2 mmol/L)	
Low-density lipoproteins (LDL): 154 mg/dL (4.0 mmol/L)	

10. A 42-year-old man has been diagnosed with primary hypertension with an average BP of 162/92 mm Hg on three consecutive clinic visits. What are four priority lifestyle modifications that should be explored in the initial treatment of the patient?

    a.

    b.

    c.

    d.

11. What is the primary BP effect of β-adrenergic blockers such as atenolol (Tenormin)?
    a. Vasodilation of arterioles by blocking movement of calcium into cells
    b. Decrease Na$^+$ and water reabsorption by blocking the effect of aldosterone
    c. Decrease CO by decreasing rate and strength of the heart and renin secretion by the kidneys
    d. Vasodilation caused by inhibiting sympathetic outflow from the central nervous system (CNS)

12. Which classification of drugs used to treat hypertension prevents the action of angiotensin II and promotes increased salt and water excretion?
    a. Thiazide diuretics
    b. Direct vasodilators
    c. Angiotensin II receptor blockers (ARBs)
    d. Angiotensin-converting enzyme (ACE) inhibitors

13. Dietary teaching that includes dietary sources of potassium is indicated for the hypertensive patient taking which drug?
    a. Enalapril (Vasotec)
    b. Labetalol (Normodyne)
    c. Spironolactone (Aldactone)
    d. Hydrochlorothiazide (HydroDiuril)
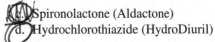

14. *Priority Decision:* A patient with stage 2 hypertension who is taking hydrochlorothiazide (HydroDiuril) and lisinopril (Prinivil) has prazosin (Minipress) added to the medication regimen. What is most important for the nurse to teach the patient to do?
    a. Weigh every morning to monitor for fluid retention
    b. Change position slowly and avoid prolonged standing
    c. Use sugarless gum or candy to help relieve dry mouth
    d. Take the pulse daily to note any slowing of the heart rate

15. A 38-year-old man is treated for hypertension with triamterene and hydrochlorothiazide (Maxzide) and metoprolol (Lopressor). Four months after his last clinic visit, his BP returns to pretreatment levels and he admits he has not been taking his medication regularly. What is the nurse's best response to this patient?
    a. "Try always to take your medication when you carry out another daily routine so you do not forget to take it."
    b. "You probably would not need to take medications for hypertension if you would exercise more and stop smoking."
    c. "The drugs you are taking cause sexual dysfunction in many patients. Are you experiencing any problems in this area?"
    d. "You need to remember that hypertension can be only controlled with medication, not cured, and you must always take your medication."

16. A 78-year-old patient is admitted with a BP of 180/98 mm Hg. Which age-related physical changes may contribute to this patient's hypertension (*select all that apply*)?
    a. Decreased renal function
    b. Increased baroreceptor reflexes
    c. Increased peripheral vascular resistance
    d. Increased adrenergic receptor sensitivity
    e. Increased collagen and stiffness of the myocardium
    f. Loss of elasticity in large arteries from arteriosclerosis

17. What should the nurse emphasize when teaching a patient who is newly prescribed clonidine (Catapres)?
    a. The drug should never be stopped abruptly.
    b. The drug should be taken early in the day to prevent nocturia.
    c. The first dose should be taken when the patient is in bed for the night.
    d. Because aspirin will decrease the drug's effectiveness, Tylenol should be used instead.

18. What is included in the correct technique for BP measurements?
    a. Always take the BP in both arms.
    b. Position the patient supine for all readings.
    c. Place the cuff loosely around the upper arm.
    d. Take readings at least two times at least 1 minute apart.

19. ***Delegation Decision:*** The unit is very busy and short staffed. What could be delegated to the unlicensed assistive personnel (UAP)?
    a. Administer antihypertensive medications to stable patients.
    b. Obtain orthostatic blood pressure (BP) readings for older patients.
    c. Check BP readings for the patient receiving IV enalapril (Vasotec).
    d. Teach about home BP monitoring and use of automatic BP monitoring equipment.

20. Which manifestation is an indication that a patient is having a hypertensive emergency?
    a. Symptoms of a stroke with an elevated BP
    b. A systolic BP >200 mm Hg and a diastolic BP >120 mm Hg
    c. A sudden rise in BP accompanied by neurologic impairment
    d. A severe elevation of BP that occurs over several days or weeks

21. Which drugs are most commonly used to treat hypertensive crises?
    a. Esmolol (Brevibloc) and captopril (Capoten)
    b. Enalaprilat (Vasotec) and minoxidil (Loniten)
    c. Labetalol (Normodyne) and bumetanide (Bumex)
    d. Fenoldopam (Corlopam) and sodium nitroprusside (Nipride)

22. During treatment of a patient with a BP of 222/148 mm Hg and confusion, nausea, and vomiting, the nurse initially titrates the medications to achieve which goal?
    a. Decrease the mean arterial pressure (MAP) to 129 mm Hg
    b. Lower the BP to the patient's normal within the second to third hour
    d. Reduce the systolic BP (SBP) to 158 mm Hg and the diastolic BP (DBP) to 111 mm Hg within the first 2 hours
    c. Decrease the SBP to 160 mm Hg and the DBP to between 100 and 110 mm Hg as quickly as possible

23. What does the nursing responsibility in the management of the patient with hypertensive urgency often include?
    a. Monitoring hourly urine output for drug effectiveness
    b. Titrating IV drug dosages based on BP measurements every 2 to 3 minutes
    c. Providing continuous electrocardiographic (ECG) monitoring to detect side effects of the drugs
    d. Instructing the patient to follow up with a health care professional within 24 hours after outpatient treatment

---

CASE STUDY

Isolated Systolic Hypertension

Patient Profile

K.J. is a 73-year-old African American woman with no history of hypertension. She came to the doctor's office for a flu shot.

Subjective Data

- Says she has gained 20 lb over the past year since her husband died
- Has never smoked and uses no alcohol
- Only medication is one multivitamin per day
- Eats a lot of canned food
- Does not exercise

Objective Data

- Height: 5 ft, 4 in (162.6 cm)
- Weight: 170 lb (77.1 kg)
- BP: 170/82
- Physical examination shows no abnormalities
- Serum potassium: 3.3 mEq/L (3.3 mmol/L)

The health care provider diagnosed isolated systolic hypertension (ISH) and prescribed lifestyle modifications.

Discussion Questions

Using a separate sheet of paper, answer the following questions:

1. What contributing factors to the development of ISH are present in K.J.?
2. What additional risk factors are present?
3. What specific dietary changes would the nurse recommend for K.J.?
4. If drug therapy became necessary to treat K.J.'s hypertension, what diuretic would be indicated based on her laboratory results?
5. *Priority Decision:* What other priority teaching measures should be instituted by the nurse?
6. *Priority Decision:* Based on the assessment data presented, what are the priority nursing diagnoses? Are there any collaborative problems?

CHAPTER 34

Nursing Management: Coronary Artery Disease and Acute Coronary Syndrome

1. Which patient is most likely to be in the fibrous stage of development of coronary artery disease (CAD)?
   a. Age 40, thrombus adhered to the coronary artery wall
   b. Age 50, rapid onset of disease with hypercholesterolemia
   c. Age 32, thickened coronary arterial walls with narrowed vessel lumen
   d. Age 19, elevated low-density lipoprotein (LDL) cholesterol, lipid-filled smooth muscle cells

2. What accurately describes the pathophysiology of CAD?
   a. Partial or total occlusion of the coronary artery occurs during the stage of raised fibrous plaque
   b. Endothelial alteration may be caused by chemical irritants such as hyperlipidemia or by tobacco use
   c. Collateral circulation in the coronary circulation is more likely to be present in the young patient with CAD
   d. The leading theory of atherogenesis proposes that infection and fatty dietary intake are the basic underlying causes of atherosclerosis

3. While obtaining patient histories, which patient does the nurse identify as having the highest risk for CAD?
   a. A white man, age 54, who is a smoker and has a stressful lifestyle
   b. A white woman, age 68, with a BP of 172/100 mm Hg and who is physically inactive
   c. An Asian woman, age 45, with a cholesterol level of 240 mg/dL and a BP of 130/74 mm Hg
   d. An obese African American man, age 65, with a cholesterol level of 195 mg/dL and a BP of 128/76 mm Hg

4. *Priority Decision:* While teaching women about the risks and incidence of CAD, what does the nurse emphasize?
   a. Smoking is not as significant a risk factor for CAD in women as it is in men.
   b. Women seek treatment sooner than men when they have symptoms of CAD.
   c. Estrogen replacement therapy in postmenopausal women decreases the risk for CAD.
   d. CAD is the leading cause of death in women, with a higher mortality rate after MI than in men.

5. Which characteristics are associated with LDLs (*select all that apply*)?
   a. Increases with exercise
   b. Contains the most cholesterol
   c. Has an affinity for arterial walls
   d. Carries lipids away from arteries to liver
   e. High levels correlate most closely with CAD
   f. The higher the level, the lower the risk for CAD

6. Which serum lipid elevation, along with elevated LDL, is strongly associated with CAD?
   a. Apolipoproteins
   b. Fasting triglycerides
   c. Total serum cholesterol
   d. High-density lipoprotein (HDL)

7. The laboratory tests for four patients show the following results. Which patient should the nurse teach first about preventing CAD because the patient is at the greatest risk for CAD even without other risk factors?
   a. Total cholesterol: 152 mg/dL, triglycerides: 148 mg/dL, LDL: 148 mg/dL, HDL: 52 mg/dL
   b. Total cholesterol: 160 mg/dL, triglycerides: 102 mg/dL, LDL: 138 mg/dL, HDL: 56 mg/dL
   c. Total cholesterol: 200 mg/dL, triglycerides: 150 mg/dL, LDL: 160 mg/dL, HDL: 48 mg/dL
   d. Total cholesterol: 250 mg/dL, triglycerides: 164 mg/dL, LDL: 172 mg/dL, HDL: 32 mg/dL

8. The nurse is encouraging a sedentary patient with major risks for CAD to perform physical exercise on a regular basis. In addition to decreasing the risk factor of physical inactivity, the nurse tells the patient that exercise will also directly contribute to reducing which risk factors?
   a. Hyperlipidemia and obesity
   b. Diabetes mellitus and hypertension
   c. Elevated serum lipids and stressful lifestyle
   d. Hypertension and elevated serum homocysteine

9. During a routine health examination, a 48-year-old patient is found to have a total cholesterol level of 224 mg/dL (5.8 mmol/L) and an LDL level of 140 mg/dL (3.6 mmol/L). What does the nurse teach the patient based on the Therapeutic Lifestyle Changes diet (*select all that apply*)?
   a. Use fat-free milk
   b. Abstain from alcohol use
   c. Reduce red meat in the diet
   d. Eliminate intake of simple sugars
   e. Avoid egg yolks and foods prepared with whole eggs

10. To which patients should the nurse teach the Therapeutic Lifestyle Changes diet to reduce the risk of coronary artery disease (CAD)?
    a. All patients to reduce CAD risk
    b. Patients who have experienced an MI
    c. Individuals with two or more risk factors for CAD
    d. Individuals with a cholesterol level >200 mg/dL (5.2 mmol/L)

11. A 62-year-old woman has prehypertension (BP 142/90 mm Hg) and smokes a pack of cigarettes per day. She has no symptoms of CAD but a recent LDL level was 154 mg/dL (3.98 mmol/L). Based on these findings, the nurse would expect that which treatment plan would be used first for this patient?
    a. Diet and drug therapy
    b. Exercise instruction only
    c. Diet therapy and smoking cessation
    d. Drug therapy and smoking cessation

12. What are manifestations of acute coronary syndrome (ACS) (*select all that apply*)?
    a. Dysrhythmia
    b. Stable angina
    c. Unstable angina
    d. ST-segment-elevation myocardial infarction (STEMI)
    e. Non–ST-segment-elevation myocardial infarction (NSTEMI)

13. Myocardial ischemia occurs as a result of increased oxygen demand and decreased oxygen supply. What factors and disorders result in increased oxygen demand (*select all that apply*)?
    a. Hypovolemia or anemia
    b. Increased cardiac workload with aortic stenosis
    c. Narrowed coronary arteries from atherosclerosis
    d. Angina in the patient with atherosclerotic coronary arteries
    e. Left ventricular hypertrophy caused by chronic hypertension
    f. Sympathetic nervous system stimulation by drugs, emotions, or exertion

14. What causes the pain that occurs with myocardial ischemia?
    a. Death of myocardial tissue
    b. Dysrhythmias caused by cellular irritability
    c. Lactic acid accumulation during anaerobic metabolism
    d. Elevated pressure in the ventricles and pulmonary vessels

15. What types of angina can occur in the absence of CAD (*select all that apply*)?
    a. Silent ischemia
    b. Nocturnal angina
    c. Prinzmetal's angina
    d. Microvascular angina
    e. Chronic stable angina

16. Which characteristics describe unstable angina (*select all that apply*)?
    a. Usually precipitated by exertion
    b. Unpredictable and unrelieved by rest
    c. Characterized by progressive severity
    d. Occurs only when the person is recumbent
    e. Usually occurs in response to coronary artery spasm

17. Tachycardia that is a response of the sympathetic nervous system to the pain of ischemia is detrimental because it increases oxygen demand and
    a. increases cardiac output.
    b. causes reflex hypotension.
    c. may lead to atrial dysrhythmias.
    d. impairs perfusion of the coronary arteries.

18. Which effects contribute to making nitrates the first-line therapy for the treatment of angina (*select all that apply*)?
    a. Decrease heart rate (HR)
    b. Decrease preload
    c. Decrease afterload
    d. Dilate coronary arteries
    e. Prevent thrombosis of plaques
    f. Decrease myocardial contractility

19. The patient has used sublingual nitroglycerin and various long-acting nitrates but now has an ejection fraction of 38% and is considered at a high risk for a cardiac event. Which medication would first be added for vasodilation and to reduce ventricular remodeling?
    a. Clopidogrel (Plavix)
    b. Captopril (Capoten)
    c. Diltiazem (Cardizem)
    d. Metoprolol (Lopressor)

20. When instructing the patient with angina about taking sublingual nitroglycerin tablets, what should the nurse teach the patient?
    a. To lie or sit and place one tablet under the tongue when chest pain occurs
    b. To take the tablet with a large amount of water so it will dissolve right away
    c. That if one tablet does not relieve the pain in 15 minutes, the patient should go to the hospital
    d. That if the tablet causes dizziness and a headache, stop the medication and call the doctor or go to the hospital

21. When teaching an older adult with CAD how to manage the treatment program for angina, which guidelines does the nurse use to teach the patient?
    a. To sit for 2 to 5 minutes before standing when getting out of bed
    b. To exercise only twice a week to avoid unnecessary strain on the heart
    c. That lifestyle changes are not as necessary as they would be in a younger person
    d. That aspirin therapy is contraindicated in older adults because of the risk for bleeding

22. When a patient reports chest pain, why must unstable angina be identified and rapidly treated?
    a. The pain may be severe and disabling.
    b. ECG changes and dysrhythmias may occur during an attack.
    c. Atherosclerotic plaque deterioration may cause complete thrombus of the vessel lumen.
    d. Spasm of a major coronary artery may cause total occlusion of the vessel with progression to MI.

23. The nurse suspects stable angina rather than MI pain in the patient who reports that his chest pain
    a. is relieved by nitroglycerin.
    b. is a sensation of tightness or squeezing.
    c. does not radiate to the neck, back, or arms.
    d. is precipitated by physical or emotional exertion.

24. A patient admitted to the hospital for evaluation of chest pain has no abnormal serum cardiac markers 4 hours after the onset of pain. What noninvasive diagnostic test can be used to differentiate angina from other types of chest pain?
    a. 12-lead ECG
    b. Exercise stress test
    c. Coronary angiogram
    d. Transesophageal echocardiogram

25. A 52-year-old man is admitted to the emergency department with severe chest pain. On what basis would the nurse suspect an MI?
    a. He has pale, cool, clammy skin.
    b. He reports nausea and vomited once at home.
    c. He says he is anxious and has a feeling of impending doom.
    d. He reports he has had no relief of the pain with rest or position change.

26. At what point in the healing process of the myocardium following an infarct does early scar tissue result in an unstable heart wall?
    a. 2 to 3 days after MI
    b. 4 to 10 days after MI
    c. 10 to 14 days after MI
    d. 6 weeks after MI

27. To detect and treat the most common complication of MI, what should the nurse do?
    a. Measure hourly urine output.
    b. Auscultate the chest for crackles.
    c. Use continuous cardiac monitoring.
    d. Take vital signs every 2 hours for the first 8 hours.

28. During the assessment, the nurse identifies crackles in the lungs and an S_3 heart sound. Which complication of MI should the nurse suspect and further investigate?
    a. Pericarditis
    b. Heart failure
    c. Ventricular aneurysm
    d. Papillary muscle dysfunction

29. In the patient with chest pain, which results can differentiate unstable angina from an MI?
    a. ECG changes present at the onset of the pain
    b. A chest x-ray indicating left ventricular hypertrophy
    c. Appearance of troponin in the blood 48 hours after the infarct
    d. Creatine kinase (CK)-MB enzyme elevations that peak 18 hours after the infarct

30. A second 12-lead ECG performed on a patient 4 hours after the onset of chest pain reveals ST segment elevation. What does the nurse recognize that this finding indicates?
    a. Transient ischemia typical of unstable angina
    b. Lack of permanent damage to myocardial cells
    c. MI associated with prolonged and complete coronary thrombosis
    d. MI associated with transient or incomplete coronary artery occlusion

31. What describes transmyocardial laser revascularization (TMR)?
    a. Structure applied to hold vessels open
    b. Requires anticoagulation following the procedure
    c. Laser-created channels between left ventricular cavity and coronary circulation
    d. Surgical construction of new vessels to carry blood beyond obstructed coronary artery

32. Which treatment is used first for the patient with a confirmed MI to open the blocked artery within 90 minutes of arrival to the facility?
    a. Stent placement
    b. Coronary artery bypass graft (CABG)
    c. Percutaneous coronary intervention (PCI)
    d. Transmyocardial laser revascularization (TMR)

33. ***Delegation Decision:*** In planning care for a patient who has just returned to the unit following a PCI, the nurse may delegate which activity to unlicensed assistive personnel (UAP)?
    a. Monitor the IV fluids and measure urine output.
    b. Check vital signs and report changes in HR, BP, or pulse oximetry.
    c. Explain to the patient the need for frequent vital signs and pulse checks.
    d. Assess circulation to the extremity used by checking pulses, skin temperature, and color.

34. A patient is scheduled to have CABG surgery. What does the nurse explain to him that is involved with the procedure?
    a. A synthetic graft will be used as a tube for blood flow from the aorta to a coronary artery distal to an obstruction.
    b. A stenosed coronary artery will be resected and a synthetic arterial tube graft will be inserted to replace the diseased artery.
    c. The internal mammary artery will be detached from the chest wall and attached to a coronary artery distal to the stenosis.
    d. Reversed segments of a saphenous artery from the aorta will be anastomosed to the coronary artery distal to an obstruction.

35. Collaborative care of the patient with NSTEMI differs from that of a patient with STEMI in that NSTEMI is more frequently initially treated with what?
    a. PCI
    b. CABG
    c. Acute intensive drug therapy
    d. Reperfusion therapy with thrombolytics

36. During treatment with reteplase (Retavase) for a patient with a STEMI, which finding should most concern the nurse?
    a. Oozing of blood from the IV site
    b. BP of 102/60 mm Hg with an HR of 78 bpm
    c. Decrease in the responsiveness of the patient
    d. Presence of intermittent accelerated idioventricular dysrhythmias

37. The nurse recognizes that thrombolytic therapy for the treatment of an MI has not been successful when the patient displays which manifestation?
    a. Continues to have chest pain
    b. Has a marked increase in CK enzyme levels within 3 hours of therapy
    c. Develops major gastrointestinal (GI) or genitourinary (GU) bleeding during treatment
    d. Develops premature ventricular contractions and ventricular tachycardia during treatment

38. When the patient who is diagnosed with an MI is not relieved of chest pain with IV nitroglycerin, which medication will the nurse expect to be used?
    a. IV morphine sulfate
    b. Calcium channel blockers
    c. IV amiodarone (Cordarone)
    d. Angiotensin-converting enzyme (ACE) inhibitors

39. What is the rationale for using docusate sodium (Colace) for a patient after an MI?
    a. Controls ventricular dysrhythmias
    b. Relieves anxiety and cardiac workload
    c. Minimizes bradycardia from vagal stimulation
    d. Prevents the binding of fibrinogen to platelets

40. The patient has hypertension and just experienced an MI. Which type of medication would be expected to be added to decrease the workload on his heart?
    a. ACE inhibitor
    b. β-adrenergic blocker
    c. Calcium channel blocker
    d. Angiotensin II receptor blocker (ARB)

41. A patient with an MI is exhibiting anxiety while being taught about possible lifestyle changes. The nurse evaluates that the anxiety is relieved when the patient states
    a. "I'm going to take this recovery one step at a time."
    b. "I feel much better and am ready to get on with my life."
    c. "How soon do you think I will be able to go back to work?"
    d. "I know you are doing everything possible to save my life."

42. *Priority Decision:* A patient hospitalized for evaluation of unstable angina experiences severe chest pain and calls the nurse. Prioritize the interventions below from 1 (highest priority) to 6 (lowest priority). The appropriate medical orders and protocols are available to the nurse.
    _____ a.   Notify the physician
    _____ b.   Obtain a 12-lead ECG
    _____ c.   Check the patient's vital signs
    _____ d.   Administer oxygen per nasal cannula
    _____ e.   Perform a focused assessment of the chest
    _____ f.   Assess pain (PQRST) and medicate as ordered

43. Which statement indicates the patient is experiencing anger as the psychologic response to his acute MI?
    a. "Yes, I'm having a little chest pain. It's no big deal."
    b. "I don't think I can take care of myself at home yet."
    c. "What's going to happen if I have another heart attack?"
    d. "I hope my wife is happy now after harping at me about my eating habits all these years."

44. The nurse and patient set a patient outcome that at the time of discharge after an MI the patient will be able to tolerate moderate-energy activities that are similar to which activity?
    a. Golfing
    b. Walking at 5 mph
    c. Cycling at 13 mph
    d. Mowing the lawn by hand

45. A 58-year-old patient is in a cardiac rehabilitation program. The nurse teaches the patient to stop exercising if what occurs?
    a. Pain or dyspnea develop
    b. The HR exceeds 150 bpm
    c. The respiratory rate increases to 30
    d. The HR is 30 bpm over the resting HR

46. In counseling the patient about sexual activity following an MI, what should the nurse do?
    a. Wait for the patient to ask about resuming sexual activity
    b. Discuss sexual activity while teaching about other physical activity
    c. Have the patient ask the health care provider when sexual activity can be resumed
    d. Inform the patient that impotence is a common long-term complication following MI

47. What advice about sexual activity should the nurse give to a male patient who has had an MI?
    a. The patient should use the superior position.
    b. Foreplay may cause too great an increase in heart rate.
    c. Prophylactic nitroglycerin may be used if angina occurs.
    d. Performance can be enhanced with the use of sildenafil (Viagra).

48. *Priority Decision:* A patient is hospitalized after a successful resuscitation of an episode of sudden cardiac death (SCD). During the care of the patient, what nursing intervention is most important?
    a. Continuous ECG monitoring
    b. Auscultation of the carotid arteries
    c. Frequent assessment of heart sounds
    d. Monitoring of airway status and respiratory patterns

CASE STUDY

Coronary Artery Disease

Patient Profile

H.C., a 47-year-old Navajo woman, comes to the emergency department with a burning sensation in her epigastric area extending into her sternum.

Subjective Data

- Has had chest pain with activity that is relieved with rest for the past 3 months
- Has had type 2 diabetes mellitus since she was age 35
- Has a smoking history of one pack a day for 27 years
- Is more than 30% over her ideal body weight
- Has no regular exercise program
- Expresses frustration with physical problems
- Is reluctant to get medical therapy because it will interfere with her life
- Has no health insurance

Objective Data

Physical Examination
- Anxious, clutching fists
- Appears overweight and withdrawn

Diagnostic Studies
- 12-lead ECG
- Cholesterol: 248 mg/dL (6.41 mmol/L)
- LDL: 160 mg/dL (4.14 mmol/L)
- Glucose: 210 mg/dL (11.7 mmol/L)

Collaborative Care

- Metoprolol (Toprol) XL 100 mg PO daily
- Nifedipine (Procardia) 10 mg tid
- Nitroglycerin 0.4 mg sublingual PRN for chest pain
- Exercise treadmill testing

Discussion Questions

Using a separate sheet of paper, answer the following questions:

1. What are H.C.'s risk factors for CAD?
2. What symptoms should lead the nurse to suspect the pain may be angina?
3. What nursing actions should be taken for H.C.'s discomfort?
4. What kind of ECG changes would indicate myocardial ischemia?
5. What information should the nurse provide for H.C. before the treadmill testing?
6. *Priority Decision:* What are the priority nursing measures that should be instituted to help H.C. decrease her risk factors?
7. Should H.C.'s angina become chronic stable angina, explain the treatment that would be used using the mnemonic A, B, C, D, E, and F.
8. *Priority Decision:* Based on the assessment data presented, what are the priority nursing diagnoses? Are there any collaborative problems?

35 Nursing Management: Heart Failure

1. Which statements accurately describe heart failure (*select all that apply*)?
   a. A common cause of diastolic failure is left ventricular hypertrophy.
   b. A primary risk factor for heart failure is coronary artery disease (CAD).
   c. Systolic heart failure results in a normal left ventricular ejection fraction.
   d. Systolic failure is characterized by abnormal resistance to ventricular filling.
   e. Hypervolemia precipitates heart failure by decreasing cardiac output and increasing oxygen consumption.

2. Describe the primary ways in which each of the following compensatory mechanisms of heart failure increases cardiac output (CO) and identify at least one effect of the mechanism that is detrimental to cardiac function.

Compensatory Mechanism	↑ Cardiac Output	Detrimental Effect
Cardiac dilation		
Cardiac hypertrophy		
Sympathetic nervous system stimulation		
Neurohormonal response		
• Renin-angiotensin-aldosterone system		
• Antidiuretic hormone (ADH)		

3. What describes the action of the natriuretic peptides and nitric oxide in their counterregulatory processes in response to heart failure (HF)?
   a. Excretion of potassium
   b. Increased release of ADH
   c. Vasodilation and decreased blood pressure
   d. Decreased glomerular filtration rate and edema

4. The acronym FACES is used to help educate patients to identify symptoms of heart failure. What does this acronym mean?
   a. **F**requent **a**ctivity leads to **c**ough in the **e**lderly and **s**welling
   b. **F**actors of risk: **a**ctivity, **c**ough, **e**motional upsets, **s**alt intake
   c. **F**ollow **a**ctivity plan, **c**ontinue **e**xercise, and know **s**igns of problems
   d. **F**atigue, limitation of **a**ctivities, chest **c**ongestion/cough, **e**dema, **s**hortness of breath

5. What is the pathophysiologic mechanism that results in the pulmonary edema of left-sided heart failure?
   a. Increased right ventricular preload
   b. Increased pulmonary hydrostatic pressure
   c. Impaired alveolar oxygen and carbon dioxide exchange
   d. Increased lymphatic flow of pulmonary extravascular fluid

6. Which initial physical assessment finding would the nurse expect to be present in a patient with acute left-sided heart failure?
   a. Bubbling crackles and tachycardia
   b. Hepatosplenomegaly and tachypnea
   c. Peripheral edema and cool, diaphoretic skin
   d. Frothy blood-tinged sputum and distended jugular veins

7. The nurse assesses the patient with chronic biventricular heart failure for paroxysmal nocturnal dyspnea (PND) by questioning the patient regarding
   a. the presence of difficulty breathing at night.
   b. frequent awakening to void during the night.
   c. the presence of a dry, hacking cough when resting.
   d. the use of two or more pillows to help breathing during sleep.

8. ***Priority Decision:*** The nurse reviews the following vital signs recorded by an unlicensed assistive personnel (UAP) on a patient with acute decompensated heart failure: BP 98/60, HR 102 bpm, RR 24, Temp 98.2°F (36.7° C), SpO_2 84% on 2 L/min via nasal cannula.
   a. Which of these findings is of highest priority?
   b. What should the nurse do next?

9. A patient with chronic heart failure has atrial fibrillation and a left ventricular ejection fraction (LVEF) of 18%. To decrease the risk of complications from these conditions, what drug does the nurse anticipate giving?
   a. Diuretics
   b. Anticoagulants
   c. β-Adrenergic blockers
   d. Potassium supplements

10. Which diagnostic test is most useful in differentiating dyspnea related to pulmonary effects of heart failure from dyspnea related to pulmonary disease?
   a. Exercise stress testing
   b. Cardiac catheterization
   c. B-type natriuretic peptide (BNP) levels
   d. Determination of blood urea nitrogen (BUN)

11. Which medication is currently approved only for use with African American patients for hypertension and angina?
   a. Captopril (Capoten)
   b. Nitroglycerin (Nitro-Bid)
   c. Spironolactone (Aldactone)
   d. Isosorbide dinitrate and hydralazine (BiDil)

12. ***Priority Decision:*** A patient is admitted to the emergency department with acute decompensated heart failure (ADHF). Which IV medication would the nurse expect to administer first?
   a. Digoxin (Lanoxin)
   b. Morphine sulfate
   c. Nesiritide (Natrecor)
   d. Bumetanide (Bumex)

13. The patient with chronic heart failure is being discharged with a diuretic, a renin-angiotensin-aldosterone system (RAAS) inhibitor, and a β-adrenergic blocker. When received from the pharmacy, which medication should not be included for this patient?
   a. Losartan (Cozaar)
   b. Carvedilol (Coreg)
   c. Dopamine (Intropin)
   d. Hydrochlorothiazide (HCTZ)

14. When caring for the patient with heart failure, which medications or treatments require careful monitoring of the patient's serum potassium level to prevent further cardiac dysfunction (*select all that apply*)?
   a. Enalapril (Vasotec)
   b. Furosemide (Lasix)
   c. Inamrinone (Inocor)
   d. Spironolactone (Aldactone)
   e. Metoprolol CR/XL (Toprol XL)

15. ***Priority Decision:*** A patient with chronic heart failure is treated with hydrochlorothiazide, digoxin, and lisinopril (Prinivil). To prevent the risk of digitalis toxicity with these drugs, what is most important that the nurse monitor for this patient?
   a. Heart rate (HR)
   b. Potassium levels
   c. Blood pressure (BP)
   d. Gastrointestinal function

16. The health care provider prescribes spironolactone (Aldactone) for the patient with chronic heart failure. What diet modifications related to the use of this drug should the nurse include in the patient teaching?
   a. Decrease both sodium and potassium intake
   b. Increase calcium intake and decrease sodium intake
   c. Decrease sodium intake and increase potassium intake
   d. Decrease sodium intake and the use of salt substitutes for seasoning

17. The nurse monitors the patient receiving treatment for acute decompensated heart failure with the knowledge that marked hypotension is most likely to occur with the IV administration of which medication?
    a. Furosemide (Lasix)
    b. Nitroglycerin (Tridil)
    c. Milrinone (Primacor)
    d. Nitroprusside (Nipride)

18. A 2400-mg sodium diet is prescribed for a patient with chronic heart failure. The nurse recognizes that additional teaching is necessary when the patient makes which statement?
    a. "I should limit my milk intake to 2 cups a day."
    b. "I can eat fresh fruits and vegetables without worrying about sodium content."
    c. "I can eat most foods as long as I do not add salt when cooking or at the table."
    d. "I need to read the labels on prepared foods and medicines for their sodium content."

19. List four cardiovascular conditions that may lead to HF and what can be done to prevent the development of HF in each condition.

Cardiovascular Condition Leading to HF	Preventive Measures

20. The nurse determines that treatment of heart failure has been successful when the patient experiences
    a. weight loss and diuresis.
    b. warm skin and less fatigue.
    c. clear lung sounds and decreased HR.
    d. absence of chest pain and improved level of consciousness (LOC).

21. Which statement by the patient with chronic heart failure should cause the nurse to determine that additional discharge teaching is needed?
    a. "I will call my health clinic if I wake up breathless at night."
    b. "I will look for sodium content on labels of foods and over-the-counter medicines."
    c. "I plan to organize my household tasks so I don't have to constantly go up and down the stairs."
    d. "I should weigh myself every morning and go on a diet if I gain more than 2 or 3 pounds in 2 days."

22. The evaluation team for cardiac transplantation is evaluating patients. Which patient is most likely to receive the most benefit from a new heart?
    a. A 24-year-old man with Down syndrome who has received excellent care from parents in their 60s
    b. A 46-year-old single woman with a limited support system who has alcohol-induced cardiomyopathy
    c. A 60-year-old man with inoperable coronary artery disease who has not been compliant with lifestyle changes and rehabilitation programs
    d. A 52-year-old woman with end-stage coronary artery disease who has limited financial resources but is emotionally stable and has strong social support

23. The nurse plans long-term goals for the patient who has had a heart transplant with the knowledge that what is the most common cause of death in heart transplant patients during the first year?
    a. Infection
    b. Heart failure
    c. Embolization
    d. Malignant conditions

CASE STUDY

Acute Decompensated Heart Failure

Patient Profile

L.J. is a 63-year-old man who has a history of hypertension, chronic HF, and sleep apnea. He has been smoking two packs of cigarettes a day for 40 years and has refused to quit. Three days ago he had an onset of flu with fever, pharyngitis, and malaise. He has not taken his antihypertensive medications or his medications to control his HF for 4 days. Today he has been admitted to the hospital intensive care area with ADHF.

Subjective Data

- Is very anxious and asks, "Am I going to die?"
- Denies pain but says that he feels like he cannot get enough air
- Says that his heart feels like it is "running away"
- After being weighed, he reports, "That is more than I usually weigh."
- Reports that he is so exhausted he can't eat or drink by himself

Objective Data

- Height: 5 ft, 10 in (175 cm)
- Weight: 210 lb (95.5 kg)
- Vital signs: Temp 99.6°F (37.6°C), HR 118 bpm and irregular, RR 34, BP 90/58
- Cardiovascular: Distant S_1, S_2; S_3, S_4 present; PMI at sixth ICS and faint; bilateral jugular vein distention; all peripheral pulses are 1+ and there is peripheral edema; initial cardiac monitoring indicates atrial fibrillation with a ventricular rate of 132 bpm
- Respiratory: Pulmonary crackles, decreased breath sounds right lower lobe, coughing frothy blood-tinged sputum; SpO_2 82% on room air
- Gastrointestinal: Bowel sounds present; hepatomegaly 4 cm below costal margin
- Laboratory work and diagnostic testing are scheduled

Discussion Questions

Using a separate sheet of paper, answer the following questions:

1. What signs and symptoms of right-sided and left-sided heart failure is L.J. experiencing?
2. *Priority Decision:* What priority nursing interventions are appropriate for L.J. at the time of his admission?
3. What diagnostic procedures and findings would help to establish a diagnosis of ADHF with pulmonary edema?
4. What monitoring will be used to evaluate L.J.'s condition?
5. During L.J.'s hospitalization, basic standards of evidence-based care for patients with HF are set forth in three core measures by The Joint Commission. Which of these measures should be implemented by the nurse?
6. The physician mentions the possibility of inserting a pacemaker called cardiac resynchronization therapy (CRT). L.J. asks the nurse what CRT is. What response would be appropriate from the nurse?
7. What information should be included in L.J.'s discharge teaching?
8. *Priority Decision:* Based on the assessment data presented, what are the priority nursing diagnoses for L.J.? Are there any collaborative problems?

1. What accurately describes electrocardiographic (ECG) monitoring?
   a. Depolarization of the cells in the ventricles produces the T wave on the ECG.
   b. An abnormal cardiac impulse that arises in the atria, ventricles, or atrioventricular (AV) junction can create a premature beat that is known as an artifact.
   c. Lead placement for V_1 includes one lead each for right arm, right leg, left arm, and left leg with the fifth lead on the fourth intercostal space to the right of the sternal border.
   d. If the sinoatrial (SA) node fails to discharge an impulse or discharges very slowly, a secondary pacemaker in the AV node is able to discharge at a rate of 30 to 40 times per minute.

2. What accurately describes the PR interval (*select all that apply*)?
   a. 0.16 seconds
   b. <0.12 seconds
   c. 0.06 to 0.12 seconds
   d. 0.12 to 0.20 seconds
   e. Time of depolarization and repolarization of ventricles
   f. Measured from beginning of P wave to beginning of QRS complex

3. A patient with a regular heart rate (HR) has four QRS complexes between every 3-second marker on the ECG paper. Calculate the patient's heart rate.
   __80__ bpm

4. The ECG pattern of a patient with a regular HR reveals 20 small squares between each R-R interval. What is the patient's heart rate?
   __75__ bpm

5. What describes the SA node's ability to discharge an electrical impulse spontaneously?
   a. Excitability
   b. Contractility
   c. Conductivity
   d. Automaticity

6. What describes refractoriness?
   a. Abnormal electrical impulses
   b. Period in which heart tissue cannot be stimulated
   c. Areas of the heart do not repolarize at the same rate because of depressed conduction
   d. Sodium migrates rapidly into the cell so it is positive compared to the outside of the cell

7. The patient's PR interval comprises six small boxes on the ECG graph. What does the nurse determine that this indicates?
   a. A normal finding
   b. A problem with ventricular depolarization
   c. A disturbance in the repolarization of the atria
   d. A problem with conduction from the SA node to the ventricular cells

8. The nurse plans close monitoring for the patient during electrophysiologic testing because this test
   a. requires the use of dyes that irritate the myocardium.
   b. causes myocardial ischemia, resulting in dysrhythmias.
   c. involves the use of anticoagulants to prevent thrombus and embolism.
   d. induces dysrhythmias that may require cardioversion or defibrillation to correct.

9. What should the nurse reading the monitor strip call a rhythm with a regular PR interval but a blocked QRS complex?
   a. Asystole
   b. Atrial fibrillation
   c. First-degree AV block
   d. Type II second-degree AV block

10. After defibrillation, the advanced cardiac life support (ACLS) nurse says that the patient has pulseless electrical activity (PEA). What is most important for the nurse to understand about this rhythm?
    a. The heart rate is 40 to 60 bpm.
    b. Hypoxemia and hypervolemia are common with PEA.
    c. There is dissociated activity of the ventricle and atrium.
    d. There is electrical activity with no mechanical response.

11. The nurse is evaluating the telemetry ECG rhythm strip. How should the nurse document the distorted P wave causing an irregular rhythm?
    a. Atrial flutter
    b. Sinus bradycardia
    c. Premature atrial contraction (PAC)
    d. Paroxysmal supraventricular tachycardia (PSVT)

12. A patient with an acute myocardial infarction (MI) develops the following ECG pattern: atrial rate of 82 and regular; ventricular rate of 46 and regular; P wave and QRS complex are normal but there is no relationship between the P wave and the QRS complex. What dysrhythmia does the nurse identify this as and what treatment is expected?
    a. Sinus bradycardia treated with atropine
    b. Third-degree heart block treated with a pacemaker
    c. Atrial fibrillation treated with electrical cardioversion
    d. Type I second-degree AV block treated with observation

13. Which rhythm abnormality has an increased risk of ventricular tachycardia and ventricular fibrillation?
    a. PAC
    b. PVC on the T wave
    c. Accelerated idioventricular rhythm
    d. Premature ventricular contraction (PVC) couplet

14. A patient with an acute MI has sinus tachycardia of 126 bpm. The nurse recognizes that if this dysrhythmia is not treated, the patient is likely to experience
    a. hypertension.
    b. escape rhythms.
    c. ventricular tachycardia.
    d. an increase in infarct size.

15. A patient with no history of heart disease has a rhythm strip that shows an occasional distorted P wave followed by normal AV and ventricular conduction. What should the nurse question the patient about?
    a. The use of caffeine
    b. The use of sedatives
    c. Any aerobic training
    d. Holding of breath during exertion

16. *Priority Decision:* A patient's rhythm strip indicates a normal HR and rhythm with normal P waves and QRS complexes, but the PR interval is 0.26 second. What is the most appropriate action by the nurse?
    a. Continue to assess the patient.
    b. Administer atropine per protocol.
    c. Prepare the patient for synchronized cardioversion.
    d. Prepare the patient for placement of a temporary pacemaker.

17. In the patient with a dysrhythmia, which assessment indicates decreased cardiac output (CO)?
    a. Hypertension and bradycardia
    b. Chest pain and decreased mentation
    c. Abdominal distention and hepatomegaly
    d. Bounding pulses and a ventricular heave

18. *Priority Decision:* A patient with an acute MI is having multifocal PVCs and ventricular couplets. He is alert and has a BP of 118/78 mm Hg with an irregular pulse of 86 bpm. What is the priority nursing action at this time?
    a. Continue to assess the patient.
    b. Ask the patient to perform Valsalva maneuver.
    c. Prepare to administer antidysrhythmic drugs per protocol.
    d. Be prepared to administer cardiopulmonary resuscitation (CPR).

19. Which rhythm pattern finding is indicative of PVCs?
    a. A QRS complex ≥0.12 second followed by a P wave
    b. Continuous wide QRS complexes with a ventricular rate of 160 bpm
    c. P waves hidden in QRS complexes with a regular rhythm of 120 bpm
    d. Saw-toothed P waves with no measurable PR interval and an irregular rhythm

20. In the patient experiencing ventricular fibrillation (VF), what is the rationale for using cardiac defibrillation?
    a. Enhance repolarization and relaxation of ventricular myocardial cells
    b. Provide an electrical impulse that stimulates normal myocardial contractions
    c. Depolarize the cells of the myocardium to allow the SA node to resume pacemaker function
    d. Deliver an electrical impulse to the heart at the time of ventricular contraction to convert the heart to a sinus rhythm

21. What action is included in the nurse's responsibilities in preparing to administer defibrillation?
    a. Applying gel pads to the patient's chest
    b. Setting the defibrillator to deliver 50 joules
    c. Setting the defibrillator to a synchronized mode
    d. Sedating the patient with midazolam (Versed) before defibrillation

22. While providing discharge instructions to the patient who has had an implantable cardioverter-defibrillator (ICD) inserted, the nurse teaches the patient that if the ICD fires, he or she should do what?
    a. Lie down.
    b. Call the cardiologist.
    c. Push the reset button on the pulse generator.
    d. Immediately take his or her antidysrhythmic medication.

23. A patient with a sinus node dysfunction has a permanent pacemaker inserted. Before discharge, what should the nurse include when teaching the patient?
    a. Avoid cooking with microwave ovens.
    b. Avoid standing near antitheft devices in doorways.
    c. Use mild analgesics to control the chest spasms caused by the pacing current.
    d. Start lifting the arm above the shoulder right away to prevent a "frozen shoulder."

24. *Priority Decision:* A patient on the cardiac telemetry unit goes into ventricular fibrillation and is unresponsive. Following initiation of the emergency call system (Code Blue), what is the next priority for the nurse in caring for this patient?
    a. Begin CPR.
    b. Get the crash cart.
    c. Administer amiodarone IV.
    d. Defibrillate with 360 joules.

25. The use of catheter ablation therapy to "burn" areas of the cardiac conduction system is indicated for the treatment of
    a. sinus arrest.
    b. heart blocks.
    c. tachydysrhythmias.
    d. premature ventricular tachycardia.

26. A patient with chest pain that is unrelieved by nitroglycerin is admitted to the coronary care unit for observation and diagnosis. While the patient has continuous ECG monitoring, what finding would most concern the nurse?
    a. Occasional PVCs
    b. An inverted T wave
    c. ST segment elevation
    d. A PR interval of 0.18 second

27. A 54-year-old patient who has no structural heart disease has an episode of syncope. An upright tilt table test is performed to rule out neurocardiogenic syncope. The nurse explains to the patient that if neurocardiogenic syncope is the problem, the patient will experience what?
    a. No change in HR or BP
    b. Palpitations and dizziness
    c. Tachydysrhythmias and chest pain
    d. Marked bradycardia and hypotension

28. The patient is brought to the emergency department with acute coronary syndrome (ACS). What changes should the nurse expect to see on the ECG if only myocardial injury has occurred?
    a. Absent P wave
    b. A wide Q wave
    c. Inverted T wave
    d. ST segment elevation

29. Identify the following cardiac rhythms using the systematic approach to assessing cardiac rhythms found in Table 36-5 in the textbook. All rhythm strips are 6 seconds.

a.

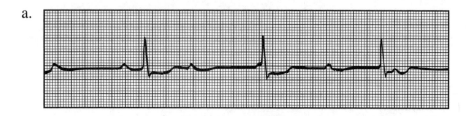

b.

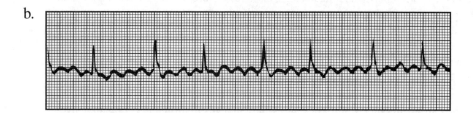

c.

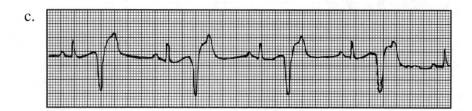

d.

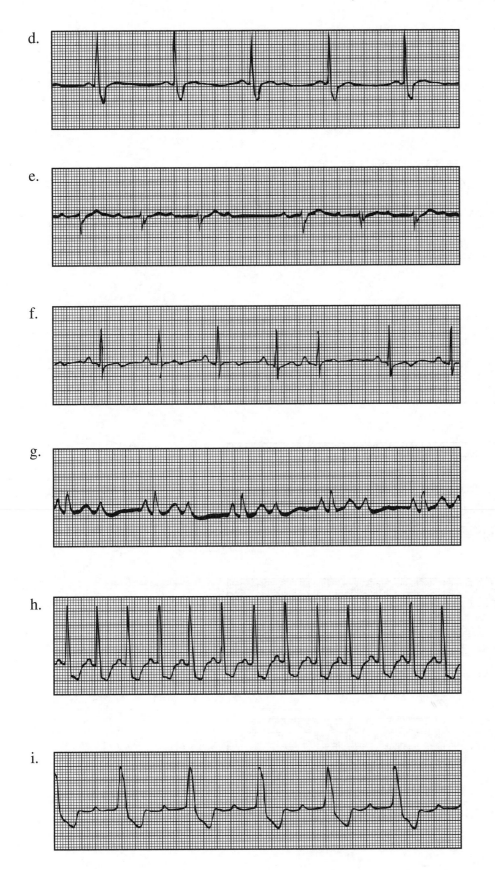

e.

f.

g.

h.

i.

j.

k.

l.

m.

n.

o.

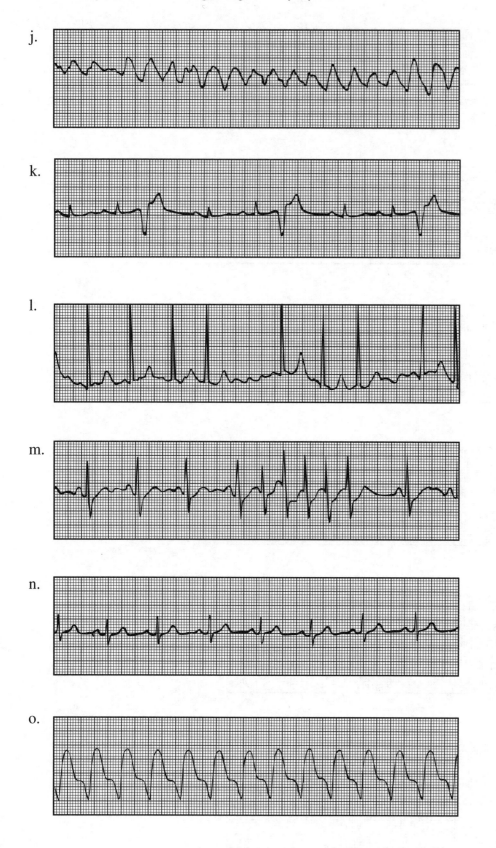

CASE STUDY
Dysrhythmia
Patient Profile

R.S. is a 75-year-old woman who is admitted to the telemetry unit with a diagnosis of new-onset atrial fibrillation.

Subjective Data

- Has a history of hypothyroidism and hypertension
- Has no history of atrial fibrillation
- Is taking levothyroxine (Synthroid) 0.125 mg PO daily and enalapril (Vasotec) 5 mg PO bid
- Experiences palpitations, dizziness, shortness of breath, and mild chest pressure
- Has been drinking more coffee since her husband died last month

Objective Data

Physical Examination
- Alert, anxious, older woman
- Vital signs: BP 100/70, HR 150 bpm, RR 32
- Lungs: Bibasilar crackles
- Heart: S_1 and S_2, irregular

Diagnostic Study
- 12-lead ECG: Atrial fibrillation with an uncontrolled ventricular response

Collaborative Care

- Discontinue enalapril (Vasotec)
- IV diltiazem (Cardizem) bolus and then IV drip
- Digoxin 0.25 mg PO daily
- Enoxaparin (Lovenox) subcutaneous bid
- Warfarin (Coumadin) 5 mg PO daily

Discussion Questions

Using a separate sheet of paper, answer the following questions:

1. What risk factors for atrial fibrillation does R.S. have?
2. What nursing interventions should be included in the initial emergency management of R.S.?
3. Explain the pathophysiology of R.S.'s symptoms on admission to the telemetry unit.
4. Describe the characteristics of R.S.'s ECG waveform.
5. What is the immediate goal of antidysrhythmic drug therapy for R.S.?
6. Explain the rationale for use of the medications ordered for R.S.
7. What nondrug therapy may be used to treat the dysrhythmia?
8. ***Priority Decision:*** Based on the assessment data presented, what are the priority nursing diagnoses? Are there any collaborative problems?

Nursing Management: Inflammatory and Structural Heart Disorders

1. A 20-year-old patient has acute infective endocarditis. While obtaining a nursing history, what should the nurse ask the patient about (*select all that apply*)?
   a. Renal dialysis
   b. IV drug abuse
   c. Recent dental work
   d. Cardiac catheterization
   e. Recent urinary tract infection

2. A patient has an admitting diagnosis of acute left-sided infective endocarditis. What is the best test to confirm this diagnosis?
   a. Blood cultures
   b. Complete blood count
   c. Cardiac catheterization
   d. Transesophageal echocardiogram

3. Which manifestation of infective endocarditis is a result of fragmentation and microembolization of vegetative lesions?
   a. Petechiae
   b. Roth's spots
   c. Osler's nodes
   d. Splinter hemorrhages

4. What describes Janeway's lesions that are manifestations of infective endocarditis?
   a. Hemorrhagic retinal lesions
   b. Black longitudinal streaks in nail beds
   c. Painful red or purple lesions on fingers or toes
   d. Flat, red, painless spots on the palms of hands and soles of feet

5. A patient with infective endocarditis of a prosthetic mitral valve develops a left hemiparesis and visual changes. What should the nurse expect to be included in collaborative management of the patient?
   a. Embolectomy
   b. Surgical valve replacement
   c. Administration of anticoagulants
   d. Higher than usual antibiotic dosages

6. A patient with aortic valve endocarditis develops dyspnea, crackles in the lungs, and restlessness. What should the nurse suspect that the patient is experiencing?
   a. Pulmonary embolization from valve vegetations
   b. Vegetative embolization to the coronary arteries
   c. Valvular incompetence with resulting heart failure
   d. Nonspecific manifestations that accompany infectious diseases

7. *Priority Decision:* A patient hospitalized for 1 week with subacute infective endocarditis is afebrile and has no signs of heart damage. Discharge with outpatient antibiotic therapy is planned. During discharge planning with the patient, what is it most important for the nurse to do?
   a. Plan how his needs will be met while he continues on bed rest.
   b. Encourage the use of diversional activities to relieve boredom and restlessness.
   c. Teach the patient to avoid crowds and exposure to upper respiratory infections.
   d. Assess the patient's home environment in terms of family assistance and hospital access.

8. When instructing a patient with endocarditis how to prevent recurrence of the infection, what should the nurse teach the patient?
   a. Start on antibiotic therapy when exposed to persons with infections.
   b. Take one aspirin a day to prevent vegetative lesions from forming around the valves.
   c. Always maintain continuous antibiotic therapy to prevent the development of any systemic infection.
   d. Obtain prophylactic antibiotic therapy before certain invasive medical or dental procedures (e.g., dental cleaning).

9. A patient is admitted to the hospital with a suspected acute pericarditis. To establish the presence of a pericardial friction rub, how should the nurse listen to the patient's chest?
   a. While timing the sound with the respiratory pattern
   b. With the bell of the stethoscope at the apex of the heart
   c. With the diaphragm of the stethoscope at the lower left sternal border of the chest
   d. With the diaphragm of the stethoscope to auscultate a high-pitched continuous rumbling sound

10. A patient with acute pericarditis has markedly distended jugular veins, decreased BP, tachycardia, tachypnea, and muffled heart sounds. The nurse recognizes that these symptoms occur when what happens?
    a. The pericardial space is obliterated with scar tissue and thickened pericardium
    b. Excess pericardial fluid compresses the heart and prevents adequate diastolic filling
    c. The parietal and visceral pericardial membranes adhere to each other, preventing normal myocardial contraction
    d. Fibrin accumulation on the visceral pericardium infiltrates into the myocardium, creating generalized myocardial dysfunction

11. What explains the measurement of pulsus paradoxus with cardiac tamponade (*select all that apply*)?
    a. A difference of less than 10 mm Hg occurs.
    b. A difference of greater than 10 mm Hg occurs.
    c. It is measured with an automatic sphygmomanometer.
    d. Rapidly inflate the cuff until you hear sounds throughout the respiratory cycle.
    e. Subtract the number when sounds are heard in the respiratory cycle from the number when the first Korotkoff sound during expiration is heard.

12. The patient with acute pericarditis is having a pericardiocentesis. Postoperatively what complication should the nurse monitor the patient for?
    a. Pneumonia
    b. Pneumothorax
    c. Myocardial infarction (MI)
    d. Cerebrovascular accident (CVA)

13. *Priority Decision:* A patient with acute pericarditis has a nursing diagnosis of pain *related to* pericardial inflammation. What is the best nursing intervention for the patient?
    a. Administer opioids as prescribed on an around-the-clock schedule.
    b. Promote progressive relaxation exercises with the use of deep, slow breathing.
    c. Position the patient on the right side with the head of the bed elevated 15 degrees.
    d. Position the patient in Fowler's position with a padded over-the-bed table for the patient to lean on.

14. When obtaining a nursing history for a patient with myocarditis, what should the nurse specifically question the patient about?
    a. Prior use of digoxin for treatment of cardiac problems
    b. Recent symptoms of a viral illness, such as fever and malaise
    c. A history of coronary artery disease (CAD) with or without an MI
    d. A recent streptococcal infection requiring treatment with penicillin

15. *Priority Decision:* What is the most important role of the nurse in preventing rheumatic fever?
    a. Teach patients with infective endocarditis to adhere to antibiotic prophylaxis.
    b. Identify patients with valvular heart disease who are at risk for rheumatic fever.
    c. Encourage the use of antibiotics for treatment of all infections involving a sore throat.
    d. Promote the early diagnosis and immediate treatment of group A streptococcal pharyngitis.

16. What manifestations most strongly support a diagnosis of acute rheumatic fever?
    a. Carditis, polyarthritis, and erythema marginatum
    b. Polyarthritis, chorea, and decreased antistreptolysin O titer
    c. Organic heart murmurs, fever, and elevated erythrocyte sedimentation rate (ESR)
    d. Positive C-reactive protein, elevated white blood cells (WBCs), and subcutaneous nodules

17. When teaching the patient with acute rheumatic fever, identify the rationale for the use of each of the following drugs in the patient's treatment plan.

Drug	Rationale for Use
Antibiotics	
Aspirin	
Corticosteroids	
Nonsteroidal antiinflammatory drugs (NSAIDs)	

18. A patient with rheumatic heart disease with carditis asks the nurse how long his activity will be restricted. What is the best answer by the nurse?
    a. "Full activity will be allowed as soon as acute symptoms have subsided."
    b. "Bed rest will be continued until symptoms of heart failure are controlled."
    c. "Nonstrenuous activities can be performed as soon as antibiotics are started."
    d. "Bed rest must be maintained until antiinflammatory therapy has been discontinued."

19. What is an effect of valvular regurgitation?
    a. It causes a pressure gradient difference across an open valve.
    b. A pericardial friction rub is heard on the right sternal border of the chest.
    c. It leads to decreased flow of blood and hypertrophy of the preceding chamber.
    d. There is a backward flow of blood and volume overload in the preceding chamber.

20. *Delegation Decision:* An RN is working with a licensed practical nurse (LPN) in caring for a group of patients on a cardiac telemetry unit. A patient with aortic stenosis has the nursing diagnosis of activity intolerance *related to* fatigue and exertional dyspnea. Which nursing activity could be delegated to the LPN?
    a. Explain the reason for planning frequent periods of rest.
    b. Evaluate the patient's understanding of his disease process.
    c. Monitor BP, HR, RR, and SpO_2 before, during, and after ambulation.
    d. Teach the patient which activities to choose that will gradually increase endurance.

21. What accurately describes mitral valve prolapse?
    a. Rapid onset prevents left chamber dilation
    b. May be caused by pulmonary hypertension
    c. Ballooning of valve into left atrium during ventricular systole
    d. Rapid development of pulmonary edema and cardiogenic shock

22. What causes a sudden onset of cardiovascular collapse?
    a. Mitral stenosis
    b. Tricuspid valve disease
    c. Pulmonic valve stenosis
    d. Acute aortic regurgitation

23. The patient is admitted with angina, syncope, and dyspnea on exertion. In the assessment, the nurse notes a systolic murmur with a prominent S_4. What will the nurse suspect is occurring with this patient?
    a. Mitral valve stenosis
    b. Aortic valve stenosis
    c. Acute mitral valve regurgitation
    d. Chronic mitral valve regurgitation

24. Which drugs would the nurse expect to be included in those prescribed for patients with a mechanical valve replacement?
    a. Oral nitrates
    b. Anticoagulants
    c. Atrial antidysrhythmics
    d. β-adrenergic blocking agents

25. *Priority Decision:* A patient with symptomatic mitral valve prolapse has atrial and ventricular dysrhythmias. In addition to monitoring for decreased cardiac output related to the dysrhythmias, what is an important nursing intervention related to the dysrhythmias identified by the nurse?
    a. Monitor breathing pattern related to hypervolemia.
    b. Encourage calling for assistance when getting out of bed.
    c. Give sleeping pills to decrease paroxysmal nocturnal dyspnea.
    d. Teach the patient exercises to prevent recurrence of dysrhythmias.

26. A patient is scheduled for a percutaneous transluminal balloon valvuloplasty. The nurse understands that this procedure is indicated for which patient?
    a. Any patient with aortic regurgitation
    b. Older patients with aortic regurgitation
    c. Older patients with stenosis of any valve
    d. Young adult patients with mild mitral valve stenosis

27. A patient is scheduled for an open surgical valvuloplasty of the mitral valve. In preparing the patient for surgery, what should the nurse know about this surgery?
    a. Cardiopulmonary bypass is not required with this procedure.
    b. Valve repair is a palliative measure, whereas valve replacement is curative.
    c. The operative mortality rate is lower in valve repair than in valve replacement.
    d. Patients with valve repair do not require postoperative anticoagulation as do those who have valve replacement.

28. In which patient would a mechanical prosthetic valve be preferred over a biologic valve for valve replacement?
    a. 41-year-old man with peptic ulcer disease
    b. 22-year-old woman who desires to have children
    c. 35-year-old man with a history of seasonal asthma
    d. 62-year-old woman with early Alzheimer's disease

29. When performing discharge teaching for the patient following a mechanical valve replacement, the nurse determines that further instruction is needed when the patient says which statement?
    a. "I may begin an exercise program to gradually increase my cardiac tolerance."
    b. "I will always need to have my blood checked once a month for its clotting function."
    c. "I should take prophylactic antibiotics before I have dental or invasive medical procedures."
    d. "The biggest risk I have during invasive health procedures is bleeding because of my anticoagulants."

30. The patient is admitted post–radiation therapy with symptoms of cardiomyopathy (CMP). Which type of CMP should the nurse suspect that the patient is experiencing?
    a. Dilated
    b. Restrictive
    c. Takotsubo
    d. Hypertrophic

31. What accurately describes dilated CMP (*select all that apply*)?
    a. Characterized by ventricular stiffness
    b. The least common type of cardiomyopathy
    c. The hyperdynamic systolic function creates a diastolic failure
    d. Echocardiogram reveals cardiomegaly with thin ventricular walls
    e. Often follows an infective myocarditis or exposure to toxins or drugs
    f. Differs from chronic heart failure in that there is no ventricular hypertrophy

32. When planning care for the patient with hypertrophic CMP, what should the nurse include?
    a. Ventricular pacing
    b. Administration of vasodilators
    c. Teach the patient to avoid strenuous activity and dehydration
    d. Surgery for cardiac transplantation will need to be done soon

33. When performing discharge teaching for a patient with any type of CMP, what should the nurse instruct the patient to do (*select all that apply*)?
    a. Eat a low-sodium diet.
    b. Go to the gym every day.
    c. Engage in stress reduction activities.
    d. Abstain from alcohol and caffeine intake.
    e. Avoid strenuous activity and allow for periods of rest.
    f. Suggest that caregivers learn cardiopulmonary resuscitation (CPR).

CASE STUDY

Infective Endocarditis

Patient Profile

N.B. is a 60-year-old man who is hospitalized with a suspected stroke.

Subjective Data

• Had a laparoscopic cholecystectomy a few weeks ago

Objective Data

• Neurologic signs typical of a stroke (paralysis on right side involving right arm and leg, slurred speech)
• Petechiae over the chest
• Crescendo-decrescendo murmur present
• Rectal temp: 103°F (39.4°C)

Discussion Questions

Using a separate sheet of paper, answer the following questions:

1. Why is N.B. at risk for infective endocarditis?
2. What asymptomatic underlying cardiac conditions might have contributed to his infective endocarditis?
3. Explain the cause of N.B.'s assessment findings.
4. What is the relevance of the endoscopic surgery that N.B. had a few weeks before this hospital admission?
5. What diagnostic tests should the nurse expect to be ordered and what will the results show?
6. What treatment should the nurse anticipate for N.B.?
7. Discuss how N.B.'s infective endocarditis could have been prevented.
8. *Priority Decision:* Based on the assessment data presented, what are the priority nursing diagnoses? Are there any collaborative problems?

Nursing Management:
Vascular Disorders

1. When obtaining a health history from a 72-year-old man with peripheral arterial disease (PAD) of the lower extremities, the nurse asks about a history of related conditions, including
   a. venous thrombosis.
   b. venous stasis ulcers.
   c. pulmonary embolism.
   d. coronary artery disease (CAD).

2. A 45-year-old patient with chronic arterial disease has a brachial systolic blood pressure (SBP) of 132 mm Hg and an ankle SBP of 102 mm Hg. The ankle-brachial index is _____ and indicates _____ (mild/moderate/severe) arterial disease.

3. Following teaching about medications for PAD, the nurse determines that additional instruction is necessary when the patient makes which statement?
   a. "I should take one aspirin a day to prevent clotting in my legs."
   b. "The lisinopril I use for my blood pressure may help me walk further without pain."
   c. "I will need to have frequent blood tests to evaluate the effect of the Coumadin I will be taking."
   d. "Pletal should help me increase my walking distance and help prevent clots from forming in my legs."

4. A patient with PAD has a nursing diagnosis of ineffective peripheral tissue perfusion. What should be included in the teaching plan for this patient (*select all that apply*)?
   a. Keep legs and feet warm.
   b. Apply cold compresses when the legs become swollen.
   c. Walk at least 30 minutes per day to the point of discomfort.
   d. Use nicotine replacement therapy as a substitute for smoking.
   e. Inspect lower extremities for pulses, temperature, and any injury.

5. When teaching the patient with PAD about modifying risk factors associated with the condition, what should the nurse emphasize?
   a. Amputation is the ultimate outcome if the patient does not alter lifestyle behaviors.
   b. Modifications will reduce the risk of other atherosclerotic conditions such as stroke.
   c. Risk-reducing behaviors initiated after angioplasty can stop the progression of the disease.
   d. Maintenance of normal body weight is the most important factor in controlling arterial disease.

6. *Priority Decision:* During care of the patient following femoral bypass graft surgery, the nurse immediately notifies the health care provider if the patient experiences
   a. fever and redness at the incision site.
   b. 2+ edema of the extremity and pain at the incision site.
   c. a loss of palpable pulses and numbness and tingling of the feet.
   d. increasing ankle-brachial indices and serous drainage from the incision.

7. *Priority Decision:* A patient has atrial fibrillation and develops an acute arterial occlusion at the iliac artery bifurcation. What are the six Ps of acute arterial occlusion the nurse may assess in this patient that require immediate notification of the physician?

   a.

   b.

   c.

   d.

   e.

   f.

8. Which conditions characterize critical limb ischemia (*select all that apply*)?
   a. Cold feet
   b. Arterial leg ulcers
   c. Venous leg ulcers
   d. Gangrene of the leg
   e. No palpable peripheral pulses
   f. Rest pain lasting more than 2 weeks

9. What are characteristic of arteriospastic disease (Raynaud's phenomenon) (*select all that apply*)?
   a. Predominant in young females
   b. May be associated with autoimmune disorders
   c. Precipitated by exposure to cold, caffeine, and tobacco
   d. Involves small cutaneous arteries of the fingers and toes
   e. Inflammation of small and medium-sized arteries and veins
   f. Episodes involve white, blue, and red color changes of fingertips

10. Which aneurysm is uniform in shape and a circumferential dilation of the artery?
    a. False aneurysm
    b. Pseudoaneurysm
    c. Saccular aneurysm
    d. Fusiform aneurysm

11. A surgical repair is planned for a patient who has a 5.5-cm abdominal aortic aneurysm (AAA). On physical assessment of the patient, what should the nurse expect to find?
    a. Hoarseness and dysphagia
    b. Severe back pain with flank ecchymosis
    c. Presence of a bruit in the periumbilical area
    d. Weakness in the lower extremities progressing to paraplegia

12. A thoracic aortic aneurysm is found when a patient has a routine chest x-ray. The nurse anticipates that additional diagnostic testing to determine the size and structure of the aneurysm will include which test?
    a. Angiography
    b. Ultrasonography
    c. Echocardiography
    d. Computed tomography (CT) scan

13. A patient with a small AAA is not a good surgical candidate. What should the nurse teach the patient is one of the best ways to prevent expansion of the lesion?
    a. Avoid strenuous physical exertion.
    b. Control hypertension with prescribed therapy.
    c. Comply with prescribed anticoagulant therapy.
    d. Maintain a low-calcium diet to prevent calcification of the vessel.

14. During preoperative preparation of the patient scheduled for an AAA, why should the nurse establish baseline data for the patient?
    a. All physiologic processes will be altered postoperatively.
    b. The cause of the aneurysm is a systemic vascular disease.
    c. Surgery will be canceled if any physiologic function is not normal.
    d. BP and HR will be maintained well below baseline levels during the postoperative period.

15. Which surgical therapy for AAA is most likely to have the postoperative complication of renal injury?
    a. Open aneurysm repair (OAR) above the level of the renal arteries
    b. Excising only the weakened area of the artery and suturing the artery closed
    c. Bifurcated graft used in aneurysm repair when the AAA extends into the iliac arteries
    d. Endovascular graft procedure with an aortic graft inside the aneurysm via the femoral artery

16. In preparation for AAA repair surgery, what should the nurse include in patient teaching?
    a. Prepare the bowel on the night before surgery with laxatives or an enema.
    b. Use moisturizing soap to clean the skin three times the day before surgery.
    c. Eat a high-protein and high-carbohydrate breakfast to help with healing postoperatively.
    d. Take the prescribed oral antibiotic the morning of surgery before going to the operating room.

17. During the patient's acute postoperative period following repair of an AAA, the nurse should ensure that which goal is achieved?
    a. Hypothermia is maintained to decrease oxygen need.
    b. BP and all peripheral pulses are evaluated at least every hour.
    c. IV fluids are administered at a rate to maintain urine output of 100 mL/hr.
    d. The patient's BP is kept lower than baseline to prevent leaking at the incision line.

18. *Priority Decision:* Following an ascending aortic aneurysm repair, what is an important finding that the nurse should report immediately to the health care provider?
    a. Shallow respirations and poor coughing
    b. Decreased drainage from the chest tubes
    c. A change in level of consciousness (LOC) and inability to speak
    d. Lower extremity pulses that are decreased from the preoperative baseline

19. Which observation made by the nurse should indicate the presence of the complication of graft thrombosis after aortic aneurysm repair?
    a. Cardiac dysrhythmias or chest pain
    b. Absent bowel sounds, abdominal distention, or diarrhea
    c. Increased temperature and increased white blood cell count
    d. Decreased pulses and cool, painful extremities below the level of repair

20. *Priority Decision*: A patient who is postoperative following repair of an AAA has been receiving IV fluids at 125 mL/hr continuously for the last 12 hours. Urine output for the last 4 hours has been 60 mL, 42 mL, 28 mL, and 20 mL, respectively. What is the priority action that the nurse should take?
    a. Monitor for a couple more hours.
    b. Contact the physician and report the decrease in urine output.
    c. Send blood for electrolytes, blood urea nitrogen (BUN), and creatinine.
    d. Decrease the rate of infusion to prevent blood leakage at the suture line.

21. Following discharge teaching with a male patient with an AAA repair, the nurse determines that further instruction is needed when the patient makes which statement?
    a. "I should avoid heavy lifting."
    b. "I may have some sexual dysfunction as a result of the surgery."
    c. "I should maintain a low-fat and low-cholesterol diet to help keep the new graft open."
    d. "I should take the pulses in my extremities and let the doctor know if they get too fast or too slow."

22. During the nursing assessment of the patient with a distal descending aortic dissection, what should the nurse expect the patient to manifest?
    a. Altered LOC with dizziness and weak carotid pulses
    b. A cardiac murmur characteristic of aortic valve insufficiency
    c. Severe "ripping" back or abdominal pain with decreasing urine output
    d. Severe hypertension and orthopnea and dyspnea of pulmonary edema

23. A patient with a dissection of the arch of the aorta has a decreased LOC and weak carotid pulses. What should the nurse anticipate that initial treatment of the patient will include?
    a. Immediate surgery to replace the torn area with a graft
    b. Administration of anticoagulants to prevent embolization
    c. Administration of packed red blood cells (RBCs) to replace blood loss
    d. Administration of antihypertensives to maintain a mean arterial pressure of 70 to 80 mm Hg

24. The nurse evaluates that treatment for the patient with an uncomplicated aortic dissection is successful when what happens?
    a. Pain is relieved.
    b. Surgical repair is completed.
    c. BP is increased to normal range.
    d. Renal output is maintained at 30 mL/hr.

25. What are characteristics of arterial disease (*select all that apply*)?
    a. Pruritus
    b. Thickened, brittle nails
    c. Dull ache in calf or thigh
    d. Decreased peripheral pulses
    e. Pallor on elevation of the legs
    f. Ulcers over bony prominences on toes and feet

26. The patient is diagnosed with a superficial vein thrombosis (SVT). Which characteristic should the nurse know about SVT?
    a. Embolization to lungs may result in death.
    b. Clot may extend to deeper veins if untreated.
    c. Vein is tender to pressure and there is edema.
    d. Typically found in the iliac, inferior, or superior vena cava.

27. The surgery area calls the transfer report for a 68-year-old, postmenopausal, female patient who smokes and takes hormone therapy. She is returning to the floor after a lengthy hip replacement surgery. Which factors present in this patient increase her risk for developing venous thromboembolism (VTE) related to Virchow's triad (*select all that apply*)?
    a. Smoking
    b. IV therapy
    c. Dehydration
    d. Estrogen therapy
    e. Orthopedic surgery
    f. Prolonged immobilization

28. The patient is admitted with pain, edema, and warm skin on her lower left leg. What test should the nurse expect to be ordered first?
    a. Duplex ultrasound
    b. Complete blood count (CBC)
    c. Magnetic resonance imaging (MRI)
    d. Computed venography (phlebogram)

29. *Delegation Decision:* The nursing care area is very busy with new surgical patients. Which care could the RN delegate to the unlicensed assistive personnel (UAP) for a patient with VTE?
    a. Assess the patient's use of herbs.
    b. Measure the patient for elastic compression stockings.
    c. Remind the patient to flex and extend the legs and feet every 2 hours
    d. Teach the patient to call emergency medical services (EMS) with signs of pulmonary embolus

30. To help prevent embolization of the thrombus in a patient with a VTE, what should the nurse teach the patient to do?
    a. Dangle the feet over the edge of the bed q2-3hr.
    b. Ambulate around the bed three to four times a day.
    c. Keep the affected leg elevated above the level of the heart.
    d. Maintain bed rest until edema is relieved and anticoagulation is established.

31. Which indirect thrombin inhibitor is only administered subcutaneously and does not need routine coagulation tests?
    a. Warfarin (Coumadin)
    b. Unfractionated heparin (Heparin)
    c. Hirudin derivatives (lepirudin [Refludan])
    d. Low-molecular-weight heparin (nadroparin [Fraxiparine])

32. Which characteristics describe the anticoagulant warfarin (Coumadin) (*select all that apply*)?
    a. Vitamin K is the antidote
    b. Protamine sulfate is the antidote → hep-lock
    c. May be administered orally or subcutaneously
    d. May be administered intravenously or subcutaneously
    e. Dosage monitored using international normalized ratio (INR)
    f. Dosage monitored using activated partial thromboplastin time (aPTT)

33. The patient with VTE is receiving therapy with heparin and asks the nurse whether the drug will dissolve the clot in her leg. What is the best response by the nurse?
    a. "This drug will break up and dissolve the clot so that circulation in the vein can be restored."
    b. "The purpose of the heparin is to prevent growth of the clot or formation of new clots where the circulation is slowed."
    c. "Heparin won't dissolve the clot but it will inhibit the inflammation around the clot and delay the development of new clots."
    d. "The heparin will dilate the vein, preventing turbulence of blood flow around the clot that may cause it to break off and travel to the lungs."

34. A patient with VTE is to be discharged on long-term warfarin (Coumadin) therapy and is taught about prevention and continuing treatment of VTE. The nurse determines that discharge teaching for the patient has been effective when the patient makes which statement?
    a. "I should expect that Coumadin will cause my stools to be somewhat black."
    b. "I should avoid all dark green and leafy vegetables while I am taking Coumadin."
    c. "Massaging my legs several times a day will help increase my venous circulation."
    d. "Swimming is a good activity to include in my exercise program to increase my circulation."

35. The nurse teaches the patient with any venous disorder that the best way to prevent venous stasis and increase venous return is to
    a. walk.
    b. sit with the legs elevated.
    c. frequently rotate the ankles.
    d. continuously wear elastic compression stockings.

36. Number in sequence the processes that occur as venous stasis leads to varicose veins and to venous stasis ulcers.

_____ a. Veins dilate

_____ b. Edema forms

_____ c. Ulceration occurs

_____ d. Venous pressure increases

_____ e. Capillary pressure increases

_____ f. Venous blood flow backs up

_____ g. Additional venous distention occurs

_____ h. Venous valves become incompetent

_____ i. Blood supply to local tissues decreases

37. What is the most important measure in the treatment of venous stasis ulcers?

a. Elevation of the limb

b. Elastic compression stockings

c. Application of moist dressings

d. Application of topical antibiotics

CASE STUDY

Abdominal Aortic Aneurysm

Patient Profile

C.S. is a 73-year-old man who was brought to the local emergency department complaining of severe back pain.

Subjective Data

- Has a known AAA, which has been followed with yearly abdominal ultrasound testing
- Has smoked a pack of cigarettes per day for 52 years
- Has had occasional bouts of angina for the past 3 years

Objective Data

- Has a pulsating abdominal mass
- HR 114 bpm, BP 88/68
- Extremities are cool and clammy

Discussion Questions

Using a separate sheet of paper, answer the following questions:

1. What are C.S.'s risk factors for AAA?
2. What is the etiology of an AAA?
3. Which signs or symptoms make the nurse suspect that C.S.'s AAA has ruptured?
4. *Priority Decision:* What is the first priority in C.S.'s care?
5. What is the nurse's role in assisting the family in this critical situation?
6. What steps, if any, could have been taken to prevent the rupture of the AAA?
7. What discharge teaching should be included for this patient after the AAA repair?
8. *Priority Decision:* Based on the assessment data presented, what are the priority nursing diagnoses? Are there any collaborative problems?

1. Identify the structures in the following illustration:

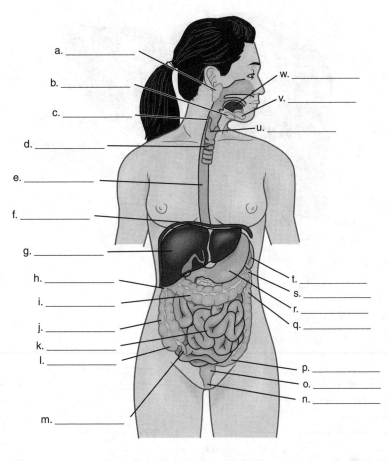

a. _____

b. _____

c. _____

d. _____

e. _____

f. _____

g. _____

h. _____

i. _____

j. _____

k. _____

l. _____

m. _____

n. _____

o. _____

p. _____

q. _____

r. _____

s. _____

t. _____

u. _____

v. _____

w. _____

2. Identify the structures in the following illustration using the terms listed below.

Terms

Ampulla of Vater	Duodenum	Pancreas (body)
Common bile duct	Gallbladder	Pancreas (head)
Common hepatic duct	Left hepatic duct	Pancreas (tail)
Cystic duct	Main pancreatic duct	Right hepatic duct

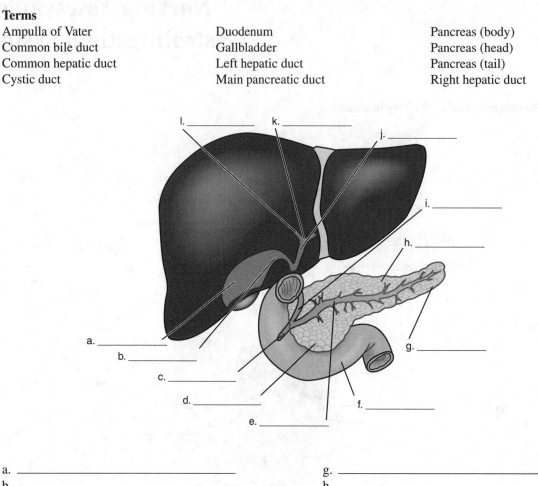

a. _____   g. _____
b. _____   h. _____
c. _____   i. _____
d. _____   j. _____
e. _____   k. _____
f. _____   l. _____

3. A patient receives atropine, an anticholinergic drug, in preparation for surgery. The nurse expects this drug to affect the GI tract by doing what?
   a. Increasing gastric emptying
   b. Relaxing pyloric and ileocecal sphincters
   c. Decreasing secretions and peristaltic action
   d. Stimulating the nervous system of the GI tract

4. After eating, a patient with an inflamed gallbladder experiences pain caused by contraction of the gallbladder. What is the mechanism responsible for this action?
   a. Production of bile by the liver
   b. Production of secretin by the duodenum
   c. Release of gastrin from the stomach antrum
   d. Production of cholecystokinin by the duodenum

5. *Priority Decision:* When caring for a patient who has had most of the stomach surgically removed, what is important for the nurse to teach the patient?
   a. Extra iron will need to be taken to prevent anemia.
   b. Avoid foods with lactose to prevent bloating and diarrhea.
   c. Lifelong supplementation of cobalamin (vitamin B$_{12}$) will be needed.
   d. Because of the absence of digestive enzymes, protein malnutrition is likely.

6. A 68-year-old patient is in the office for a physical. She notes that she no longer has regular bowel movements. Which suggestion by the nurse would be most helpful to the patient?
   a. Take an additional laxative to stimulate defecation.
   b. Eat less acidic foods to enable the gastrointestinal system to increase peristalsis.
   c. Eat less food at each meal to prevent feces from backing up related to slowed peristalsis.
   d. Attempt defecation after breakfast because gastrocolic reflexes increase colon peristalsis at that time.

7. Which digestive substances are active or activated in the stomach (*select all that apply*)?
   a. Bile
   b. Pepsin
   c. Gastrin
   d. Maltase
   e. Secretin
   f. Amylase

8. What problem should the nurse assess the patient for if the patient was on prolonged antibiotic therapy?
   a. Coagulation problems
   b. Elevated serum ammonia levels
   c. Impaired absorption of amino acids
   d. Increased mucus and bicarbonate secretion

9. How will an obstruction at the ampulla of Vater affect the digestion of all nutrients?
   a. Bile is responsible for emulsification of all nutrients and vitamins.
   b. Intestinal digestive enzymes are released through the ampulla of Vater.
   c. Both bile and pancreatic enzymes enter the duodenum at the ampulla of Vater.
   d. Gastric contents can only pass to the duodenum when the ampulla of Vater is open.

10. A patient experiences increased red blood cell (RBC) destruction from a mechanical heart valve prosthesis. Describe what happens to the bilirubin that is released from the breakdown of hemoglobin (Hgb) from the RBCs.

11. What is a clinical manifestation of age-related changes in the GI system that the nurse may find in an older patient?
    a. Gastric hyperacidity
    b. Intolerance to fatty foods
    c. Yellowish tinge to the skin
    d. Reflux of gastric contents into the esophagus

12. Identify one specific finding identified by the nurse during assessment of each of the patient's functional health patterns that indicates a risk factor for GI problems or the response of the patient to a GI disorder.

Functional Health Pattern	Risk Factor for or Response to GI Problem
Health perception–health management	
Nutritional-metabolic	
Elimination	
Activity-exercise	
Sleep-rest	
Cognitive-perceptual	
Self-perception–self-concept	
Role-relationship	
Sexuality-reproductive	
Coping–stress tolerance	
Value-belief	

13. What is a normal finding during physical assessment of the mouth?
    a. A red, slick appearance of the tongue
    b. Uvular deviation to the side on saying "Ahh"
    c. A thin, white coating of the dorsum of the tongue
    d. Scattered red, smooth areas on the dorsum of the tongue

14. What is a normal finding on physical examination of the abdomen?
    a. Auscultation of bruits
    b. Observation of visible pulsations
    c. Percussion of liver dullness in the left midclavicular line
    d. Palpation of the spleen 1 to 2 cm below the left costal margin

15. A patient is admitted to the hospital with left upper quadrant (LUQ) pain. What may be a possible source of the pain?
    a. Liver
    b. Pancreas
    c. Appendix
    d. Gallbladder

16. What characterizes auscultation of the abdomen?
    a. The presence of borborygmi indicates hyperperistalsis.
    b. The bell of the stethoscope is used to auscultate high-pitched sounds.
    c. High-pitched, rushing, and tinkling bowel sounds are heard after eating.
    d. Absence of bowel sounds for 1 minute in each quadrant is reported as abnormal.

17. *Priority Decision:* Following auscultation of the abdomen, what should the nurse's next action be?
    a. Lightly percuss over all four quadrants
    b. Have the patient empty his or her bladder
    c. Inspect perianal and anal areas for color, masses, rashes, and scars
    d. Perform deep palpation to delineate abdominal organs and masses

18. Complete the table below by indicating with an X which preparations are required for each of the diagnostic procedures listed.
    (1) NPO up to 8 or more hours
    (2) Bowel emptying with laxatives, enemas, or both
    (3) Informed consent
    (4) Allergy to iodine assessed

Procedure	(1) NPO	(2) Bowel	(3) Consent	(4) Allergy
Upper GI series				
Barium enema				
Percutaneous transhepatic cholangiogram				
Gallbladder ultrasound				
Hepatobiliary scintigraphy				
Upper GI endoscopy				
Colonoscopy				
Endoscopic retrograde cholangiopancreatography (ERCP)				

19. A patient's serum liver enzyme tests reveal an elevated aspartate aminotransferase (AST). The nurse recognizes what about the elevated AST?
    a. It eliminates infection as a cause of liver damage.
    b. It is diagnostic for liver inflammation and damage.
    c. Tissue damage in organs other than the liver may be identified.
    d. Nervous system symptoms related to hepatic encephalopathy may be the cause.

20. Which nursing actions are indicated for a liver biopsy (*select all that apply*)?
    a. Observe for white stools
    b. Monitor for rectal bleeding
    c. Monitor for internal bleeding
    d. Position to right side after test
    e. Ensure bowel preparation was done
    f. Check coagulation status before test

21. Checking for the return of the gag reflex and monitoring for LUQ pain, nausea and vomiting are necessary nursing actions after which diagnostic procedure?
    a. ERCP
    b. Colonoscopy
    c. Barium swallow
    d. Esophagogastroduodenoscopy (EGD)

CHAPTER 40

Nursing Management: Nutritional Problems

1. A 30-year-old man's diet consists of 3000 calories with 120 g of protein, 160 g of fat, and 270 g of carbohydrate. He weighs 176 lb and is 5 ft, 11 in tall.
   a. In the table below, indicate what percentage of total calories each of the nutrients contributes to this man's diet.

Nutrient	Percentage of Total Calories from Nutrient
Protein	
Fat	
Carbohydrates	

   b. How many calories would be recommended for him as an average adult?
   c. Using MyPlate as a guide, what changes could the nurse suggest to bring the man's diet more in line with nutrition recommendations?

2. Which statement accurately describes vitamin deficiencies?
   a. The two nutrients most often lacking in the diet of a vegan are vitamin B_6 and folic acid.
   b. Vitamin imbalances occur frequently in the United States because of excessive fat intake.
   c. Surgery on the GI tract may contribute to vitamin deficiencies because of impaired absorption.
   d. Vitamin deficiencies in adults most commonly are clinically manifested by disorders of the skin.

3. What is the most common cause of secondary protein-calorie malnutrition in the United States?
   a. The unavailability of foods high in protein
   b. A lack of knowledge about nutritional needs
   c. A lack of money to purchase high-protein foods
   d. An alteration in ingestion, digestion, absorption, or metabolism

4. Describe the metabolism of nutrients used for energy during starvation within the given approximate time frames.

Time Frame	Metabolism of Nutrients
First 18 hours	
18 hours to 5 to 9 days	
9 days to 6 weeks	
Over 6 weeks	

5. What may occur with failure of the sodium-potassium pump during severe protein depletion?
   a. Ascites
   b. Anemia
   c. Hyperkalemia
   d. Hypoalbuminemia

6. What contributes to increased protein-calorie needs?
   a. Surgery
   b. Vegan diet
   c. Lowered temperature
   d. Cultural or religious beliefs

7. During assessment of the patient with protein-calorie malnutrition, what should the nurse expect to find (*select all that apply*)?
   a. Frequent cold symptoms
   b. Decreased bowel sounds
   c. Cool, rough, dry, scaly skin
   d. A flat or concave abdomen
   e. Prominent bony structures
   f. Decreased reflexes and lack of attention

8. Which patient has the highest risk for poor nutritional balance related to decreased ingestion?
   a. Tuberculosis infection
   b. Malabsorption syndrome
   c. Draining decubitus ulcers
   d. Severe anorexia resulting from radiation therapy

9. The nurse monitors the laboratory results of the patient with protein-calorie malnutrition during treatment. Which result is an indication of improvement in the patient's condition?
   a. Decreased lymphocytes
   b. Increased serum potassium
   c. Increased serum transferrin
   d. Decreased serum prealbumin

10. To evaluate the effect of nutritional interventions for a patient with protein-calorie malnutrition, what is the best indicator for the nurse to use?
    a. Height and weight
    b. Body mass index (BMI)
    c. Weight in relation to ideal body weight
    d. Mid-upper arm circumference and triceps skinfold

11. The nurse evaluates that patient teaching about a high-calorie, high-protein diet has been effective when the patient selects which breakfast option from the hospital menu?
    a. Two poached eggs, hash brown potatoes, and whole milk
    b. Two slices of toast with butter and jelly, orange juice, and skim milk
    c. Three pancakes with butter and syrup, two slices of bacon, and apple juice
    d. Cream of wheat with 2 tbsp of skim milk powder, one half grapefruit, and a high-protein milkshake

12. When teaching the older adult about nutritional needs during aging, what does the nurse emphasize?
    a. Need for all nutrients decreases as one ages.
    b. Fewer calories, but the same or slightly increased amount of protein, are required as one ages.
    c. Fats, carbohydrates, and protein should be decreased, but vitamin and mineral intake should be increased.
    d. High-calorie oral supplements should be taken between meals to ensure that recommended nutrient needs are met.

13. When planning nutritional interventions for a healthy 83-year-old man, the nurse recognizes what factor is most likely to affect his nutritional status?
    a. Living alone on a fixed income
    b. Changes in cardiovascular function
    c. An increase in GI motility and absorption
    d. Snacking between meals, resulting in obesity

14. When considering tube feedings for a patient with severe protein-calorie malnutrition, what is an advantage of a gastrostomy tube versus a nasogastric (NG) tube?
    a. There is less irritation to the nasal and esophageal mucosa.
    b. The patient experiences the sights and smells associated with eating.
    c. Aspiration resulting from reflux of formulas into the esophagus is less common.
    d. Routine checking for placement is not required because gastrostomy tubes do not become displaced.

15. Identify one nursing intervention indicated for each of the following desired outcomes of tube feeding.

Desired Outcome	Nursing Intervention
Prevention of aspiration	
Prevention of diarrhea	
Maintenance of tube patency	
Maintenance of tube placement	
Administration of medication	

16. *Priority Decision:* Before administering a bolus of intermittent tube feeding to a patient with a percutaneous endoscopic gastrostomy (PEG), the nurse aspirates 220 mL of gastric contents. How should the nurse respond?
    a. Return the aspirate to the stomach and recheck the volume of aspirate in an hour.
    b. Return the aspirate to the stomach and continue with the tube feeding as planned.
    c. Discard the aspirate to prevent overdistending the stomach when the new feeding is given.
    d. Notify the health care provider that the feedings have been scheduled too frequently to allow for stomach emptying.

17. **Delegation Decision:** Indicate whether the following nursing actions must be performed by the RN or if they can be delegated to unlicensed assistive personnel (UAP).

_____ a. Insert NG tube for stable patients.

_____ b. Weigh the patient receiving enteral feedings.

_____ c. Teach the patient about home gastric tube care.

_____ d. Remove an NG tube.

_____ e. Provide oral care to the patient with an NG tube.

_____ f. Position patient receiving enteral feedings.

_____ g. Monitor a patient with continuous feeding for complications.

_____ h. Respond to infusion pump alarm by reporting it to an RN or licensed practical nurse (LPN).

18. Indicate whether the following characteristics of parenteral nutrition apply more to central parenteral nutrition (CPN) or peripheral parenteral nutrition (PPN).

_____ a. Limited to 20% glucose

_____ b. Tonicity of 1600 mOsm/L

_____ c. Nutrients can be infused using smaller volumes

_____ d. Supplements oral feedings

_____ e. Long-term nutritional support

_____ f. Phlebitis more common

_____ g. May use peripherally inserted central catheter (PICC)

19. What is an indication for parenteral nutrition that is not an appropriate indication for enteral tube feedings?
a. Head and neck cancer
b. Hypermetabolic states
c. Malabsorption syndrome
d. Protein-calorie malnutrition

20. What nursing interventions are indicated during parenteral nutrition to prevent the following complications?

Complication	Preventive Measure
Infection	
Hyperglycemia	
Air embolism	

21. **Priority Decision:** The nurse is caring for a patient receiving 1000 mL of parenteral nutrition solution over 24 hours. When it is time to change the solution, 150 mL remain in the bottle. What is the most appropriate action by the nurse?
a. Hang the new solution and discard the unused solution.
b. Open the IV line and rapidly infuse the remaining solution.
c. Notify the health care provider for instructions regarding the infusion rate.
d. Wait to change the solution until the remaining solution infuses at the prescribed rate.

22. Identify the following characteristics of eating disorders as being associated with anorexia nervosa (A), bulimia (B), or both (AB).

_____ a. Treated with psychotherapy

_____ b. Ignores feelings of hunger

_____ c. Binge eating with purging

_____ d. Conceals abnormal eating habits

_____ e. Concerned about body image

_____ f. Self-induced starvation

_____ g. Compulsive exerciser

_____ h. Broken blood vessels in the eyes

23. *Priority Decision:* An 18-year-old female patient with anorexia nervosa is admitted to the hospital for treatment. On admission she weighs 82 lb (37 kg) and is 5 ft, 3 in (134.6 cm). Her laboratory test results include the following: K^+ 2.8 mEq/L (2.8 mmol/L), Hgb 8.9 g/dL (89 g/L), and BUN 64 mg/dL (22.8 mmol/L). In planning care for the patient, the nurse gives the highest priority to which of the following nursing diagnoses?
   a. Risk for injury *related to* dizziness and weakness resulting from anemia
   b. Imbalanced nutrition: less than body requirements *related to* inadequate food intake
   c. Risk for impaired urinary elimination *related to* elevated BUN resulting from renal failure
   d. Risk for decreased cardiac output (CO) *related to* dysrhythmias resulting from hypokalemia

---

CASE STUDY

Malnutrition

Patient Profile

R.M., a 62-year-old Hispanic widow, recently underwent radiation and chemotherapy following surgery for breast cancer. On a follow-up visit to the clinic, the nurse notes that R.M. appears thinner and more tired than usual.

Subjective Data

- Says she has not had an appetite since the treatment for cancer was started
- Feels "weak" and "worn out"
- Thinks the treatment for cancer has not been effective
- Lives alone in an apartment in the inner city
- Is a naturalized citizen from Honduras
- Speaks English but does not read English very well

Objective Data

Physical Examination
- Height: 5 ft, 2 in (155 cm)
- Weight: 92 lb (41.8 kg)
- Vital signs: BP 98/60, HR 60 bpm, RR 12
- Ulcerations of her buccal mucosal membranes and tongue

Laboratory Tests
- Serum albumin: 2.8 g/dL (28 g/L)
- Hgb: 10 g/dL (100 g/L)
- Hct: 32%

Discussion Questions

Using a separate sheet of paper, answer the following questions:

1. What additional assessment data should the nurse obtain from R.M. related to her nutritional status?
2. What physical and psychosocial factors have contributed to R.M.'s malnutrition?
3. What additional symptoms would the nurse expect to see based on R.M.'s laboratory test results?
4. What complications of malnutrition are most likely to occur in R.M. because of her history and clinical manifestations?
5. *Priority Decision:* What are the priority teaching instructions that the nurse should give to R.M. regarding her diet that would be most therapeutic?
6. *Priority Decision:* Based on the assessment data presented, what are the priority nursing diagnoses? Are there any collaborative problems?

CHAPTER 41

Nursing Management: Obesity

1. Using the body mass index (BMI) chart (Figure 41-2) in the textbook or the BMI formula:

$$\text{BMI (kg/m}^2) = \frac{\text{Weight (pounds)} \times 703}{\text{Height (inches)}^2}$$

   a. Determine the BMI for a patient who is 5 ft, 5 in (164 cm) and weighs 202 lb (91.8 kg). What is the patient's weight classification?
   b. Calculate the waist-to-hip ratio of a woman who has a waist measurement of 32 in and a hip measurement of 36 in. What does this value indicate?

2. Which statement about obesity is explained by genetics?
   a. Older obese patients have exacerbated changes of aging.
   b. Android body shape and weight gain are influenced by genetics.
   c. White Americans have a higher incidence of obesity than African Americans.
   d. Men have a harder time losing weight, as they have more muscle mass than women.

3. Which patient is at highest risk for complications of obesity?
   a. A 30-year-old woman who is 5 ft (151 cm) tall, weighs 140 lb (63.6 kg), and carries weight in her thighs
   b. A 56-year-old woman with a BMI of 38 kg/m^2, a waist measurement of 38 in (96 cm), and a hip measurement of 36 in (91 cm)
   c. A 42-year-old man with a waist measurement of 36 in (91 cm) and a hip measurement of 36 in (91 cm) who is 5 ft, 6 in (166 cm) tall and weighs 150 lb (68.2 kg)
   d. A 68-year-old man with a waist measurement of 38 in (96 cm) and a hip measurement of 42 in (76 cm) who is 5 ft, 11 in (179 cm) tall and weighs 200 lb (90.9 kg)

4. A woman is 5 ft, 6 in (166 cm) tall and weighs 200 lb (90.9 kg) with a waist-to-hip ratio of 0.7. The nurse counsels the patient with the knowledge that the patient is at greatest risk for
   a. heart disease.
   b. osteoporosis.
   c. diabetes mellitus.
   d. endometrial cancer.

5. *Priority Decision:* Before selecting a weight reduction plan with an obese patient, what is most important for the nurse to first assess?
   a. The patient's motivation to lose weight
   b. The length of time that the patient has been obese
   c. Whether financial considerations will affect the patient's choices
   d. The patient's anthropometric measures of height, weight, BMI, waist-to-hip ratio, and skinfold thickness

6. Normally, which hormones and peptides affect appetite (*select all that apply*)?
   a. Leptin
   b. Insulin
   c. Ghrelin
   d. Peptide YY
   e. Neuropeptide Y
   f. Cholecystokinin

7. *Priority Decision:* The nurse is teaching a moderately obese woman interventions for the management of obesity. Initially, which strategies will support restricting dietary intake to below energy requirements (*select all that apply*)?
   a. Limit alcohol
   b. Rest when fatigued
   c. Determine portion sizes
   d. 1800- to 2200-calorie diet
   e. Attend Overeaters Anonymous

8. Which explanation about weight reduction should be included when teaching the obese patient and her obese husband?
   a. Weight gain is caused by psychologic factors.
   b. Daily weighing is recommended to monitor weight loss.
   c. Fat is not burned until the glycogen-water pool is depleted.
   d. Men lose weight less quickly than women because they have a higher percentage of metabolically less-active fat.

9. A patient has been on a 1000-calorie diet with a daily exercise routine. In 2 months, the patient has lost 20 lb (9 kg) toward a goal of 50 lb (23 kg) but is now discouraged that no weight has been lost in the last 2 weeks. What should the nurse tell the patient about this?
   a. Plateaus where no weight is lost normally occur during a weight-loss program.
   b. A weight considered by the body to be most efficient for functioning has been reached.
   c. A return to former eating habits is the most common cause of not continuing to lose weight.
   d. A steady weight may be due to water gain from eating foods high in sodium.

10. When teaching a patient about weight reduction diets, the nurse teaches the patient that an appropriate single serving of a food is
    a. a 6-inch bagel.
    b. 1 cup of chopped vegetables.
    c. a piece of cheese the size of three dice.
    d. a chicken breast the size of a deck of cards.

11. *Priority Decision:* When medications are used in the treatment of obesity, what is most important for the nurse to teach the patient?
    a. Over-the-counter (OTC) diet aids are safer than other agents and can be useful in controlling appetite.
    b. Drugs should be used only as adjuncts to a diet and exercise program as treatment for a chronic condition.
    c. All drugs used for weight control are capable of altering central nervous system (CNS) function and should be used with caution.
    d. The primary effect of the medications is psychologic, controlling the urge to eat in response to stress or feelings of rejection.

12. A patient asks the nurse about taking phentermine and topiramate (Qsymia) for weight loss. To avoid side effects, it is important for the nurse to determine whether the patient has a history of
    a. glaucoma.
    b. hypertension.
    c. valvular heart disease.
    d. irritable bowel disease.

13. The nurse has completed initial instruction with a patient regarding a weight-loss program. Which patient comment indicates to the nurse that the teaching has been effective?
    a. "I will keep a diary of daily weight to illustrate my weight loss."
    b. "I plan to lose 4 lb a week until I have lost the 60 lb I want to lose."
    c. "I should not exercise more than what is required so I don't increase my appetite."
    d. "I plan to join a behavior modification group to help establish long-term behavior changes."

14. A 40-year-old severely obese female patient with type 2 diabetes wants to lose weight. After learning about the surgical procedures, she thinks a combination of restrictive and malabsorptive surgery would be best. Which procedure should the nurse teach her about?
    a. Lipectomy
    b. Roux-en-Y gastric bypass
    c. Adjustable gastric banding
    d. Vertical sleeve gastrectomy

15. What characteristics describe adjustable gastric banding (*select all that apply*)?
    a. 85% of the stomach is removed.
    b. Stomach restriction can be reversed.
    c. Eliminates hormones that stimulate hunger.
    d. Malabsorption of fat-soluble vitamins occurs.
    e. Inflatable band allows for modification of gastric stoma size.
    f. Stomach with a gastric pouch surgically anastomosed to the jejunum.

16. ***Priority Decision:*** During care of the severely obese patient, what is most important for the nurse to do?
    a. Avoid reference to the patient's weight to avoid embarrassing the patient.
    b. Emphasize to the patient how important it is to lose weight to maintain health.
    c. Plan for necessary modifications in equipment and nursing techniques before initiating care.
    d. Recognize that a full assessment of each body system might not be possible because of numerous layers of skinfolds.

17. In preparing to care for the obese patient with cancer, what physiologic problems is this patient at a greater risk for having (*select all that apply*)?
    a. Tinnitus
    b. Fractures
    c. Sleep apnea
    d. Trousseau's sign
    e. Type 2 diabetes mellitus
    f. Gastroesophageal reflux disease (GERD)

18. ***Priority Decision:*** The nurse admitting a patient for bariatric surgery obtains the following information from the patient. Which finding should be brought to the surgeon's attention before proceeding with further patient preparation?
    a. History of hypertension
    b. History of untreated depression
    c. History of multiple attempts at weight loss
    d. History of sleep apnea treated with continuous positive airway pressure (CPAP)

19. What is a postoperative nursing intervention for the obese patient who has undergone bariatric surgery?
    a. Irrigating and repositioning the nasogastric (NG) tube as needed
    b. Delaying ambulation until the patient has enough strength to support self
    c. Keeping the patient positioned on the side to facilitate respiratory function
    d. Providing adequate support to the incision during coughing, deep breathing, and turning

20. What information should be included in the dietary teaching for the patient following a Roux-en-Y gastric bypass?
    a. Avoid sugary foods and limit fluids to prevent dumping syndrome.
    b. Gradually increase the amount of food ingested to preoperative levels.
    c. Maintain a long-term liquid diet to prevent damage to the surgical site.
    d. Consume foods high in complex carbohydrates, protein, and fiber to add bulk to contents.

21. Which female patient is most likely to have metabolic syndrome?
    a. BP 128/78 mm Hg, triglycerides 160 mg/dL, fasting blood glucose 102 mg/dL
    b. BP 142/90 mm Hg, high-density lipoproteins 45 mg/dL, fasting blood glucose 130 mg/dL
    c. Waist circumference 36 in, triglycerides 162 mg/dL, high-density lipoproteins 55 mg/dL
    d. Waist circumference 32 in, high-density lipoproteins 38 mg/dL, fasting blood glucose 122 mg/dL

22. Which teaching points are important when providing information to a patient with metabolic syndrome (*select all that apply*)?
    a. Stop smoking.
    b. Monitor weight daily.
    c. Increase level of activity.
    d. Decrease saturated fat intake.
    e. Reduce weight and maintain lower weight.
    f. Check blood glucose each morning prior to eating.

23. What is the main underlying risk factor for metabolic syndrome?
    a. Age
    b. Heart disease
    c. Insulin resistance
    d. High cholesterol levels

CASE STUDY

Severe Obesity

Patient Profile

L.C., a 32-year-old single man, is seeking information at the outpatient center regarding possible bariatric surgery for his obesity. He reports that he has always been heavy, even as a small child, but he has gained about 100 lb in the last 2 to 3 years. Previous medical evaluations have not indicated any metabolic disease but he says he has sleep apnea and high BP, which he tries to control with sodium restriction. He currently works at a catalog telephone center.

Subjective Data

- Says he is constantly dieting but eventually hunger takes over and he eats to satisfy his appetite
- Reports that he used fenfluramine (Pondimin) for about 2 months before it was taken off the market but he lost only about 5 lb
- Admits to being treated for depression when he felt that he had no quality of life
- Lives alone in an apartment and has several good friends in the building but rarely socializes with them outside of the complex because of his size

Objective Data

Physical Examination
- Height: 68 in (171 cm)
- Weight: 296 lb (134.5 kg)
- Vital signs: BP 172/96, HR 88 bpm, RR 24
- Waist measure: 56 in (141 cm)

Laboratory Tests
- Fasting blood glucose: 146 mg/dL (8.1 mmol/L)
- Total cholesterol: 250 mg/dL (6.5 mmol/L)
- Triglycerides: 312 mg/dL (3.5 mmol/L)
- High-density lipoprotein (HDL): 30 mg/dL (0.77 mmol/L)

Discussion Questions

Using a separate sheet of paper, answer the following questions:

1. What is L.C.'s estimated BMI?
2. What health risks associated with obesity does L.C. have?
3. Does L.C. qualify for bariatric surgery? Why or why not?
4. L.C. says that he has read about Roux-en-Y gastric bypass surgery and the adjustable gastric banding surgery and asks which is best. What advantages and disadvantages of these procedures should the nurse explain to L.C.?

Surgical Procedure	Advantages	Disadvantages
Roux-en-Y gastric bypass		
Adjustable gastric banding		

5. *Priority Decision:* After an extensive workup by the health care provider, L.C. is scheduled for Roux-en-Y bypass surgery. What priority preoperative teaching should the nurse provide for L.C. before he is admitted to the hospital?
6. What discharge teaching should be provided for this patient?
7. *Priority Decision:* Based on the assessment data presented, what are the priority nursing diagnoses? Are there any collaborative problems?

1. What physiologically occurs with vomiting?
   a. The acid-base imbalance most commonly associated with persistent vomiting is metabolic acidosis caused by loss of bicarbonate.
   b. Stimulation of the vomiting center by the chemoreceptor trigger zone (CTZ) is commonly caused by stretch and distention of hollow organs.
   c. Vomiting requires the coordination of activities of structures including the glottis, respiratory expiration, relaxation of the pylorus, and closure of the lower esophageal sphincter.
   d. Immediately before the act of vomiting, activation of the parasympathetic nervous system causes increased salivation, increased gastric motility, and relaxation of the lower esophageal sphincter.

2. Which laboratory findings should the nurse expect in the patient with persistent vomiting?
   a. ↓ pH, ↑ sodium, ↓ hematocrit
   b. ↑ pH, ↓ chloride, ↓ hematocrit
   c. ↑ pH, ↓ potassium, ↑ hematocrit
   d. ↓ pH, ↓ potassium, ↑ hematocrit

3. A patient who has been vomiting for several days from an unknown cause is admitted to the hospital. What should the nurse anticipate will be included in collaborative care?
   a. Oral administration of broth and tea
   b. IV replacement of fluid and electrolytes
   c. Administration of parenteral antiemetics
   d. Insertion of a nasogastric (NG) tube for suction

4. *Priority Decision:* A patient treated for vomiting is to begin oral intake when the symptoms have subsided. To promote rehydration, the nurse plans to administer which fluid first?
   a. Water
   b. Hot tea
   c. Gatorade
   d. Warm broth

5. Ondansetron (Zofran) is prescribed for a patient with cancer chemotherapy–induced vomiting. What should the nurse understand about this drug?
   a. It is a derivative of cannabis and has a potential for abuse.
   b. It has a strong antihistamine effect that provides sedation and induces sleep.
   c. It is used only when other therapies are ineffective because of side effects of anxiety and hallucinations.
   d. It relieves vomiting centrally by action in the vomiting center and peripherally by promoting gastric emptying.

6. *Priority Decision:* Older patients may have cardiac or renal insufficiency and may be more susceptible to problems from vomiting and antiemetic drug side effects. What nursing intervention is most important to implement with these patients?
   a. Keep the patient flat in bed to decrease dizziness.
   b. Keep the patient NPO until nausea and vomiting has stopped.
   c. Do hourly visual checks or use a sitter to keep the patient safe.
   d. Administer IV fluids as rapidly as possible to prevent dehydration.

7. What are characteristics of gingivitis?
   a. Formation of abscesses with loosening of teeth
   b. Caused by upper respiratory tract viral infection
   c. Shallow, painful vesicular ulcerations of lips and mouth
   d. Infectious ulcers of mouth and lips as a result of systemic disease

8. Which infection or inflammation is found related to systemic disease and cancer chemotherapy?
   a. Parotitis
   b. Stomatitis
   c. Oral candidiasis
   d. Vincent's infection

9. A patient is scheduled for biopsy of a painful tongue ulcer. Based on knowledge of risk factors for oral cancer, what should the nurse specifically ask the patient about during a history?
   a. Excessive exposure to sunlight
   b. Recurrent herpes simplex infections
   c. Use of any type of tobacco products
   d. Difficulty swallowing and pain in the ear

10. *Priority Decision:* When caring for a patient following a glossectomy with dissection of the floor of the mouth and a radical neck dissection for cancer of the tongue, what is the nurse's primary concern?
   a. Relief of pain
   b. Patent airway
   c. Positive body image
   d. Tube feedings to provide nutrition

11. A patient with oral cancer has a history of heavy smoking, excessive alcohol intake, and personal neglect. During the patient's early postoperative course, what does the nurse anticipate that the patient may need?
   a. Oral nutritional supplements
   b. Drug therapy to prevent substance withdrawal symptoms
   c. Counseling about lifestyle changes to prevent recurrence of the tumor
   d. Less pain medication because of cross-tolerance with central nervous system (CNS) depressants

12. The nurse is planning to teach the patient with gastroesophageal reflux disease (GERD) about foods or beverages that decrease lower esophageal sphincter (LES) pressure. What should be included in this list (*select all that apply*)?
   a. Alcohol
   b. Root beer
   c. Chocolate
   d. Citrus fruits
   e. Fatty foods
   f. Cola sodas

13. How should the nurse teach the patient with a hiatal hernia or GERD to control symptoms?
   a. Drink 10 to 12 oz of water with each meal.
   b. Space six small meals a day between breakfast and bedtime.
   c. Sleep with the head of the bed elevated on 4- to 6-inch blocks
   d. Perform daily exercises of toe-touching, sit-ups, and weight lifting.

14. *Priority Decision:* A patient with esophageal cancer is scheduled for a partial esophagectomy. Which nursing intervention is likely to be of highest priority preoperatively?
   a. Practice turning and deep breathing.
   b. Brush the teeth and mouth well each day.
   c. Encourage a high-calorie, high-protein diet.
   d. Teach about postoperative tubes and cares.

15. *Priority Decision:* Following a patient's esophagogastrostomy for cancer of the esophagus, what is most important for the nurse to do?
   a. Report any bloody drainage from the NG tube.
   b. Maintain the patient in semi-Fowler's or Fowler's position.
   c. Monitor for abdominal distention that may disrupt the surgical site.
   d. Expect to find decreased breath sounds bilaterally because of the surgical approach.

16. Which esophageal disorder is described as a precancerous lesion associated with GERD?
   a. Achalasia
   b. Barrett's esophagus
   c. Esophageal strictures
   d. Esophageal diverticula

17. What is an accurate description of eosinophilic esophagitis?
   a. Adenocarcinoma or squamous cell tumors of the esophagus
   b. Dilated veins in the esophagus caused by portal hypertension
   c. Inflammation of the esophagus from irritants or gastric reflux
   d. Swelling of the esophagus caused by an allergic response to food or environmental triggers

18. Which type of gastritis is most likely to occur in a college student who has an isolated drinking binge?
   a. Acute gastritis
   b. Chronic gastritis
   c. *Helicobacter pylori* gastritis
   d. Autoimmune metaplastic atrophic gastritis

19. Nursing management of the patient with chronic gastritis includes teaching the patient to
    a. take antacids before meals to decrease stomach acidity.
    b. maintain a nonirritating diet with six small meals a day.
    c. eliminate alcohol and caffeine from the diet when symptoms occur.
    d. use nonsteroidal antiinflammatory drugs (NSAIDs) instead of aspirin for minor pain relief.

20. Duodenal and gastric ulcers have similar as well as differentiating features. What are characteristics unique to duodenal ulcers (*select all that apply*)?
    a. Pain is relieved with eating food.
    b. They have a high recurrence rate.
    c. Increased gastric secretion occurs.
    d. Associated with *Helicobacter pylori* infection.
    e. Hemorrhage, perforation, and obstruction may result.
    f. There is burning and cramping in the midepigastric area.

21. Which patient is at highest risk for having a gastric ulcer?
    a. 55-year-old female, smoker, with nausea and vomiting
    b. 45-year-old female admitted for illicit drug detoxification
    c. 37-year-old male, smoker, who fell while looking for a job
    d. 27-year old male who is being divorced and has back pain

22. Corticosteroid medications are associated with the development of peptic ulcers because of which probable pathophysiologic mechanism?
    a. The enzyme urease is produced.
    b. Secretion of hydrochloric acid is increased.
    c. The rate of mucous cell renewal is decreased.
    d. The synthesis of mucus and prostaglandins is inhibited.

23. Regardless of the precipitating factor, what causes the injury to mucosal cells in peptic ulcers?
    a. Acid back diffusion into the mucosa
    b. The release of histamine from GI cells
    c. Ammonia formation in the mucosal wall
    d. Breakdown of the gastric mucosal barrier

24. What type of pain does the nurse expect a patient with an ulcer of the posterior portion of the duodenum to experience?
    a. Pain that occurs after not eating all day
    b. Back pain that occurs 2 to 4 hours following meals
    c. Midepigastric pain that is unrelieved with antacids
    d. High epigastric burning that is relieved with food intake

25. What does the nurse include when teaching a patient with newly diagnosed peptic ulcer disease?
    a. Maintain a bland, soft, low-residue diet.
    b. Use alcohol and caffeine in moderation and always with food.
    c. Eat as normally as possible, eliminating foods that cause pain or discomfort.
    d. Avoid milk and milk products because they stimulate gastric acid production.

26. What is the rationale for treating acute exacerbation of peptic ulcer disease with NG intubation?
    a. Stop spillage of GI contents into the peritoneal cavity
    b. Remove excess fluids and undigested food from the stomach
    c. Feed the patient the nutrients missing from the lack of ingestion
    d. Remove stimulation for hydrochloric acid and pepsin secretion by keeping the stomach empty

27. Which statements are characteristic of the uses of antacids for peptic ulcer disease (*select all that apply*)?
    a. Used in patients with verified *H. pylori*
    b. Patients frequently noncompliant with use
    c. Prevent conversion of pepsinogen to pepsin
    d. Cover the ulcer, protecting it from erosion by acids
    e. High incidence of side effects and contraindications
    f. High dose and frequency stimulate release of gastrin

28. Which medications are used to decrease gastric or hydrochloric acid secretion (*select all that apply*)?
    a. Famotidine (Pepcid)
    b. Sucralfate (Carafate)
    c. Omeprazole (Prilosec)
    d. Misoprostol (Cytotec)
    e. Amoxicillin/clarithromycin/omeprazole

29. The nurse determines that teaching for the patient with peptic ulcer disease has been effective when the patient makes which statement?
    a. "I should stop all my medications if I develop any side effects."
    b. "I should continue my treatment regimen as long as I have pain."
    c. "I have learned some relaxation strategies that decrease my stress."
    d. "I can buy whatever antacids are on sale because they all have the same effect."

30. A patient with a history of peptic ulcer disease is hospitalized with symptoms of a perforation. During the initial assessment, what should the nurse expect the patient to report?
    a. Vomiting of bright-red blood
    b. Projectile vomiting of undigested food
    c. Sudden, severe upper abdominal pain and back pain
    d. Hyperactive stomach sounds and upper abdominal swelling

31. *Priority Decision:* A patient with a gastric outlet obstruction has been treated with NG decompression. After the first 24 hours, the patient develops nausea and increased upper abdominal bowel sounds. What is the best action by the nurse?
    a. Check the patency of the NG tube.
    b. Place the patient in a recumbent position.
    c. Assess the patient's vital signs and circulatory status.
    d. Encourage the patient to deep breathe and consciously relax.

32. *Priority Decision:* When caring for a patient with an acute exacerbation of a peptic ulcer, the nurse finds the patient doubled up in bed with shallow, grunting respirations. Which action should the nurse take first?
    a. Irrigate the patient's NG tube.
    b. Notify the health care provider.
    c. Place the patient in high-Fowler's position.
    d. Assess the patient's abdomen and vital signs.

33. Match the descriptions with the following surgical procedures used to treat peptic ulcer disease.
    _____ a. Often performed with a vagotomy to increase gastric emptying
    _____ b. Severing of a parasympathetic nerve to decrease gastric secretion
    _____ c. Removal of distal two thirds of stomach with anastomosis to jejunum
    _____ d. Removal of distal two thirds of stomach with anastomosis to duodenum

    1. Billroth I
    2. Billroth II
    3. Pyloroplasty
    4. Vagotomy

34. Following a Billroth II procedure, a patient develops dumping syndrome. The nurse should explain that the symptoms associated with this problem are caused by
    a. distention of the smaller stomach by too much food and fluid intake.
    b. hyperglycemia caused by uncontrolled gastric emptying into the small intestine.
    c. irritation of the stomach lining by reflux of bile salts because the pylorus has been removed.
    d. movement of fluid into the small bowel because concentrated food and fluids move rapidly into the intestine.

35. Which statement by a patient with dumping syndrome should lead the nurse to determine that further dietary teaching is needed?
    a. "I should eat bread and jam with every meal."
    b. "I should avoid drinking fluids with my meals."
    c. "I should eat smaller meals about six times a day."
    d. "I need to lie down for 30 to 60 minutes after my meals."

36. *Priority Decision:* While caring for a patient following a subtotal gastrectomy with a gastroduodenostomy anastomosis, the nurse determines that the NG tube is obstructed. Which action should the nurse take first?
    a. Replace the tube with a new one.
    b. Irrigate the tube until return can be aspirated.
    c. Reposition the tube and then attempt irrigation.
    d. Notify the surgeon to reposition or replace the tube.

37. A patient with cancer of the stomach at the lesser curvature undergoes a total gastrectomy with an esophagojejunostomy. Postoperatively, what should the nurse teach the patient to expect?
    a. Rapid healing of the surgical wound
    b. Lifelong administration of cobalamin
    c. To be able to return to normal dietary habits
    d. Close follow-up for development of peptic ulcers in the jejunum

38. What type of bleeding will a patient with peptic ulcer disease with a slow upper GI source of bleeding have?
    a. Melena
    b. Occult blood
    c. Coffee-ground emesis
    d. Profuse bright-red hematemesis

39. *Priority Decision:* A patient is admitted to the emergency department with profuse bright-red hematemesis. During the initial care of the patient, what is the nurse's first priority?
    a. Establish two IV sites with large-gauge catheters
    b. Perform a focused nursing assessment of the patient's status
    c. Obtain a thorough health history to assist in determining the cause of the bleeding
    d. Perform a gastric lavage with cool tap water in preparation for endoscopic examination

40. A patient with upper GI bleeding is treated with several drugs. Which drug should the nurse recognize as an agent that is used to decrease bleeding and decrease gastric acid secretions?
    a. Nizatidine (Axid)
    b. Omeprazole (Prilosec)
    c. Vasopressin (Pitressin)
    d. Octreotide (Sandostatin)

41. What should the nurse emphasize when teaching patients at risk for upper GI bleeding to prevent bleeding episodes?
    a. All stools and vomitus must be tested for the presence of blood.
    b. The use of over-the-counter (OTC) medications of any kind should be avoided.
    c. Antacids should be taken with all prescribed medications to prevent gastric irritation.
    d. Misoprostol (Cytotec) should be used to protect the gastric mucosa in individuals with peptic ulcers.

42. The nurse evaluates that management of the patient with upper GI bleeding is effective when assessment and laboratory findings reveal which result?
    a. Hematocrit (Hct) of 35%
    b. Urinary output of 20 mL/hr
    c. Urine specific gravity of 1.030
    d. Decreasing blood urea nitrogen (BUN)

43. A large number of children at a public school have developed profuse diarrhea and bloody stools. The school nurse suspects food poisoning related to food from the school cafeteria and requests analysis and culture of which food?
    a. Chicken
    b. Ground beef
    c. Commercially canned fish
    d. Salads with mayonnaise dressing

CASE STUDY
Gastric Cancer

Patient Profile

S.E. is a 75-year-old retired garment worker who was diagnosed with gastric cancer 2 weeks ago. The home health nurse assigned to her case reads the following information on her medical record.

Subjective Data

- 6-month history of epigastric discomfort, anorexia, nausea, vomiting, and a 25-lb weight loss
- Stated she has had "stomach problems" for a long time and was diagnosed with gastritis 20 years ago
- Stated she was told that the tumor could not be removed because it was too advanced
- Stated: "I've always been a strong person but now I'm just too tired to eat or do anything."

Objective Data

Physical Examination
- Palpable mass in left upper quadrant of the abdomen

Diagnostic Studies
- Barium swallow, gastroscopy, and biopsy/cytology all confirmed the presence of a well-advanced tumor in the fundus of the stomach

Laboratory Tests
- Decreased hemoglobin and hematocrit
- Serum albumin: 2.4 g/dL (24 g/L)
- Appears emaciated, with areas of skin discoloration on her forearms

When the nurse visits S.E., she has just returned from a radiation treatment and is holding a plastic emesis basin and tissues in her lap.

Discussion Questions

Using a separate sheet of paper, answer the following questions:
1. What pathophysiologic changes occur in gastric cancer that led to the symptoms experienced by S.E.?
2. What subjective and objective data indicate that S.E. has the presence of malnutrition?
3. What other factors might be contributing to S.E.'s malnutrition besides those described?
4. What other complications may develop as a result of S.E.'s malnutrition?
5. *Priority Decision:* What priority interventions should the nurse include in the treatment plan for S.E. and her family?
6. S.E. asks the nurse if anyone with her stage of gastric cancer has ever recovered. What is the nurse's best response to S.E.?
7. *Priority Decision:* Based on the assessment data presented, what are the priority nursing diagnoses? Are there any collaborative problems?

1. The nurse identifies a need for additional teaching when a patient with acute infectious diarrhea makes which statement?
   a. "I can use A&D ointment or Vaseline jelly around the anal area to protect my skin."
   b. "Gatorade is a good liquid to drink because it replaces the fluid and salts I have lost."
   c. "I may use over-the-counter Imodium or Parepectolin when I need to control the diarrhea."
   d. "I must wash my hands after every bowel movement to prevent spreading the diarrhea to my family."

2. *Priority Decision:* What is the most important thing the nurse should do when caring for a patient who has contracted *Clostridium difficile*?
   a. Clean the entire room with ammonia.
   b. Feed the patient yogurt with probiotics.
   c. Wear gloves and wash hands with soap and water.
   d. Teach the family to use alcohol-based hand cleaners.

3. *Priority Decision:* In instituting a bowel training program for a patient with fecal incontinence, what should the nurse first plan to do?
   a. Teach the patient to use a perianal pouch.
   b. Insert a rectal suppository at the same time every morning.
   c. Place the patient on a bedpan 30 minutes before breakfast.
   d. Assist the patient to the bathroom at the time of the patient's normal defecation.

4. A nurse is doing a nursing assessment on a patient with chronic constipation. What data obtained during the interview may be a factor contributing to the constipation?
   a. Taking methylcellulose (Citrucel) daily
   b. High dietary fiber with high fluid intake
   c. History of hemorrhoids and hypertension
   d. Suppressing the urge to defecate while at work

5. The nurse should teach the patient with chronic constipation that which food has the highest dietary fiber?
   a. Peach
   b. Popcorn
   c. Dried beans
   d. Shredded wheat

6. Which method is preferred for immediate treatment of an acute episode of constipation?
   a. An enema
   b. Increased fluid
   c. Stool softeners
   d. Bulk-forming medication

7. *Priority Decision:* A patient is admitted to the emergency department with acute abdominal pain. What nursing intervention should the nurse implement first?
   a. Measurement of vital signs
   b. Administration of prescribed analgesics
   c. Assessment of the onset, location, intensity, duration, and character of the pain
   d. Physical assessment of the abdomen for distention, bowel sounds, and pigmentation changes

8. When considering the following causes of acute abdomen, the nurse should know that surgery would be indicated for (*select all that apply*)?
   a. pancreatitis
   b. acute ischemic bowel
   c. foreign-body perforation
   d. pelvic inflammatory disease
   e. ruptured ectopic pregnancy
   f. ruptured abdominal aneurysm

9. ***Priority Decision:*** A patient returns to the surgical unit with a nasogastric (NG) tube to low intermittent suction, IV fluids, and a Jackson-Pratt drain at the surgical site following an exploratory laparotomy and repair of a bowel perforation. Four hours after admission, the patient experiences nausea and vomiting. What is a priority nursing intervention for the patient?
   a. Assess the abdomen for distention and bowel sounds.
   b. Inspect the surgical site and drainage in the Jackson-Pratt.
   c. Check the amount and character of gastric drainage and the patency of the NG tube.
   d. Administer prescribed prochlorperazine (Compazine) to control the nausea and vomiting.

10. ***Priority Decision:*** A postoperative patient has a nursing diagnosis of pain *related to* effects of medication and decreased GI motility *as evidenced by* abdominal pain and distention and inability to pass flatus. Which nursing intervention is most appropriate for this patient?
    a. Ambulate the patient more frequently.
    b. Assess the abdomen for bowel sounds.
    c. Place the patient in high Fowler's position.
    d. Withhold opioids because they decrease bowel motility.

11. A 22-year-old patient calls the outpatient clinic complaining of nausea and vomiting and right lower abdominal pain. What should the nurse advise the patient to do?
    a. Use a heating pad to relax the muscles at the site of the pain.
    b. Drink at least 2 quarts of juice to replace the fluid lost in vomiting.
    c. Take a laxative to empty the bowel before examination at the clinic.
    d. Have the symptoms evaluated by a health care provider right away.

12. ***Priority Decision:*** When caring for a patient with irritable bowel syndrome (IBS), what is most important for the nurse to do?
    a. Recognize that IBS is a psychogenic illness that cannot be definitively diagnosed.
    b. Develop a trusting relationship with the patient to provide support and symptomatic care.
    c. Teach the patient that a diet high in fiber will relieve the symptoms of both diarrhea and constipation.
    d. Inform the patient that new medications for IBS are available and effective for treatment of IBS manifested by either diarrhea or constipation.

13. ***Priority Decision:*** A patient with a gunshot wound to the abdomen complains of increasing abdominal pain several hours after surgery to repair the bowel. What action should the nurse take first?
    a. Take the patient's vital signs.
    b. Notify the health care provider.
    c. Position the patient with the knees flexed.
    d. Determine the patient's IV intake since the end of surgery.

14. The patient has persistent and continuous pain at McBurney's point. The nursing assessment reveals rebound tenderness and muscle guarding with the patient preferring to lie still with the right leg flexed. What should the nursing interventions for this patient include?
    a. Laxatives to move the constipated bowel
    b. NPO status in preparation for possible appendectomy
    c. Parenteral fluids and antibiotic therapy for 6 hours before surgery
    d. NG tube inserted to decompress the stomach and prevent aspiration

15. The patient has peritonitis, which is a major complication of appendicitis. What treatment will the nurse plan to include?
    a. Peritoneal lavage
    b. Peritoneal dialysis
    c. IV fluid replacement
    d. Increased oral fluid intake

16. A 20-year old patient with a history of Crohn's disease comes to the clinic with persistent diarrhea. What are characteristics of Crohn's disease (*select all that apply*)?
    a. Weight loss
    b. Rectal bleeding
    c. Abdominal pain
    d. Toxic megacolon
    e. Has segmented distribution
    f. Involves the entire thickness of the bowel wall

17. What laboratory findings are expected in ulcerative colitis as a result of diarrhea and vomiting?
    a. Increased albumin
    b. Elevated white blood cells (WBCs)
    c. Decreased Na^+, K^+, Mg^+, Cl^-, and HCO_3^-
    d. Decreased hemoglobin (Hgb) and hematocrit (Hct)

18. What extraintestinal manifestations are seen in both ulcerative colitis and Crohn's disease?
    a. Celiac disease and gallstones
    b. Peptic ulcer disease and uveitis
    c. Conjunctivitis and colonic dilation
    d. Erythema nodosum and osteoporosis

19. For the patient hospitalized with inflammatory bowel disease (IBD), which treatments would be used to rest the bowel (*select all that apply*)?
    a. NPO
    b. IV fluids
    c. Bed rest
    d. Sedatives
    e. Nasogastric suction
    f. Parenteral nutrition

20. The medications prescribed for the patient with inflammatory bowel disease include cobalamin and iron injections. What is the rationale for using these drugs?
    a. Alleviate stress
    b. Combat infection
    c. Correct malnutrition
    d. Improve quality of life

21. The patient is receiving the following medications. Which one is prescribed to relieve symptoms rather than treat a disease?
    a. Corticosteroids
    b. 6-Mercaptopurine
    c. Antidiarrheal agents
    d. Sulfasalazine (Azulfidine)

22. A patient with ulcerative colitis undergoes the first phase of a total proctocolectomy with ileal pouch and anal anastomosis. On postoperative assessment of the patient, what should the nurse expect to find?
    a. A rectal tube set to low continuous suction
    b. A loop ileostomy with a plastic rod to hold it in place
    c. A colostomy stoma with an NG tube in place to provide pouch irrigations
    d. A permanent ileostomy stoma in the right lower quadrant of the abdomen

23. ***Priority Decision:*** A patient with ulcerative colitis has a total proctocolectomy with formation of a terminal ileum stoma. What is the most important nursing intervention for this patient postoperatively?
    a. Measure the ileostomy output to determine the status of the patient's fluid balance.
    b. Change the ileostomy appliance every 3 to 4 hours to prevent leakage of drainage onto the skin.
    c. Emphasize that the ostomy is temporary and the ileum will be reconnected when the large bowel heals.
    d. Teach the patient about the high-fiber, low-carbohydrate diet required to maintain normal ileostomy drainage.

24. A patient with inflammatory bowel disease has a nursing diagnosis of imbalanced nutrition: less than body requirements *related to* decreased nutritional intake and decreased intestinal absorption. Which assessment data support this nursing diagnosis?
    a. Pallor and hair loss
    b. Frequent diarrhea stools
    c. Anorectal excoriation and pain
    d. Hypotension and urine output below 30 mL/hr

25. A physician just told a patient that she has a volvulus. When the patient asks the nurse what this is, what is the best description for the nurse to give her?
    a. Bowel folding on itself
    b. Twisting of bowel on itself
    c. Emboli of arterial supply to the bowel
    d. Protrusion of bowel in weak or abnormal opening

26. The patient comes to the emergency department with intermittent crampy abdominal pain, nausea, projectile vomiting, and dehydration. The nurse suspects a GI obstruction. Based on the manifestations, what area of the bowel should the nurse suspect is obstructed?
    a. Large intestine
    b. Esophageal sphincter
    c. Upper small intestine
    d. Lower small intestine

27. An important nursing intervention for a patient with a small intestinal obstruction who has an NG tube is to
    a. offer ice chips to suck PRN.
    b. provide mouth care every 1 to 2 hours.
    c. irrigate the tube with normal saline every 8 hours.
    d. keep the patient supine with the head of the bed elevated 30 degrees.

28. During a routine screening colonoscopy on a 56-year-old patient, a rectosigmoidal polyp was identified and removed. The patient asks the nurse if his risk for colon cancer is increased because of the polyp. What is the best response by the nurse?
    a. "It is very rare for polyps to become malignant but you should continue to have routine colonoscopies."
    b. "Individuals with polyps have a 100% lifetime risk of developing colorectal cancer and at an earlier age than those without polyps."
    c. "All polyps are abnormal and should be removed but the risk for cancer depends on the type and if malignant changes are present."
    d. "All polyps are premalignant and a source of most colon cancer. You will need to have a colonoscopy every 6 months to check for new polyps."

29. When obtaining a nursing history from the patient with colorectal cancer, the nurse should specifically ask the patient about
    a. dietary intake.
    b. sports involvement.
    c. environmental exposure to carcinogens.
    d. long-term use of nonsteroidal antiinflammatory drugs (NSAIDs).

30. When a patient returns to the clinical unit after an abdominal-perineal resection (APR), what should the nurse expect?
    a. An abdominal dressing
    b. An abdominal wound and drains
    c. A temporary colostomy and drains
    d. A perineal wound, drains, and a stoma

31. The patient with a new ileostomy needs discharge teaching. What should the nurse plan to include in this teaching?
    a. The pouch can be worn for up to 2 weeks before changing it.
    b. Decrease the amount of fluid intake to decrease the amount of drainage.
    c. The pouch can be removed when bowel movements have been regulated.
    d. If leakage occurs, promptly remove the pouch, clean the skin, and apply a new pouch.

32. On examining a patient 8 hours after having surgery to create a colostomy, what should the nurse expect to find?
    a. Hyperactive, high-pitched bowel sounds
    b. A brick-red, puffy stoma that oozes blood
    c. A purplish stoma, shiny and moist with mucus
    d. A small amount of liquid fecal drainage from the stoma

33. **Delegation Decision:** The RN coordinating the care for a patient who is 2 days postoperative following an anterior-posterior resection with colostomy may delegate which interventions to the licensed practical nurse (LPN) (*select all that apply*)?
    a. Irrigate the colostomy.
    b. Teach ostomy and skin care.
    c. Assess and document stoma appearance.
    d. Monitor and record the volume, color, and odor of the drainage.
    e. Empty the ostomy bag and measure and record the amount of drainage.

34. A male patient who has undergone an anterior-posterior repair is worried about his sexuality. What is an appropriate nursing intervention for this patient?
    a. Have the patient's sexual partner reassure the patient that he is still desirable.
    b. Reassure the patient that sexual function will return when healing is complete.
    c. Remind the patient that affection can be expressed in ways other than through sexual intercourse.
    d. Explain that physical and emotional factors can affect sexual function but not necessarily the patient's sexuality.

35. In report, the nurse learns that the patient has a transverse colostomy. What should the nurse expect when providing care for this patient?
    a. Semiliquid stools with increased fluid requirements
    b. Liquid stools in a pouch and increased fluid requirements
    c. Formed stools with a pouch, needing irrigation, but no fluid needs
    d. Semiformed stools in a pouch with the need to monitor fluid balance

36. The nurse plans teaching for the patient with a colostomy but the patient refuses to look at the nurse or the stoma, stating, "I just can't see myself with this thing." What is the best nursing intervention for this patient?
    a. Encourage the patient to share concerns and ask questions.
    b. Refer the patient to a chaplain to help cope with this situation.
    c. Explain that there is nothing the patient can do about it and must take care of it.
    d. Tell the patient that learning about it will prevent stool leaking and the sounds of flatus.

37. What information should be included when the nurse teaches a patient about colostomy irrigation?
    a. Infuse 1500 to 2000 mL of warm tap water as irrigation fluid.
    b. Allow 30 to 45 minutes for the solution and feces to be expelled.
    c. Insert a firm plastic catheter 3 to 4 inches into the stoma opening.
    d. Hang the irrigation bag on a hook about 36 inches above the stoma.

38. What should the nurse teach the patient with diverticulosis to do?
    a. Use anticholinergic drugs routinely to prevent bowel spasm.
    b. Have an annual colonoscopy to detect malignant changes in the lesions.
    c. Maintain a high-fiber diet and use bulk laxatives to increase fecal volume.
    d. Exclude whole grain breads and cereals from the diet to prevent irritating the bowel.

39. An 82-year-old man is admitted with an acute attack of diverticulitis. What should the nurse include in his care?
    a. Monitor for signs of peritonitis.
    b. Treat with daily medicated enemas.
    c. Prepare for surgery to resect the involved colon.
    d. Provide a heating pad to apply to the left lower quadrant.

40. The patient calls the clinic and describes a bump at the site of a previous incision that disappears when he lies down. The nurse suspects that this is which type of hernia (*select all that apply*)?
    a. Ventral   d. Reducible
    b. Inguinal   e. Incarcerated
    c. Femoral   f. Strangulated

41. The patient asks the nurse why she needs to have surgery for a femoral, strangulated hernia. What is the best explanation the nurse can give the patient?
    a. The surgery will relieve her constipation.
    b. The abnormal hernia must be replaced into the abdomen.
    c. The surgery is needed to allow intestinal flow and prevent necrosis.
    d. The hernia is because the umbilical opening did not close after birth as it should have.

42. What is a nursing intervention that is indicated for a male patient following an inguinal herniorrhaphy?
    a. Applying heat to the inguinal area   c. Applying a truss to support the operative site
    b. Elevating the scrotum with a scrotal support   d. Encouraging the patient to cough and deep breathe

43. How is the most common form of malabsorption syndrome treated?
    a. Administration of antibiotics
    b. Avoidance of milk and milk products
    c. Supplementation with pancreatic enzymes
    d. Avoidance of gluten found in wheat, barley, oats, and rye

44. A patient is diagnosed with celiac disease following a workup for iron-deficiency anemia and decreased bone density. The nurse identifies that additional teaching about disease management is needed when the patient makes which statement?
    a. "I should ask my close relatives to be screened for celiac disease."
    b. "If I do not follow the gluten-free diet, I might develop a lymphoma."
    c. "I don't need to restrict gluten intake because I don't have diarrhea or bowel symptoms."
    d. "It is going to be difficult to follow a gluten-free diet because it is found in so many foods."

45. Which patient is most likely to be diagnosed with short bowel syndrome?
    a. History of ulcerative colitis
    b. Had extensive resection of the ileum
    c. Diagnosed with irritable bowel syndrome
    d. Had colectomy performed for cancer of the bowel

46. The patient asks the nurse to explain what the physician meant when he said the patient had an anorectal abscess. Which description should the nurse use to explain this to the patient?
    a. Ulcer in anal wall
    b. Collection of perianal pus
    c. Sacrococcygeal hairy tract
    d. Tunnel leading from the anus or rectum

47. A 60-year-old African American patient is afraid she might have anal cancer. What assessment finding puts her at high risk for anal cancer?
    a. Alcohol use
    b. Only one sexual partner
    c. Human papillomavirus (HPV)
    d. Use of a condom with sexual intercourse

48. Following a hemorrhoidectomy, what should the nurse advise the patient to do?
    a. Use daily laxatives to facilitate bowel emptying.
    b. Use ice packs to the perineum to prevent swelling.
    c. Avoid having a bowel movement for several days until healing occurs.
    d. Take warm sitz baths several times a day to promote comfort and cleaning.

CASE STUDY
Cancer of the Rectum
Patient Profile

C.D., a 63-year-old married insurance salesman, has undergone an abdominal-perineal resection for stage III cancer of the rectum. He is 1 day postoperative on the general surgical unit.

Subjective Data

- Complains of pain in his abdominal and perineal incisions that is not well controlled even with his patient-controlled analgesia (PCA) machine
- Jokes about his stoma winking at him when the dressings are removed the first time and a temporary colostomy bag is applied
- Refers to his stoma as "Jake"
- Tells his wife that "Jake" will be watching her

Objective Data

- Bright-red stoma on left lower quadrant of abdomen; colostomy bag has small amount of pink mucus drainage
- Midline abdominal incision; no signs of infection; sutures intact
- Perineal incision partially closed; two Penrose drains with bulky dressings with a large amount of serosanguineous drainage
- All vital signs normal
- PCA orders of 1 mg morphine sulfate every 10 minutes, with 17 attempts in the past hour

Discussion Questions

Using a separate sheet of paper, answer the following questions:

1. What symptoms may have alerted C.D. to seek medical care for his cancer of the rectum?
2. What care is indicated for C.D.'s perineal wound?
3. What are the primary goals of care for C.D.'s colostomy?
4. What would be the nurse's evaluation of C.D.'s adjustment to his colostomy?
5. What factors may be influencing the pain that C.D. is experiencing?
6. Will C.D. need adjuvant chemotherapy or biologic and targeted therapy? If so, which medications would be used?
7. *Priority Decision:* What are the priority teaching needs for C.D. before his discharge?
8. *Priority Decision:* Based on the assessment data presented, what are the priority nursing diagnoses? Are there any collaborative problems?

Nursing Management: Liver, Pancreas, and Biliary Tract Problems

1. The patient has a diagnosis of a biliary obstruction from gallstones. What type of jaundice is the patient experiencing and what serum bilirubin results would be expected?
   a. Hemolytic jaundice with normal conjugated bilirubin
   b. Posthepatic icteris with decreased unconjugated bilirubin
   c. Obstructive jaundice with elevated unconjugated and conjugated bilirubin
   d. Hepatocellular jaundice with altered conjugated bilirubin in severe disease

2. The patient experienced a blood transfusion reaction. How should the nurse explain to the patient the cause of the hemolytic jaundice that occurred?
   a. Results from hepatocellular disease
   b. Due to a malaria parasite breaking apart red blood cells (RBCs)
   c. Results from decreased flow of bile through the liver or biliary system
   d. Due to increased breakdown of RBCs that caused elevated serum unconjugated bilirubin

3. The patient returned from a 6-week mission trip to Somalia with complaints of nausea, malaise, fatigue, and achy muscles. Which type of hepatitis is this patient most likely to have contracted?
   a. Hepatitis B (HBV)   c. Hepatitis D (HDV)
   b. Hepatitis C (HCV)   d. Hepatitis E (HEV)

4. Which type of hepatitis is a DNA virus, can be transmitted via exposure to infectious blood or body fluids, is required for HDV to replicate, and increases the risk of the chronic carrier for hepatocellular cancer?
   a. Hepatitis A (HAV)   c. Hepatitis C (HCV)
   b. Hepatitis B (HBV)   d. Hepatitis E (HEV)

5. Serologic findings in viral hepatitis include both the presence of viral antigens and antibodies produced in response to the viruses. What laboratory result indicates that the nurse is immune to HBV after vaccination?
   a. Anti-HBcIgG   c. Surface antibody Anti-HBs
   b. Surface antigen HBsAg   d. Core antigen Anti-HBcIgM

6. The patient asks why the serologic test of HBV DNA quantitation is being done. What is the best rationale for the nurse to explain the test to the patient?
   a. Indicates ongoing infection with HBV
   b. Indicates co-infection with HBV and HDV
   c. Indicates previous infection or immunization to HBV
   d. Indicates viral replication and effectiveness of therapy for chronic HBV

7. Although HAV antigens are not tested in the blood, they stimulate specific immunoglobulin M (IgM) and immunoglobulin G (IgG) antibodies. Which antibody indicates there is acute HAV infection?
   a. Anti-HBc IgG   c. Anti-HAV IgG
   b. Anti-HBc IgM   d. Anti-HAV IgM

8. What test will be done before prescribing treatment for the patient with positive testing for HCV?
   a. Anti-HCV   c. HCV RNA quantitation
   b. HCV genotyping   d. Recombinant immunoblot assay (RIBA)

9. What causes the systemic effects of viral hepatitis?
   a. Cholestasis
   b. Impaired portal circulation
   c. Toxins produced by the infected liver
   d. Activation of the complement system by antigen-antibody complexes

10. During the incubation period of viral hepatitis, what should the nurse expect the patient to report?
    a. Pruritus and malaise
    b. Dark urine and easy fatigability
    c. Anorexia and right upper quadrant discomfort
    d. Constipation or diarrhea with light-colored stools

11. The occurrence of acute liver failure is most common in which situation?
    a. An individual with hepatitis A
    b. An individual with hepatitis C
    c. Antihypertensive medication use
    d. Use of acetaminophen with alcohol abuse

12. Following a needle stick, what is used as prophylaxis against HBV?
    a. Interferon
    b. HBV vaccine
    c. Hepatitis B immune globulin (HBIG)
    d. HBV vaccine and HBIG

13. The family members of a patient with hepatitis A ask if there is anything that will prevent them from developing the disease. What is the best response by the nurse?
    a. "No immunization is available for hepatitis A, nor are you likely to get the disease."
    b. "All family members should receive the hepatitis A vaccine to prevent or modify the infection."
    c. "Those who have had household or close contact with the patient should receive immune globulin."
    d. "Only those individuals who have had sexual contact with the patient should receive immunization."

14. A patient diagnosed with chronic hepatitis B asks about drug therapy to treat the disease. What is the most appropriate response by the nurse?
    a. "Only chronic hepatitis C is treatable and primarily with antiviral agents and interferon."
    b. "There are no specific drug therapies that are effective for treating acute viral hepatitis."
    c. "Interferon combined with lamivudine (Epivir) will decrease viral load and prevent complications."
    d. "There are no drugs used for the treatment of viral hepatitis because of the risk of additional liver damage."

15. The nurse identifies a need for further teaching when the patient with hepatitis B makes which statement?
    a. "I should avoid alcohol completely for as long as a year."
    b. "I must avoid all physical contact with my family until the jaundice is gone."
    c. "I should use a condom to prevent spread of the disease to my sexual partner."
    d. "I will need to rest several times a day, gradually increasing my activity as I tolerate it."

16. What is one of the most challenging nursing interventions to promote healing in the patient with viral hepatitis?
    a. Providing adequate nutritional intake
    b. Promoting strict bed rest during the icteric phase
    c. Providing pain relief without using liver-metabolized drugs
    d. Providing quiet diversional activities during periods of fatigue

17. When caring for a patient with autoimmune hepatitis, the nurse understands that what in this patient is different from the patient who has viral hepatitis?
    a. Does not manifest hepatomegaly or jaundice
    b. Experiences less liver inflammation and damage
    c. Is treated with corticosteroids or other immunosuppressive agents
    d. Is usually an older adult who has used a wide variety of prescription and over-the-counter drugs

18. The patient has been newly diagnosed with Wilson's disease and D-penicillamine, a chelating agent, has been prescribed. What assessment finding should the nurse expect?
    a. Pruritus
    b. Acute kidney injury
    c. Corneal Fleischer rings
    d. Elevated serum iron levels

19. The patient presents with jaundice and itching, steatorrhea, and liver enlargement. This patient has also had ulcerative colitis for several years. What diagnosis should the nurse expect for this patient?
    a. Cirrhosis
    b. Acute liver failure
    c. Hepatorenal syndrome
    d. Primary sclerosing cholangitis

20. The patient is an older woman with cirrhosis who also has anemia. What pathophysiologic changes may contribute to this patient's anemia (*select all that apply*)?
    a. Vitamin B deficiencies
    b. Stretching of liver capsule
    c. Vascular congestion of spleen
    d. Decreased prothrombin production
    e. Decreased bilirubin conjugation and excretion

21. A patient was diagnosed with nonalcoholic fatty liver disease (NAFLD). What treatment measures should the nurse plan to teach the patient about (*select all that apply*)?
    a. Weight loss
    b. Diabetes management
    c. Ulcerative colitis dietary changes
    d. Dietary management of hyperlipidemia
    e. Maintaining blood pressure with increased sodium and fluid intake

22. Which manifestations may be seen in the patient with cirrhosis related to esophageal varices?
    a. Jaundice, peripheral edema, and ascites from increased intrahepatic pressure and dysfunction
    b. Loss of the small bile ducts and cholestasis and cirrhosis in patients with other autoimmune disorders
    c. Development of collateral channels of circulation in inelastic, fragile esophageal veins as a result of portal hypertension
    d. Scarring and nodular changes in the liver lead to compression of the veins and sinusoids, causing resistance of blood flow through the liver from the portal vein

23. Which conditions contribute to the formation of abdominal ascites?
    a. Esophageal varices contribute to 80% of variceal hemorrhages
    b. Increased colloidal oncotic pressure caused by decreased albumin production
    c. Hypoaldosteronism causes increased sodium reabsorption by the renal tubules
    d. Blood flow through the portal system is obstructed, which causes portal hypertension

24. What laboratory test results should the nurse expect to find in a patient with cirrhosis?
    a. Serum albumin: 7.0 g/dL (70 g/L)
    b. Total bilirubin: 3.2 mg/dL (54.7 mmol/L)
    c. Serum cholesterol: 260 mg/dL (6.7 mmol/L)
    d. Aspartate aminotransferase (AST): 6.0 U/L (0.1 mkat/L)

25. Malnutrition can be a big problem for patients with cirrhosis. Which nursing intervention can help to improve nutrient intake?
    a. Oral hygiene before meals and snacks
    b. Provide all foods the patient likes to eat
    c. Improve oral intake by feeding the patient
    d. Limit snack offers to when the patient is hungry

26. The patient being treated with diuretics for ascites from cirrhosis must be monitored for (*select all that apply*)?
    a. GI bleeding
    b. Hypokalemia
    c. Renal function
    d. Body image disturbances
    e. Increased clotting tendencies

27. What manifestation in the patient does the nurse recognize as an early sign of hepatic encephalopathy?
    a. Manifests asterixis
    b. Becomes unconscious
    c. Has increasing oliguria
    d. Is irritable and lethargic

28. To treat a cirrhotic patient with hepatic encephalopathy, lactulose (Cephulac), rifaximin (Xifaxan), and a proton pump inhibitor are ordered. The patient's family wants to know why the laxative is ordered. What is the best explanation the nurse can give to the patient's family?
    a. It reduces portal venous pressure.
    b. It eliminates blood from the GI tract.
    c. It traps ammonia and eliminates it in the feces.
    d. It decreases bacteria to decrease ammonia formation.

29. ***Priority Decision:*** The patient has hepatic encephalopathy. What is a priority nursing intervention to keep the patient safe?
    a. Turn the patient every 3 hours.
    b. Encourage increasing ambulation.
    c. Assist the patient to the bathroom.
    d. Prevent constipation to reduce ammonia production.

30. A patient with advanced cirrhosis has a nursing diagnosis of imbalanced nutrition: less than body requirements *related to* anorexia and inadequate food intake. What would be an appropriate midday snack for the patient?
    a. Peanut butter and salt-free crackers
    b. A fresh tomato sandwich with salt-free butter
    c. Popcorn with salt-free butter and herbal seasoning
    d. Canned chicken noodle soup with low-protein bread

31. The patient with liver failure has had a liver transplant. What should the nurse teach the patient about care after the transplant?
    a. Alcohol intake is now okay.
    b. HBIG will be required to prevent rejection.
    c. Elevate the head 30 degrees to improve ventilation when sleeping.
    d. Monitor closely for infection because of the immunosuppressive medication.

32. ***Priority Decision:*** During the treatment of the patient with bleeding esophageal varices, what is the most important thing the nurse should do?
    a. Prepare the patient for immediate portal shunting surgery.
    b. Perform guaiac testing on all stools to detect occult blood.
    c. Maintain the patient's airway and prevent aspiration of blood.
    d. Monitor for the cardiac effects of IV vasopressin and nitroglycerin.

33. A patient with cirrhosis that is refractory to other treatments for esophageal varices undergoes a portacaval shunt. As a result of this procedure, what should the nurse expect the patient to experience?
    a. An improved survival rate
    b. Decreased serum ammonia levels
    c. Improved metabolism of nutrients
    d. Improved hemodynamic function and renal perfusion

34. In discussing long-term management with the patient with alcoholic cirrhosis, what should the nurse advise the patient?
    a. A daily exercise regimen is important to increase the blood flow through the liver.
    b. Cirrhosis can be reversed if the patient follows a regimen of proper rest and nutrition.
    c. Abstinence from alcohol is the most important factor in improvement of the patient's condition.
    d. The only over-the-counter analgesic that should be used for minor aches and pains is acetaminophen.

35. A patient is hospitalized with metastatic cancer of the liver. The nurse plans care for the patient based on what knowledge?
    a. Chemotherapy is highly successful in the treatment of liver cancer.
    b. The patient will undergo surgery to remove the involved portions of the liver.
    c. Supportive care that is appropriate for all patients with severe liver damage is indicated.
    d. Metastatic cancer of the liver is more responsive to treatment than primary carcinoma of the liver.

36. A patient with cirrhosis asks the nurse about the possibility of a liver transplant. What is the best response by the nurse?
    a. "Liver transplants are indicated only in young people with irreversible liver disease."
    b. "If you are interested in a transplant, you really should talk to your doctor about it."
    c. "Rejection is such a problem in liver transplants that it is seldom attempted in patients with cirrhosis."
    d. "Cirrhosis is an indication for transplantation in some cases. Have you talked to your doctor about this?"

37. Which complication of acute pancreatitis requires prompt surgical drainage to prevent sepsis?
    a. Tetany
    b. Pseudocyst
    c. Pleural effusion
    d. Pancreatic abscess

38. When assessing a patient with acute pancreatitis, the nurse would expect to find
    a. hyperactive bowel sounds.
    b. hypertension and tachycardia.
    c. a temperature greater than 102°F (38.9°C).
    d. severe midepigastric or left upper quadrant (LUQ) pain.

39. Combined with clinical manifestations, what is the laboratory finding that is most commonly used to diagnose acute pancreatitis?
    a. Increased serum calcium
    b. Increased serum amylase
    c. Increased urinary amylase
    d. Decreased serum glucose

40. What treatment measure is used in the management of the patient with acute pancreatitis?
    a. Surgery to remove the inflamed pancreas
    b. Pancreatic enzyme supplements administered with meals
    c. Nasogastric (NG) suction to prevent gastric contents from entering the duodenum
    d. Endoscopic pancreatic sphincterotomy using endoscopic retrograde cholangiopancreatography (ERCP)

41. A patient with acute pancreatitis has a nursing diagnosis of pain *related to* distention of the pancreas and peritoneal irritation. In addition to effective use of analgesics, what should the nurse include in this patient's plan of care?
    a. Provide diversional activities to distract the patient from the pain.
    b. Provide small, frequent meals to increase the patient's tolerance to food.
    c. Position the patient on the side with the head of the bed elevated 45 degrees for pain relief.
    d. Ambulate the patient every 3 to 4 hours to increase circulation and decrease abdominal congestion.

42. The nurse determines that further discharge instruction is needed when the patient with acute pancreatitis makes which statement?
    a. "I should observe for fat in my stools."
    b. "I must not use alcohol to prevent future attacks of pancreatitis."
    c. "I shouldn't eat any salty foods or foods with high amounts of sodium."
    d. "I will need to continue to monitor my blood glucose levels until my pancreas is healed."

43. What is the patient with chronic pancreatitis more likely to have than the patient with acute pancreatitis?
    a. The need to abstain from alcohol
    b. Experience acute abdominal pain
    c. Malabsorption and diabetes mellitus
    d. Require a high-carbohydrate, high-protein, low-fat diet

44. The nurse is instructing a patient with chronic pancreatitis on measures to prevent further attacks. What information should be provided (*select all that apply*)?
    a. Avoid nicotine.
    b. Eat bland foods.
    c. Observe stools for steatorrhea.
    d. Eat high-fat, low-protein, high-carbohydrate meals.
    e. Take prescribed pancreatic enzymes immediately following meals.

45. What is a risk factor associated with cancer of the pancreas?
    a. Alcohol intake
    b. Cigarette smoking
    c. Exposure to asbestos
    d. Increased dietary intake of spoiled milk products

46. In a radical pancreaticoduodenectomy (Whipple procedure) for treatment of cancer of the pancreas, what anatomic structure is completely resected that will affect the patient's nutritional status?
    a. Stomach
    b. Pancreas
    c. Common bile duct
    d. Duodenum adjoining the pancreas

47. Of the following characteristics, identify those that are most commonly associated with cholelithiasis (*select all that apply*).
    a. Obesity
    b. Age over 40
    c. Multiparous female
    d. History of excessive alcohol intake
    e. Family history of gallbladder disease
    f. Use of estrogen or oral contraceptives

48. Acalculous cholecystitis is diagnosed in an older, critically ill patient. Which factors may be associated with this condition (*select all that apply*)?
    a. Fasting
    b. Hypothyroidism
    c. Parenteral nutrition
    d. Prolonged immobility
    e. *Streptococcus pneumoniae*
    f. Absence of bile in the intestine

49. A patient with an obstruction of the common bile duct has clay-colored fatty stools, among other manifestations. What is the pathophysiologic change that causes this clinical manifestation?
    a. Soluble bilirubin in the blood excreted into the urine
    b. Absence of bile salts in the intestine and duodenum, preventing fat emulsion and digestion
    c. Contraction of the inflamed gallbladder and obstructed ducts, stimulated by cholecystokinin when fats enter the duodenum
    d. Obstruction of the common duct prevents bile drainage into the duodenum, resulting in congestion of bile in the liver and subsequent absorption into the blood

50. The patient with suspected gallbladder disease is scheduled for an ultrasound of the gallbladder. What should the nurse explain to the patient about this test?
    a. It is noninvasive and is a very reliable method of detecting gallstones.
    b. It is used only when other tests cannot be used because of allergy to contrast media.
    c. It will outline the gallbladder and the ductal system to enable visualization of stones.
    d. It is an adjunct to liver function tests to determine whether the gallbladder is inflamed.

51. What treatment for acute cholecystitis will prevent further stimulation of the gallbladder?
    a. NPO with NG suction   c. Administration of antiemetics
    b. Incisional cholecystectomy   d. Administration of anticholinergics

52. Following a laparoscopic cholecystectomy, what should the nurse expect to be part of the plan of care?
    a. Return to work in 2 to 3 weeks
    b. Be hospitalized for 3 to 5 days postoperatively
    c. Have a T-tube placed in the common bile duct to provide bile drainage
    d. Have up to four small abdominal incisions covered with small dressings

53. A patient with chronic cholecystitis asks the nurse whether she will need to continue a low-fat diet after she has a cholecystectomy. What is the best response by the nurse?
    a. "A low-fat diet will prevent the development of further gallstones and should be continued."
    b. "Yes; because you will not have a gallbladder to store bile, you will not be able to digest fats adequately."
    c. "A low-fat diet is recommended for a few weeks after surgery until the intestine adjusts to receiving a continuous flow of bile."
    d. "Removal of the gallbladder will eliminate the source of your pain associated with fat intake, so you may eat whatever you like."

54. What must the nurse do to care for a T-tube in a patient following a cholecystectomy?
    a. Keep the tube supported and free of kinks.
    b. Attach the tube to low, continuous suction.
    c. Clamp the tube when ambulating the patient.
    d. Irrigate the tube with 10-mL sterile saline every 2 to 4 hours.

55. During discharge instructions for a patient following a laparoscopic cholecystectomy, what should the nurse include in the teaching?
    a. Keep the incision areas clean and dry for at least a week.
    b. Report the need to take pain medication for shoulder pain.
    c. Report any bile-colored or purulent drainage from the incisions.
    d. Expect some postoperative nausea and vomiting for a few days.

CASE STUDY

Acute Pancreatitis

Patient Profile

V.A. is a 55-year-old man admitted to the hospital with acute pancreatitis.

Subjective Data

- Has severe abdominal pain in the LUQ radiating to the back
- States that he is nauseated and has been vomiting

Objective Data

Physical Examination
- Vital signs: Temp 101°F (38.3°C), HR 114 bpm, RR 26, BP 92/58
- Jaundice noted in sclera

Laboratory Tests
- Serum amylase: 400 U/L (6.67 mkat/L)
- Serum lipase: 600 U/L
- Urinary amylase: 3800 U/day
- WBC count: 20,000/µL
- Blood glucose: 180 mg/dL (10 mmol/L)
- Serum calcium: 7 mg/dL (1.7 mmol/L)

Collaborative Care

- NPO status
- NG tube to low, intermittent suction
- IV therapy with lactated Ringer's solution
- Morphine PCA
- Pantoprazole (Protonix) IV

Discussion Questions

Using a separate sheet of paper, answer the following questions:

1. Explain the pathophysiology of acute pancreatitis.
2. What are the most common causes of acute pancreatitis?
3. How do the results of V.A.'s laboratory values relate to the pathophysiology of acute pancreatitis?
4. What causes hypocalcemia in acute pancreatitis? How does the nurse assess for hypocalcemia?
5. Describe the characteristics of the pain that occurs in acute pancreatitis.
6. What complications can occur with acute pancreatitis?
7. Why is V.A. NPO? What is the purpose of the NG tube?
8. Identify the purpose of each medication prescribed for this patient.
9. *Priority Decision:* Based on the assessment data presented, what are the priority nursing diagnoses? Are there any collaborative problems?

Nursing Assessment: Urinary System

1. Using the following list of terms, identify the structures in the illustrations below (some of the terms may be used in both illustrations).

Terms

Adrenal gland	Hilus	Right renal artery
Aorta	Kidney	Right renal vein
Bladder	Medulla	Ureter
Calyx	Papilla	Urethra
Cortex	Pyramid	Vena cava
Fibrous capsule	Renal pelvis	

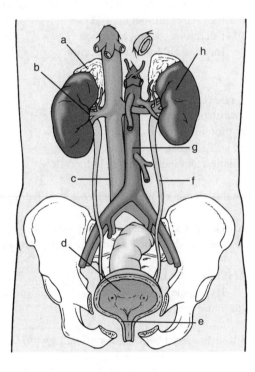

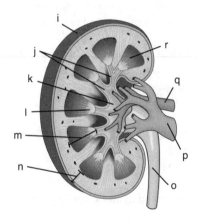

a. _____	j. _____
b. _____	k. _____
c. _____	l. _____
d. _____	m. _____
e. _____	n. _____
f. _____	o. _____
g. _____	p. _____
h. _____	q. _____
i. _____	r. _____

2. Number the following physiologic occurrences in the order they occur in the formation of urine. Begin with 1 for the first occurrence and number through 6 for the last occurrence in the formation of urine.
   - _1_ a. Blood is filtered in the glomerulus.
   - _4_ b. Reabsorption of water in the loop of Henle.
   - _3_ c. Reabsorption of electrolytes, glucose, amino acids, and small proteins in the tubules.
   - _6_ d. Acid-base regulation with conservation of bicarbonate (HCO_3^-) and secretion of excess H^+ in the distal tubule.
   - _5_ e. Active reabsorption of chloride (Cl^-) ions and passive reabsorption of sodium (Na^+) ions in the ascending loop of Henle.
   - _2_ f. Ultrafiltrate flows from Bowman's capsule and passes down the tubules without blood cells, platelets, or large plasma proteins.

3. Which important functions of regulation of water balance and acid-base balance occur in the distal convoluted tubes of the nephron (*select all that apply*)?
   - a. Secretion of H^+ into filtrate
   - b. Reabsorption of water without ADH
   - c. Reabsorption of Na^+ in exchange for K^+
   - d. Reabsorption of glucose and amino acids
   - e. Reabsorption of water under ADH influence
   - f. Reabsorption of Ca^{+2} under parathormone influence

4. The right atrium myocytes secrete atrial natriuretic peptide (ANP) when there is increased plasma volume. What actions does ANP take to produce a large volume of dilute urine (*select all that apply*)?
   - a. Inhibits renin
   - b. Increases ADH
   - c. Inhibits angiotensin II action
   - d. Decreases sodium excretion
   - e. Increases aldosterone secretion

5. Which statement accurately describes glomerular filtration rate (GFR)?
   - a. The primary function of GFR is to excrete nitrogenous waste products.
   - b. Decreased permeability in the glomerulus causes loss of proteins into the urine.
   - c. The GFR is primarily dependent on adequate blood flow and adequate hydrostatic pressure.
   - d. The GFR is decreased when prostaglandins cause vasodilation and increased renal blood flow.

6. A patient with an obstruction of the renal artery causing renal ischemia exhibits hypertension. What is one factor that may contribute to the hypertension?
   - a. Increased renin release
   - b. Increased ADH secretion
   - c. Decreased aldosterone secretion
   - d. Increased synthesis and release of prostaglandins

7. In which clinical situation would the increased release of erythropoietin be expected?
   - a. Hypoxemia
   - b. Hypotension
   - c. Hyperkalemia
   - d. Fluid overload

8. What are common diagnostic studies done for a patient with severe renal colic (*select all that apply*)?
   - a. CT scan
   - b. Urinalysis
   - c. Cystoscopy
   - d. Ureteroscopy
   - e. Abdominal ultrasound

9. Which volume of urine in the bladder would cause discomfort and require urinary catheterization?
   - a. 250 mL
   - b. 500 mL
   - c. 1200 mL
   - d. 1500 mL

10. What is a factor that contributes to an increased incidence of urinary tract infections in aging women?
    - a. Length of the urethra
    - b. Larger capacity of bladder
    - c. Relaxation of pelvic floor and bladder muscles
    - d. Tight muscular support at the urinary sphincter

11. A 78-year-old man asks the nurse why he has to urinate so much at night. The nurse should explain to the patient that as an older adult, what may contribute to his nocturia?
    - a. Decreased renal mass
    - b. Decreased detrusor muscle tone
    - c. Decreased ability to conserve sodium
    - d. Decreased ability to concentrate urine

12. List one specific finding identified by the nurse during assessment of each of the patient's functional health patterns that indicates a risk factor for urinary problems or a patient response to a urinary disorder.

Functional Health Pattern	Risk Factor for or Response to Urinary Problem
Health perception–health management	
Nutritional-metabolic	
Elimination	
Activity-exercise	
Sleep-rest	
Cognitive-perceptual	
Self-perception–self-concept	
Role-relationship	
Sexuality-reproductive	
Coping–stress tolerance	
Value-belief	

13. What accurately describes a normal physical assessment of the urinary system by the nurse?
    a. Auscultates the lower abdominal quadrants for fluid sounds
    b. Palpates an empty bladder at the level of the symphysis pubis
    c. Percusses the kidney with a firm blow at the posterior costovertebral angle
    d. Positions the patient prone to palpate the kidneys with a posterior approach

14. The patient complains of "wetting when she sneezes." How should the nurse document this information?
    a. Nocturia
    b. Micturition
    c. Urge incontinence
    d. Stress incontinence

15. The physician documented that the patient has urinary retention. How should the nurse explain this when the nursing student asks what it is?
    a. Inability to void
    b. No urine formation
    c. Large amount of urine output
    d. Increased incidence of urination

16. The male patient is admitted with a diagnosis of benign prostatic hyperplasia (BPH). What urination characteristics should the nurse expect to assess in this patient?
    a. Oliguria
    b. Hesitancy
    c. Hematuria
    d. Pneumaturia

17. The mother of an 8-year-old girl has brought her child to the clinic because she is wetting the bed at night. What terminology should the nurse use when documenting this situation?
    a. Ascites
    b. Dysuria
    c. Enuresis
    d. Urgency

18. A urinalysis of a urine specimen that is not processed within 1 hour may result in erroneous measurement of
    a. glucose.
    b. bacteria.
    c. specific gravity.
    d. white blood cells.

19. Which urinalysis results most likely indicate a urinary tract infection (UTI)?
    a. Yellow; protein 6 mg/dL; pH 6.8; 10^2/mL bacteria
    b. Cloudy, yellow; WBC >5/hpf; pH 8.2; numerous casts
    c. Cloudy, brown; ammonia odor; specific gravity 1.030; RBC 3/hpf
    d. Clear; colorless; glucose: trace; ketones: trace; osmolality 500 mOsm/kg (500 mmol/kg)

→ how concentrated your urine is 1.003-1.030

20. Which urine specific gravity value would indicate to the nurse that the patient is receiving excessive IV fluid therapy?
    a. 1.002
    b. 1.010
    c. 1.025
    d. 1.030

21. *Priority Decision:* After a patient had a renal arteriogram and is back on the clinical unit, what is the most important action by the nurse?
    a. Observe for gross bleeding in the urine.
    b. Place the patient in high Fowler's position.
    c. Monitor the patient for signs of allergy to the contrast medium.
    d. Assess peripheral pulses in the involved leg every 30 to 60 minutes.

22. Which test is most specific for renal function?
    a. Renal scan
    b. Serum creatinine
    c. Creatinine clearance
    d. Blood urea nitrogen (BUN)

23. What is the most likely reason that the BUN would be increased in a patient?
    a. Has impaired renal function
    b. Has not eaten enough protein
    c. Has decreased urea in the urine
    d. May have nonrenal tissue destruction

24. What impairment in kidney function would cause the following laboratory findings in a patient with kidney disease?

Laboratory Finding	Impaired Kidney Function
Serum Ca²⁺: 7.2 mg/dL (1.8 mmol/L)	
Hgb: 9.6 g/dL (96 g/L)	
Serum creatinine: 3.2 mg/dL (283 mmol/L)	

25. *Priority Decision:* Following a renal biopsy, what is the nurse's priority?
    a. Offer warm sitz baths to relieve discomfort.
    b. Test urine for microscopic bleeding with a dipstick.
    c. Expect the patient to experience burning on urination.
    d. Monitor the patient for symptoms of a urinary infection.

26. What nursing responsibilities are done to obtain a clean-catch urine specimen from a patient (*select all that apply*)?
    a. Use sterile container.
    b. Must start the test with full bladder.
    c. Insert catheter immediately after voiding.
    d. Have the patient void, stop, and void in container.
    e. Have the patient clean the meatus before voiding.

27. Which diagnostic study would include assessing for iodine sensitivity, teaching the patient to take a cathartic the night before the procedure, and telling the patient that a salty taste may occur during the procedure?
    a. Cystometrogram
    b. Renal arteriogram
    c. Intravenous pyelogram (IVP)
    d. Kidneys, ureters, bladder (KUB)

46

Nursing Management: Renal and Urologic Problems

1. Which classification of urinary tract infection (UTI) is described as infection of the renal parenchyma, renal pelvis, and ureters?
   - a. Upper UTI
   - b. Lower UTI
   - c. Complicated UTI
   - d. Uncomplicated UTI

2. While caring for a 77-year-old woman who has a urinary catheter, the nurse monitors the patient for the development of a UTI. What clinical manifestations is the patient most likely to experience?
   - a. Cloudy urine and fever
   - b. Urethral burning and bloody urine
   - c. Vague abdominal discomfort and disorientation
   - d. Suprapubic pain and slight decline in body temperature

3. A woman with no history of UTIs who is experiencing urgency, frequency, and dysuria comes to the clinic, where a dipstick and microscopic urinalysis indicate bacteriuria. What should the nurse anticipate for this patient?
   - a. Obtaining a clean-catch midstream urine specimen for culture and sensitivity
   - b. No treatment with medication unless she develops fever, chills, and flank pain
   - c. Empirical treatment with trimethoprim-sulfamethoxazole (TMP-SMX, Bactrim) for 3 days
   - d. Need to have a blood specimen drawn for a complete blood count (CBC) and kidney function tests

4. A female patient with a UTI has a nursing diagnosis of risk for infection *related to* lack of knowledge regarding prevention of recurrence. What should the nurse include in the teaching plan instructions for this patient?
   - a. Empty the bladder at least 4 times a day.
   - b. Drink at least 2 quarts of water every day.
   - c. Wait to urinate until the urge is very intense.
   - d. Clean the urinary meatus with an antiinfective agent after voiding.

5. What is the most common cause of acute pyelonephritis resulting from an ascending infection from the lower urinary tract?
   - a. The kidney is scarred and fibrotic.
   - b. The organism is resistant to antibiotics.
   - c. There is a preexisting abnormality of the urinary tract.
   - d. The patient does not take all of the antibiotics for treatment of a UTI.

6. Which characteristic is more likely with acute pyelonephritis than with a lower UTI?
   - a. Fever
   - b. Dysuria
   - c. Urgency
   - d. Frequency

7. Which test is required for a diagnosis of pyelonephritis?
   - a. Renal biopsy
   - b. Blood culture
   - c. Intravenous pyelogram (IVP)
   - d. Urine for culture and sensitivity

8. A patient with suprapubic pain and symptoms of urinary frequency and urgency has two negative urine cultures. What is one assessment finding that would indicate interstitial cystitis?
   - a. Residual urine greater than 200 mL
   - b. A large, atonic bladder on urodynamic testing
   - c. A voiding pattern that indicates psychogenic urinary retention
   - d. Pain with bladder filling that is transiently relieved by urination

9. When caring for the patient with interstitial cystitis, what can the nurse teach the patient to do?
    a. Avoid foods that make the urine more alkaline.
    b. Use high-potency vitamin therapy to decrease the autoimmune effects of the disorder.
    c. Always keep a voiding diary to document pain, voiding frequency, and patterns of nocturia.
    d. Use the dietary supplement calcium glycerophosphate (Prelief) to decrease bladder irritation.

10. Glomerulonephritis is characterized by glomerular damage caused by
    a. growth of microorganisms in the glomeruli.
    b. release of bacterial substances toxic to the glomeruli.
    c. accumulation of immune complexes in the glomeruli.
    d. hemolysis of red blood cells circulating in the glomeruli.

11. What manifestation in the patient will indicate the need for restriction of dietary protein in management of acute poststreptococcal glomerulonephritis (APSGN)?
    a. Hematuria
    b. Proteinuria
    c. Hypertension
    d. Elevated blood urea nitrogen (BUN)

12. The nurse plans care for the patient with APSGN based on what knowledge?
    a. Most patients with APSGN recover completely or rapidly improve with conservative management.
    b. Chronic glomerulonephritis leading to renal failure is a common sequela to acute glomerulonephritis.
    c. Pulmonary hemorrhage may occur as a result of antibodies also attacking the alveolar basement membrane.
    d. A large percentage of patients with APSGN develop rapidly progressive glomerulonephritis, resulting in kidney failure.

13. What results in the edema associated with nephrotic syndrome?
    a. Hypercoagulability
    b. Hyperalbuminemia
    c. Decreased plasma oncotic pressure
    d. Decreased glomerular filtration rate

14. Number in sequence the following ascending pathologic changes that occur in the urinary tract in the presence of a bladder outlet obstruction.
    _____ a. Hydronephrosis
    _____ b. Reflux of urine into ureter
    _____ c. Bladder detrusor muscle hypertrophy
    _____ d. Ureteral dilation
    _____ e. Renal atrophy
    _____ f. Vesicoureteral reflux
    _____ g. Large residual urine in bladder
    _____ h. Chronic pyelonephritis

15. Which infection is asymptomatic in the male patient at first and then progresses to cystitis, frequent urination, burning on voiding, and epididymitis?
    a. Urosepsis
    b. Renal tuberculosis
    c. Urethral diverticula
    d. Goodpasture syndrome

16. What can patients at risk for renal lithiasis do to prevent the stones in many cases?
    a. Lead an active lifestyle
    b. Limit protein and acidic foods in the diet
    c. Drink enough fluids to produce dilute urine
    d. Take prophylactic antibiotics to control UTIs

17. Which type of urinary tract calculi are the most common and frequently obstruct the ureter?
    a. Cystine
    b. Uric acid
    c. Calcium oxalate
    d. Calcium phosphate

18. The female patient with a UTI also has renal calculi. The nurse knows that these are most likely which type of stone?
    a. Cystine
    b. Struvite
    c. Uric acid
    d. Calcium phosphate

19. The male patient is Jewish, has a history of gout, and has been diagnosed with renal calculi. Which treatment will be used with this patient (*select all that apply*)?
    a. Reduce dietary oxalate
    b. Administer allopurinol
    c. Administer α-penicillamine
    d. Administer thiazide diuretics
    e. Reduce animal protein intake
    f. Reduce intake of milk products

20. Besides being mixed with struvite or oxalate stones, what characteristic is associated with calcium phosphate calculi?
    a. Associated with alkaline urine
    b. Genetic autosomal recessive defect
    c. Three times as common in women as in men
    d. Defective gastrointestinal (GI) and kidney absorption

21. On assessment of the patient with a renal calculus passing down the ureter, what should the nurse expect the patient to report?
    a. A history of chronic UTIs
    b. Dull, costovertebral flank pain
    c. Severe, colicky back pain radiating to the groin
    d. A feeling of bladder fullness with urgency and frequency

22. Prevention of calcium oxalate stones would include dietary restriction of which foods or drinks?
    a. Milk and milk products
    b. Dried beans and dried fruits
    c. Liver, kidney, and sweetbreads
    d. Spinach, cabbage, and tomatoes

23. *Priority Decision:* Following electrohydraulic lithotripsy for treatment of renal calculi, the patient has a nursing diagnosis of risk for infection *related to* the introduction of bacteria following manipulation of the urinary tract. What is the most appropriate nursing intervention for this patient?
    a. Monitor for hematuria.
    b. Encourage fluid intake of 3 L/day.
    c. Apply moist heat to the flank area.
    d. Strain all urine through gauze or a special strainer.

24. With which diagnosis will the patient benefit from being taught to do self-catheterization?
    a. Renal trauma
    b. Urethral stricture
    c. Renal artery stenosis
    d. Accelerated nephrosclerosis

25. In providing care for the patient with adult-onset polycystic kidney disease, what should the nurse do?
    a. Help the patient to cope with the rapid progression of the disease
    b. Suggest genetic counseling resources for the children of the patient
    c. Expect the patient to have polyuria and poor concentration ability of the kidneys
    d. Implement measures for the patient's deafness and blindness in addition to the renal problems

26. Which disease causes connective tissue changes that cause glomerulonephritis?
    a. Gout
    b. Amyloidosis
    c. Diabetes mellitus
    d. Systemic lupus erythematosus

27. When obtaining a nursing history from a patient with cancer of the urinary system, what does the nurse recognize as a risk factor associated with both kidney cancer and bladder cancer?
    a. Smoking
    b. Family history of cancer
    c. Chronic use of phenacetin
    d. Chronic, recurrent nephrolithiasis

28. Thirty percent of patients with kidney cancer have metastasis at the time of diagnosis. Why does this occur?
    a. The only treatment modalities for the disease are palliative.
    b. Diagnostic tests are not available to detect tumors before they metastasize.
    c. Classic symptoms of hematuria and palpable mass do not occur until the disease is advanced.
    d. Early metastasis to the brain impairs the patient's ability to recognize the seriousness of symptoms.

29. Which characteristics are associated with urge incontinence (*select all that apply*)?
    a. Treated with Kegel exercises
    b. Found following prostatectomy
    c. Common in postmenopausal women
    d. Involuntary urination preceded by urgency
    e. Caused by overactivity of the detrusor muscle
    f. Bladder contracts by reflex, overriding central inhibition

30. The patient has a thoracic spinal cord lesion and incontinence that occurs equally during the day and night. What type of incontinence is this patient experiencing?
    a. Reflex incontinence
    b. Overflow incontinence
    c. Functional incontinence
    d. Incontinence after trauma

31. Which drugs are used to treat overflow incontinence (*select all that apply*)?
    a. Baclofen (Lioresal)
    b. Anticholinergic drugs
    c. α-Adrenergic blockers
    d. 5α-reductase inhibitors
    e. Bethanechol (Urecholine)

32. To assist the patient with stress incontinence, what is the best thing the nurse should teach the patient to do?
    a. Void every 2 hours to prevent leakage.
    b. Use absorptive perineal pads to contain urine.
    c. Perform pelvic floor muscle exercises 40 to 50 times per day.
    d. Increase intraabdominal pressure during voiding to empty the bladder completely.

33. What is included in nursing care that applies to the management of all urinary catheters in hospitalized patients?
    a. Measuring urine output every 1 to 2 hours to ensure patency
    b. Turning the patient frequently from side to side to promote drainage
    c. Using strict sterile technique during irrigation and obtaining culture specimens
    d. Daily cleaning of the catheter insertion site with soap and water and application of lotion

34. A patient has a right ureteral catheter placed following a lithotripsy for a stone in the ureter. In caring for the patient after the procedure, what is an appropriate nursing action?
    a. Milk or strip the catheter every 2 hours.
    b. Measure ureteral urinary drainage every 1 to 2 hours.
    c. Irrigate the catheter with 30-mL sterile saline every 4 hours.
    d. Encourage ambulation to promote urinary peristaltic action.

35. During assessment of the patient who has a nephrectomy, what should the nurse expect to find?
    a. Shallow, slow respirations
    b. Clear breath sounds in all lung fields
    c. Decreased breath sounds in the lower left lobe
    d. Decreased breath sounds in the right and left lower lobes

36. Which urinary diversion is a continent diversion created by formation of an ileal pouch with a stoma for catheterization?
    a. Kock pouch
    b. Ileal conduit
    c. Orthotopic neobladder
    d. Cutaneous ureterostomy

37. A patient with bladder cancer undergoes cystectomy with formation of an ileal conduit. During the patient's first postoperative day, what should the nurse plan to do?
    a. Measure and fit the stoma for a permanent appliance.
    b. Encourage high oral intake to flush mucus from the conduit.
    c. Teach the patient to self-catheterize the stoma every 4 to 6 hours.
    d. Empty the drainage bag every 2 to 3 hours and measure the urinary output.

38. A teaching plan developed by the nurse for the patient with a new ileal conduit includes instructions to do what?
    a. Clean the skin around the stoma with alcohol every day.
    b. Use a wick to keep the skin dry during appliance changes.
    c. Use sterile supplies and technique during care of the stoma.
    d. Change the appliance every day and wash it with soap and warm water.

39. ***Delegation Decision:*** Which nursing interventions could be delegated to unlicensed assistive personnel (UAP) (*select all that apply*)?
    a. Assess the need for catheterization.
    b. Use bladder scanner to estimate residual urine.
    c. Teach patient pelvic floor muscle (Kegel) exercises.
    d. Insert indwelling catheter for uncomplicated patient.
    e. Assist incontinent patient to commode at regular intervals.
    f. Provide perineal care with soap and water around a urinary catheter.

CASE STUDY
Bladder Cancer
Patient Profile

P.G., a male patient, is a married, 55-year-old mechanic who has been healthy all of his life until he passed some blood in his urine and saw a urologist at his wife's insistence. A urine specimen for cytology revealed atypical cells, and a diagnosis of bladder cancer was made following a cystoscopy with biopsy of bladder tissue. The tumor was removed with a transurethral resection and laser cauterization. Intravesical therapy with bacille Calmette-Guérin (BCG), a weakened strain of *Mycobacterium bovis*, is planned.

Subjective Data

- Has smoked a pack of cigarettes a day since he was a teenager
- Says he dreads having the chemotherapy because he has heard cancer drugs cause severe side effects

Objective Data

- Cystoscopy and biopsy results: Moderately differentiated stage II tumor on the left lateral bladder wall, with T1N0M0 pathologic stage
- Continues to have gross hematuria

Discussion Questions

Using a separate sheet of paper, answer the following questions:

1. What does staging of bladder tumors indicate?
2. What care will the nurse provide for P.G. postoperatively?
3. What information and instructions would the nurse provide for P.G. about the intravesical therapy?
4. How can P.G. help to prevent future bladder tumors from occurring?
5. How should the nurse explain the importance of follow-up cystoscopies?
6. What surgery might be indicated if the chemotherapy is not effective?
7. If surgery is needed, what elements will be considered in deciding the type of surgery?
8. ***Priority Decision:*** Based on the assessment data presented, what are the priority nursing diagnoses? Are there any collaborative problems?

47 Nursing Management: Acute Kidney Injury and Chronic Kidney Disease

1. What are intrarenal causes of acute kidney injury (AKI) (*select all that apply*)?
   a. Anaphylaxis
   b. Renal stones
   c. Bladder cancer
   d. Nephrotoxic drugs
   e. Acute glomerulonephritis
   f. Tubular obstruction by myoglobin

2. An 83-year-old female patient was found lying on the bathroom floor. She said she fell 2 days ago and has not been able to take her heart medicine or eat or drink anything since then. What conditions could be causing prerenal AKI in this patient (*select all that apply*)?
   a. Anaphylaxis
   b. Renal calculi
   c. Hypovolemia
   d. Nephrotoxic drugs
   e. Decreased cardiac output

3. Acute tubular necrosis (ATN) is the most common cause of intrarenal AKI. Which patient is most likely to develop ATN?
   a. Patient with diabetes mellitus
   b. Patient with hypertensive crisis
   c. Patient who tried to overdose on acetaminophen
   d. Patient with major surgery who required a blood transfusion

4. ***Priority Decision:*** A dehydrated patient is in the Injury stage of the RIFLE staging of AKI. What would the nurse first anticipate in the treatment of this patient?
   a. Assess daily weight
   b. IV administration of fluid and furosemide (Lasix)
   c. IV administration of insulin and sodium bicarbonate
   d. Urinalysis to check for sediment, osmolality, sodium, and specific gravity

5. What indicates to the nurse that a patient with oliguria has prerenal oliguria?
   a. Urine testing reveals a low specific gravity.
   b. Causative factor is malignant hypertension.
   c. Urine testing reveals a high sodium concentration.
   d. Reversal of oliguria occurs with fluid replacement.

6. In a patient with AKI, which laboratory urinalysis result indicates tubular damage?
   a. Hematuria
   b. Specific gravity fixed at 1.010
   c. Urine sodium of 12 mEq/L (12 mmol/L)
   d. Osmolality of 1000 mOsm/kg (1000 mmol/kg)

7. Metabolic acidosis occurs in the oliguric phase of AKI as a result of impairment of
   a. ammonia synthesis. $\rightarrow NH_3$
   b. excretion of sodium.
   c. excretion of bicarbonate.
   d. conservation of potassium.

8. What indicates to the nurse that a patient with AKI is in the recovery phase?
   a. A return to normal weight
   b. A urine output of 3700 mL/day
   c. Decreasing sodium and potassium levels
   d. Decreasing blood urea nitrogen (BUN) and creatinine levels

9. While caring for the patient in the oliguric phase of AKI, the nurse monitors the patient for associated collaborative problems. When should the nurse notify the health care provider?
   a. Urine output is 300 mL/day.
   b. Edema occurs in the feet, legs, and sacral area.
   c. Cardiac monitor reveals a depressed T wave and elevated ST segment.
   d. The patient experiences increasing muscle weakness and abdominal cramping.

10. In caring for the patient with AKI, what should the nurse be aware of?
    a. The most common cause of death in AKI is irreversible metabolic acidosis.
    b. During the oliguric phase of AKI, daily fluid intake is limited to 1000 mL plus the prior day's measured fluid loss.
    c. Dietary sodium and potassium during the oliguric phase of AKI are managed according to the patient's urinary output.
    d. One of the most important nursing measures in managing fluid balance in the patient with AKI is taking accurate daily weights.

11. A 68-year-old man with a history of heart failure resulting from hypertension has AKI as a result of the effects of nephrotoxic diuretics. Currently his serum potassium is 6.2 mEq/L (6.2 mmol/L) with cardiac changes, his BUN is 108 mg/dL (38.6 mmol/L), his serum creatinine is 4.1 mg/dL (362 mmol/L), and his serum HCO_3^- is 14 mEq/L (14 mmol/L). He is somnolent and disoriented. Which treatment should the nurse expect to be used for him?
    a. Loop diuretics
    b. Renal replacement therapy
    c. Insulin and sodium bicarbonate
    d. Sodium polystyrene sulfonate (Kayexalate)

12. Prevention of AKI is important because of the high mortality rate. Which patients are at increased risk for AKI (*select all that apply*)?
    a. An 86-year-old woman scheduled for a cardiac catheterization
    b. A 48-year-old man with multiple injuries from a motor vehicle accident
    c. A 32-year-old woman following a C-section delivery for abruptio placentae
    d. A 64-year-old woman with chronic heart failure admitted with bloody stools
    e. A 58-year-old man with prostate cancer undergoing preoperative workup for prostatectomy

13. *Priority Decision:* A patient on a medical unit has a potassium level of 6.8 mEq/L. What is the priority action that the nurse should take?
    a. Place the patient on a cardiac monitor.
    b. Check the patient's blood pressure (BP).
    c. Instruct the patient to avoid high-potassium foods.
    d. Call the lab and request a redraw of the lab to verify results.

14. A patient with AKI has a serum potassium level of 6.7 mEq/L (6.7 mmol/L) and the following arterial blood gas results: pH 7.28, $PaCO_2$ 30 mm Hg, PaO_2 86 mm Hg, HCO_3^- 18 mEq/L (18 mmol/L). The nurse recognizes that treatment of the acid-base problem with sodium bicarbonate would cause a decrease in which value?
    a. pH
    b. Potassium level
    c. Bicarbonate level
    d. Carbon dioxide level

15. In replying to a patient's questions about the seriousness of her chronic kidney disease (CKD), the nurse knows that the stage of CKD is based on what?
    a. Total daily urine output
    b. Glomerular filtration rate
    c. Degree of altered mental status
    d. Serum creatinine and urea levels

16. The patient with CKD is receiving dialysis, and the nurse observes excoriations on the patient's skin. What pathophysiologic changes in CKD can contribute to this finding (*select all that apply*)?
    a. Dry skin
    b. Sensory neuropathy
    c. Vascular calcifications
    d. Calcium-phosphate skin deposits
    e. Uremic crystallization from high BUN

17. What causes the gastrointestinal (GI) manifestation of stomatitis in the patient with CKD?
    a. High serum sodium levels
    b. Irritation of the GI tract from creatinine
    c. Increased ammonia from bacterial breakdown of urea
    d. Iron salts, calcium-containing phosphate binders, and limited fluid intake

18. The patient with CKD is brought to the emergency department with Kussmaul respirations. What does the nurse know about CKD that could cause this patient's Kussmaul respirations?
    a. Uremic pleuritis is occurring.
    b. There is decreased pulmonary macrophage activity.
    c. They are caused by respiratory compensation for metabolic acidosis.
    d. Pulmonary edema from heart failure and fluid overload is occurring.

19. Which serum laboratory value indicates to the nurse that the patient's CKD is getting worse?
    a. Decreased BUN
    b. Decreased sodium
    c. Decreased creatinine
    d. Decreased calculated glomerular filtration rate (GFR)

20. What is the most serious electrolyte disorder associated with kidney disease?
    a. Hypocalcemia
    b. Hyperkalemia
    c. Hyponatremia
    d. Hypermagnesemia

21. For a patient with CKD the nurse identifies a nursing diagnosis of risk for injury: fracture *related to* alterations in calcium and phosphorus metabolism. What is the pathologic process directly related to the increased risk for fractures?
    a. Loss of aluminum through the impaired kidneys
    b. Deposition of calcium phosphate in soft tissues of the body
    c. Impaired vitamin D activation resulting in decreased GI absorption of calcium
    d. Increased release of parathyroid hormone in response to decreased calcium levels

22. *Priority Decision:* What is the most appropriate snack for the nurse to offer a patient with stage 4 CKD?
    a. Raisins
    b. Ice cream
    c. Dill pickles
    d. Hard candy

23. Which complication of chronic kidney disease is treated with erythropoietin (EPO)?
    a. Anemia
    b. Hypertension
    c. Hyperkalemia
    d. Mineral and bone disorder

24. The patient with CKD asks why she is receiving nifedipine (Procardia) and furosemide (Lasix). The nurse understands that these drugs are being used to treat the patient's
    a. anemia.
    b. hypertension.
    c. hyperkalemia.
    d. mineral and bone disorder.

25. Which drugs will be used to treat the patient with CKD for mineral and bone disorder (*select all that apply*)?
    a. Cinacalcet (Sensipar)
    b. Sevelamer (Renagel)
    c. IV glucose and insulin
    d. Calcium acetate (PhosLo)
    e. IV 10% calcium gluconate

26. What accurately describes the care of the patient with CKD?
    a. A nutrient that is commonly supplemented for the patient on dialysis because it is dialyzable is iron.
    b. The syndrome that includes all of the signs and symptoms seen in the various body systems in CKD is azotemia.
    c. The use of morphine is contraindicated in the patient with CKD because accumulation of its metabolites may cause seizures.
    d. The use of calcium-based phosphate binders in the patient with CKD is contraindicated when serum calcium levels are increased.

27. During the nursing assessment of the patient with renal insufficiency, the nurse asks the patient specifically about a history of
    a. angina.
    b. asthma.
    c. hypertension.
    d. rheumatoid arthritis.

28. The patient with chronic kidney disease is considering whether to use peritoneal dialysis (PD) or hemodialysis (HD). What are advantages of PD when compared to HD (*select all that apply*)?
    a. Less protein loss
    b. Rapid fluid removal
    c. Less cardiovascular stress
    d. Decreased hyperlipidemia
    e. Requires fewer dietary restrictions

29. What does the dialysate for PD routinely contain?
    a. Calcium in a lower concentration than in the blood
    b. Sodium in a higher concentration than in the blood
    c. Dextrose in a higher concentration than in the blood
    d. Electrolytes in an equal concentration to that of the blood

30. Number the following in the order of the phases of exchange in PD. Begin with 1 and end with 3.
    ___3___ a. Drain
    ___2___ b. Dwell
    ___1___ c. Inflow

31. In which type of dialysis does the patient dialyze during sleep and leave the fluid in the abdomen during the day?
    a. Long nocturnal hemodialysis
    b. Automated peritoneal dialysis (APD)
    c. Continuous venovenous hemofiltration (CVVH)
    d. Continuous ambulatory peritoneal dialysis (CAPD)

32. To prevent the most common serious complication of PD, what is important for the nurse to do?
    a. Infuse the dialysate slowly.
    b. Use strict aseptic technique in the dialysis procedures.
    c. Have the patient empty the bowel before the inflow phase.
    d. Reposition the patient frequently and promote deep breathing.

peritonitis (handwritten)

33. A patient on hemodialysis develops a thrombus of a subcutaneous arteriovenous (AV) graft, requiring its removal. While waiting for a replacement graft or fistula, the patient is most likely to have what done for treatment?
    a. Peritoneal dialysis
    b. Peripheral vascular access using radial artery
    c. Silastic catheter tunneled subcutaneously to the jugular vein
    d. Peripherally inserted central catheter (PICC) line inserted into subclavian vein

34. A man with end-stage kidney disease is scheduled for hemodialysis following healing of an arteriovenous fistula (AVF). What should the nurse explain to him that will occur during dialysis?
    a. He will be able to visit, read, sleep, or watch TV while reclining in a chair.
    b. He will be placed on a cardiac monitor to detect any adverse effects that might occur.
    c. The dialyzer will remove and hold part of his blood for 20 to 30 minutes to remove the waste products.
    d. A large catheter with two lumens will be inserted into the fistula to send blood to and return it from the dialyzer.

35. What is the primary way that a nurse will evaluate the patency of an AVF?
    a. Palpate for pulses distal to the graft site.
    b. Auscultate for the presence of a bruit at the site.
    c. Evaluate the color and temperature of the extremity.
    d. Assess for the presence of numbness and tingling distal to the site.

36. A patient with AKI is a candidate for continuous renal replacement therapy (CRRT). What is the most common indication for use of CRRT?
    a. Azotemia
    b. Pericarditis
    c. Fluid overload
    d. Hyperkalemia

37. A patient rapidly progressing toward end-stage kidney disease asks about the possibility of a kidney transplant. In responding to the patient, the nurse knows that what is a contraindication to kidney transplantation?
    a. Hepatitis C infection
    b. Coronary artery disease
    c. Refractory hypertension
    d. Extensive vascular disease

38. *Priority Decision:* During the immediate postoperative care of a recipient of a kidney transplant, what should the nurse expect to do?
    a. Regulate fluid intake hourly based on urine output.
    b. Monitor urine-tinged drainage on abdominal dressing.
    c. Medicate the patient frequently for incisional flank pain.
    d. Remove the urinary catheter to evaluate the ureteral implant.

39. A patient received a kidney transplant last month. Because of the effects of immunosuppressive drugs and CKD, what complication of transplantation should the nurse be assessing the patient for to decrease the risk of mortality?
    a. Infection
    b. Rejection
    c. Malignancy
    d. Cardiovascular disease

CASE STUDY
Kidney Transplant
Patient Profile

D.B. has CKD resulting from diabetes and hypertension. She underwent hemodialysis for 2 years and then received a deceased (cadaveric) renal transplant 1 year ago. She had one episode of acute rejection 3 months after transplant. Her baseline creatinine has been 1.2 to 1.3 mg/dL (106 to 115 mmol/L). She came to the clinic complaining of decreased urinary output, fever, and tenderness at the transplant site. She is admitted to the hospital for testing and possible kidney biopsy.

Subjective Data

- Tells the nurse that if she loses this kidney, she does not think she can stand to go back on dialysis

Objective Data

Physical Examination
- BP: 150/90 mm Hg
- Flank area tender to palpation

Laboratory Tests
- Serum creatinine: 3.0 mg/dL (265 mmol/L)
- BUN: 70 mg/dL (25 mmol/L)
- Glucose: 404 mg/dL (22.4 mmol/L)
- K^+: 5.1 mEq/L (5.1 mmol/L)
- HCO_3^-: 18 mEq/L (18 mmol/L)

Collaborative Care

- Metformin
- IV insulin
- Furosemide (Lasix)
- Nifedipine (Procardia)
- Sodium bicarbonate
- Mycophenolate mofetil (CellCept)
- Methylprednisolone (Solu-Medrol)
- Tacrolimus (Prograf)
- Muromonab-CD3 (Orthoclone OKT3) therapy for 10 days

Discussion Questions

Using a separate sheet of paper, answer the following questions:

1. Explain the pathophysiology of acute rejection.
2. Identify the abnormal laboratory tests and explain why each would occur. What significance do the abnormal results have for nursing care?
3. Explain the rationale for D.B.'s collaborative care. How does each immunosuppressive medication work? (See Table 14-16.)
4. What clinical manifestations may develop as a result of immunosuppressive therapy? What nursing care is indicated?
5. Explain the long-term problems of a patient with a kidney transplant.
6. ***Priority Decision:*** Based on the assessment data presented, what are the priority nursing diagnoses? Are there any collaborative problems?

1. Identify the glands in the following illustration.

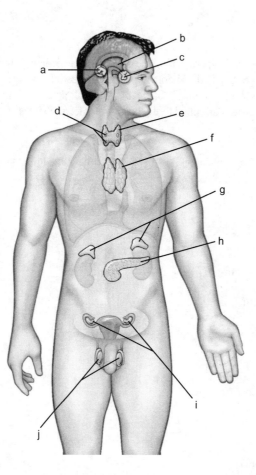

a. _____	f. _____
b. _____	g. _____
c. _____	h. _____
d. _____	i. _____
e. _____	j. _____

2. Which hormones are secreted by the anterior pituitary gland (*select all that apply*)?
    a. Prolactin
    b. Melatonin
    c. Somatostatin
    d. Parathormone
    e. Growth hormone (GH)
    f. Gonadotropic hormones
    g. Antidiuretic hormone (ADH)
    h. Melanocyte-stimulating hormone
    i. Thyroid-stimulating hormone (TSH)
    j. Adrenocorticotropic hormone (ACTH)

3. From where is the hormone glucagon secreted?
    a. F cells of the islets of Langerhans
    b. β-Cells of the islets of Langerhans
    c. α-Cells of the islets of Langerhans
    d. Delta cells of the islets of Langerhans

4. Which endocrine gland secretes cortisol?
    a. Ovaries
    b. Thyroid
    c. Adrenal cortex
    d. Adrenal medulla

5. Which statement about the adrenal medulla hormones is accurate?
    a. Overproduction of androgens may cause masculinization in women.
    b. Both the adrenal medulla and the thyroid gland have a negative feedback system to the hypothalamus.
    c. Cortisol levels would be altered in a person who normally works a night shift from 11:00 PM to 7:00 AM and sleeps from 8:00 AM to 3:00 PM.
    d. Epinephrine and norepinephrine are considered hormones when they are secreted by the adrenal medulla and neurotransmitters when they are secreted by nerve cells.

6. Match each hormone with the primary factor that stimulates its secretion and the primary factor that inhibits its secretion (factors may be used more than once).

Stimulate	Inhibit	Hormone	Primary Factor
_____	_____	a. TSH or thyrotropin	1. Increased stress
_____	_____	b. Corticotropin-releasing hormone	2. Increased serum T_3
_____	_____	c. ADH	3. Decreased serum T_3
_____	_____	d. Follicle-stimulating hormone (FSH)	4. Increased serum cortisol
_____	_____	e. Calcitonin	5. Increased serum estrogen
_____	_____	f. Aldosterone	6. Decreased serum estrogen
_____	_____	g. Glucagon	7. Increased serum glucose
_____	_____	h. Parathyroid hormone (PTH)	8. Decreased serum glucose
_____	_____	i. Insulin	9. Increased serum calcium
			10. Decreased serum calcium
			11. Decreased blood pressure (BP)
			12. Increased arterial BP
			13. Increased plasma osmolality
			14. Decreased plasma osmolality

7. The normal response to increased serum osmolality is the release of
    a. aldosterone from the adrenal cortex, which stimulates sodium excretion by the kidney.
    b. ADH from the posterior pituitary gland, which stimulates the kidney to reabsorb water.
    c. mineralocorticoids from the adrenal gland, which stimulate the kidney to excrete potassium.
    d. calcitonin from the thyroid gland, which increases bone resorption and decreases serum calcium levels.

8. What accurately demonstrates that hormones of one gland influence the function of hormones of another gland?
    a. Increased insulin levels inhibit the secretion of glucagon.
    b. Increased cortisol levels stimulate the secretion of insulin.
    c. Increased testosterone levels inhibit the release of estrogen.
    d. Increased atrial natriuretic peptide (ANP) levels inhibit the secretion of aldosterone.

9. How do hormones respond following the ingestion of a high-protein, carbohydrate-free meal?
    a. Both insulin and glucagon are inhibited because blood glucose levels are unchanged.
    b. Insulin is inhibited by low glucose levels and glucagon is released to promote gluconeogenesis.
    c. Insulin is released to facilitate the breakdown of amino acids into glucose and glucagon is inhibited.
    d. Glucagon is released to promote gluconeogenesis and insulin is released to facilitate movement of amino acids into muscle cells.

10. What are two effects of hypokalemia on the endocrine system?
    a. Decreased insulin and aldosterone release
    b. Decreased glucagon and increased cortisol release
    c. Decreased release of atrial natriuretic factor and increased ADH release
    d. Decreased release of parathyroid hormone and increased calcitonin release

11. Identify one specific finding identified by the nurse during assessment of each of the patient's functional health patterns that indicates a risk factor for endocrine problems or a patient response to an actual endocrine problem.

Functional Health Pattern	Risk Factor for or Response to Endocrine Problem
Health perception–health management	
Nutritional-metabolic	
Elimination	
Activity-exercise	
Sleep-rest	
Cognitive-perceptual	
Self-perception–self-concept	
Role-relationship	
Sexuality-reproductive	
Coping–stress tolerance	
Value-belief	

12. In a patient with an elevated serum cortisol, what would the nurse expect other laboratory findings to reveal?
    a. Hypokalemia
    b. Hyponatremia
    c. Hypoglycemia
    d. Decreased serum triglycerides

13. What manifestations of endocrine problems in the older adult are commonly attributed to the aging process?
    a. Tremors and paresthesias
    b. Fatigue and mental impairment
    c. Hyperpigmentation and oily skin
    d. Fluid retention and hypertension

14. Common nonspecific manifestations that may alert the nurse to endocrine dysfunction include
    a. goiter and alopecia.
    b. exophthalmos and tremors.
    c. weight loss, fatigue, and depression.
    d. polyuria, polydipsia, and polyphagia.

15. What is a potential adverse effect of palpation of an enlarged thyroid gland?
    a. Carotid artery obstruction
    b. Damage to the cricoid cartilage
    c. Release of excessive thyroid hormone into circulation
    d. Hoarseness from pressure on the recurrent laryngeal nerve

16. Which abnormal assessment findings are related to thyroid dysfunction (*select all that apply*)?
    a. Tetanic muscle spasms with hypofunction
    b. Heat intolerance caused by hyperfunction
    c. Exophthalmos associated with excessive secretion
    d. Hyperpigmentation associated with hypofunction
    e. A goiter with either hyperfunction or hypofunction
    f. Increase in hand and foot size associated with excessive secretion

17. A patient has a low serum T_3 level. The health care provider orders measurement of the TSH level. If the TSH level is elevated, what does this indicate?
    a. The cause of the low T_3 level is most likely primary hypothyroidism.
    b. The negative feedback system is failing to stimulate the anterior pituitary gland.
    c. The patient has an underactive thyroid gland that is not receiving TSH stimulation.
    d. Most likely there is a tumor on the anterior pituitary gland that is causing increased production of TSH.

18. To ensure accurate results of a fasting blood glucose analysis, the nurse instructs the patient to fast for at least how long?
    a. 2 hours
    b. 4 hours
    c. 8 hours
    d. 12 hours

19. A 30-year-old female patient was brought to the emergency department (ED) after a seizure at work. During the assessment she mentions hair loss and menstrual irregularities. What diagnostic tests would be helpful to determine if endocrine problems are a cause of her problem (*select all that apply*)?
    a. Thyroglobulin
    b. Luteinizing hormone (LH)
    c. Parathyroid hormone (PTH)
    d. Follicle-stimulating hormone (FSH)
    e. Magnetic resonance imaging (MRI) of the head
    f. Adrenal corticotropic hormone (ACTH) suppression

20. The female patient is admitted with a new diagnosis of Cushing syndrome with elevated serum and urine cortisol levels. Which assessment findings should the nurse expect to see in this patient?
    a. Hair loss and moon face
    b. Decreased weight and hirsutism
    c. Decreased muscle mass and thick skin
    d. Elevated blood pressure and blood glucose

21. The patient with type 1 diabetes mellitus is in the clinic to check his long-term glycemic control. Which test should be used?
    a. Water deprivation test
    b. Fasting blood glucose test
    c. Oral glucose tolerance test
    d. Glycosylated hemoglobin (A1C)

49

Nursing Management: Diabetes Mellitus

1. In addition to promoting the transport of glucose from the blood into the cell, what does insulin do?
   a. Enhances the breakdown of adipose tissue for energy
   b. Stimulates hepatic glycogenolysis and gluconeogenesis
   c. Prevents the transport of triglycerides into adipose tissue
   d. Accelerates the transport of amino acids into cells and their synthesis into protein

2. Which tissues require insulin to enable movement of glucose into the tissue cells (*select all that apply*)?
   a. Liver
   b. Brain
   c. Adipose
   d. Blood cells
   e. Skeletal muscle

3. Why are the hormones cortisol, glucagon, epinephrine, and growth hormone referred to as counter regulatory hormones?
   a. Decrease glucose production
   b. Stimulate glucose output by the liver
   c. Increase glucose transport into the cells
   d. Independently regulate glucose level in the blood

4. What characterizes type 2 diabetes (*select all that apply*)?
   a. β-Cell exhaustion
   b. Insulin resistance
   c. Genetic predisposition
   d. Altered production of adipokines
   e. Inherited defect in insulin receptors
   f. Inappropriate glucose production by the liver

5. Which laboratory results would indicate that the patient has prediabetes?
   a. Glucose tolerance result of 132 mg/dL
   b. Glucose tolerance result of 240 mg/dL
   c. Fasting blood glucose result of 80 mg/dL
   d. Fasting blood glucose result of 120 mg/dL

6. The nurse is teaching the patient with prediabetes ways to prevent or delay the development of type 2 diabetes. What information should be included (*select all that apply*)?
   a. Maintain a healthy weight.
   b. Exercise for 60 minutes each day.
   c. Have blood pressure checked regularly.
   d. Assess for visual changes on monthly basis.
   e. Monitor for polyuria, polyphagia, and polydipsia.

7. In type 1 diabetes there is an osmotic effect of glucose when insulin deficiency prevents the use of glucose for energy. Which classic symptom is caused by the osmotic effect of glucose?
   a. Fatigue
   b. Polydipsia
   c. Polyphagia
   d. Recurrent infections

8. Which patient should the nurse plan to teach how to prevent or delay the development of diabetes?
   a. An obese 50-year-old Hispanic woman
   b. A child whose father has type 1 diabetes
   c. A 34-year-old woman whose parents both have type 2 diabetes
   d. A 12-year-old boy whose father has maturity onset diabetes of the young (MODY)

9. *Priority Decision:* When caring for a patient with metabolic syndrome, what should the nurse give the highest priority to teaching the patient about?
   a. Achieving a normal weight
   b. Performing daily aerobic exercise
   c. Eliminating red meat from the diet
   d. Monitoring the blood glucose periodically

normal weight is most important

10. During routine health screening, a patient is found to have fasting plasma glucose (FPG) of 132 mg/dL (7.33 mmol/L). At a follow-up visit, a diagnosis of diabetes would be made based on which laboratory results (*select all that apply*)?
    a. A1C of 7.5%
    b. Glycosuria of 3+
    c. FPG ≥126 mg/dL (7.0 mmol/L).
    d. Random blood glucose of 126 mg/dL (7.0 mmol/L)
    e. A 2-hour oral glucose tolerance test (OGTT) of 190 mg/dL (10.5 mmol/L)

11. The nurse determines that a patient with a 2-hour OGTT of 152 mg/dL has
    a. diabetes.
    b. elevated A1C.
    c. impaired fasting glucose.
    d. impaired glucose tolerance.

12. When teaching the patient with diabetes about insulin administration, the nurse should include which instruction for the patient?
    a. Pull back on the plunger after inserting the needle to check for blood.
    b. Consistently use the same size of insulin syringe to avoid dosing errors.
    c. Clean the skin at the injection site with an alcohol swab before each injection.
    d. Rotate injection sites from arms to thighs to abdomen with each injection to prevent lipodystrophies.

13. A patient with type 1 diabetes uses 20 U of 70/30 neutral protamine Hagedorn (NPH/regular) in the morning and at 6:00 PM. When teaching the patient about this regimen, what should the nurse emphasize?
    a. Hypoglycemia is most likely to occur before the noon meal.
    b. Flexibility in food intake is possible because insulin is available 24 hours a day.
    c. A set meal pattern with a bedtime snack is necessary to prevent hypoglycemia.
    d. Premeal glucose checks are required to determine needed changes in daily dosing.

14. Lispro insulin (Humalog) with NPH insulin is ordered for a patient with newly diagnosed type 1 diabetes. The nurse knows that when lispro insulin is used, when should it be administered? *↳ rapid*
    a. Only once a day
    b. 1 hour before meals
    c. 30 to 45 minutes before meals
    d. At mealtime or within 15 minutes of meals

15. A patient with diabetes is learning to mix regular insulin and NPH insulin in the same syringe. The nurse determines that additional teaching is needed when the patient does what?
    a. Withdraws the NPH dose into the syringe first
    b. Injects air equal to the NPH dose into the NPH vial first
    c. Removes any air bubbles after withdrawing the first insulin
    d. Adds air equal to the insulin dose into the regular vial and withdraws the dose

16. *Delegation Decision:* The following interventions are planned for a diabetic patient. Which intervention can the nurse delegate to unlicensed assistive personnel (UAP)?
    a. Discuss complications of diabetes.
    b. Check that the bath water is not too hot.
    c. Check the patient's technique for drawing up insulin.
    d. Teach the patient to use a meter for self-monitoring of blood glucose.

17. The home care nurse should intervene to correct a patient whose insulin administration includes
    a. warming a prefilled refrigerated syringe in the hands before administration.
    b. storing syringes prefilled with NPH and regular insulin needle-up in the refrigerator.
    c. placing the insulin bottle currently in use in a small container on the bathroom countertop.
    d. mixing an evening dose of regular insulin with insulin glargine in one syringe for administration.

↓
Lantus
long-acting insulins cannot be mixed w/ anything!

18. When teaching the patient with type 1 diabetes, what should the nurse emphasize as the major advantage of using an insulin pump?
    a. Tight glycemic control can be maintained.
    b. Errors in insulin dosing are less likely to occur.
    c. Complications of insulin therapy are prevented.
    d. Frequent blood glucose monitoring is unnecessary.

19. *Priority Decision:* A patient taking insulin has recorded fasting glucose levels above 200 mg/dL (11.1 mmol/L) on awakening for the last five mornings. What should the nurse advise the patient to do first?
    a. Increase the evening insulin dose to prevent the dawn phenomenon.
    b. Use a single-dose insulin regimen with an intermediate-acting insulin.
    c. Monitor the glucose level at bedtime, between 2:00 AM and 4:00 AM, and on arising.
    d. Decrease the evening insulin dosage to prevent night hypoglycemia and the Somogyi effect.

20. Which class of oral glucose-lowering agents is most commonly used for people with type 2 diabetes because it reduces hepatic glucose production and enhances tissue uptake of glucose?
    a. Insulin
    b. Biguanide
    c. Meglitinide
    d. Sulfonylurea

21. The patient with type 2 diabetes is being put on acarbose (Precose) and wants to know why she is taking it. What should the nurse include in this patient's teaching (*select all that apply*)?
    a. Take it with the first bite of each meal.
    b. It is not used in patients with heart failure.
    c. Endogenous glucose production is decreased.
    d. Effectiveness is measured by 2-hour postprandial glucose.
    e. It delays glucose absorption from the gastrointestinal (GI) tract.

22. *Priority Decision:* The nurse is assessing a newly admitted diabetic patient. Which observation should be addressed as the priority by the nurse?
    a. Bilateral numbness of both hands
    b. Stage II pressure ulcer on the right heel
    c. Rapid respirations with deep inspiration
    d. Areas of lumps and dents on the abdomen

23. Individualized nutrition therapy for patients using conventional, fixed insulin regimens should include teaching the patient to
    a. eat regular meals at regular times.
    b. restrict calories to promote moderate weight loss.
    c. eliminate sucrose and other simple sugars from the diet.
    d. limit saturated fat intake to 30% of dietary calorie intake.

24. What should the goals of nutrition therapy for the patient with type 2 diabetes include?
    a. Ideal body weight
    b. Normal serum glucose and lipid levels
    c. A special diabetic diet using dietetic foods
    d. Five small meals per day with a bedtime snack

25. To prevent hyperglycemia or hypoglycemia related to exercise, what should the nurse teach the patient using glucose-lowering agents about the best time for exercise?
    a. Only after a 15-g carbohydrate snack is eaten
    b. About 1 hour after eating when blood glucose levels are rising
    c. When glucose monitoring reveals that the blood glucose is in the normal range
    d. When blood glucose levels are high, because exercise always has a hypoglycemic effect

26. The nurse assesses the diabetic patient's technique of self-monitoring of blood glucose (SMBG) 3 months after initial instruction. Which error in the performance of SMBG noted by the nurse requires intervention?
    a. Doing the SMBG before and after exercising
    b. Puncturing the finger on the side of the finger pad
    c. Cleaning the puncture site with alcohol before the puncture
    d. Holding the hand down for a few minutes before the puncture

27. A nurse working in an outpatient clinic plans a screening program for diabetes. What recommendations for screening should be included?
    a. OGTT for all minority populations every year
    b. FPG for all individuals at age 45 and then every 3 years
    c. Testing people under the age of 21 for islet cell antibodies
    d. Testing for type 2 diabetes in all overweight or obese individuals

28. ***Priority Decision:*** A patient with diabetes calls the clinic because she is experiencing nausea and flu-like symptoms. Which advice from the nurse will be the best for this patient?
    a. Administer the usual insulin dosage.
    b. Hold fluid intake until the nausea subsides.
    c. Come to the clinic immediately for evaluation and treatment.
    d. Monitor the blood glucose every 1 to 2 hours and call if it rises over 150 mg/dL (8.3 mmol/L).

29. The nurse should observe the patient for symptoms of ketoacidosis when
    a. illnesses causing nausea and vomiting lead to bicarbonate loss with body fluids.
    b. glucose levels become so high that osmotic diuresis promotes fluid and electrolyte loss.
    c. an insulin deficit causes the body to metabolize large amounts of fatty acids rather than glucose for energy.
    d. the patient skips meals after taking insulin, leading to rapid metabolism of glucose and breakdown of fats for energy.

30. What are manifestations of diabetic ketoacidosis (DKA) (*select all that apply*)?
    a. Thirst
    b. Ketonuria
    c. Dehydration
    d. Metabolic acidosis
    e. Kussmaul respirations
    f. Sweet, fruity breath odor

31. What describes the primary difference in treatment for diabetic ketoacidosis (DKA) and hyperosmolar hyperglycemic syndrome (HHS)?
    a. DKA requires administration of bicarbonate to correct acidosis.
    b. Potassium replacement is not necessary in management of HHS.
    c. HHS requires greater fluid replacement to correct the dehydration.
    d. Administration of glucose is withheld in HHS until the blood glucose reaches a normal level.

32. The patient with newly diagnosed diabetes is displaying shakiness, confusion, irritability, and slurred speech. What should the nurse suspect is happening?
    a. DKA
    b. HHS
    c. Hypoglycemia
    d. Hyperglycemia

33. The patient with diabetes has a blood glucose level of 248 mg/dL. Which manifestations in the patient would the nurse understand as being related to this blood glucose level (*select all that apply*)?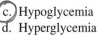
    a. Headache
    b. Unsteady gait
    c. Abdominal cramps
    d. Emotional changes
    e. Increase in urination
    f. Weakness and fatigue

34. A diabetic patient is found unconscious at home and a family member calls the clinic. After determining that a glucometer is not available, what should the nurse advise the family member to do?
    a. Have the patient drink some orange juice.
    b. Administer 10 U of regular insulin subcutaneously.
    c. Call for an ambulance to transport the patient to a medical facility.
    d. Administer glucagon 1 mg intramuscularly (IM) or subcutaneously.

35. The patient with diabetes is brought to the emergency department by his family members, who say that he is not acting like himself and he is more tired than usual. Number the nursing actions in the order of priority for this patient.
    _____3_____ a. Establish IV access.
    _____2_____ b. Check blood glucose.
    _____1_____ c. Ensure patent airway.
    _____5_____ d. Begin continuous regular insulin drip.
    _____4_____ e. Administer 0.9% NaCl solution at 1L/hr.
    _____6_____ f. Establish time of last food and medication(s).

36. *Priority Decision:* Two days following a self-managed hypoglycemic episode at home, the patient tells the nurse that his blood glucose levels since the episode have been between 80 and 90 mg/dL. Which is the best response by the nurse?
    a. "That is a good range for your glucose levels."
    b. "You should call your health care provider because you need to have your insulin increased."
    c. "That level is too low in view of your recent hypoglycemia and you should increase your food intake."
    d. "You should take only half your insulin dosage for the next few days to get your glucose level back to normal."

37. Which statement best describes atherosclerotic disease affecting the cerebrovascular, cardiovascular, and peripheral vascular systems in patients with diabetes?
    a. It can be prevented by tight glucose control.
    b. It occurs with a higher frequency and earlier onset than in the nondiabetic population.
    c. It is caused by the hyperinsulinemia related to insulin resistance common in type 2 diabetes.
    d. It cannot be modified by reduction of risk factors such as smoking, obesity, and high fat intake.

38. What disorders and diseases are related to macrovascular complications of diabetes (*select all that apply*)?
    a. Chronic kidney disease
    b. Coronary artery disease
    c. Microaneurysms and destruction of retinal vessels
    d. Ulceration and amputation of the lower extremities
    e. Capillary and arteriole membrane thickening specific to diabetes

39. The patient with diabetes has been diagnosed with autonomic neuropathy. What problems should the nurse expect to find in this patient (*select all that apply*)?
    a. Painless foot ulcers
    b. Erectile dysfunction
    c. Burning foot pain at night
    d. Loss of fine motor control
    e. Vomiting undigested food
    f. Painless myocardial infarction

40. Following the teaching of foot care to a diabetic patient, the nurse determines that additional instruction is needed when the patient makes which statement?
    a. "I should wash my feet daily with soap and warm water."
    b. "I should always wear shoes to protect my feet from injury."
    c. "If my feet are cold, I should wear socks instead of using a heating pad."
    d. "I'll know if I have sores or lesions on my feet because they will be painful."

41. A 72-year-old woman is diagnosed with diabetes. What does the nurse recognize about the management of diabetes in the older adult?
    a. It is more difficult to achieve strict glucose control than in younger patients.
    b. It usually is not treated unless the patient becomes severely hyperglycemic.
    c. It does not include treatment with insulin because of limited dexterity and vision.
    d. It usually requires that a younger family member be responsible for care of the patient.

CASE STUDY
Hypoglycemia

Patient Profile

After running in a half marathon, F.W., a 24-year-old woman with type 1 diabetes, was brought to the first aid tent provided for participants in a charity run. She is well maintained on a regimen of self-monitoring of blood glucose, insulin, and diet.

Subjective Data

- States that she feels cold and has a headache; her fingers feel numb
- She took her usual insulin dose this morning but was unable to eat her entire breakfast because of a lack of time
- Completed the half marathon in a personal-best time

Objective Data

- Has slurred speech and unsteady gait
- HR: 120 bpm
- Appears confused
- Capillary blood glucose level: 48 mg/dL (2.7 mmol/L)

Discussion Questions

Using a separate sheet of paper, answer the following questions:

1. Describe what F.W. could have done to prevent this hypoglycemic event.
2. What is the etiology of the manifestations that the patient displays?
3. How would you expect to treat F.W.'s hypoglycemia?
4. *Priority Decision:* What are the priority teaching needs for this patient once her condition has stabilized?
5. What adjustments in her diabetic regimen could F.W. make to allow her to continue with her exercise habits?
6. *Priority Decision:* Based on the assessment data presented, what are the priority nursing diagnoses? Are there any collaborative problems?

50 Nursing Management: Endocrine Problems

1. A patient suspected of having acromegaly has an elevated plasma growth hormone (GH) level. In acromegaly, what would the nurse also expect the patient's diagnostic results to indicate?
   a. Hyperinsulinemia
   b. Plasma glucose of <70 mg/dL (3.9 mmol/L)
   c. Decreased GH levels with an oral glucose challenge test
   d. Elevated levels of plasma insulin-like growth factor-1 (IGF-1)

2. During assessment of the patient with acromegaly, what should the nurse expect the patient to report?
   a. Infertility
   b. Dry, irritated skin
   c. Undesirable changes in appearance
   d. An increase in height of 2 to 3 inches a year

3. A patient with acromegaly is treated with a transsphenoidal hypophysectomy. What should the nurse do postoperatively?
   a. Ensure that any clear nasal drainage is tested for glucose.
   b. Maintain the patient flat in bed to prevent cerebrospinal fluid (CSF) leakage.
   c. Assist the patient with toothbrushing every 4 hours to keep the surgical area clean.
   d. Encourage deep breathing, coughing, and turning to prevent respiratory complications.

4. What findings are commonly found in a patient with a prolactinoma?
   a. Gynecomastia in men
   b. Profuse menstruation in women
   c. Excess follicle-stimulating hormone (FSH) and luteinizing hormone (LH)
   d. Signs of increased intracranial pressure, including headache, nausea, and vomiting

5. An African American woman with a history of breast cancer has panhypopituitarism from radiation therapy for primary pituitary tumors. Which medications should the nurse teach her about needing for the rest of her life (*select all that apply*)?
   a. Cortisol
   b. Vasopressin
   c. Sex hormones
   d. Levothyroxine (Synthroid)
   e. Growth hormone (somatropin [Omnitrope])
   f. Dopamine agonists (bromocriptine [Parlodel])

6. The patient is diagnosed with syndrome of inappropriate antidiuretic hormone (SIADH). What manifestation should the nurse expect to find?
   a. Decreased body weight
   b. Decreased urinary output
   c. Increased plasma osmolality
   d. Increased serum sodium levels

7. During care of the patient with SIADH, what should the nurse do?
   a. Monitor neurologic status at least every 2 hours.
   b. Teach the patient receiving treatment with diuretics to restrict sodium intake.
   c. Keep the head of the bed elevated to prevent antidiuretic hormone (ADH) release.
   d. Notify the health care provider if the patient's blood pressure decreases more than 20 mm Hg from baseline.

8. A patient with SIADH is treated with water restriction. What does the patient experience when the nurse determines that treatment has been effective?
   a. Increased urine output, decreased serum sodium, and increased urine specific gravity
   b. Increased urine output, increased serum sodium, and decreased urine specific gravity
   c. Decreased urine output, increased serum sodium, and decreased urine specific gravity
   d. Decreased urine output, decreased serum sodium, and increased urine specific gravity

9. The patient with diabetes insipidus is brought to the emergency department with confusion and dehydration after excretion of a large volume of urine today even though several liters of fluid were drunk. What is a diagnostic test that the nurse should expect to be done to help make a diagnosis?
   a. Blood glucose
   c. Urine specific gravity
   b. Serum sodium level
   d. Computed tomography (CT) of the head

10. In a patient with central diabetes insipidus, what will the administration of ADH during a water deprivation test result in?
   a. Decrease in body weight
   c. Decrease in blood pressure
   b. Increase in urinary output
   d. Increase in urine osmolality

11. A patient with diabetes insipidus is treated with nasal desmopressin acetate (DDAVP). The nurse determines that the drug is not having an adequate therapeutic effect when the patient experiences
   a. headache and weight gain.
   c. a urine specific gravity of 1.002.
   b. nasal irritation and nausea.
   d. an oral intake greater than urinary output.

12. When caring for a patient with nephrogenic diabetes insipidus, what should the nurse expect the treatment to include?
   a. Fluid restriction
   c. A high-sodium diet
   b. Thiazide diuretics
   d. Chlorpropamide (Diabinese)

13. What characteristic is related to Hashimoto's thyroiditis?
   a. Enlarged thyroid gland
   b. Viral-induced hyperthyroidism
   c. Bacterial or fungal infection of thyroid gland
   d. Chronic autoimmune thyroiditis with antibody destruction of thyroid tissue

14. Which statement accurately describes Graves' disease?
   a. Exophthalmos occurs in Graves' disease.
   b. It is an uncommon form of hyperthyroidism.
   c. Manifestations of hyperthyroidism occur from tissue desensitization to the sympathetic nervous system.
   d. Diagnostic testing in the patient with Graves' disease will reveal an increased thyroid-stimulating hormone (TSH) level.

15. A patient with Graves' disease asks the nurse what caused the disorder. What is the best response by the nurse?
   a. "The cause of Graves' disease is not known, although it is thought to be genetic."
   b. "It is usually associated with goiter formation from an iodine deficiency over a long period of time."
   c. "Antibodies develop against thyroid tissue and destroy it, causing a deficiency of thyroid hormones."
   d. "In genetically susceptible persons, antibodies are formed that cause excessive thyroid hormone secretion."

16. A patient is admitted to the hospital with thyrotoxicosis. On physical assessment of the patient, what should the nurse expect to find?
   a. Hoarseness and laryngeal stridor
   b. Bulging eyeballs and dysrhythmias
   c. Elevated temperature and signs of heart failure
   d. Lethargy progressing suddenly to impairment of consciousness

17. What medication is used with thyrotoxicosis to block the effects of the sympathetic nervous stimulation of the thyroid hormones?
   a. Potassium iodide
   c. Propylthiouracil (PTU)
   b. Atenolol (Tenormin)
   d. Radioactive iodine (RAI)

18. Which characteristics describe the use of RAI (*select all that apply*)?
    a. Often causes hypothyroidism over time
    b. Decreases release of thyroid hormones
    c. Blocks peripheral conversion of T_4 to T_3
    d. Treatment of choice in nonpregnant adults
    e. Decreases thyroid secretion by damaging thyroid gland
    f. Often used with iodine to produce euthyroid before surgery

19. What preoperative instruction should the nurse give to the patient scheduled for a subtotal thyroidectomy?
    a. How to support the head with the hands when turning in bed
    b. Coughing should be avoided to prevent pressure on the incision
    c. Head and neck will need to remain immobile until the incision heals
    d. Any tingling around the lips or in the fingers after surgery is expected and temporary

20. As a precaution for vocal cord paralysis from damage to the recurrent laryngeal nerve during thyroidectomy surgery, what equipment should be in the room in case it is needed for this emergency situation?
    a. Tracheostomy tray
    b. Oxygen equipment
    c. IV calcium gluconate
    d. Paper and pencil for communication

21. When providing discharge instructions to a patient who had a subtotal thyroidectomy for hyperthyroidism, what should the nurse teach the patient?
    a. Never miss a daily dose of thyroid replacement therapy.
    b. Avoid regular exercise until thyroid function is normalized.
    c. Use warm saltwater gargles several times a day to relieve throat pain.
    d. Substantially reduce caloric intake compared to what was eaten before surgery.

22. What is a cause of primary hypothyroidism in adults?
    a. Malignant or benign thyroid nodules
    b. Surgical removal or failure of the pituitary gland
    c. Surgical removal or radiation of the thyroid gland
    d. Autoimmune-induced atrophy of the thyroid gland

23. The nurse has identified the nursing diagnosis of fatigue for a patient who is hypothyroid. What should the nurse do while caring for this patient?
    a. Monitor for changes in orientation, cognition, and behavior.
    b. Monitor for vital signs and cardiac rhythm response to activity.
    c. Monitor bowel movement frequency, consistency, shape, volume, and color.
    d. Assist in developing well-balanced meal plans consistent with level of energy expenditure.

24. *Priority Decision:* When replacement therapy is started for a patient with long-standing hypothyroidism, what is most important for the nurse to monitor the patient for?
    a. Insomnia
    b. Weight loss
    c. Nervousness
    d. Dysrhythmias

25. A patient with hypothyroidism is treated with levothyroxine (Synthroid). What should the nurse include when teaching the patient about this therapy?
    a. Explain that alternate-day dosage may be used if side effects occur.
    b. Provide written instruction for all information related to the drug therapy.
    c. Assure the patient that a return to normal function will occur with replacement therapy.
    d. Inform the patient that the drug must be taken until the hormone balance is reestablished.

26. A patient who recently had a calcium oxalate renal stone had a bone density study, which showed a decrease in her bone density. What endocrine problem could this patient have?
    a. SIADH
    b. Hypothyroidism
    c. Cushing syndrome
    d. Hyperparathyroidism

27. What is an appropriate nursing intervention for the patient with hyperparathyroidism?
    a. Pad side rails as a seizure precaution.
    b. Increase fluid intake to 3000 to 4000 mL daily.
    c. Maintain bed rest to prevent pathologic fractures.
    d. Monitor the patient for Trousseau's and Chvostek's signs.

28. A patient has been diagnosed with hypoparathyroidism. What manifestations should the nurse expect to observe (*select all that apply*)?
    a. Skeletal pain
    b. Dry, scaly skin
    c. Personality changes
    d. Abdominal cramping
    e. Cardiac dysrhythmias
    f. Muscle spasms and stiffness

29. When the patient with parathyroid disease experiences symptoms of hypocalcemia, what is a measure that can be used to temporarily raise serum calcium levels?
    a. Administer IV normal saline.
    b. Have patient rebreathe in a paper bag.
    c. Administer furosemide (Lasix) as ordered.
    d. Administer oral phosphorus supplements.

30. A patient with hypoparathyroidism resulting from surgical treatment of hyperparathyroidism is preparing for discharge. What should the nurse teach the patient?
    a. Milk and milk products should be increased in the diet.
    b. Parenteral replacement of parathyroid hormone will be required for life.
    c. Calcium supplements with vitamin D can effectively maintain calcium balance.
    d. Bran and whole-grain foods should be used to prevent GI effects of replacement therapy.

31. A patient is admitted to the hospital with a diagnosis of Cushing syndrome. On physical assessment of the patient, what should the nurse expect to find?
    a. Hypertension, peripheral edema, and petechiae
    b. Weight loss, buffalo hump, and moon face with acne
    c. Abdominal and buttock striae, truncal obesity, and hypotension
    d. Anorexia, signs of dehydration, and hyperpigmentation of the skin

32. A patient is scheduled for a bilateral adrenalectomy. During the postoperative period, what should the nurse expect related to the administration of corticosteroids?
    a. Reduced to promote wound healing
    b. Withheld until symptoms of hypocortisolism appear
    c. Increased to promote an adequate response to the stress of surgery
    d. Reduced because excessive hormones are released during surgical manipulation of adrenal glands

33. A patient with Addison's disease comes to the emergency department with complaints of nausea, vomiting, diarrhea, and fever. What collaborative care should the nurse expect?
    a. IV administration of vasopressors
    b. IV administration of hydrocortisone
    c. IV administration of D$_5$W with 20 mEq KCl
    d. Parenteral injections of adrenocorticotropic hormone (ACTH)

34. During discharge teaching for the patient with Addison's disease, which statement by the patient indicates that the nurse needs to do additional teaching?
    a. "I should always call the doctor if I develop vomiting or diarrhea."
    b. "If my weight goes down, my dosage of steroid is probably too high."
    c. "I should double or triple my steroid dose if I undergo rigorous physical exercise."
    d. "I need to carry an emergency kit with injectable hydrocortisone in case I can't take my medication by mouth."

35. A patient who is on corticosteroid therapy for treatment of an autoimmune disorder has the following additional drugs ordered. Which one is used to prevent corticosteroid-induced osteoporosis?
    a. Potassium
    b. Furosemide (Lasix)
    c. Alendronate (Fosamax)
    d. Pantoprazole (Protonix)

36. A patient with mild iatrogenic Cushing syndrome is on an alternate-day regimen of corticosteroid therapy. What does the nurse explain to the patient about this regimen?
    a. It maintains normal adrenal hormone balance.
    b. It prevents ACTH release from the pituitary gland.
    c. It minimizes hypothalamic-pituitary-adrenal suppression.
    d. It provides a more effective therapeutic effect of the drug.

37. When caring for a patient with primary hyperaldosteronism, the nurse would question a health care provider's prescription for which drug?
    a. Furosemide (Lasix)
    b. Amiloride (Midamor)
    c. Spironolactone (Aldactone)
    d. Aminoglutethimide (Cytadren)

38. *Priority Decision:* What is the priority nursing intervention during the management of the patient with pheochromocytoma?
    a. Administering IV fluids
    b. Monitoring blood pressure
    c. Administering β-adrenergic blockers
    d. Monitoring intake and output and daily weights

CASE STUDY
Cushing Syndrome
Patient Profile

T.H. is a 26-year-old elementary school teacher. He seeks the advice of his health care provider because of changes in his appearance over the past year.

Subjective Data

- Reports weight gain (particularly through his midsection), easy bruising, and edema of his feet, lower legs, and hands
- Has been having increasing weakness and insomnia

Objective Data

- Physical examination: BP 150/110; 2+ edema of lower extremities; purplish striae on abdomen; thin extremities with thin, friable skin; severe acne of the face and neck
- Blood analysis: Glucose 167 mg/dL (9.3 mmol/L); white blood cell (WBC) count 13,600/μL; lymphocytes 12%; red blood cell (RBC) count 6.6×10^6/μL; K$^+$ 3.2 mEq/L (3.2 mmol/L)

Discussion Questions

Using a separate sheet of paper, answer the following questions:

1. Discuss the probable causes of the alterations in T.H.'s laboratory results.
2. Explain the pathophysiology of Cushing syndrome.
3. What diagnostic testing would identify the cause of T.H.'s Cushing syndrome?
4. What is the usual treatment of Cushing syndrome?
5. What is meant by a "medical adrenalectomy"?
6. *Priority Decision:* What are the priority nursing responsibilities in the care of this patient?
7. *Priority Decision:* Based on the assessment data presented, what are the priority nursing diagnoses? Are there any collaborative problems?

Nursing Assessment: Reproductive System

1. Identify the structures in the following illustrations by filling in the blanks on the next page with the correct answers from the list of terms below (some terms will be used in both illustrations).

Terms

Anus
Bladder
Body of uterus
Cervix
Cowper's gland
Ductus deferens
Ejaculatory duct
Epididymis

Fallopian tube
Fornix of vagina
Fundus of uterus
Glans
Ovary
Penis
Prostate gland
Rectum

Scrotum
Seminal vesicle
Testis
Ureter
Urethra
Vagina
Vaginal introitus

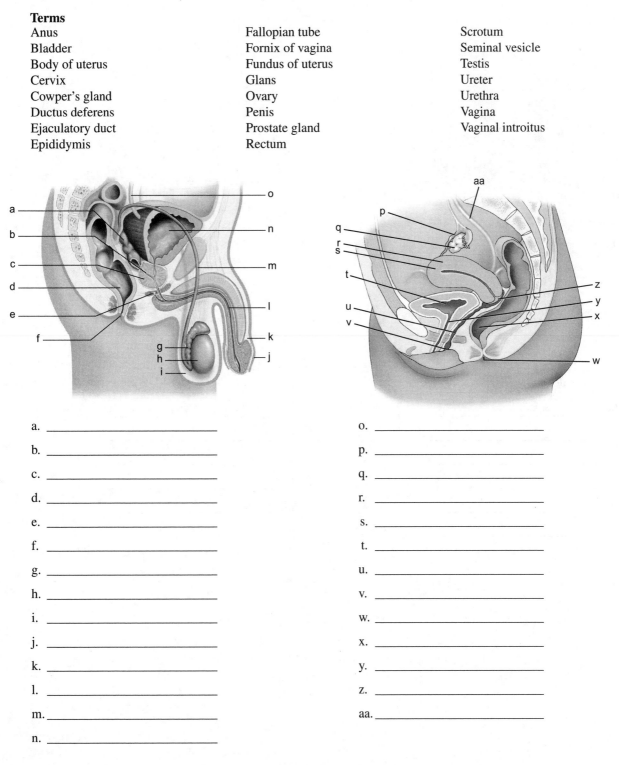

a. _____

b. _____

c. _____

d. _____

e. _____

f. _____

g. _____

h. _____

i. _____

j. _____

k. _____

l. _____

m. _____

n. _____

o. _____

p. _____

q. _____

r. _____

s. _____

t. _____

u. _____

v. _____

w. _____

x. _____

y. _____

z. _____

aa. _____

2. Using the list of terms below, identify the structures in the following illustrations.

Terms

Alveoli	Labia minora	Prepuce
Anus	Mons pubis	Urethral meatus
Areola	Nipple	Vaginal introitus
Clitoris	Pectoralis major muscle	Vestibule
Labia majora	Perineum	

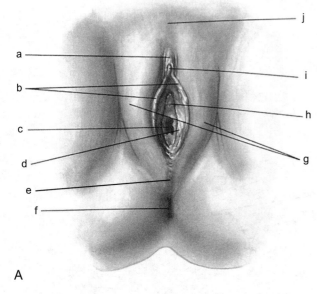

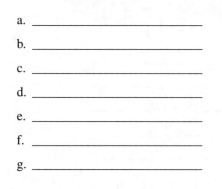

A

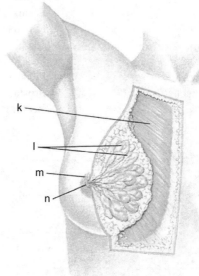

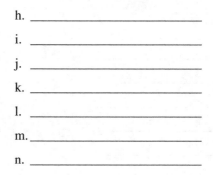

B

a. _____

b. _____

c. _____

d. _____

e. _____

f. _____

g. _____

h. _____

i. _____

j. _____

k. _____

l. _____

m. _____

n. _____

3. Number in sequence from 1 to 8 the passage of sperm through, and the formation of semen in, the structures of the male reproductive system.
   _____ a. Ductus deferens
   _____ b. Urethra
   _____ c. Epididymis
   _____ d. Prostate gland
   _____ e. Seminiferous tubules
   _____ f. Cowper's glands
   _____ g. Seminal vesicles
   _____ h. Ejaculatory duct

4. Which structure of the female breast carries milk from the alveoli to the lactiferous sinuses?
   a. Ducts
   b. Areola
   c. Nipple
   d. Adipose tissue

5. What describes Montgomery's tubercles in the female breast?
   a. Store milk during lactation
   b. Secrete milk during lactation
   c. Sebaceous-like glands on areola
   d. Erectile tissues containing pores

6. Which statement accurately describes the female reproductive system?
   a. Fertilization of an ovum by sperm occurs in the uterus.
   b. Only the ectocervix is used for obtaining Papanicolaou (Pap) tests.
   c. A middle-aged woman is considered to be in menopause when she has not had a menstrual period for 1 year.
   d. The normal process of reabsorption of immature oocytes throughout the female life span is caused by follicle-stimulating hormone (FSH) and luteinizing hormone (LH).

7. What are characteristics of LH (*select all that apply*)?
   a. Maintains implanted egg
   b. Completes follicle maturation
   c. Stimulates testosterone production
   d. Required for female sex characteristics
   e. Needed for growth of mammary glands
   f. Called interstitial cell-stimulating hormone (ICSH) in men

8. FSH is secreted by the anterior pituitary gland in both women and men. Which characteristics describe FSH (*select all that apply*)?
   a. Produced by testes
   b. Elevated at onset of menopause
   c. Responsible for spermatogenesis
   d. Needed for male sex characteristics
   e. Stimulated by elevated estrogen levels
   f. Stimulates growth and maturity of ovarian follicles

9. A 72-year-old man asks the nurse whether it is normal for him to become impotent at his age. The best response by the nurse includes what information?
   a. Most decreased sexual function in older adults is due to psychologic stress.
   b. Physiologic changes of aging may require increased stimulation for an erection to occur.
   c. Although the penis decreases in size in older men, there should be no change in sexual function.
   d. Benign changes in the prostate gland that occur with aging can cause a decreased ability to attain an erection.

10. List one problem associated with each of these factors that may be identified during assessment of the reproductive system.

Factor	Problem Identified During Assessment
Rubella	
Mumps	
Diabetes mellitus	
Antihypertensive agents	

11. A 58-year-old man has difficulty starting a urinary stream and benign prostatic hyperplasia (BPH) is suspected. What is involved in the assessment of the patient for the presence of BPH?
    a. Palpating the scrotum and testes for a mass
    b. Palpating the base of the penis for enlargement
    c. Palpating the inguinal ring while the patient bears down
    d. A digital rectal examination to palpate the prostate gland

12. When assessing an aging adult man, what does the nurse note as a normal finding?
    a. Decreased penis size
    b. Decreased pubic hair
    c. A decrease in scrotal color
    d. Unilateral breast enlargement

13. When assessing an aging adult woman, what does the nurse note as a normal finding?
    a. Rectocele
    b. Larger breasts
    c. Vaginal dryness
    d. Severe osteoporosis

14. Identify one specific finding identified by the nurse during assessment of each of the patient's functional health patterns that indicates a risk factor for reproductive problems or a patient response to an actual reproductive problem.

Functional Health Pattern	Risk Factor for or Patient Response to Reproductive Problem
Health perception–health management	
Nutritional-metabolic	
Elimination	
Activity-exercise	
Sleep-rest	
Cognitive-perceptual	
Self-perception–self-concept	
Role-relationship	
Sexuality-reproductive	
Coping–stress tolerance	
Value-belief	

15. A 25-year-old female patient is at the clinic and says that she has white vaginal drainage and itching. Which etiology would be suspected?
    a. Cancer
    b. Candidiasis
    c. Trichomonas vaginalis
    d. Bacterial vaginosis infection

16. During examination of the female reproductive system, the nurse would note which finding as abnormal?
    a. Clear vaginal discharge
    b. Perineal episiotomy scars
    c. Nonpalpable Skene's glands
    d. Reddened base of the vulva

17. Which laboratory tests are used to diagnose *Chlamydia* (*select all that apply*)?
    a. Pap test
    b. Gram stain
    c. Rapid plasma reagin (RPR)
    d. Nucleic acid amplified test (NAAT)
    e. Venereal Disease Research Laboratory (VDRL)
    f. Fluorescent treponemal antibody absorption (FTA-Abs)

18. What is the serum estradiol laboratory test used for?
    a. Detect pregnancy
    b. Detect prostate cancer
    c. Measure ovarian function
    d. Identify secondary gonadal failure

19. ***Priority Decision:*** Following a dilation and curettage (D&C), what complication is most important for the nurse to assess the patient for?
    a. Infection
    b. Hemorrhage
    c. Urinary retention
    d. Perforation of the bladder

20. Which diagnostic tests of the female reproductive system are operative procedures requiring surgical anesthesia (*select all that apply*)?
    a. D&C
    b. Conization
    c. Culdoscopy
    d. Colposcopy
    e. Laparoscopy
    f. Endometrial biopsy

21. What is the fertility test that requires a couple to have sexual intercourse at the time of ovulation and come for testing 2 to 8 hours after intercourse?
    a. Huhner test
    b. Semen analysis
    c. Endometrial biopsy
    d. Hysterosalpingogram

CHAPTER 52

Nursing Management: Breast Disorders

1. A woman at the health clinic tells the nurse that she does not do breast self-examination (BSE) because it just seems too much of a bother. What is the best response by the nurse about BSE?
   a. It reduces mortality from breast cancer in women under the age of 50.
   b. It is useful to help women learn how their breasts normally look and feel.
   c. BSE has little value in detection of cancer and is not recommended anymore.
   d. BSE is the most common way that malignant tumors of the breast are discovered.

2. Identify the four screening guidelines for breast cancer accepted by organizations involved with breast cancer.
   a.

   b.

   c.

   d.

3. When teaching a 24-year-old woman who desires to learn BSE, the nurse knows that it is important to do what?
   a. Provide time for a return demonstration.
   b. Emphasize the statistics related to breast cancer survival and mortality.
   c. Have the woman set a consistent monthly date for performing the examination.
   d. Inform the woman that professional examinations are not necessary unless she finds an abnormality.

4. Which diagnostic test is most accurate and advantageous in terms of time and expense in diagnosing malignant breast disorders?
   a. Surgical biopsy
   b. Mammography
   c. Fine-needle aspiration
   d. Core (core needle) biopsy

5. A 24-year-old female patient has breast cancer with estrogen receptor–negative cells. Which genomic assay test can be used to provide information about the likely recurrence and need for chemotherapy?
   a. CA 27-29
   b. TNM system
   c. Oncotype DX
   d. MammaPrint

6. While examining a patient's breasts, the nurse notes multiple, bilateral mobile lumps. To assess the patient further, what is the most appropriate question by the nurse?
   a. "Do you have a high caffeine intake?"
   b. "When did you last have a mammogram?"
   c. "Is there a history of breast cancer in your mother or sisters?"
   d. "Do the size and tenderness of the lumps change with your menstrual cycle?"

7. A patient has fibrocystic changes in her breast. The nurse explains to the patient that this condition is significant because it
   a. commonly becomes malignant over time.
   b. can be controlled with hormone therapy (HT).
   c. makes it more difficult to examine the breasts.
   d. will eventually cause atrophy of normal breast tissue.

8. Which characteristics describe an intraductal papilloma (*select all that apply*)?
   a. Associated with breast trauma
   b. Occurs in 10% of women ages 15 to 40
   c. Has multicolored, sticky nipple discharge
   d. Is associated with an increased cancer risk
   e. Is more common in women ages 40 to 60
   f. Has wartlike growth in mammary ducts near nipple

9. Which benign breast disorder occurs most often during lactation and is commonly caused by *Staphylococcus aureus*?
   a. Mastitis
   b. Ductal ectasia
   c. Fibroadenoma
   d. Senescent gynecomastia

10. Which patient probably has the highest risk of breast cancer?
    a. 60-year-old obese man
    b. 58-year-old woman with sedentary lifestyle
    c. 55-year-old woman with fibrocystic breast changes
    d. 65-year-old woman with a sister diagnosed with breast cancer

11. The nurse would be most concerned when the patient's breast examination reveals which finding?
    a. A large, tender, moveable mass in the upper inner quadrant
    b. An immobile, hard, nontender lesion in the upper outer quadrant
    c. A 2- to 3-cm, firm, defined, mobile mass in the lower outer quadrant
    d. A painful, immobile mass with reddened skin in the upper outer quadrant

12. The best prognosis is indicated in the patient with breast cancer when diagnostic studies reveal
    a. negative axillary lymph nodes.
    b. aneuploid DNA tumor content.
    c. cells with high S-phase fractions.
    d. an estrogen receptor- and progesterone receptor–negative tumor.

13. The health care provider of a patient with a positive biopsy of a 2-cm breast tumor has recommended a lumpectomy with radiation therapy or a modified radical mastectomy as treatment. The patient says that she does not know how to choose and asks the female nurse what she would do if she had to make the choice. What is the best response by the nurse to this patient?
    a. "It doesn't matter what I would do. It is a decision you have to make for yourself."
    b. "There are advantages and disadvantages of both procedures. What do you know about these procedures?"
    c. "I would choose the modified radical mastectomy because it would ensure that the entire tumor was removed."
    d. "The lumpectomy maintains a nearly normal breast but the survival rate is not as good as it is with a mastectomy."

14. A patient undergoing either a mastectomy or a lumpectomy for treatment of breast cancer can also usually expect to undergo what other treatment?
    a. Chemotherapy
    b. Radiation therapy
    c. Hormonal therapy
    d. Sentinel lymph node dissection

15. Lymphatic mapping with sentinel lymph node dissection (SLND) is planned for a patient undergoing a modified radical mastectomy for breast cancer. What does the nurse teach the patient and her family?
    a. If one sentinel lymph node is positive for malignant cells, all of the sentinel lymph nodes will be removed.
    b. If malignant cells are found in any sentinel nodes, a complete axillary lymph node dissection will be done.
    c. Lymphatic mapping indicates which lymph nodes are most likely to have metastasis and all of those nodes are removed.
    d. Lymphatic mapping with SLND provides metastatic lymph nodes to test for responsiveness to chemotherapy.

16. What describes the use of high-dose brachytherapy radiation (*select all that apply*)?
    a. May be completed in 5 days
    b. Follows local excision of tumor
    c. Alternative to traditional radiation therapy for early-stage breast cancer
    d. Used to treat possible local residual cancer cells following a mastectomy
    e. Used to reduce tumor size and stabilize metastatic lesions for pain relief

17. A patient with a positive breast biopsy tells the nurse that she read about tamoxifen (Nolvadex) on the Internet and asks about its use. The best response by the nurse includes which information?
    a. Tamoxifen is the primary treatment for breast cancer if axillary lymph nodes are positive for cancer.
    b. Tamoxifen is used only to prevent the development of new primary tumors in women with high risk for breast cancer.
    c. Tamoxifen is the treatment of choice after surgery if the tumor has receptors for estrogen and progesterone on its cells.
    d. Because tamoxifen has been shown to increase the risk for uterine cancer, it is used only when other treatment has not been successful.

18. During the immediate postoperative period following a mastectomy, the nurse initially institutes which exercises for the affected arm?
    a. Have the patient brush or comb her hair with the affected arm.
    b. Perform full passive range-of-motion (ROM) exercises to the affected arm.
    c. Ask the patient to flex and extend the fingers and wrist of the operative side.
    d. Have the patient crawl her fingers up the wall, raising her arm above her head.

19. Following a modified radical mastectomy, a patient develops lymphedema of the affected arm. What does the nurse teach the patient to do?
    a. Avoid skin-softening agents on the arm.
    b. Protect the arm from any type of trauma.
    c. Abduct and adduct the arm at the shoulder hourly.
    d. Keep the arm positioned so that it is in straight and dependent alignment.

20. A patient undergoing surgery and radiation for treatment of breast cancer has a nursing diagnosis of disturbed body image *related to* absence of the breast. What is an appropriate nursing intervention for this patient?
    a. Provide the patient with information about surgical breast reconstruction.
    b. Restrict visitors and phone calls until the patient feels better about herself.
    c. Arrange for a Reach to Recovery visitor or similar resource available in the community.
    d. Encourage the patient to obtain a permanent breast prosthesis as soon as she is discharged from the hospital.

21. A 56-year-old patient is undergoing a mammoplasty for breast reconstruction following a mastectomy 1 year ago. During the preoperative preparation of the patient, what is important for the nurse to do?
    a. Determine why the patient is choosing reconstruction surgery rather than the use of an external prosthesis.
    b. Ensure that the patient has realistic expectations about the outcome and possible complications of the surgery.
    c. Inform the patient that implants used for breast reconstruction have been shown to cause immune-related diseases.
    d. Let the patient know that although the shape will be different from the other breast, the nipple can be reconstructed from other erectile tissue.

22. A patient undergoing a modified radical mastectomy for cancer of the breast is going to use tissue expansion and an implant for breast reconstruction. What should the nurse teach the patient about tissue expansion?
    a. Weekly injections of water or saline into the expander will be required.
    b. The expander cannot be placed until healing from the mastectomy is complete.
    c. This method of breast reconstruction uses the patient's own tissue to replace breast tissue.
    d. The nipple from the affected breast will be saved to be grafted onto the reconstructed breast.

23. The patient's breast cancer has metastasized. Which medication for metastasis is better tolerated and has fewer and milder side effects than other chemotherapy medications?
    a. Capecitabine (Xeloda)
    b. Vinorelbine (Navelbine)
    c. Doxorubicin (Adriamycin)
    d. Eribulin mesylate (Halaven)

CASE STUDY
Metastatic Breast Cancer

Patient Profile

P.T., a 57-year-old married lawyer, was found to have a 4- × 6-cm firm, fixed mass in the upper, outer quadrant of the right breast during a routine physical examination. A core (core needle) biopsy indicated a malignant tumor. Although the surgeon recommended a mastectomy because of the size of the tumor, P.T. chose to have a lumpectomy. Now 3 weeks postoperative, she is scheduled for chemotherapy.

Subjective Data

- Never had a routine mammogram
- Never practiced BSE
- States that she deserves to have breast cancer for being so careless about her health
- Chose to have a lumpectomy to remove the tumor despite its large size because she believes that her breasts are critical in her relationship with her husband

Objective Data

- Physical examination
- Right breast: Healed lumpectomy breast incision and right axillary incision
- Limited ROM of right arm
- Groshong catheter in place on left upper chest

Diagnostic Studies

- Pathology: Estrogen receptor–positive infiltrating ductal carcinoma; 8 of 12 lymph nodes positive for malignant cells
- Staging: Stage IIIA carcinoma of the right breast
- Lumpectomy performed to remove tumor 3 weeks ago
- Chemotherapy with CAF protocol planned: cyclophosphamide (Cytoxan), doxorubicin (Adriamycin), and 5-fluorouracil (5-FU)

Discussion Questions

Using a separate sheet of paper, answer the following questions:

1. Why is chemotherapy indicated for P.T.?
2. Compare the three chemotherapeutic agents planned for P.T. with respect to classification type, cell specificity, and common side effects.
3. What can the nurse do to help P.T. reduce or manage the common physical effects of the chemotherapy?
4. What does the finding that P.T.'s tumor is estrogen receptor–positive mean? What additional treatment modalities might this suggest?
5. How could the nurse help P.T. cope with her feelings of guilt and maintain a positive relationship with her husband?
6. What are some possible reasons that P.T. did not perform BSE or have mammography performed?
7. P.T's husband asks the nurse about his wife's problems concentrating during their conversations. How should the nurse respond?
8. *Priority Decision:* What are the teaching priorities for P.T. regarding follow-up care related to recurrence of the breast cancer?
9. *Priority Decision:* Based on the assessment data presented, what are the priority nursing diagnoses? Are there any collaborative problems?

53

Nursing Management: Sexually Transmitted Infections

1. The current incidence of sexually transmitted infections (STIs) is related in part to what?
   a. Increased social acceptance of homosexuality
   b. Increased virulence of organisms causing STIs
   c. The use of oral agents rather than condoms as contraceptives
   d. Development of resistance of microorganisms to common antibiotics

2. In establishing screening programs for populations at high risk for STIs, the nurse recognizes that which microorganism causes nongonococcal urethritis in men and cervicitis in women?
   a. Herpes simplex virus
   b. *Treponema pallidum*
   c. *Chlamydia trachomatis*
   d. *Neisseria gonorrhoeae*

3. The laboratory result of a specimen from a 20-year-old female patient shows human papillomavirus (HPV). What would the nurse suspect the patient's diagnosis to be?
   a. Syphilis
   b. Gonorrhea
   c. Genital warts
   d. Genital herpes

4. A female patient with a purulent vaginal discharge is seen at an outpatient clinic. The nurse suspects a diagnosis of gonorrhea. How would this STI be treated?
   a. Oral acyclovir (Zovirax)   Herpes
   b. Benzathine penicillin G given IM
   c. Ceftriaxone (Rocephin) IM or oral cefixime (Suprax)
   d. Would need a second confirmatory test result before treatment

5. A 22-year-old woman with multiple sexual partners seeks care after several weeks of experiencing painful and frequent urination and vaginal discharge. Although the results of a culture of cervical secretions are not yet available, the nurse explains to the patient that she will be treated as if she has gonorrhea and chlamydia to prevent
   a. obstruction of the fallopian tubes.
   b. endocarditis and aortic aneurysms.   Syphillis
   c. disseminated gonococcal infection.
   d. polyarthritis and generalized adenopathy.

6. *Priority Decision:* During evaluation and treatment of gonorrhea in a young man at the health clinic, what is most important for the nurse to question the patient about?
   a. A prior history of STIs
   b. When the symptoms began
   c. The date of his last sexual activity
   d. The names of his recent sexual partners

7. Which manifestations are characteristic of the late or tertiary stage of syphilis (*select all that apply*)?
   a. Heart failure
   b. Tabes dorsalis
   c. Saccular aneurysms
   d. Mental deterioration
   e. Generalized cutaneous rash
   f. Destructive skin, bone, and soft tissue lesions

8. Which stage of syphilis is identified by the absence of clinical manifestations and a positive fluorescent treponemal antibody absorption (FTA-Abs) test?
   a. Latent
   b. Primary
   c. Secondary
   d. Late (tertiary)

9. A premarital blood test for syphilis reveals that a woman has a positive Venereal Disease Research Laboratory (VDRL) test. How should the nurse advise the patient?
   a. A single dose of penicillin will cure the syphilis.
   b. She should question her fiancé about prior sexual contacts.
   c. Additional testing to detect specific antitreponemal antibodies is necessary.
   d. A lumbar puncture to evaluate cerebrospinal fluid (CSF) is necessary to rule out active syphilis.

10. Why should the nurse encourage serologic testing for human immunodeficiency virus (HIV) in the patient with syphilis?
    a. Syphilis is more difficult to treat in patients with HIV infection.
    b. The presence of HIV infection increases the risk of contracting syphilis.
    c. The incidence of syphilis is increased in those with high rates of sexual promiscuity and drug abuse.
    d. Central nervous system (CNS) involvement is more common in patients with HIV infection and syphilis.

11. A male patient returns to the clinic with a recurrent urethral discharge after being treated for a chlamydial infection 2 weeks ago. Which statement by the patient indicates the most likely cause of the recurrence of his infection?
    a. "I took the Vibramycin twice a day for a week."
    b. "I haven't told my girlfriend about my infection yet."
    c. "I had a couple of beers while I was taking the medication."
    d. "I've only had sexual intercourse once since my medication was finished."

12. What is the most common way to determine a diagnosis of chlamydial infection in a male patient?
    a. Cultures for chlamydial organisms are positive.
    b. The nucleic acid amplification test (NAAT) is positive.
    c. Gram stain smears and cultures are negative for gonorrhea.
    d. Signs and symptoms of epididymitis or proctitis are also present.

13. What are characteristics of a herpes simplex virus infection (*select all that apply*)?
    a. Treatment with acyclovir can cure genital herpes.
    b. Herpes simplex virus type 2 (HSV-2) is capable of causing only genital lesions.
    c. Recurrent symptomatic genital herpes may be precipitated by sexual activity and stress.
    d. To prevent transmission of genital herpes, condoms should be used when lesions are present.
    e. The primary symptom of genital herpes is painful vesicular lesions that rupture and ulcerate.

14. During the physical assessment of a female patient with HPV infection, what should the nurse expect to find?
    a. Purulent vaginal discharge
    b. A painless, indurated lesion on the vulva
    c. Painful perineal vesicles and ulcerations
    d. Multiple coalescing gray warts in the perineal area

15. ***Priority Decision:*** What is most important for the nurse to teach the female patient with genital warts?
    a. Have an annual Papanicolaou (Pap) test.
    b. Apply topical acyclovir faithfully as directed.
    c. Have her sexual partner treated for the condition.
    d. Use a contraceptive to prevent pregnancy, which might exacerbate the disease.

16. Which STI actively occurring at the time of delivery would indicate the need for a cesarean section delivery of the woman's baby?
    a. Syphilis
    b. Chlamydia
    c. Gonorrhea
    d. Genital herpes

17. Although an 18-year-old girl knows that abstinence is one way to prevent STIs, she does not consider that as an alternative. She asks the nurse at the clinic if there are other measures for preventing STIs. What should the nurse teach her?
    a. Abstinence is the only way to prevent STIs.
    b. Voiding immediately after intercourse will decrease the risk for infection.
    c. A vaccine can prevent genital warts and cervical cancer caused by some strains of HPV.
    d. Thorough hand washing after contact with genitals can prevent oral-genital spread of STIs.

18. Patients with which STI are most likely to avoid obtaining and following treatment measures for their infection?
    a. Syphilis
    b. Gonorrhea
    c. HPV infection
    d. Genital herpes

CASE STUDY

Gonorrhea

Patient Profile

C.J., a 20-year-old male college student, had intercourse with a prostitute while he was on vacation. He returns home 3 days later and has intercourse with his fiancée, Ms. A. The next day he begins to experience symptoms of an STI.

Subjective Data

- Experiences pain and burning on urination
- Has a yellowish-white discharge from his penis
- Expresses concern over the possibility of having gonorrhea and what this diagnosis would mean in his relationship with his fiancée

Objective Data

- Positive Gram stain for *N. gonorrhoeae*

Discussion Questions

Using a separate sheet of paper, answer the following questions:

1. C.J. asks the nurse's advice on how to tell his fiancée about the diagnosis. What should the nurse's advice be?
2. What symptoms will Ms. A. have if she becomes infected?
3. What physical examinations and laboratory procedures are required to establish a diagnosis of gonorrhea in C.J. and Ms. A.?
4. What measures can be used to assist the couple in coping with the psychologic implications of the infection?
5. What treatment will be prescribed for C.J. and Ms. A.?
6. What are the possible complications of untreated gonorrhea in men and in women?
7. *Priority Decision:* Based on the assessment data presented, what are the priority nursing diagnoses? Are there any collaborative problems?

CHAPTER

54

Nursing Management: Female Reproductive Problems

1. A couple seeks assistance from an infertility specialist for evaluation of their infertility. What does the nurse inform the couple they can expect during the initial visit?
   a. Physical and psychosocial functioning examinations
   b. Assessment of tubal patency with a hysterosalpingogram
   c. Pelvic ultrasound for the woman and semen analysis for the man
   d. Postcoital testing to evaluate sperm numbers and motility in cervical and vaginal secretions

2. An infertile couple has used at-home ovulation testing using basal body temperature without conceiving. The nurse understands that what will be used first to treat this infertile couple?
   a. Surgery to reduce endometriosis
   b. Intrauterine insemination with sperm from the husband
   c. Selective estrogen receptor modulator (clomiphene [Clomid])
   d. Assisted reproductive technologies (e.g., in vitro fertilization [IVF])

3. A patient with a 10-week pregnancy is admitted to the emergency department with vaginal bleeding and abdominal cramping. What does the nurse recognize about this situation?
   a. The patient will recover quickly when the bleeding stops.
   b. The patient is most likely experiencing a spontaneous abortion.
   c. The patient will be scheduled for an immediate dilation and curettage (D&C).
   d. Treatment of the patient with bed rest is usually successful in preventing further bleeding.

4. The patient is a perimenopausal woman who has an unexpected and unwanted pregnancy. She wants an abortion. What should the nurse teach her about the effects of an abortion?
   a. D&C will be needed.
   b. She will feel much better afterwards.
   c. The products of conception will pass immediately.
   d. She will need someone to support her through her loss.

5. Premenstrual syndrome (PMS) is most likely to be diagnosed in a woman with which occurrence?
   a. Symptoms can be controlled with the use of progesterone.
   b. The woman has symptoms only when oral contraceptives are used.
   c. Symptoms can be correlated with altered serum levels of estrogen and progesterone.
   d. The woman has the same symptom pattern following ovulation for two or three consecutive menstrual cycles.

6. When teaching a patient with PMS about management of the disorder, the nurse includes the need to
   a. supplement the diet with vitamins C and E.
   b. limit dietary intake of caffeine and refined sugar.
   c. use estrogen supplements during the luteal phase.
   d. limit exercise and physical activity when symptoms are present.

7. What is the rationale for the regular use of nonsteroidal antiinflammatory drugs (NSAIDs) during the first several days of the menstrual period for women who have primary dysmenorrhea?
   a. They suppress ovulation and the production of prostaglandins that occur with ovulation.
   b. They cause uterine relaxation and small vessel constriction, preventing cramping and abdominal congestion.
   c. They inhibit the production of prostaglandins believed to be responsible for menstrual pain and associated symptoms.
   d. They block the release of luteinizing hormone, preventing the increase in progesterone associated with maturation of the corpus luteum.

8. A 20-year-old woman is a college softball player who participates in strenuous practices and a heavy class schedule. She is describing an absence of menses. What could be contributing to her amenorrhea?
   a. Decreased sexual activity
   b. Excess prostaglandin production
   c. Strenuous exercise or lack of calories
   d. Endometrial cancer or uterine fibroids

9. A young woman who runs vigorously as a form of exercise has not had a menstrual period in more than 6 months. What should the nurse teach her?
   a. Normal periods will return when she stops running.
   b. Uterine balloon therapy may be necessary to promote uterine sloughing of the overgrown endometrium.
   c. Progesterone or birth control pills should be used to prevent persistent overgrowth of the endometrium.
   d. Unopposed progesterone production causes an overgrowth of the endometrium that increases her risk for endometrial cancer.

10. A 29-year-old woman is at the clinic with menorrhagia. What finding would the nurse expect in this patient's assessment?
    a. Pain with each menstrual period
    b. Excessive bleeding at irregular intervals
    c. Bleeding or spotting between menstrual periods
    d. Increased duration or amount of menstrual bleeding

11. **Priority Decision:** A patient with abdominal pain and irregular vaginal bleeding is admitted to the hospital with a suspected ectopic pregnancy. Before actual diagnosis, what is the most appropriate action by the nurse?
    a. Provide analgesics for pain relief.
    b. Monitor vital signs, pain, and bleeding frequently.
    c. Explain the need for frequent blood samples for β-human chorionic gonadotropin monitoring.
    d. Offer support for the patient's emotional response to the loss of the pregnancy.

12. Which manifestations of menopause are related to estrogen deficiency (*select all that apply*)?
    a. Cessation of menses
    b. Breast engorgement
    c. Vasomotor instability - 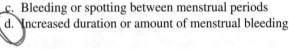 hot flashes, night sweats
    d. Reduction of bone fractures
    e. Decreased cardiovascular risk

13. A patient is 51 years old and suffered a wrist fracture when she slipped on the ice. She has her uterus and is interested in starting hormone therapy (HT), as she is also experiencing menopause symptoms. What should the nurse include when discussing the risks and benefits of HT with this patient?
    a. Taking only progestin is suggested for a woman with a uterus.
    b. Taking both estrogen and progestin may decrease her bone loss.
    c. The risk of breast cancer and cardiovascular disease is decreased with HT.
    d. Taking estrogen and progestin will increase the risk of endometrial cancer.

14. The patient arrives at the urgent care facility worried about the fishy smell of her vaginal discharge. What does the nurse suspect will be diagnosed?
    a. Cervicitis
    b. Trichomoniasis
    c. Bacterial vaginosis
    d. Vulvovaginal candidiasis

15. The patient calls the office and says that she thinks she has a "yeast infection." What signs or symptoms should the nurse expect in this patient (*select all that apply*)?
    a. Intense itching and dysuria
    b. Hemorrhagic cervix and vagina
    c. Pruritic, frothy greenish or gray discharge
    d. Thick, white, cottage cheese–like discharge
    e. Mucopurulent discharge and postcoital spotting

16. A patient is diagnosed and treated for a *Gardnerella vaginalis* infection at a clinic. For her treatment to be effective, what does the nurse tell the patient?
    a. Her sexual partner should also be examined and treated.
    b. Her sexual partner must use a condom during intercourse.
    c. She should wear minipads to prevent reinfection as long as she has vaginal drainage.
    d. The vaginal suppository should be used in the morning so it will be fighting the infection all day.

17. A young woman is admitted to the hospital with acute pelvic inflammatory disease (PID). During the nursing history, the nurse notes which risk factor as being significant for this patient?
    a. Lack of any method of birth control
    b. Sexual activity with multiple partners
    c. Use of a vaginal sponge for contraception
    d. Recent antibiotic-induced monilial vaginitis

18. What should the nurse include when implementing care for the patient with acute PID?
    a. Perform vaginal irrigations every 4 hours.
    b. Promote bed rest in semi-Fowler's position.
    c. Instruct the patient to use tampons to control vaginal drainage.
    d. Ambulate the patient frequently to promote drainage of exudate.

19. A 20-year-old patient with PID is crying and tells the nurse that she is afraid she will not be able to have children as a result of the infection. What is the nurse's best response to the patient?
    a. "I would not worry about that right now. Our immediate concern is to cure the infection you have."
    b. "Sterility following PID is possible but not common and it is too soon to know what the effects will be."
    c. "The possibility of infertility following PID is increased. Would you like to talk about what it means to you?"
    d. "The infection can cause more serious complications, such as abscesses and shock, that you should be more concerned about."

20. The patient is suspected of having endometriosis and/or uterine leiomyoma. What best describes what is found with these conditions?
    a. Endometriosis and uterine leiomyoma are two gynecologic conditions that increase with the onset of menopause.
    b. Danazol (Danacrine) and Lupron (GnRH analog) are used to treat endometriosis and leiomyomas to create a pseudopregnancy.
    c. Treatment of endometriosis and leiomyomas depends on the severity of symptoms and the woman's desire to maintain fertility.
    d. The presence of ectopic uterine tissue that bleeds and causes pelvic and abdominal adhesions, cysts, and pain is known as uterine leiomyoma.

21. An 18-year-old patient with irregular menstrual periods, hirsutism, and obesity has been diagnosed with polycystic ovary syndrome (PCOS). What is an accurate rationale for the expected treatment?
    a. Hirsutism may be treated with leuprolide to decrease an altered body image.
    b. The medication used will cure the hormonal abnormality of excess testosterone.
    c. The loss of weight will improve all of the symptoms, so this will be the first treatment tried.
    d. The progression of PCOS leads to cardiovascular disease and possibly to type 2 diabetes mellitus if untreated.

22. A patient with a stage 0 cervical cancer identified from a Papanicolaou (Pap) test asks the nurse what this finding means. The nurse's response should include which information?
    a. Malignant cells have extended beyond the cervix to the upper vagina.
    b. Abnormal cells are present but are confined to the epithelial layer of the cervix.
    c. Atypical cells characteristic of inflammation but not necessarily malignancy are present.
    d. This is a common finding on Pap testing and she will be examined frequently to see whether the abnormal cells spread beyond the cervix.

23. Fertility and normal reproductive function can be maintained when a cancer of the cervix is successfully treated with which therapy?
    a. External radiation therapy
    b. Internal radiation implants
    c. Conization or laser surgery
    d. Cryotherapy or subtotal hysterectomy

24. A woman who has been postmenopausal for 10 years calls the clinic because of vaginal bleeding. The nurse schedules a visit for the patient and informs her to expect to have which diagnostic procedure?
    a. An endometrial biopsy
    b. Abdominal radiography
    c. A laser treatment to the cervix
    d. Only a routine pelvic examination and Pap test

25. A patient has been diagnosed with cancer of the ovary. In planning care for the patient, what does the nurse recognize that treatment of the patient depends on?
    a. Results of a direct-needle biopsy of the ovary
    b. Results of a laparoscopy with multiple biopsies
    c. Whether the patient desires to maintain fertility
    d. The findings of metastasis by ultrasound or computed tomography (CT) scan

26. Which cancer is associated with intrauterine exposure to diethylstilbestrol (DES) or metastasis from another gynecologic cancer?
    a. Vaginal
    b. Ovarian
    c. Cervical
    d. Endometrial

27. Which factors are associated with endometrial cancer (*select all that apply*)?
    a. Obesity
    b. Smoking
    c. Family history
    d. Early sexual activity
    e. Early menarche and late menopause
    f. Unopposed estrogen-only replacement therapy

28. During assessment of the patient with vulvar cancer, what should the nurse expect to find?
    a. Soreness and itching of the vulva
    b. Labial lesions with purulent exudate
    c. Severe excoriation of the labia and perineum
    d. Painless, firm nodules embedded in the labia

29. A 44-year-old woman undergoing a total abdominal hysterectomy asks whether she will need to take estrogen until she reaches the age of menopause. What is the best response by the nurse?
    a. "Yes, it will help to prevent the more intense symptoms caused by surgically induced menopause."
    b. "You are close enough to normal menopause that you probably won't need additional estrogen."
    c. "Because your ovaries won't be removed, they will continue to secrete estrogen until your normal menopause."
    d. "There are so many risks associated with estrogen replacement therapy that it is best to begin menopause now."

30. A disturbed body image needing nursing interventions to assist the patient and family to cope may be seen in any patient undergoing gynecologic surgery. With which surgery will this most likely be expected to occur?
    a. Vaginectomy
    b. Hemivulvectomy
    c. Pelvic exenteration
    d. Radical hysterectomy

31. What occurs during treatment of the patient with an intrauterine radioactive implant?
    a. All care should be provided by the same nurse.
    b. The patient may ambulate in the room as desired.
    c. There can be unlimited number and duration of visitors.
    d. The patient is restricted to bed rest with turning from side to side.

32. When teaching a patient with problems of pelvic support to perform Kegel exercises, what should the nurse tell the patient to do?
    a. Contract her muscles as if trying to stop the flow of urine.
    b. Tighten the lower abdominal muscles over the bladder area.
    c. Squeeze all of the perineal muscles as if trying to close the vagina.
    d. Lie on the floor and do leg lifts to strengthen the abdominal muscles.

33. The patient is describing a feeling of something coming down her vagina and having a backache. What is most likely the cause of this discomfort?
    a. Cystocele
    b. Dysmenorrhea
    c. Uterine prolapse
    d. Abdominal distention

34. *Priority Decision:* The patient's diagnosis is a large rectocele requiring surgery. What nursing interventions will be the priority postoperatively?
    a. An ice pack to relieve swelling
    b. An enema each day to relieve constipation
    c. Administration of a stool softener each night
    d. Perineal care after each urination or defecation

35. What is an appropriate outcome for a patient who undergoes an anterior colporrhaphy?
    a. Maintain normal bowel patterns   ↳surgery to fix recto or cystocele
    b. Adjust to temporary ileal conduit
    c. Urinate within 8 hours postoperatively
    d. Experience healing of excoriated vaginal and vulvar tissue

36. *Priority Decision:* On admission of a victim of sexual assault to the emergency department, what should be the first priority of the nurse?
    a. Contact a rape support person for the patient.
    b. Assess the patient for urgent medical problems.
    c. Question the patient about the details of the assault.
    d. Inform the patient what procedures and treatments will be performed.

37. *Priority Decision:* To prepare a woman who has been raped for physical examination, what should the nurse do first?
    a. Ensure that a signed informed consent is obtained from the patient.
    b. Provide a private place for the patient to talk about what happened to her.
    c. Instruct the patient not to wash, eat, drink, or urinate before the examination.
    d. Administer prophylaxis for sexually transmitted infections (STIs) and tetanus.

CASE STUDY
Acute Pelvic Inflammatory Disease
Patient Profile

A.R. is a 23-year-old unmarried woman. For the past 2 weeks she has had a heavy purulent vaginal discharge, lower abdominal pain, and general malaise. Concerned that her symptoms appear to be worsening, A.R. makes an appointment at the gynecologic clinic.

Subjective Data

- Experiences an increase in lower abdominal pain during vaginal examination
- Expresses concern over worsening of her condition and the effect this will have on future childbearing ability

Objective Data

- Vital signs: Temp 101°F (38.3°C), HR 90 bpm, RR 18, BP 110/58
- Physical examination: Heavy, purulent vaginal discharge
- Diagnostic studies: Vaginal discharge positive for *Neisseria gonorrhoeae*
- Admitted to the hospital for monitoring, IV fluids, and antibiotic therapy

---

Discussion Questions

Using a separate sheet of paper, answer the following questions:

1. What route does the gonococcus take in the development of PID?
2. What are the clinical manifestations of acute PID?
3. How would A.R.'s infection be managed if the decision is made to treat her as an outpatient? What instructions should she receive?
4. How is chronic pelvic pain related to acute PID?
5. *Priority Decision:* What priority measures should the nurse take to prevent complications of the infection?
6. How should the nurse respond to A.R.'s concern over the effect of this infection on her future childbearing ability?
7. *Priority Decision:* Based on the assessment data presented, what are the priority nursing diagnoses? Are there any collaborative problems?

1. A patient asks the nurse what the difference is between benign prostatic hyperplasia (BPH) and prostate cancer. The best response by the nurse includes what information about BPH?
   a. BPH is a benign tumor that does not spread beyond the prostate gland.
   b. BPH is a precursor to prostate cancer but does not yet show any malignant changes.
   c. BPH is an enlargement of the gland caused by an increase in the size of existing cells.
   d. BPH is a benign enlargement of the gland caused by an increase in the number of normal cells.

2. When taking a nursing history from a patient with BPH, the nurse would expect the patient to report
   a. nocturia, dysuria, and bladder spasms.
   b. urinary frequency, hematuria, and perineal pain.
   c. urinary hesitancy, postvoid dribbling, and weak urinary stream.
   d. urinary urgency with a forceful urinary stream and cloudy urine.

3. The extent of urinary obstruction caused by BPH can be determined by which diagnostic study?
   a. A cystometrogram
   b. Transrectal ultrasound
   c. Urodynamic flow studies
   d. Postvoiding catheterization

4. What is the effect of finasteride (Proscar) in the treatment of BPH?
   a. A reduction in the size of the prostate gland
   b. Relaxation of the smooth muscle of the urethra
   c. Increased bladder tone that promotes bladder emptying
   d. Relaxation of the bladder detrusor muscle promoting urine flow

5. On admission to the ambulatory surgical center, a patient with BPH informs the nurse that he is going to have a laser treatment of his enlarged prostate. The nurse plans patient teaching with the knowledge that the patient will need to know what?
   a. The effects of general anesthesia
   b. The possibility of short-term incontinence
   c. Home management of an indwelling catheter
   d. Monitoring for postoperative urinary retention

6. What is the most common screening intervention for detecting BPH in men over age 50?
   a. PSA level
   b. Urinalysis
   c. Cystoscopy
   d. Digital rectal examination

7. Which treatment for BPH uses a low-wave radiofrequency to precisely destroy prostate tissue?
   a. Laser prostatectomy
   b. Transurethral needle ablation (TUNA)
   c. Transurethral microwave thermotherapy (TUMT)
   d. Transurethral electrovaporization of prostate (TUVP)

8. Which characteristics describe transurethral resection of the prostate (TURP) (*select all that apply*)?
   a. Best used for a very large prostate gland
   b. Inappropriate for men with rectal problems
   c. Involves an external incision prostatectomy
   d. Uses transurethral incisions into the prostate
   e. Most common surgical procedure to treat BPH
   f. Resectoscopic excision and cauterization of prostate tissue

9. Which therapies for BPH are done on an outpatient basis (*select all that apply*)?
   a. Intraprostatic urethral stents
   b. Transurethral needle ablation (TUNA)
   c. Transurethral incision of prostate (TUIP)
   d. Transurethral microwave therapy (TUMT)
   e. Visual laser ablation of the prostate (VLAP)

10. Before undergoing a TURP, what should the patient be taught?
    a. Some degree of urinary incontinence is likely to occur.
    b. This surgery results in some degree of retrograde ejaculation.
    c. Erectile dysfunction is a common complication of this prostate surgery.
    d. An indwelling catheter will be used to maintain urinary output until healing is complete.

11. Following a TURP, a patient has continuous bladder irrigation. Four hours after surgery, the catheter is draining thick, bright red clots and tissue. What should the nurse do?
    a. Release the traction on the catheter.
    b. Manually irrigate the catheter until the drainage is clear.
    c. Increase the rate of the irrigation and take the patient's vital signs.
    d. Clamp the drainage tube and notify the patient's health care provider.

12. **Priority Decision:** A patient with continuous bladder irrigation following a prostatectomy tells the nurse that he has bladder spasms and leaking of urine around the catheter. What should the nurse do first?
    a. Slow the rate of the irrigation.
    b. Assess the patency of the catheter.
    c. Encourage the patient to try to urinate around the catheter.
    d. Administer a belladonna and opium (B&O) suppository as prescribed.

13. The nurse provides discharge teaching to a patient following a TURP and determines that the patient understands the instructions when he makes which statement?
    a. "I should use daily enemas to avoid straining until healing is complete."
    b. "I should avoid heavy lifting, climbing, and driving until my follow-up visit."
    c. "At least I don't have to worry about developing cancer of the prostate now."
    d. "Every day I should drink 10 to 12 glasses of liquids such as coffee, tea, or soft drinks."

14. A 55-year-old man with a history of prostate cancer in his family asks the nurse what he can do to decrease the risk of prostate cancer. What should the nurse teach him about prostate cancer risks?
    a. Nothing can decrease the risk because prostate cancer is primarily a disease of aging.
    b. Treatment of any enlargement of the prostate gland will help to prevent prostate cancer.
    c. Substituting fresh fruits and vegetables for high-fat foods in the diet may lower the risk of prostate cancer.
    d. Using a natural herb, saw palmetto, has been found to be an effective protection against prostate cancer.

15. **Priority Decision:** When caring for a patient following a radical prostatectomy with a perineal approach, what is the priority nursing intervention the nurse should use to prevent complications?
    a. Use chemotherapeutic agents to prevent metastasis.
    b. Administer sildenafil (Viagra) as needed for erectile dysfunction.
    c. Provide wound care after each bowel movement to prevent infection.
    d. Insert a smaller indwelling urinary catheter to prevent urinary retention.

16. What accurately describes prostate cancer detection and/or treatment (*select all that* apply)?
    a. The symptoms of pelvic or perineal pain, fatigue, and malaise may be present.
    b. Palpation of the prostate reveals hard and asymmetric enlargement with areas of induration or nodules.
    c. Orchiectomy is a treatment option for all patients with prostatic cancer except those with stage IV tumors.
    d. The preferred hormonal therapy for treatment of prostate cancer includes estrogen and androgen receptor blockers.
    e. Early detection of cancer of the prostate is increased with annual rectal examinations and serum prostatic acid phosphatase (PAP) measurements.
    f. An annual prostate examination is recommended starting at age 45 for African American men because of the increased mortality rate from prostatic cancer in this population.

17. What occurs with chronic bacterial prostatitis but not with acute prostatitis?
    a. Postejaculatory pain
    b. Frequency, urgency, and dysuria
    c. Symptoms of a urinary tract infection
    d. Enlarged, boggy prostate on palpation

18. What describes hypospadias?
    a. Scrotal lymphedema
    b. Undescended testicle
    c. Ventral urinary meatus
    d. Inflammation of the prepuce

19. What is an explanation that the nurse should give to the patient who asks what his diagnosis of paraphimosis means?
    a. Painful, prolonged erection
    b. Inflammation of the epididymis
    c. Painful downward curvature of an erect penis
    d. Retracted tight foreskin preventing return over the glans

20. The cremasteric reflex is absent in which problem of the scrotum and testes?
    a. Hydrocele
    b. Varicocele
    c. Spermatocele
    d. Testicular torsion

21. Serum tumor markers that may be elevated on diagnosis of testicular cancer and used to monitor the response to therapy include
    a. tumor necrosis factor (TNF) and C-reactive protein (CRP).
    b. α-fetoprotein (AFP) and human chorionic gonadotropin (hCG).
    c. prostate-specific antigen (PSA) and prostate acid phosphatase (PAP).
    d. carcinoembryonic antigen (CEA) and antinuclear antibody (ANA).

22. When teaching a patient testicular self-examination, the nurse instructs the patient to report which finding?
    a. An irregular-feeling epididymis
    b. One testis larger than the other
    c. The spermatic cord within the testicle
    d. A firm, nontender nodule on the testis

23. The nurse teaches the patient having a vasectomy that what occurs after the procedure?
    a. The amount of ejaculate will be noticeably decreased.
    b. He may have difficulty maintaining an erection for several months.
    c. An alternative form of contraception must be used for 6 to 8 weeks.
    d. The testes will gradually decrease production of sperm and testosterone.

24. A patient is seeking medical intervention for erectile dysfunction. Why should he be thoroughly evaluated?
    a. Treatment of erectile dysfunction is based on the cause of the problem.
    b. Psychologic counseling can reverse the problem in 80% to 90% of the cases.
    c. New invasive and experimental techniques currently used have unknown risks.
    d. Most treatments for erectile dysfunction are contraindicated in patients with systemic diseases.

25. A 66-year-old male patient is experiencing erectile dysfunction (ED). He and his wife have used tadalafil (Cialis) but because he experienced priapism, they have decided to change their treatment option to an intraurethral device. How should the nurse explain how this device works?
    a. The device relaxes smooth muscle in the penis.
    b. Blood is drawn into corporeal bodies and held with a ring.
    c. The device is implanted into corporeal bodies to firm the penis.
    d. The device directly applies drugs that increase blood flow in the penis.

26. A 47-year-old patient who is experiencing andropause has decided to try the testosterone gel Testim. What should the nurse teach the patient and his wife about this gel?
    a. Wash the hands with soap and water after applying it.
    b. His wife should apply it to help him feel better about using it.
    c. Do not wear clothing over the area until it has been absorbed.
    d. The gel may be taken buccally if it is not effective on the abdomen.

27. The couple has not been able to become pregnant. The wife has not been diagnosed with any infertility problems. Which treatment will the nurse expect to teach the couple about if the problem is the most common testicular problem causing male infertility?
    a. Antibiotics
    b. Semen analysis
    c. Avoidance of scrotal heat
    d. Surgery to correct the problem

CASE STUDY
Testicular Cancer
Patient Profile

Following a shower last evening, C.E., who is 19 years old, was performing his routine testicular self-examination when he discovered a firm lump on his left testis. After a medical examination, he was admitted to the hospital for a left orchiectomy and lymph node resection.

Subjective Data

- Has a history of an undescended left testis, which was surgically corrected at age 2
- Expresses concern about surgery and how it will affect him
- Asks about his prognosis and chances for recovery after the surgery
- Denies back pain

Objective Data

- Very firm, nontender nodule on left testis
- Local lymph node enlargement
- No gynecomastia noted
- Biopsy revealed seminoma germ cell tumor

Discussion Questions

Using a separate sheet of paper, answer the following questions:

1. Explain the development and risk factors for cancer of the testis.
2. How does cancer of the testis differ from a spermatocele on examination?
3. What is C.E.'s prognosis if the malignancy is in early stages?
4. What blood tests for tumor markers should be done preoperatively and are indicated for long-term follow-up care and why?
5. How can the nurse help C.E. to deal with the psychologic components of his illness?
6. What effect will this surgery have on C.E.'s sexual functioning?
7. Will he need any further treatment?
8. He tells the nurse that he is not married yet but would like to have children someday. What should the nurse explain to him?
9. *Priority Decision:* Based on the assessment data presented, what are the priority nursing diagnoses?

Nursing Assessment: Nervous System

1. Using the list of terms below, identify the structures of the neuron in the following illustration.

Terms

Axon
Collateral axon
Dendrites
Mitochondrion

Myelin sheath
Neuron cell body
Node of Ranvier
Nucleolus

Nucleus
Schwann cell
Synaptic knobs
Telodendria (presynaptic terminal)

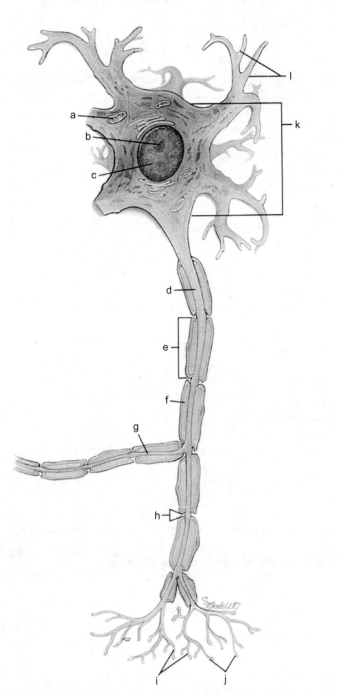

a. _____

b. _____

c. _____

d. _____

e. _____

f. _____

g. _____

h. _____

i. _____

j. _____

k. _____

l. _____

2. Using the following list of terms, identify the structures in the illustration below.

Terms

Anterior horn	Dura mater	Spinal nerves
Arachnoid	Gray matter	Sympathetic ganglion
Body of vertebra	Pia mater	Transverse process of vertebra
Central canal	Spinal cord	Ventral root
Dorsal root	Spinal ganglia	White matter

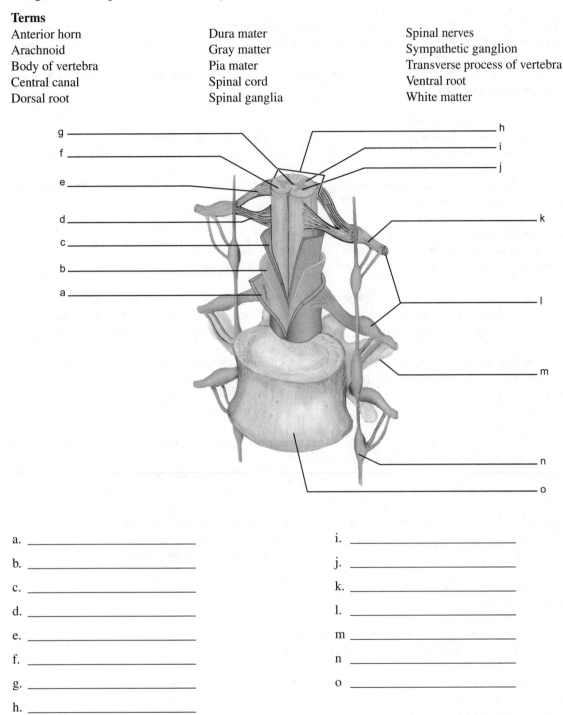

a. _____		i. _____
b. _____		j. _____
c. _____		k. _____
d. _____		l. _____
e. _____		m _____
f. _____		n _____
g. _____		o _____
h. _____		

3. What is the protective fluid of the central nervous system (CNS)?
   a. Synaptic cleft
   b. Limbic system
   c. Myelin sheath
   d. Cerebrospinal fluid (CSF)

4. Which type of macroglial cells myelinate peripheral nerve fibers?
   a. Neurons
   b. Astrocytes
   c. Schwann cells
   d. Ependymal cells

5. What happens at the synapse?
   a. The synapse physically joins two neurons.
   b. The nerve impulse is transmitted only from one neuron to another neuron.
   c. The presynaptic terminal submits a nerve impulse through the synaptic cleft to the receptor site on the postsynaptic cell.
   d. When a presynaptic cell releases excitatory neurotransmitters, the postsynaptic cell depolarizes enough to generate an action potential.

6. What is the function of the dendrite?
   a. A gap in the peripheral nerve axons
   b. Carries impulses to the nerve cell body
   c. Carries impulses from the nerve cell body
   d. May occur with damage to peripheral axons

7. A patient has a lesion involving the fasciculus gracilis and fasciculus cuneatus of the spinal cord. What should the nurse expect the patient to experience the loss of?
   a. Pain and temperature sensations
   b. Touch, deep pressure, vibration, and position sense
   c. Subconscious information about body position and muscle tension
   d. Voluntary muscle control from the cerebral cortex to the peripheral nerves

8. What is different when a lesion occurs in a lower motor neuron compared to in an upper motor neuron?
   a. Causes hyporeflexia and flaccidity
   b. Affects motor control of the lower body
   c. Arises in structures above the spinal cord
   d. Interferes with reflex arcs in the spinal cord

9. The patient is admitted to the emergency department having difficulty with respiratory, vasomotor, and cardiac function. Which portion of the brain is affected to cause these manifestations?
   a. Medulla
   b. Cerebellum
   c. Parietal lobe
   d. Wernicke's area

10. A 28-year-old female patient has been diagnosed with occipital lobe damage after a car accident. What should the nurse expect the patient to need help with?
    a. Being able to feel heat
    b. Processing visual images
    c. Identifying smells appropriately
    d. Being able to say what she means

11. Which area of the brain regulates endocrine and autonomic nervous system (ANS) functions?
    a. Basal ganglia
    b. Temporal lobe
    c. Hypothalamus
    d. Reticular activating system

12. What functions does the thalamus have?
    a. Registers auditory input
    b. Integrates past experiences
    c. Relays sensory and motor input to and from the cerebrum
    d. Controls and facilitates learned and automatic movements

13. How do spinal nerves of the peripheral nervous system (PNS) differ from cranial nerves (CNs)?
    a. Only spinal nerves occur in pairs.
    b. CNs affect only the sensory and motor functions of the head and neck.
    c. Cell bodies of all CNs are located in the brain whereas cell bodies of spinal nerves are located in the spinal cord.
    d. All spinal nerves contain both afferent sensory and efferent motor fibers whereas CNs contain one or the other or both.

14. Which descriptions are characteristic of the sympathetic nervous system (SNS) (*select all that apply*)?
    a. Necessary for male erection
    b. Necessary for male ejaculation
    c. Increases heart rate (HR) and dilates coronary arteries
    d. Norepinephrine released by most postganglionic fibers
    e. Preganglionic cell bodies located in spinal segments T1–L2
    f. Responsible for conservation and restoration of energy stores

15. A patient has an atherosclerotic plaque in the middle cerebral artery. What does the nurse recognize about this patient's situation?
    a. Assessment will reveal distended jugular veins.
    b. Cerebral circulation may be maintained through the circle of Willis.
    c. The patient will develop a loss of temporal and parietal lobe function.
    d. Increased pressure in the middle cerebral artery will back up into the vertebral arteries.

16. When the patient has a rapidly growing brain tumor, what slows expansion of cerebral brain tissue into the adjacent hemisphere?
    a. Ventricles
    b. Falx cerebri
    c. Arachnoid layer
    d. Tentorium cerebella

17. After talking with the health care provider, the patient asks what the blood-brain barrier does. What is the best description that the nurse can give the patient?
    a. Protects the brain from external trauma
    b. Protects against harmful blood-borne agents
    c. Provides for flexibility while protecting the spinal cord
    d. Forms the outer layer of protective membranes around the brain and spinal cord

18. During neurologic assessment of the older adult, what should the nurse expect to find?
    a. Absent deep tendon reflexes
    b. Below-average intelligence score
    c. Decreased sensation of touch and temperature
    d. Decreased frequency of spontaneous awakening

19. What factors should be considered when taking the history of a patient with a neurologic problem (*select all that apply*)?
    a. Avoid suggesting symptoms.
    b. Include the CN assessment as the first assessment.
    c. Mental status must be accurately assessed to ensure that the reported history is factual.
    d. Do a focused assessment of the neurologic system, as other body systems will not be affected.
    e. The mode of onset and course of illness are especially important aspects of the nursing history.

20. Identify one specific finding identified by the nurse during assessment of each of the patient's functional health patterns that indicates a risk factor for neurologic problems or a patient response to an actual neurologic problem.

Functional Health Pattern	Risk Factor for or Patient Response to Neurologic Problem
Health perception–health management	
Nutritional-metabolic	
Elimination	
Activity-exercise	
Sleep-rest	
Cognitive-perceptual	
Self-perception–self-concept	
Role-relationship	
Sexuality-reproductive	
Coping–stress tolerance	
Value-belief	

21. Which CNs are involved with oblique eye movements (*select all that apply*)?
    a. Optic (CN II)
    b. Trochlear (CN IV)
    c. Trigeminal (CN V)
    d. Abducens (CN VI)
    e. Oculomotor (CN III)

22. Which CN responds to the corneal reflex test?
    a. Optic (CN II)
    b. Vagus (CN X)
    c. Trigeminal (CN V)
    d. Spinal accessory (CN XI)

23. What methods are used to assess the facial (CN VII) nerve (*select all that apply*)?
    a. Gag reflex
    b. Confrontation
    c. Corneal reflex test
    d. Light touch to the face
    e. Smile, frown, and close eyes
    f. Salt and sugar discrimination

24. Which CN is tested with tongue protrusion?
    a. Vagus (CN X)
    b. Olfactory (CN I)
    c. Hypoglossal (CN XII)
    d. Glossopharyngeal (CN IX)

25. In the neurologic nursing assessment of the patient, he is unable to hear a ticking watch. What neurologic problem could be the cause of this finding?
    a. The patient is distracted.
    b. The patient is hard of hearing.
    c. The vagus (CN X) nerve is malfunctioning.
    d. The cochlear branch of the acoustic (CN VIII) nerve is damaged.

26. During an assessment of the motor system, the nurse finds that the patient has a staggering gait and an abnormal arm swing. What should the nurse use this information to do?
    a. Assist the patient to cope with the disability.
    b. Plan a rehabilitation program for the patient.
    c. Protect the patient from injury caused by falls.
    d. Help to establish a diagnosis of cerebellar dysfunction.

27. When using the heel-to-shin test, for what abnormality is the nurse assessing the patient?
    a. Hypertonia
    b. Lack of coordination
    c. Extension of the toes
    d. Loss of proprioception

28. What method is used to assess for extinction?
    a. Cotton wisp
    b. Sharp and dull end of a pin
    c. Tuning fork to bony prominences
    d. Simultaneously stimulating both sides of the body

29. What is demonstrated when the patient stands with the feet close together and eyes closed and the patient sways or falls?
    a. Pronator drift
    b. Absent patellar reflex
    c. Positive Romberg test
    d. Absence of two-point discrimination

30. What is the normal response to striking the triceps tendon with a reflex hammer?
    a. Forearm pronation
    b. Extension of the arm
    c. Flexion of the arm at the elbow
    d. Flexion and supination of the elbow

31. The patellar tendon is struck and the leg extends with contraction of the quadriceps. What grade should this response be given?
    a. 1/5
    b. 2/5
    c. 3/5
    d. 4/5

32. What should the nurse do to prepare a patient for a lumbar puncture?
    a. Sedate the patient with medication before the test.
    b. Withhold beverages containing caffeine for 8 hours.
    c. Have the patient sit on the side of the bed, leaning on a padded over-the-bed table.
    d. Position the patient in a lateral recumbent position with the hips, knees, and neck flexed.

33. Following a lumbar puncture, what should the nurse assess the patient for?
    a. Headache
    b. Lower limb paralysis
    c. Allergic reactions to the dye
    d. Hemorrhage from the puncture site

34. The patient has just had a myelogram. What should be included in the nursing care for this patient?
    a. Restrict fluids until the patient is ambulatory.
    b. Keep the patient positioned flat in bed for several hours.
    c. Position the patient with the head of the bed elevated 30 degrees.
    d. Provide mild analgesics for pain associated with the insertion of needles.

35. What is the neurologic diagnostic test that has the highest risk of complications and requires frequent monitoring of neurologic and vital signs following the procedure?
    a. Myelogram
    b. Cerebral angiography
    c. Electroencephalogram
    d. Transcranial Doppler sonography

36. In noting the results of an analysis of CSF, what should the nurse identify as an abnormal finding?
    a. pH of 7.35
    b. Clear, colorless appearance
    c. WBC count of 5/mL (0.005/L)
    d. Glucose level of 30 mg/dL (1.7 mmol/L)

CHAPTER 57

Nursing Management: Acute Intracranial Problems

1. Which components are able to change to adapt to small increases in intracranial pressure (ICP) (*select all that apply*)?
   a. **Blood**
   b. Skull bone
   c. **Brain tissue**
   d. Scalp tissue
   e. **Cerebrospinal fluid (CSF)**

2. The cerebral perfusion pressure (CPP) is the pressure needed to ensure blood flow to the brain. Normal CPP is 60 to 100 mm Hg. Calculate the CPP of a patient whose blood pressure (BP) is 106/52 mm Hg and ICP is 14 mm Hg.

   56 _____ mm Hg

3. Calculate the CPP for the patient with an ICP of 34 mm Hg and a systemic BP of 108/64 mm Hg.

   44.7 or 45 _____ mm Hg $\frac{SYS + (2 \times dys) - ICP}{3}$

4. Which factors decrease cerebral blood flow (*select all that apply*)?
   a. Increased ICP
   b. PaO_2 of 45 mm Hg
   c. **$PaCO_2$ of 30 mm Hg**
   d. Arterial blood pH of 7.3
   e. **Decreased mean arterial pressure (MAP)**

5. What are causes of vasogenic cerebral edema (*select all that apply*)?
   a. Hydrocephalus
   b. **Ingested toxins**
   c. Destructive lesions or trauma
   d. Local disruption of cell membranes
   e. **Fluid flowing from intravascular to extravascular space**

6. Which events cause increased ICP (*select all that apply*)?
   a. **Vasodilation**
   b. **Necrotic tissue edema**
   c. Blood vessel compression
   d. **Edema from initial brain insult**
   e. Brainstem compression and herniation

7. An early sign of increased ICP that the nurse should assess for is
   a. Cushing's triad.
   b. unexpected vomiting.
   c. **decreasing level of consciousness (LOC).**
   d. dilated pupil with sluggish response to light.

8. The nurse recognizes the presence of Cushing's triad in the patient with which vital sign changes?
   a. Increased pulse, irregular respiration, increased BP
   b. Decreased pulse, increased respiration, decreased systolic BP
   c. **Decreased pulse, irregular respiration, widened pulse pressure**
   d. Increased pulse, decreased respiration, widened pulse pressure

9. Increased ICP in the left cerebral cortex caused by intracranial bleeding causes displacement of brain tissue to the right hemisphere beneath the falx cerebri. The nurse knows that this is referred to as what?
   a. Uncal herniation
   b. Tentorial herniation
   c. **Cingulate herniation**
   d. Temporal lobe herniation

10. ***Priority Decision:*** A patient has ICP monitoring with an intraventricular catheter. What is a priority nursing intervention for the patient?
    a. Aseptic technique to prevent infection
    b. Constant monitoring of ICP waveforms
    c. Removal of CSF to maintain normal ICP
    d. Sampling CSF to determine abnormalities

11. When using intraventricular ICP monitoring, what should the nurse be aware of to prevent inaccurate readings?
    a. The P2 wave is higher than the P1 wave.
    b. CSF is leaking around the monitoring device.
    c. The transducer of the ventriculostomy monitor is at the level of the upper ear.
    d. The drain of the CSF drainage device was closed for 6 minutes before taking the reading.

12. The patient is being monitored long-term with a brain tissue oxygenation catheter. What range for the pressure of oxygen in brain tissue (PbtO$_2$) will maintain cerebral oxygen supply and demand?
    a. 55% to 75%
    b. 20 to 40 mm Hg
    c. 70 to 150 mm Hg
    d. 80 to 100 mm Hg

13. Which drug treatment helps to decrease ICP by expanding plasma and the osmotic effect to move fluid?
    a. Oxygen administration
    b. Pentobarbital (Nembutal)
    c. Mannitol (Osmitrol) (25%)
    d. Dexamethasone (Decadron)

14. How are the metabolic and nutritional needs of the patient with increased ICP best met?
    a. Enteral feedings that are low in sodium
    b. Simple glucose available in D$_5$W IV solutions
    c. Fluid restriction that promotes a moderate dehydration
    d. Balanced, essential nutrition in a form that the patient can tolerate

15. Why is the Glasgow Coma Scale (GCS) used?
    a. To quickly assess the LOC
    b. To assess the patient's ability to communicate
    c. To assess the patient's ability to respond to commands
    d. To assess the patient's coordination with motor responses

16. A patient with an intracranial problem does not open his eyes to any stimulus, has no verbal response except moaning and muttering when stimulated, and flexes his arm in response to painful stimuli. What should the nurse record as the patient's GCS score?
    a. 6
    b. 7
    c. 9
    d. 11

17. ***Priority Decision:*** When assessing the body functions of a patient with increased ICP, what should the nurse assess first?
    a. Corneal reflex testing
    b. Pupillary reaction to light
    c. Extremity strength testing
    d. Circulatory and respiratory status

18. How is cranial nerve (CN) III, originating in the midbrain, assessed by the nurse for an early indication of pressure on the brainstem?
    a. Assess for nystagmus
    b. Test the corneal reflex
    c. Test pupillary reaction to light
    d. Test for oculocephalic (doll's eyes) reflex

19. A patient has a nursing diagnosis of risk for ineffective cerebral tissue perfusion *related to* cerebral edema. What is an appropriate nursing intervention for the patient?
    a. Avoid positioning the patient with neck and hip flexion.
    b. Maintain hyperventilation to a PaCO$_2$ of 15 to 20 mm Hg.
    c. Cluster nursing activities to provide periods of uninterrupted rest.
    d. Routinely suction to prevent accumulation of respiratory secretions.

20. An unconscious patient with increased ICP is on ventilatory support. The nurse notifies the health care provider when arterial blood gas (ABG) measurement results reveal what?
    a. pH of 7.43
    b. SaO$_2$ of 94%
    c. PaO$_2$ of 70 mm Hg (normal = 100
    d. PaCO$_2$ of 35 mm Hg

21. The nurse is monitoring a patient for increased ICP following a head injury. What are manifestations of increased ICP (*select all that apply*)?
    a. Fever
    b. Oriented to name only
    c. Narrowing pulse pressure
    d. Right pupil dilated greater than left pupil
    e. Decorticate posturing to painful stimulus

22. *Priority Decision:* While the nurse performs range of motion (ROM) on an unconscious patient with increased ICP, the patient experiences severe decerebrate posturing reflexes. What should the nurse do first?
    a. Use restraints to protect the patient from injury.
    b. Perform the exercises less frequently because posturing can increase ICP.
    c. Administer central nervous system (CNS) depressants to lightly sedate the patient.
    d. Continue the exercises because they are necessary to maintain musculoskeletal function.

23. The patient has been diagnosed with a cerebral concussion. What should the nurse expect to see in this patient?
    a. Deafness, loss of taste, and CSF otorrhea
    b. CSF otorrhea, vertigo, and Battle's sign with a dural tear
    c. Boggy temporal muscle because of extravasation of blood
    d. Headache, retrograde amnesia, and transient reduction in LOC

24. The patient comes to the emergency department (ED) with cortical blindness and visual field defects. Which type of head injury does the nurse suspect?
    a. Cerebral contusion
    b. Orbital skull fracture
    c. Posterior fossa fracture
    d. Frontal lobe skull fracture

25. The patient has a depressed skull fracture and scalp lacerations with communication to the intracranial cavity. Which type of injury should the nurse record?
    a. Linear skull fracture
    b. Depressed skull fracture
    c. Compound skull fracture
    d. Comminuted skull fracture

26. A patient with a head injury has bloody drainage from the ear. What should the nurse do to determine if CSF is present in the drainage?
    a. Examine the tympanic membrane for a tear.
    b. Test the fluid for a halo sign on a white dressing.
    c. Test the fluid with a glucose-identifying strip or stick.
    d. Collect 5 mL of fluid in a test tube and send it to the laboratory for analysis.

27. The nurse suspects the presence of an arterial epidural hematoma in the patient who experiences
    a. failure to regain consciousness following a head injury.
    b. a rapid deterioration of neurologic function within 24 to 48 hours following a head injury.
    c. nonspecific, nonlocalizing progression of alteration in LOC occurring over weeks or months.
    d. unconsciousness at the time of a head injury with a brief period of consciousness followed by a decrease in LOC.

28. Skull x-rays and a computed tomography (CT) scan provide evidence of a depressed parietal fracture with a subdural hematoma in a patient admitted to the ED following an automobile accident. In planning care for the patient, what should the nurse anticipate?
    a. The patient will receive life support measures until the condition stabilizes.
    b. Immediate burr holes will be made to rapidly decompress the intracranial cavity.
    c. The patient will be treated conservatively with close monitoring for changes in neurologic status.
    d. The patient will be taken to surgery for a craniotomy for evacuation of blood and decompression of the cranium.

29. ***Priority Decision:*** When a patient is admitted to the ED following a head injury, what should be the nurse's first priority in management of the patient once a patent airway is confirmed?
    a. Maintain cervical spine precautions.
    b. Monitor for changes in neurologic status.
    c. Determine the presence of increased ICP.
    d. Establish IV access with a large-bore catheter.

30. A 54-year-old man is recovering from a skull fracture with a subacute subdural hematoma that caused unconsciousness. He has return of motor control and orientation but appears apathetic and has reduced awareness of his environment. When planning discharge of the patient, what should the nurse explain to the patient and the family?
    a. The patient is likely to have long-term emotional and mental changes that may require professional help.
    b. Continuous improvement in the patient's condition should occur until he has returned to pretrauma status.
    c. The patient's complete recovery may take years and the family should plan for his long-term dependent care.
    d. Role changes in family members will be necessary because the patient will be dependent on his family for care and support.

31. The patient is suspected of having a new brain tumor. Which test will the nurse expect to be ordered to detect a small tumor?
    a. CT scan
    b. Angiography
    c. Electroencephalography (EEG)
    d. Positron emission tomography (PET) scan

32. Assisting the family to understand what is happening to the patient is an especially important role of the nurse when the patient has a tumor in which part of the brain?
    a. Ventricles
    b. Frontal lobe
    c. Parietal lobe
    d. Occipital lobe

33. Which cranial surgery would require the patient to learn how to protect the surgical area from trauma?
    a. Burr holes
    b. Craniotomy
    c. Cranioplasty
    d. Craniectomy

34. What is the best explanation of stereotactic radiosurgery?
    a. Radioactive seeds are implanted in the brain.
    b. Very precisely focused radiation destroys tumor cells.
    c. Tubes are placed to redirect CSF from one area to another.
    d. The cranium is opened with removal of a bone flap to open the dura.

35. For the patient undergoing a craniotomy, when should the nurse provide information about the use of wigs and hairpieces or other methods to disguise hair loss?
    a. During preoperative teaching
    b. If the patient asks about their use
    c. In the immediate postoperative period
    d. When the patient expresses negative feelings about his or her appearance

36. Successful achievement of patient outcomes for the patient with cranial surgery would best be indicated by what?
    a. Ability to return home in 6 days
    b. Ability to meet all self-care needs
    c. Acceptance of residual neurologic deficits
    d. Absence of signs and symptoms of increased ICP

37. On physical examination of a patient with headache and fever, the nurse should suspect a brain abscess when the patient has
    a. seizures.
    b. nuchal rigidity.
    c. focal symptoms.
    d. signs of increased ICP.

38. Which of the following descriptions are characteristic of encephalitis (*select all that apply*)?
    a. CSF production is increased
    b. Almost always has a viral cause
    c. Is an inflammation of the brain
    d. Most frequently caused by bacteria
    e. May be transmitted by insect vectors
    f. Involves inflammation of tissues surrounding the brain and spinal cord

39. A patient is admitted to the hospital with possible bacterial meningitis. During the initial assessment, the nurse questions the patient about a recent history of what?
    a. Mosquito or tick bites
    b. Chickenpox or measles
    c. Cold sores or fever blisters
    d. An upper respiratory infection

40. What are the key manifestations of bacterial meningitis?
    a. Papilledema and psychomotor seizures
    b. High fever, nuchal rigidity, and severe headache
    c. Behavioral changes with memory loss and lethargy
    d. Jerky eye movements, loss of corneal reflex, and hemiparesis

41. Vigorous control of fever in the patient with meningitis is required to prevent complications of increased cerebral edema, seizure frequency, neurologic damage, and fluid loss. What nursing care should be included?
    a. Administer analgesics as ordered.
    b. Monitor LOC related to increased brain metabolism.
    c. Rapidly decrease temperature with a cooling blanket.
    d. Assess for peripheral edema from rapid fluid infusion.

42. When teaching children about rabies, which statement tells the school nurse that the child understands the teaching?
    a. "Only dogs spread rabies."
    b. "It is okay to play with wild raccoons."
    c. "Any warm-blooded mammal can carry rabies."
    d. "It is easier to treat rabies than it is to prevent it."

CASE STUDY
Neurologic Complications
Patient Profile

J.K., a 19-year-old unrestrained driver, suffered a compound fracture of the skull and facial fractures in a motor vehicle accident. On admission to the hospital, he was immediately taken to surgery for evacuation of a right subdural hematoma in the temporal region and repair of facial fractures. On the fourth postoperative day, the nurse discovers the following findings during assessment of J.K.

Subjective Data
- Increasingly difficult to arouse

Objective Data
- GCS score decreased from 10 to 5
- Signs of nuchal rigidity
- Vital signs: Temp 102.2°F (39°C), BP 110/60, HR 114 bpm
- ICP ranges between 20 and 30 mm Hg despite CSF drainage and mannitol

---

Discussion Questions

Using a separate sheet of paper, answer the following questions:

1. What is the probable cause of J.K.'s change in neurologic status?
2. What were the contributing factors that put J.K. at risk for complications after a head injury and surgery?
3. Discuss the pathophysiologic basis for the symptoms exhibited by J.K.
4. *Priority Decision:* On the basis of the nursing assessment, what are the priority interventions?
5. Discuss the possible areas for organisms to gain access to the meninges in the case of J.K.
6. *Priority Decision:* Based on the assessment data presented, what are the priority nursing diagnoses? Are there any collaborative problems?

1. In promoting health maintenance for prevention of strokes, the nurse understands that the highest risk for the most common type of stroke is present in which people?
   a. African Americans
   b. Women who smoke
   c. Individuals with hypertension and diabetes
   d. Those who are obese with high dietary fat intake

2. A thrombus that develops in a cerebral artery does not always cause a loss of neurologic function because
   a. the body can dissolve atherosclerotic plaques as they form.
   b. some tissues of the brain do not require constant blood supply to prevent damage.
   c. circulation via the circle of Willis may provide blood supply to the affected area of the brain.
   d. neurologic deficits occur only when major arteries are occluded by thrombus formation around atherosclerotic plaque.

3. A patient comes to the emergency department immediately after experiencing numbness of the face and an inability to speak but while the patient awaits examination, the symptoms disappear and the patient requests discharge. Why should the nurse emphasize that it is important for the patient to be treated before leaving?
   a. The patient has probably experienced an asymptomatic lacunar stroke.
   b. The symptoms are likely to return and progress to worsening neurologic deficit in the next 24 hours.
   c. Neurologic deficits that are transient occur most often as a result of small hemorrhages that clot off.
   d. The patient has probably experienced a transient ischemic attack (TIA), which is a sign of progressive cerebrovascular disease.

4. What are characteristics of a stroke caused by an intracerebral hemorrhage (*select all that apply*)?
   a. Carries a poor prognosis
   b. Caused by rupture of a vessel
   c. Strong association with hypertension
   d. Commonly occurs during or after sleep
   e. Creates a mass that compresses the brain

5. Which type of stroke is associated with endocardial disorders, has a rapid onset, and is unrelated to activity?
   a. Embolic
   b. Thrombotic
   c. Intracerebral hemorrhage
   d. Subarachnoid hemorrhage

6. What primarily determines the neurologic functions that are affected by a stroke?
   a. The amount of tissue area involved
   b. The rapidity of the onset of symptoms
   c. The brain area perfused by the affected artery
   d. The presence or absence of collateral circulation

7. Indicate whether the following manifestations of a stroke are more likely to occur with right brain damage (R) or left brain damage (L).

   _____L_____ a. Aphasia
   _____R_____ b. Impaired judgment
   _____R_____ c. Quick, impulsive behavior
   _____L_____ d. Inability to remember words
   _____R_____ e. Left homonymous hemianopsia
   _____R_____ f. Neglect of the left side of the body
   _____L_____ g. Hemiplegia of the right side of the body

8. The patient has a lack of comprehension of both verbal and written language. Which type of communication difficulty does this patient have?
   a. Dysarthria
   b. Fluent dysphasia
   c. Receptive aphasia
   d. Expressive aphasia

9. A patient is admitted to the hospital with a left hemiplegia. To determine the size and location and to ascertain whether a stroke is ischemic or hemorrhagic, the nurse anticipates that the health care provider will request a
   a. lumbar puncture.
   b. cerebral arteriogram.
   c. magnetic resonance imaging (MRI).
   d. computed tomography (CT) scan with contrast.

10. A carotid endarterectomy is being considered as treatment for a patient who has had several TIAs. What should the nurse explain to the patient about this surgery?
    a. It involves intracranial surgery to join a superficial extracranial artery to an intracranial artery.
    b. It is used to restore blood circulation to the brain following an obstruction of a cerebral artery.
    c. It involves removing an atherosclerotic plaque in the carotid artery to prevent an impending stroke.
    d. It is used to open a stenosis in a carotid artery with a balloon and stent to restore cerebral circulation.

11. The incidence of ischemic stroke in patients with TIAs and other risk factors is reduced with the administration of which medication?
    a. Furosemide (Lasix)
    b. Lovastatin (Mevacor)
    c. Daily low-dose aspirin
    d. Nimodipine (Nimotop)

12. ***Priority Decision:*** What is the priority intervention in the emergency department for the patient with a stroke?
    a. Intravenous fluid replacement
    b. Administration of osmotic diuretics to reduce cerebral edema
    c. Initiation of hypothermia to decrease the oxygen needs of the brain
    d. Maintenance of respiratory function with a patent airway and oxygen administration

13. A diagnosis of a ruptured cerebral aneurysm has been made in a patient with manifestations of a stroke. The nurse anticipates which treatment option that would be considered for the patient?
    a. Hyperventilation therapy
    b. Surgical clipping of the aneurysm
    c. Administration of hyperosmotic agents
    d. Administration of thrombolytic therapy

14. During the acute phase of a stroke, the nurse assesses the patient's vital signs and neurologic status every 4 hours. What is a cardiovascular sign that the nurse would see as the body attempts to increase cerebral blood flow?
    a. Hypertension
    b. Fluid overload
    c. Cardiac dysrhythmias
    d. S_3 and S_4 heart sounds

15. During the secondary assessment of the patient with a stroke, what should be included (*select all that apply*)?
    a. Gaze
    b. Sensation
    c. Facial palsy
    d. Proprioception
    e. Current medications
    f. Distal motor function

16. What is a nursing intervention that is indicated for the patient with hemiplegia?
    a. The use of a footboard to prevent plantar flexion
    b. Immobilization of the affected arm against the chest with a sling
    c. Positioning the patient in bed with each joint lower than the joint proximal to it
    d. Having the patient perform passive range of motion (ROM) of the affected limb with the unaffected limb

17. A newly admitted patient diagnosed with a right-sided brain stroke has a nursing diagnosis of disturbed visual sensory perception related to homonymous hemianopsia. Early in the care of the patient, what should the nurse do?
    a. Place objects on the right side within the patient's field of vision.
    b. Approach the patient from the left side to encourage the patient to turn the head.
    c. Place objects on the patient's left side to assess the patient's ability to compensate.
    d. Patch the affected eye to encourage the patient to turn the head to scan the environment.

18. Four days following a stroke, a patient is to start oral fluids and feedings. Before feeding the patient, what should the nurse do first?
    a. Check the patient's gag reflex.
    b. Order a soft diet for the patient.
    c. Raise the head of the bed to a sitting position.
    d. Evaluate the patient's ability to swallow small amounts of crushed ice or ice water.

19. What is an appropriate food for a patient with a stroke who has mild dysphagia?
    - a. Fruit juices
    - b. Pureed meat
    - c. Scrambled eggs
    - d. Fortified milkshakes

20. A patient's wife asks the nurse why her husband did not receive the clot busting medication (tissue plasminogen activator [tPA]) she has been reading about. Her husband is diagnosed with a hemorrhagic stroke. What is the best response by the nurse to the patient's wife?
    - a. "He didn't arrive within the timeframe for that therapy."
    - b. "Not everyone is eligible for this drug. Has he had surgery lately?"
    - c. "You should discuss the treatment of your husband with his doctor."
    - d. "The medication you are talking about dissolves clots and could cause more bleeding in your husband's brain."

21. The rehabilitation nurse assesses the patient, caregiver, and family before planning the rehabilitation program for this patient. What needs to be included in this assessment (*select all that apply*)?
    - a. Cognitive status of the family
    - b. Patient resources and support
    - c. Rehabilitation potential of the patient
    - d. Body strength remaining after the stroke
    - e. Physical status of body systems affected by the stroke
    - f. Patient and caregiver expectations of the rehabilitation

22. What is an appropriate nursing intervention to promote communication during rehabilitation of the patient with aphasia?
    - a. Use gestures, pictures, and music to stimulate patient responses.
    - b. Talk about activities of daily living (ADLs) that are familiar to the patient.
    - c. Structure statements so that the patient does not have to respond verbally.
    - d. Use flashcards with simple words and pictures to promote recall of language.

23. A patient with a right hemisphere stroke has a nursing diagnosis of unilateral neglect *related to* sensory-perceptual deficits. During the patient's rehabilitation, what nursing intervention is important for the nurse to do?
    - a. Avoid positioning the patient on the affected side.
    - b. Place all objects for care on the patient's unaffected side.
    - c. Teach the patient to care consciously for the affected side.
    - d. Protect the affected side from injury with pillows and supports.

24. A patient with a stroke has a right-sided hemiplegia. What does the nurse teach the family to prepare them to cope with the behavior changes seen with this type of stroke?
    - a. Ignore undesirable behaviors manifested by the patient.
    - b. Provide directions to the patient verbally in small steps.
    - c. Distract the patient from inappropriate emotional responses.
    - d. Supervise all activities before allowing the patient to pursue them independently.

25. The nurse can assist the patient and family in coping with the long-term effects of a stroke by doing what?
    - a. Informing family members that the patient will need assistance with almost all ADLs
    - b. Explaining that the patient's prestroke behavior will return as improvement progresses
    - c. Encouraging the patient and family members to seek assistance from family therapy or stroke support groups
    - d. Helping the patient and family to understand the significance of residual stroke damage to promote problem solving and planning

26. ***Delegation Decision:*** Which intervention should the nurse delegate to the licensed practical nurse (LPN) when caring for a patient following an acute stroke?
    - a. Assess the patient's neurologic status.
    - b. Assess the patient's gag reflex before beginning feeding.
    - c. Administer ordered antihypertensives and platelet inhibitors.
    - d. Teach the patient's caregivers strategies to minimize unilateral neglect.

CASE STUDY

Stroke

Patient Profile

R.C., a 38-year-old married woman, was admitted to the hospital unconscious after her family could not rouse her in the morning. She was accompanied by her husband and three daughters, ages 10, 13, and 15.

Subjective Data

- Has no history of hypertension or other health problems
- Complained of a headache the day before she became unconsciousness

Objective Data

- Diagnostic tests reveal a subarachnoid hemorrhage
- Vital signs: BP 150/82, RR 16, HR 56 bpm, Temp 101°F (38.3°C)
- Glasgow Coma Scale score: 5

Discussion Questions

Using a separate sheet of paper, answer the following questions:

1. What diagnostic tests were indicated to determine the cause of R.C.'s unconsciousness?
2. What signs of increased intracranial pressure are present in R.C.?
3. What should the family be told to expect in terms of R.C.'s condition?
4. *Priority Decision:* What nursing interventions have the highest priority for R.C. at this stage of her illness?
5. What treatment modalities indicated for thrombotic strokes are contraindicated for R.C.?
6. What therapeutic options are available for the patient with a hemorrhagic stroke resulting from a ruptured aneurysm?
7. *Priority Decision:* Based on the assessment data presented, what are the priority nursing diagnoses? Are there any collaborative problems?

Nursing Management:
Chronic Neurologic Problems

1. Which type of headache is suspected when the headaches are unilateral and throbbing, preceded by a prodrome of photophobia, and associated with a family history of this type of headache?
   a. Cluster
   b. Migraine
   c. Frontal-type
   d. Tension-type

2. A patient is diagnosed with cluster headaches. The nurse knows that which characteristics are associated with this type of headache (*select all that apply*)?
   a. Family history
   b. Alcohol is the only dietary trigger
   c. Abrupt onset lasting 5 to 180 minutes
   d. Severe, sharp, penetrating head pain
   e. Bilateral pressure or tightness sensation
   f. May be accompanied by unilateral ptosis or lacrimation

3. What is the most important method of diagnosing functional headaches?
   a. CT scan
   b. Electromyography (EMG)
   c. Cerebral blood flow studies
   d. Thorough history of the headache

4. What drug therapy is included for acute migraine and cluster headaches that appears to alter the pathophysiologic process for these headaches?
   a. β-Adrenergic blockers such as propranolol (Inderal)
   b. Serotonin antagonists such as methysergide (Sansert)
   c. Tricyclic antidepressants such as amitriptyline (Elavil)
   d. Specific serotonin receptor agonists such as sumatriptan (Imitrex)

5. What is a nursing intervention that is appropriate for the patient with a nursing diagnosis of anxiety *related to* lack of knowledge of the etiology and treatment of headache?
   a. Help the patient to examine lifestyle patterns and precipitating factors.
   b. Administer medications as ordered to relieve pain and promote relaxation.
   c. Provide a quiet, dimly lit environment to reduce stimuli that increase muscle tension and anxiety.
   d. Support the patient's use of counseling or psychotherapy to enhance conflict resolution and stress reduction.

6. **Delegation Decision:** The nurse is preparing to admit a newly diagnosed patient experiencing tonic-clonic seizures. What could the nurse delegate to unlicensed assistive personnel (UAP)?
   a. Complete the admission assessment.
   b. Explain the call system to the patient.
   c. Obtain the suction equipment from the supply cabinet.
   d. Place a padded tongue blade on the wall above the patient's bed.

7. How do generalized seizures differ from focal seizures?
   a. Focal seizures are confined to one side of the brain and remain focal in nature.
   b. Generalized seizures result in loss of consciousness whereas focal seizures do not.
   c. Generalized seizures result in temporary residual deficits during the postictal phase.
   d. Generalized seizures have bilateral synchronous epileptic discharges affecting the whole brain at onset of the seizure.

8. Which type of seizure occurs in children, is also known as a petit mal seizure, and consists of a staring spell that lasts for a few seconds?
   a. Atonic
   b. Simple focal
   c. Typical absence
   d. Atypical absence

9. The patient is diagnosed with complex focal seizures. Which characteristics are related to complex focal seizures (*select all that apply*)?
   a. Formerly known as grand mal seizure
   b. Often accompanied by incontinence or tongue or cheek biting
   c. Psychomotor seizures with repetitive behaviors and lip smacking
   d. Altered memory, sexual sensations, and distortions of visual or auditory sensations
   e. Loss of consciousness and stiffening of the body with subsequent jerking of extremities
   f. Often involves behavioral, emotional, and cognitive functions with altered consciousness

10. Which type of seizure is most likely to cause death for the patient?
    a. Subclinical seizures
    b. Myoclonic seizures
    c. Psychogenic seizures
    d. Tonic-clonic status epilepticus

11. A patient admitted to the hospital following a generalized tonic-clonic seizure asks the nurse what caused the seizure. What is the best response by the nurse?
    a. "So many factors can cause epilepsy that it is impossible to say what caused your seizure."
    b. "Epilepsy is an inherited disorder. Does anyone else in your family have a seizure disorder?"
    c. "In seizures, some type of trigger causes sudden, abnormal bursts of electrical brain activity."
    d. "Scar tissue in the brain alters the chemical balance, creating uncontrolled electrical discharges."

12. A patient with a seizure disorder is being evaluated for surgical treatment of the seizures. The nurse recognizes that what is one of the requirements for surgical treatment?
    a. Identification of scar tissue that is able to be removed
    b. An adequate trial of drug therapy that had unsatisfactory results
    c. Development of toxic syndromes from long-term use of antiseizure drugs
    d. The presence of symptoms of cerebral degeneration from repeated seizures

13. The nurse teaches the patient taking antiseizure drugs that this method is most commonly used to measure compliance and monitor for toxicity.
    a. A daily seizure log
    b. Urine testing for drug levels
    c. Blood testing for drug levels
    d. Monthly electroencephalography (EEG)

14. *Priority Decision:* When teaching a patient with a seizure disorder about the medication regimen, what is it most important for the nurse to emphasize?
    a. The patient should increase the dosage of the medication if stress is increased.
    b. Most over-the-counter and prescription drugs are safe to take with antiseizure drugs.
    c. Stopping the medication abruptly may increase the intensity and frequency of seizures.
    d. If gingival hypertrophy occurs, the drug should be stopped and the health care provider notified.

15. *Priority Decision:* The nurse finds a patient in bed having a generalized tonic-clonic seizure. During the seizure activity, what actions should the nurse take (*select all that apply*)?
    a. Loosen restrictive clothing.
    b. Turn the patient to the side.
    c. Protect the patient's head from injury.
    d. Place a padded tongue blade between the patient's teeth.
    e. Restrain the patient's extremities to prevent soft tissue and bone injury.

16. Following a generalized tonic-clonic seizure, the patient is tired and sleepy. What care should the nurse provide?
    a. Suction the patient before allowing him to rest.
    b. Allow the patient to sleep as long as he feels sleepy.
    c. Stimulate the patient to increase his level of consciousness.
    d. Check the patient's level of consciousness every 15 minutes for an hour.

17. During the diagnosis and long-term management of a seizure disorder, what should the nurse recognize as one of the major needs of the patient?
    a. Managing the complicated drug regimen of seizure control
    b. Coping with the effects of negative social attitudes toward epilepsy
    c. Adjusting to the very restricted lifestyle required by a diagnosis of epilepsy
    d. Learning to minimize the effect of the condition in order to obtain employment

18. A patient at the clinic for a routine health examination mentions that she is exhausted because her legs bother her so much at night that she cannot sleep. The nurse questions the patient further about her leg symptoms with what knowledge about restless legs syndrome?
    a. The condition can be readily diagnosed with EMG.
    b. Other more serious nervous system dysfunctions may be present.
    c. Dopaminergic agents are often effective in managing the symptoms.
    d. Symptoms can be controlled by vigorous exercise of the legs during the day.

19. Which chronic neurologic disorder involves a deficiency of the neurotransmitters acetylcholine and γ-aminobutyric acid (GABA) in the basal ganglia and extrapyramidal system?
    a. Myasthenia gravis
    b. Parkinson's disease
    c. Huntington's disease
    d. Amyotrophic lateral sclerosis (ALS)

20. A 38-year-old woman has newly diagnosed multiple sclerosis (MS) and asks the nurse what is going to happen to her. What is the best response by the nurse?
    a. "You will have either periods of attacks and remissions or progression of nerve damage over time."
    b. "You need to plan for a continuous loss of movement, sensory functions, and mental capabilities."
    c. "You will most likely have a steady course of chronic progressive nerve damage that will change your personality."
    d. "It is common for people with MS to have an acute attack of weakness and then not to have any other symptoms for years."

21. During assessment of a patient admitted to the hospital with an acute exacerbation of MS, what should the nurse expect to find?
    a. Tremors, dysphasia, and ptosis
    b. Bowel and bladder incontinence and loss of memory
    c. Motor impairment, visual disturbances, and paresthesias
    d. Excessive involuntary movements, hearing loss, and ataxia

22. The nurse explains to a patient newly diagnosed with MS that the diagnosis is made primarily by
    a. spinal x-ray findings.
    b. T-cell analysis of the blood.
    c. analysis of cerebrospinal fluid.
    d. history and clinical manifestations.

23. Mitoxantrone (Novantrone) is being considered as treatment for a patient with progressive-relapsing MS. The nurse explains that a disadvantage of this drug compared with other drugs used for MS is what?
    a. It must be given subcutaneously every day.
    b. It has a lifetime dose limit because of cardiac toxicity.
    c. It is an anticholinergic agent that causes urinary incontinence.
    d. It is an immunosuppressant agent that increases the risk for infection.

24. ***Priority Decision:*** A patient with MS has a nursing diagnosis of self-care deficit *related to* muscle spasticity and neuromuscular deficits. In providing care for the patient, what is most important for the nurse to do?
    a. Teach the family members how to care adequately for the patient's needs.
    b. Encourage the patient to maintain social interactions to prevent social isolation.
    c. Promote the use of assistive devices so the patient can participate in self-care activities.
    d. Perform all activities of daily living (ADLs) for the patient to conserve the patient's energy.

25. A patient with newly diagnosed MS has been hospitalized for evaluation and initial treatment of the disease. Following discharge teaching, the nurse realizes that additional instruction is needed when the patient says what?
    a. "It is important for me to avoid exposure to people with upper respiratory infections."
    b. "When I begin to feel better, I should stop taking the prednisone to prevent side effects."
    c. "I plan to use vitamin supplements and a high-protein diet to help manage my condition."
    d. "I must plan with my family how we are going to manage my care if I become more incapacitated."

26. The classic triad of manifestations associated with Parkinson's disease is tremor, rigidity, and bradykinesia. What is a consequence related to rigidity?
    a. Shuffling gait
    b. Impaired handwriting
    c. Lack of postural stability
    d. Muscle soreness and pain

27. A patient with a tremor is being evaluated for Parkinson's disease. The nurse explains to the patient that Parkinson's disease can be confirmed by
    a. CT and MRI scans.
    b. relief of symptoms with administration of dopaminergic agents.
    c. the presence of tremors that increase during voluntary movement.
    d. cerebral angiogram that reveals the presence of cerebral atherosclerosis.

28. Which observation of the patient made by the nurse is most indicative of Parkinson's disease?
    a. Large, embellished handwriting
    b. Weakness of one leg resulting in a limping walk
    c. Difficulty rising from a chair and beginning to walk
    d. Onset of muscle spasms occurring with voluntary movement

29. A patient with Parkinson's disease is started on levodopa. What should the nurse explain about this drug?
    a. It stimulates dopamine receptors in the basal ganglia.
    b. It promotes the release of dopamine from brain neurons.
    c. It is a precursor of dopamine that is converted to dopamine in the brain.
    d. It prevents the excessive breakdown of dopamine in the peripheral tissues.

30. To reduce the risk for falls in the patient with Parkinson's disease, what should the nurse teach the patient to do?
    a. Use an elevated toilet seat.
    b. Use a walker or cane for support.
    c. Consciously lift the toes when stepping.
    d. Rock side to side to initiate leg movements.

31. A patient with myasthenia gravis is admitted to the hospital with respiratory insufficiency and severe weakness. When is a diagnosis of cholinergic crisis made?
    a. The patient's respiration is impaired because of muscle weakness.
    b. Administration of edrophonium (Tensilon) increases muscle weakness.
    c. Administration of edrophonium (Tensilon) results in improved muscle contractility.
    d. EMG reveals decreased response to repeated stimulation of muscles.

32. *Priority Decision:* During care of a patient in myasthenic crisis, maintenance of what is the nurse's first priority for the patient?
    a. Mobility
    b. Nutrition
    c. Respiratory function
    d. Verbal communication

33. When providing care for a patient with ALS, the nurse recognizes what as one of the most distressing problems experienced by the patient?
    a. Painful spasticity of the face and extremities
    b. Retention of cognitive function with total degeneration of motor function
    c. Uncontrollable writhing and twisting movements of the face, limbs, and body
    d. Knowledge that there is a 50% chance the disease has been passed to any offspring

34. In providing care for patients with chronic, progressive neurologic disease, what is the major goal of treatment that the nurse works toward?
    a. Meet the patient's personal care needs.
    b. Return the patient to normal neurologic function.
    c. Maximize neurologic functioning for as long as possible.
    d. Prevent the development of additional chronic diseases.

CASE STUDY
Multiple Sclerosis
Patient Profile

D.S., a 32-year-old white woman of European descent, born and raised in Minneapolis, is diagnosed with MS after an episode of numbness and tingling on the left side of her body that started several months ago. Two years ago she had an episode of optic neuritis in the right eye.

Subjective Data

- Difficulty seeing out of the right eye
- Numbness and tingling on the left side that worsens in hot weather
- Tires easily
- Used all sick days at work; concerned about losing her job and her ability to care for her 3-year-old son

Objective Data

- Cries softly during the interview
- Appears tense and anxious
- Results of visual evoked potential: prolonged in right eye
- MRI scan of head shows several plaques in white matter

Discussion Questions

Using a separate sheet of paper, answer the following questions:

1. What is the pathophysiology of MS?
2. What risk factors does this patient have?
3. What precipitating factors for MS are present in D.S.'s life?
4. Why did it take so long for a definitive diagnosis to be made for D.S.?
5. *Priority Decision:* What are the priority teaching needs for D.S.?
6. What treatment would be appropriate for D.S.?
7. *Priority Decision:* Based on the assessment data presented, what are the priority nursing diagnoses? Are there any collaborative problems?

60

Nursing Management: Alzheimer's Disease, Dementia, and Delirium

1. What manifestations of cognitive impairment are primarily characteristic of delirium (*select all that apply*)?
   a. Reduced awareness
   b. Impaired judgments
   c. Words difficult to find
   d. Sleep/wake cycle reversed
   e. Distorted thinking and perception
   f. Insidious onset with prolonged duration

2. Which statement accurately describes dementia?
   a. Overproduction of β-amyloid protein causes all dementias.
   b. Dementia resulting from neurodegenerative causes can be prevented.
   c. Dementia caused by hepatic or renal encephalopathy cannot be reversed.
   d. Vascular dementia can be diagnosed by brain lesions identified with neuroimaging.

3. A patient with Alzheimer's disease (AD) dementia has manifestations of depression. The nurse knows that treatment of the patient with antidepressants will most likely do what?
   a. Improve cognitive function
   b. Not alter the course of either condition
   c. Cause interactions with the drugs used to treat the dementia
   d. Be contraindicated because of the central nervous system (CNS)–depressant effect of antidepressants

4. For what purpose would the nurse use the Mini-Mental State Examination to evaluate a patient with cognitive impairment?
   a. It is a good tool to determine the etiology of dementia.
   b. It is a good tool to evaluate mood and thought processes.
   c. It can help to document the degree of cognitive impairment in delirium and dementia.
   d. It is useful for initial evaluation of mental status but additional tools are needed to evaluate changes in cognition over time.

5. During assessment of a patient with dementia, the nurse determines that the condition is potentially reversible when finding out what about the patient?
   a. Has long-standing abuse of alcohol
   b. Has a history of Parkinson's disease
   c. Recently developed symptoms of hypothyroidism
   d. Was infected with human immunodeficiency virus (HIV) 10 years ago

6. The husband of a patient is complaining that his wife's memory has been decreasing lately. When asked for examples of her memory loss, the husband says that she is forgetting the neighbors' names and forgot their granddaughter's birthday. What kind of loss does the nurse recognize this to be?
   a. Delirium
   b. Memory loss in AD
   c. Normal forgetfulness
   d. Memory loss in mild cognitive impairment

7. The wife of a patient who is manifesting deterioration in memory asks the nurse whether her husband has AD. The nurse explains that a diagnosis of AD is usually made when what happens?
   a. A urine test indicates elevated levels of isoprostanes
   b. All other possible causes of dementia have been eliminated
   c. Blood analysis reveals increased amounts of β-amyloid protein
   d. A computed tomography (CT) scan of the brain indicates brain atrophy

8. The newly admitted patient has moderate AD. What does the nurse know this patient will need help with?
   a. Eating
   b. Walking
   c. Dressing
   d. Self-care activities

9. What is one focus of collaborative care of patients with AD?
   a. Replacement of deficient acetylcholine in the brain
   b. Drug therapy for cognitive problems and undesirable behaviors
   c. The use of memory-enhancing techniques to delay disease progression
   d. Prevention of other chronic diseases that hasten the progression of AD

10. The patient is receiving donepezil (Aricept), lorazepam (Ativan), risperidone (Risperdal), and sertraline (Zoloft) for the management of AD. What benzodiazepine medication is being used to help manage this patient's behavior?
    a. Sertraline (Zoloft)
    b. Donepezil (Aricept)
    c. Lorazepam (Ativan)
    d. Risperidone (Risperdal)

11. What *N*-methyl-D-aspartate (NMDA) receptor antagonist is frequently used for a patient with AD who is experiencing decreased memory and cognition?
    a. Trazodone (Desyrel)
    b. Olanzapine (Zyprexa)
    c. Rivastigmine (Exelon)
    d. Memantine (Namenda)

12. A patient with AD in a long-term care facility is wandering the halls very agitated, asking for her "mommy" and crying. What is the best response by the nurse?
    a. Ask the patient, "Why are you behaving this way?"
    b. Tell the patient, "Let's go get a snack in the kitchen."
    c. Ask the patient, "Wouldn't you like to lie down now?"
    d. Tell the patient, "Just take some deep breaths and calm down."

13. The sister of a patient with AD asks the nurse whether prevention of the disease is possible. In responding, the nurse explains that there is no known way to prevent AD but there are ways to keep the brain healthy. What is included in the ways to keep the brain healthy (*select all that apply*)?
    a. Avoid trauma to the brain.
    b. Recognize and treat depression early.
    c. Avoid social gatherings to avoid infections.
    d. Do not overtax the brain by trying to learn new skills.
    e. Daily wine intake will increase circulation to the brain.
    f. Exercise regularly to decrease the risk for cognitive decline.

14. The son of a patient with early-onset AD asks if he will get AD. What should the nurse tell this man about the genetics of AD?
    a. The risk of early-onset AD for the children of parents with it is about 50%.
    b. Women get AD more often than men do, so his chances of getting AD are slim.
    c. The blood test for the *ApoE* gene to identify this type of AD can predict who will develop it.
    d. This type of AD is not as complex as regular AD, so he does not need to worry about getting AD.

15. A patient with moderate AD has a nursing diagnosis of impaired memory *related to* effects of dementia. What is an appropriate nursing intervention for this patient?
    a. Post clocks and calendars in the patient's environment.
    b. Establish and consistently follow a daily schedule with the patient.
    c. Monitor the patient's activities to maintain a safe patient environment.
    d. Stimulate thought processes by asking the patient questions about recent activities.

16. The family caregiver for a patient with AD expresses an inability to make decisions, concentrate, or sleep. The nurse determines what about the caregiver?
    a. The caregiver is also developing signs of AD.
    b. The caregiver is manifesting symptoms of caregiver role strain.
    c. The caregiver needs a period of respite from care of the patient.
    d. The caregiver should ask other family members to participate in the patient's care.

17. The wife of a man with moderate AD has a nursing diagnosis of social isolation *related to* diminishing social relationships and behavioral problems of the patient with AD. What is a nursing intervention that would be appropriate to provide respite care and allow the wife to have satisfactory contact with significant others?
    a. Help the wife to arrange for adult day care for the patient.
    b. Encourage permanent placement of the patient in the Alzheimer's unit of a long-term care facility.
    c. Refer the wife to a home health agency to arrange daily home nursing visits to assist with the patient's care.
    d. Arrange for hospitalization of the patient for 3 or 4 days so that the wife can visit out-of-town friends and relatives.

18. The health care provider is trying to differentiate the diagnosis of the patient between dementia and dementia with Lewy bodies (DLB). What observations by the nurse support a diagnosis of DLB (*select all that apply*)?
    a. Tremors
    b. Fluctuating cognitive ability
    c. Disturbed behavior, sleep, and personality
    d. Symptoms of pneumonia, including congested lung sounds
    e. Bradykinesia, rigidity, and postural instability without tremor

19. ***Delegation Decision:*** The RN in charge at a long-term care facility could delegate which activities to unlicensed assistive personnel (UAP) (*select all that apply*)?
    a. Assist the patient with eating.
    b. Provide personal hygiene and skin care.
    c. Check the environment for safety hazards.
    d. Assist the patient to the bathroom at regular intervals.
    e. Monitor for skin breakdown and swallowing difficulties.

20. A 72-year-old woman is hospitalized in the intensive care unit (ICU) with pneumonia resulting from chronic obstructive pulmonary disease (COPD). She has a fever, productive cough, and adventitious breath sounds throughout her lungs. In the past 24 hours her fluid intake was 1000 mL and her urine output was 700 mL. She was diagnosed with early-stage AD 6 months ago but has been able to maintain her activities of daily living (ADLs) with supervision. Identify at least six risk factors for the development of delirium in this patient.
    a. ICU
    b. age
    c. infection
    d. 1000 mL dehydration
    e. inactive
    f. AD

21. A 68-year-old man is admitted to the emergency department with multiple blunt trauma following a one-vehicle car accident. He is restless; disoriented to person, place, and time; and agitated. He resists attempts at examination and calls out the name "Janice." Why should the nurse suspect delirium rather than dementia in this patient?
    a. The fact that he wouldn't have been allowed to drive if he had dementia
    b. His hyperactive behavior, which differentiates his condition from the hypoactive behavior of dementia
    c. The report of emergency personnel that he was noncommunicative when they arrived at the accident scene
    d. The report of his family that although he has heart disease and is "very hard of hearing," this behavior is unlike him

22. What should be included in the management of a patient with delirium?
    a. The use of restraints to protect the patient from injury
    b. The use of short-acting benzodiazepines to sedate the patient
    c. Identification and treatment of underlying causes when possible
    d. Administration of high doses of an antipsychotic drug such as haloperidol (Haldol)

23. When caring for a patient in the severe stage of AD, what diversion or distraction activities would be appropriate?
    a. Watching TV
    b. Playing games
    c. Books to read
    d. Mobiles or dangling ribbons

CASE STUDY
Alzheimer's Disease
Patient Profile

G.D. is a 79-year-old man whose wife noticed that he has become increasingly forgetful over the past 3 years. Recently he was diagnosed with AD.

Subjective Data

- Wanders out of the house at night
- States that he "sees things that aren't there"
- Is able to dress, bathe, and feed himself
- Has trouble figuring out how to use his electric razor
- His wife is distressed about his cognitive decline
- His wife says that she is depressed and cannot watch him at night and get rest herself

Objective Data

- CT scan: Moderate cerebral atrophy

Discussion Questions

Using a separate sheet of paper, answer the following questions:

1. What pathophysiologic changes are associated with AD?
2. How is a diagnosis of AD made?
3. What progression of symptoms should G.D.'s wife be told to expect over the course of the disease?
4. What suggestions can the nurse make to relieve some of the stress on the wife?
5. What community resources might be available to G.D. and his wife?
6. *Priority Decision:* Based on the assessment data presented, what are the priority nursing diagnoses for G.D.? Are there any collaborative problems?
7. *Priority Decision:* Based on the assessment data presented, what are the priority nursing diagnoses for G.D.'s wife? Are there any collaborative problems?

1. A patient is diagnosed with Bell's palsy. What information should the nurse teach the patient about Bell's palsy (*select all that apply*)?
    a. Bell's palsy affects the motor branches of the facial nerve.
    b. Antiseizure drugs are the drugs of choice for treatment of Bell's palsy.
    c. Nutrition and avoidance of hot foods or beverages are special needs of this patient.
    d. Herpes simplex virus 1 is strongly associated as a precipitating factor in the development of Bell's palsy.
    e. Moist heat, gentle massage, electrical stimulation of the nerve, and exercises are prescribed to treat Bell's palsy.
    f. An inability to close the eyelid, with an upward movement of the eyeball when closure is attempted, is evident.

2. *Priority Decision:* When planning care for the patient with trigeminal neuralgia, which patient outcome should the nurse set as the highest priority?
    a. Relief of pain
    b. Protection of the cornea
    c. Maintenance of nutrition
    d. Maintenance of positive body image

3. Surgical intervention is being considered for a patient with trigeminal neuralgia. The nurse recognizes that which procedure has the least residual effects with a positive outcome?
    a. Glycerol rhizotomy
    b. Gamma knife radiosurgery
    c. Microvascular decompression
    d. Percutaneous radiofrequency rhizotomy

4. What should the nurse do when providing care for a patient with an acute attack of trigeminal neuralgia?
    a. Carry out all hygiene and oral care for the patient.
    b. Use conversation to distract the patient from pain.
    c. Maintain a quiet, comfortable, draft-free environment.
    d. Have the patient examine the mouth after each meal for residual food.

5. A patient is admitted to the hospital with Guillain-Barré syndrome. She had weakness in her feet and ankles that has progressed to weakness with numbness and tingling in both legs. During the acute phase of the illness, what should the nurse know about Guillain-Barré syndrome?
    a. The most important aspect of care is to monitor the patient's respiratory rate and depth and vital capacity.
    b. Early treatment with corticosteroids can suppress the immune response and prevent ascending nerve damage.
    c. The most serious complication of this condition is ascending demyelination of the peripheral nerves and the cranial nerves.
    d. Although voluntary motor neurons are damaged by the inflammatory response, the autonomic nervous system is unaffected by the disease.

6. A patient with Guillain-Barré syndrome asks whether he is going to die as the paralysis spreads toward his chest. In responding to the patient, what should the nurse know to be able to answer this question?
    a. Patients who require ventilatory support almost always die.
    b. Death occurs when nerve damage affects the brain and meninges.
    c. Most patients with Guillain-Barré syndrome make a complete recovery.
    d. If death can be prevented, residual paralysis and sensory impairment are usually permanent.

7. Which condition is transmitted through wound contamination, causes painful tonic spasms or seizures, and can be prevented by immunization?
   a. Tetanus
   b. Botulism
   c. Neurosyphilis
   d. Systemic inflammatory response syndrome

8. Which statements describe neurosyphilis (*select all that apply*)?
   a. Occurs 10 to 20 years after bacterial infection
   b. Infection can affect any part of the nervous system
   c. Descending paralysis with cranial nerve involvement
   d. Degenerative changes in the spinal cord and brainstem
   e. Inhibits transmission of acetylcholine at myoneural junction
   f. Initially manifests with GI symptoms with subsequent absorption of neurotoxin

9. In planning community education for prevention of spinal cord injuries, what group should the nurse target?
   a. Older men
   b. Teenage girls
   c. Elementary school–age children
   d. Adolescent and young adult men

10. A 70-year-old patient is admitted after falling from his roof. He has a spinal cord injury at the C7 level. What findings during the assessment identify the presence of spinal shock?
    a. Paraplegia with a flaccid paralysis
    b. Tetraplegia with total sensory loss
    c. Total hemiplegia with sensory and motor loss
    d. Spastic tetraplegia with loss of pressure sensation

11. Which syndrome of incomplete spinal cord lesion is described as cord damage common in the cervical region resulting in greater weakness in upper extremities than lower?
    a. Central cord syndrome
    b. Anterior cord syndrome
    c. Posterior cord syndrome
    d. Cauda equina and conus medullaris syndromes

12. The patient is diagnosed with Brown-Séquard syndrome after a knife wound to the spine. Which description accurately describes this syndrome?
    a. Damage to the most distal cord and nerve roots, resulting in flaccid paralysis of the lower limbs and areflexic bowel and bladder
    b. Spinal cord damage resulting in ipsilateral motor paralysis and contralateral loss of pain and sensation below the level of the lesion
    c. Rare cord damage resulting in loss of proprioception below the lesion level with retention of motor control and temperature and pain sensation
    d. Often caused by flexion injury with acute compression of cord resulting in complete motor paralysis and loss of pain and temperature sensation below the level of injury

13. What causes an initial incomplete spinal cord injury to result in complete cord damage?
    a. Edematous compression of the cord above the level of the injury
    b. Continued trauma to the cord resulting from damage to stabilizing ligaments
    c. Infarction and necrosis of the cord caused by edema, hemorrhage, and metabolites
    d. Mechanical transection of the cord by sharp vertebral bone fragments after the initial injury

14. A patient with a spinal cord injury has spinal shock. The nurse plans care for the patient based on what knowledge?
    a. Rehabilitation measures cannot be initiated until spinal shock has resolved.
    b. The patient will need continuous monitoring for hypotension, tachycardia, and hypoxemia.
    c. Resolution of spinal shock is manifested by spasticity, hyperreflexia, and reflex emptying of the bladder.
    d. The patient will have complete loss of motor and sensory functions below the level of the injury but autonomic functions are not affected.

15. Two days following a spinal cord injury, a patient asks continually about the extent of impairment that will result from the injury. What is the best response by the nurse?
    a. "You will have more normal function when spinal shock resolves and the reflex arc returns."
    b. "The extent of your injury cannot be determined until the secondary injury to the cord is resolved."
    c. "When your condition is more stable, MRI will be done to reveal the extent of the cord damage."
    d. "Because long-term rehabilitation can affect the return of function, it will be years before we can tell what the complete effect will be."

16. *Priority Decision:* The patient was in a traffic collision and is experiencing loss of function below C4. Which effect must the nurse be aware of to provide priority care for the patient?
    a. Respiratory diaphragmatic breathing
    b. Loss of all respiratory muscle function
    c. Decreased response of the sympathetic nervous system
    d. GI hypomotility with paralytic ileus and gastric distention

17. A patient is admitted to the emergency department with a spinal cord injury at the level of T2. Which finding is of most concern to the nurse?
    a. SpO$_2$ of 92%
    b. Heart rate of 42 bpm
    c. Blood pressure of 88/60 mm Hg
    d. Loss of motor and sensory function in arms and legs

18. The patient's spinal cord injury is at T4. What is the highest-level goal of rehabilitation that is realistic for this patient to have?
    a. Indoor mobility in manual wheelchair
    b. Ambulate with crutches and leg braces
    c. Be independent in self-care and wheelchair use
    d. Completely independent ambulation with short leg braces and canes

19. What is one indication for early surgical therapy of the patient with a spinal cord injury?
    a. There is incomplete cord lesion involvement.
    b. The ligaments that support the spine are torn.
    c. A high cervical injury causes loss of respiratory function.
    d. Evidence of continued compression of the cord is apparent.

20. *Priority Decision:* A patient is admitted to the emergency department with a possible cervical spinal cord injury following an automobile crash. During admission of the patient, what is the highest priority for the nurse?
    a. Maintaining a patent airway
    b. Maintaining immobilization of the cervical spine
    c. Assessing the patient for head and other injuries
    d. Assessing the patient's motor and sensory function

21. Without surgical stabilization, what method of immobilization for the patient with a cervical spinal cord injury should the nurse expect to be used?
    a. Kinetic beds
    b. Hard cervical collar
    c. Skeletal traction with skull tongs
    d. Sternal-occipital-mandibular immobilizer brace

22. The health care provider has ordered IV dopamine (Intropin) for a patient in the emergency department with a spinal cord injury. The nurse determines that the drug is having the desired effect when what is observed in patient assessment?
    a. Heart rate of 68 bpm
    b. Respiratory rate of 24
    c. Blood pressure of 106/82 mm Hg
    d. Temperature of 96.8°F (36.0°C)

23. ***Priority Decision:*** During assessment of a patient with a spinal cord injury, the nurse determines that the patient has a poor cough with diaphragmatic breathing. Based on this finding, what should be the nurse's first action?
    a. Institute frequent turning and repositioning.
    b. Use tracheal suctioning to remove secretions.
    c. Assess lung sounds and respiratory rate and depth.
    d. Prepare the patient for endotracheal intubation and mechanical ventilation.

24. Following a T2 spinal cord injury, the patient develops paralytic ileus. While this condition is present, what should the nurse anticipate that the patient will need?
    a. IV fluids
    b. Tube feedings
    c. Parenteral nutrition
    d. Nasogastric suctioning

25. How is urinary function maintained during the acute phase of spinal cord injury?
    a. An indwelling catheter
    b. Intermittent catheterization
    c. Insertion of a suprapubic catheter
    d. Use of incontinent pads to protect the skin

26. A week following a spinal cord injury at T2, a patient experiences movement in his leg and tells the nurse that he is recovering some function. What is the nurse's best response to the patient?
    a. "It is really still too soon to know if you will have a return of function."
    b. "That could be a really positive finding. Can you show me the movement?"
    c. "That's wonderful. We will start exercising your legs more frequently now."
    d. "I'm sorry but the movement is only a reflex and does not indicate normal function."

27. ***Priority Decision:*** A patient with a spinal cord injury suddenly experiences a throbbing headache, flushed skin, and diaphoresis above the level of injury. After checking the patient's vital signs and finding a systolic blood pressure of 210 and a heart rate of 48 bpm, number the following nursing actions in order of priority from highest to lowest (begin with number 1 as first priority).
    _____ 5 _____ a. Administer ordered prn nifedipine (Procardia).
    2 _____ 3 _____ b. Check for bladder distention.
    _____ 6 _____ c. Document the occurrence, treatment, and response.
    3 _____ 4 _____ d. Place call to physician.
    _____ 1 _____ e. Raise the head of bed (HOB) to 45 degrees or above.
    4 _____ 2 _____ f. Loosen tight clothing on the patient.

28. A patient with paraplegia has developed an irritable bladder with reflex emptying. What will be most helpful for the nurse to teach the patient?
    a. Hygiene care for an indwelling urinary catheter
    b. How to perform intermittent self-catheterization
    c. To empty the bladder with manual pelvic pressure in coordination with reflex voiding patterns
    d. That a urinary diversion, such as an ileal conduit, is the easiest way to handle urinary elimination

29. In counseling patients with spinal cord lesions regarding sexual function, how should the nurse advise a male patient with a complete lower motor neuron lesion?
    a. He is most likely to have reflexogenic erections and may experience orgasm if ejaculation occurs.
    b. He may have uncontrolled reflex erections but orgasm and ejaculation are usually not possible.
    c. He has a lesion with the greatest possibility of successful psychogenic erection with ejaculation and orgasm.
    d. He will probably be unable to have either psychogenic or reflexogenic erections and no ejaculation or orgasm.

30. During the patient's process of grieving for the losses resulting from spinal cord injury, what should the nurse do?
    a. Help the patient to understand that working through the grief will be a lifelong process.
    b. Assist the patient to move through all stages of the mourning process to acceptance.
    c. Let the patient know that anger directed at the staff or the family is not a positive coping mechanism.
    d. Facilitate the grieving process so that it is completed by the time the patient is discharged from rehabilitation.

31. A patient with a metastatic tumor of the spinal cord is scheduled for removal of the tumor by a laminectomy. In planning postoperative care for the patient, what should the nurse recognize?
    a. Most cord tumors cause autodestruction of the cord as in traumatic injuries.
    b. Metastatic tumors are commonly extradural lesions that are treated palliatively.
    c. Radiation therapy is routinely administered following surgery for all malignant spinal cord tumors.
    d. Because complete removal of intramedullary tumors is not possible, the surgery is considered palliative.

CASE STUDY
Spinal Cord Injury
Patient Profile

S.M. is an 18-year-old high school student who sustained a C7 spinal cord injury when she dove into a lake while swimming with her friends. S.M. is admitted directly to the intensive care unit (ICU).

Subjective Data

- Has patchy sensation in her upper extremities

Objective Data

- Very weak bicep and tricep strength bilaterally
- Moderate strength in both of her lower extremities
- Bladder control present
- X-rays show no fracture dislocation of the spine
- Placed on bed rest with a hard cervical collar
- Methylprednisolone administered per protocol

Discussion Questions

Using a separate sheet of paper, answer the following questions:

1. What spinal cord syndrome is S.M. experiencing?
2. What is the physiologic reason that S.M. can move her lower extremities better than her upper extremities?
3. Why does S.M. have a spinal cord injury without having sustained any spinal fracture?
4. What is the rationale for the use of the methylprednisolone?
5. What psychologic problems are anticipated?
6. What can be done to begin long-term plans for S.M.?
7. *Priority Decision:* Based on the assessment data presented, what are the priority nursing diagnoses? Are there any collaborative problems?

1. Using the terms listed below, identify the structures in the following illustration.

Terms

Articular cartilage   Epiphysis   Spongy bone
Compact bone   Medullary cavity Yellow marrow
Diaphysis   Periosteum
Epiphyseal plate   Red marrow cavities

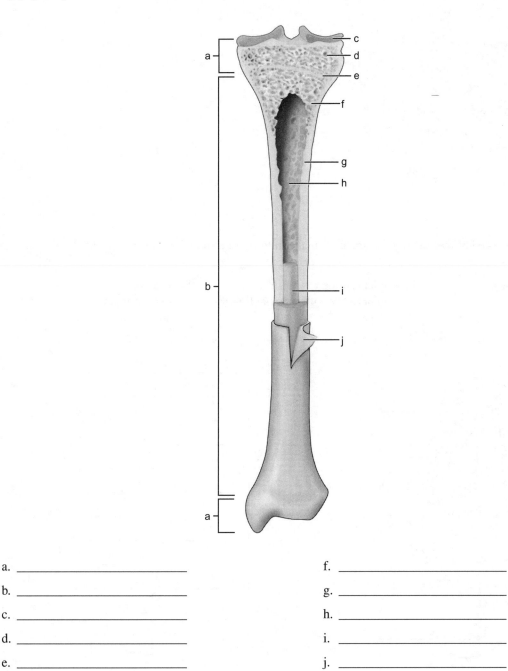

a. _____   f. _____

b. _____   g. _____

c. _____   h. _____

d. _____   i. _____

e. _____   j. _____

2. Using the terms listed below, identify the structures in the following illustration.

Terms

Blood vessels
Canaliculi
Osteon (Haversian system)
Periosteum

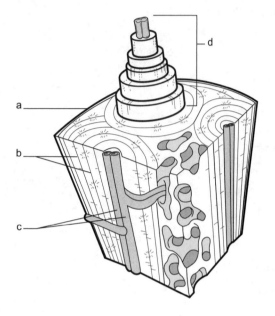

a. _____

b. _____

c. _____

d. _____

3. Using the terms listed below, identify the structures in the following illustration (terms may be used more than once).

Terms

Articular cartilage   Joint capsule   Periosteum
Blood vessel   Joint cavity with synovial fluid   Synovial membrane
Bone   Nerve   Tendon sheath
Bursa

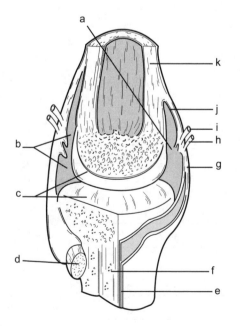

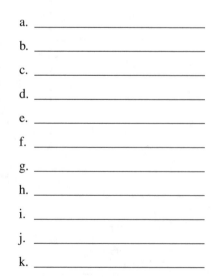

a. _____

b. _____

c. _____

d. _____

e. _____

f. _____

g. _____

h. _____

i. _____

j. _____

k. _____

4. Which type of bone cell is responsible for the formation of bone?
   a. Osteocyte
   b. Osteoclast
   c. Osteoblast
   d. Sarcomere

5. The patient is told by the health care provider that the size of the patient's muscle has decreased. How should the nurse document this occurrence?
   a. Hyaline
   b. Atrophy
   c. Isometric
   d. Hypertrophy

6. An older patient is describing increased rigidity in the shoulders, back, and hips. The loss of elasticity in what tissue contributes to this?
   a. Actin
   b. Fascia
   c. Myosin
   d. Cartilage

7. What is the best description of the periosteum?
   a. Lining of a joint capsule
   b. A characteristic of skeletal muscle
   c. Most common type of cartilage tissue
   d. Fibrous connective tissue covering bone

8. What is the function of a tendon?
   a. Attaches muscle to bone
   b. Connects bone to bone at the joint
   c. Connects cartilage to muscle in joints
   d. Attaches synovium to the joint capsule

9. In performing range of motion (ROM) with a patient, the nurse puts each joint through its full movement. Which joints are capable of abduction and adduction (*select all that apply*)?
   a. Hip
   b. Knee
   c. Wrist
   d. Elbow
   e. Thumb
   f. Shoulder

10. While having his height measured during a routine health examination, a 79-year-old man asks the nurse why he is "shrinking." How should the nurse explain the decreased height that occurs with aging?
    a. Decreased muscle mass results in a stooped posture.
    b. Loss of cartilage in the knees and hip joints causes a loss of height.
    c. Long bones become less dense and shorten as bone tissue compacts.
    d. Vertebrae become more compressed with thinning of intervertebral discs.

11. A 78-year-old woman has a physiologic change related to aging in her joints. What is an appropriate nursing intervention related to common changes of aging in the musculoskeletal system?
    a. Encourage rest to eliminate fatigue.
    b. Provide all care for the patient to ensure that care is completed.
    c. Encourage eating enough calories to avoid the risk for impaired skin integrity.
    d. Have the patient exercise to maintain muscle strength and avoid the risk for falls.

12. When obtaining information about the patient's use of medications, the nurse recognizes that both bone and muscle function may be impaired when the patient reports taking what type of drug?
    a. Corticosteroids
    b. Oral hypoglycemic agents
    c. Potassium-depleting diuretics
    d. Nonsteroidal antiinflammatory drugs (NSAIDs)

13. Identify one specific finding noted by the nurse during assessment of each of the patient's functional health patterns that indicates a risk factor for musculoskeletal problems or a patient response to an actual musculoskeletal problem.

Functional Health Pattern	Risk Factor for or Response to Musculoskeletal Problem
Health perception–health management	
Nutritional-metabolic	
Elimination	
Activity-exercise	
Sleep-rest	
Cognitive-perceptual	
Self-perception–self-concept	
Role-relationship	
Sexuality-reproductive	
Coping–stress tolerance	
Value-belief	

14. During muscle strength testing, the patient has active movement against gravity and some resistance to pressure. What score should the nurse give this finding?
    a. 2
    b. 3
    c. 4
    d. 5

15. On observation of the patient, the nurse notes the presence of a gait disturbance. How should the nurse further evaluate the patient?
    a. Palpate the hips for crepitation.
    b. Measure the length of the limbs.
    c. Evaluate the degree of leg movement.
    d. Compare the muscle mass of one leg with the other.

16. A patient with severe joint immobility is receiving physical and exercise therapy. To evaluate the effect of the treatment, the nurse may assess joint range of motion with what equipment?
    a. Ergometer
    b. Myometer
    c. Goniometer
    d. Arthrometer

17. The patient was referred to the office by the school nurse for a lateral curvature of the spine. The nurse knows this is called
    a. lordosis.
    b. scoliosis.
    c. ankylosis.
    d. kyphosis.

18. In report, the nurse is told that the patient has a contracture of the right arm. What does the nurse know this means?
    a. A fluid-filled cyst
    b. Generalized muscle pain
    c. Shortening of a muscle or ligament
    d. Grating sensation between bones with movement

19. The patient is diagnosed with torticollis. What should the nurse be prepared to provide for the patient?
    a. An immobilizer to hold the bones in place
    b. Exercises to increase the strength of the muscles
    c. A pillow to use to support the knees while sleeping
    d. Enough pillows to support the patient's head comfortably

20. The patient has a burning, sharp pain on the sole of the foot, especially in the morning. The nurse knows that this describes what common musculoskeletal problem?
    a. Pes planus
    b. Tenosynovitis
    c. Plantar fasciitis
    d. Muscle atrophy

21. When assessing the patient the nurse notices that the patient has footdrop and the foot slaps down on the floor as the patient walks. How does the nurse document this gait?
    a. Ataxic gait
    b. Spastic gait
    c. Antalgic gait
    d. Steppage gait

22. What is the most common diagnostic test used to assess musculoskeletal disorders?
    a. Myelogram
    b. Arthroscopy
    c. Standard x-ray
    d. Magnetic resonance imaging (MRI)

23. What test provides fast, precise measurement of the bone mass of the spine, forearm, and total body to evaluate osteoporosis?
    a. Bone scan
    b. Diskogram
    c. Quantitative ultrasound (QUS)
    d. Dual energy x-ray absorptiometry (DXA)

24. Which serologic tests would be done to evaluate rheumatoid arthritis (*select all that apply*)?
    a. Uric acid
    b. Anti-DNA antibody
    c. Rheumatoid factor (RF)
    d. Antinuclear antibody (ANA)
    e. Erythrocyte sedimentation rate (ESR)

63

Nursing Management: Musculoskeletal Trauma and Orthopedic Surgery

1. A 72-year-old man tells the nurse that he cannot perform most of the physical activities he could do 5 years ago because of overall joint aches and pains. What can the nurse do to assist the patient to prevent further deconditioning and decrease the risk for developing musculoskeletal problems?
   a. Limit weight-bearing exercise to prevent stress on fragile bones and possible hip fractures.
   b. Advise the patient to avoid the use of canes and walkers because they increase dependence on ambulation aids.
   c. Advise the patient to increase his activity by more frequently climbing stairs in buildings and other environments with steps.
   d. Discuss use of over-the-counter (OTC) medications to decrease inflammation and pain so that exercise can be maintained.

2. The nurse teaches individuals that one of the best ways to prevent musculoskeletal injuries during physical exercise is by doing what?
   a. Increase muscle strength with daily isometric exercise.
   b. Avoid exercising on concrete or hard pavement surfaces.
   c. Perform stretching and warm-up exercises before exercise.
   d. Wrap susceptible joints with elastic bandages or adhesive tape before exercise.

3. The patient asks, "What does the doctor mean when he says that I have an avulsion fracture in my leg? I thought I had a sprain!" What is the best response by the nurse?
   a. "It is a fracture with more than two fragments."
   b. "It means that a ligament pulled a bone fragment loose."
   c. "The line of the fracture is twisted along the shaft of the bone."
   d. "The line of the fracture is at right angles to the longitudinal axis of the bone."

4. The patient with osteoporosis had a spontaneous hip fracture. How should the nurse document this before the x-ray results return?
   a. Open fracture
   b. Oblique fracture
   c. Pathologic fracture
   d. Greenstick fracture

5. The patient works on a computer 8 hours each day. What kind of repetitive strain injury would be expected in this patient?
   a. Meniscus injury
   b. Rotator cuff injury
   c. Radial-ulnar fracture
   d. Carpal tunnel syndrome

6. The athlete comes to the clinic with bursitis. What does the nurse know happens to the tissue to cause pain when bursitis occurs?
   a. Tearing of a ligament
   b. Stretching of muscle and fascia sheath
   c. Inflammation of synovial membrane sac at friction sites
   d. Incomplete separation of articular surfaces of joint caused by ligament injury

7. Application of RICE (rest, ice, compression, and elevation) is indicated for initial management of which type of injury?
   a. Muscle spasms
   b. Sprains and strains
   c. Repetitive strain injury
   d. Dislocations and subluxations

8. What should be included in the management during the first 48 hours after an acute soft tissue injury of the ankle (*select all that apply*)?
   a. Use of elastic wrap
   b. Initial immobilization and rest
   c. Elevation of ankle above the heart
   d. Alternating the use of heat and cold
   e. Administration of antiinflammatory drugs

9. The patient had a fracture. At 3 weeks to 6 months there is clinical union, and this is the first stage of healing that is sufficient to prevent movement of the fracture site when the bones are gently stressed. How is this stage of fracture healing documented?
   a. Ossification
   b. Remodeling
   c. Consolidation
   d. Callus formation

10. The x-ray shows that the patient's fracture is at the remodeling stage. What characteristics of the fracture healing process are happening at this stage (*select all that apply*)?
    a. Radiologic union
    b. Absorption of excess cells
    c. Return to preinjury strength and shape
    d. Semisolid blood clot at the ends of fragments
    e. Deposition and absorption of bone in response to stress
    f. Unorganized network of bone woven around fracture parts

11. A patient is brought to the emergency department with an injured lower left leg following a fall while rock climbing. The nurse identifies the presence of a fracture based on what cardinal sign of fracture?
    a. Muscle spasms
    b. Obvious deformity
    c. Edema and swelling
    d. Pain and tenderness

12. A patient with a fractured femur experiences the complication of malunion. The nurse recognizes that what happens with this complication?
    a. The fracture heals in an unsatisfactory position.
    b. The fracture fails to heal properly despite treatment. –nonunion
    c. Fracture healing progresses more slowly than expected.
    d. Loss of bone substances occurs as a result of immobilization.

13. What is a disadvantage of open reduction and internal fixation of a fracture compared to closed reduction?
    a. Infection
    b. Skin irritation
    c. Nerve impairment
    d. Complications of immobility

14. A young patient with a fractured femur has a hip spica cast applied. While the cast is drying, what should the nurse do?
    a. Elevate the legs above the level of the heart for 24 hours.
    b. Turn the patient to both sides and prone to supine every 2 hours.
    c. Cover the cast with a light blanket to avoid chilling from evaporation.
    d. Assess the patient frequently for abdominal pain, nausea, and vomiting.

15. A patient is admitted with an open fracture of the tibia following a bicycle accident. During assessment of the patient, what specifically should the nurse question the patient about?
    a. Any previous injuries to the leg
    b. The status of tetanus immunization
    c. The use of antibiotics in the last month
    d. Whether the injury was exposed to dirt or gravel

16. ***Priority Decision:*** A patient has fallen in the bathroom of the hospital room and reports pain in the upper right arm and elbow. Before splinting the injury, the nurse knows that the priority management of a possible fracture should include which action?
    a. Elevation of the arm
    b. Application of ice to the site
    c. Notification of the health care provider
    d. Neurovascular checks below the site of the injury

17. To assess for neurologic status in a patient with a fractured humerus, what should the nurse ask the patient to do?
    a. Evert, invert, dorsiflex, and plantar flex the foot.
    b. Abduct, adduct, and oppose the fingers and pronate and supinate the hand.
    c. Assess the location, quality, and intensity of pain below the site of the injury.
    d. Assess the color, temperature, capillary refill, peripheral pulses, and presence of edema in the extremity.

18. A patient is discharged from the outpatient clinic following application of a synthetic fiberglass long arm cast for a fractured ulna. Before discharge, the nurse instructs the patient to do what?
    a. Never get the cast wet.
    b. Move the shoulder and fingers frequently.
    c. Place tape petals around the edges of the cast when it is dry.
    d. Use a sling to support the arm at waist level for the first 48 hours.

19. A patient with a fractured tibia accompanied by extensive soft tissue damage initially has a splint applied and held in place with an elastic bandage. What early sign should alert the nurse that the patient is developing compartment syndrome?
    a. Paralysis of the toes
    b. Absence of peripheral pulses
    c. Distal pain unrelieved by opioid analgesics
    d. Skin over the injury site is blanched when the bandage is removed

20. What surgical treatment will the nurse prepare the patient for in the presence of compartment syndrome?
    a. Fasciotomy
    b. Amputation
    c. Internal fixation
    d. Release of tendons

21. Which type of fracture occurred when there is radial nerve and brachial artery damage and the fracture is reduced with a hanging arm cast?
    a. Fractured tibia
    b. Colles' fracture
    c. Fractured humerus
    d. Femoral shaft fracture

22. The woman with osteoporosis slipped on the ice and now her wrist hurts. If there is a fracture, what type of fracture is expected?
    a. Dislocation
    b. Open fracture
    c. Colles' fracture
    d. Incomplete fracture

23. What emergency considerations must be included with facial fractures (*select all that apply*)?
    a. Airway patency
    b. Oral examination
    c. Cervical spine injury
    d. Cranial nerve assessment
    e. Immobilization of the jaw

24. In a patient with a stable vertebral fracture, what should the nurse teach the patient to do?
    a. Remain on bed rest until the pain is gone.
    b. Logroll to keep the spine straight when turning.
    c. How to use bone cement to correct the problem.
    d. Take as much analgesic as needed to relieve the pain.

25. When is a fat embolism most likely to occur? _long bones_
    a. 24 to 48 hours following a fractured tibia
    b. 36 to 72 hours following a skull fracture
    c. 4 to 5 days following a fractured femur
    d. 5 to 6 days following a pelvic fracture

26. The nurse suspects a fat embolism rather than a pulmonary embolism from a venous thrombosis when the patient with a fracture develops what?
    a. Tachycardia and dyspnea
    b. A sudden onset of chest pain
    c. Petechiae around the neck and upper chest
    d. Electrocardiographic (ECG) changes and decreased PaO$_2$

27. Which kind of hip fracture is usually repaired with a hip prosthesis?
    a. Intracapsular
    b. Extracapsular
    c. Subtrochanteric
    d. Intertrochanteric

28. An older adult woman is admitted to the emergency department after falling at home. The nurse cautions her not to put weight on the leg after finding what in the patient assessment?
    a. Inability to move the toes and ankle
    b. Edema of the thigh extending to the knee
    c. Internal rotation of the leg with groin pain
    d. Shortening and external rotation of the leg

29. A patient with an extracapsular hip fracture is admitted to the orthopedic unit and placed in Buck's traction. The nurse explains to the patient that the purpose of the traction is to do what?
    a. Pull bone fragments back into alignment
    b. Immobilize the leg until healing is complete
    c. Reduce pain and muscle spasms before surgery
    d. Prevent damage to the blood vessels at the fracture site

30. A patient with a fractured right hip has an anterior open reduction and internal fixation of the fracture. What should the nurse plan to do postoperatively?
    a. Get the patient up to the chair on the first postoperative day.
    b. Position the patient only on the back and the unoperative side.
    c. Keep the leg abductor pillow on the patient even when bathing.
    d. Ambulate the patient with partial weight bearing by discharge.

31. What should the nurse include in discharge instructions for the patient following a hip prosthesis with a posterior approach?
    a. Restrict walking for 2 to 3 months.
    b. Take a bath rather than a shower to prevent falling.
    c. Keep the leg internally rotated while sitting and standing.
    d. Have a family member put on the patient's shoes and socks.

32. When preparing a patient for discharge following fixation of a mandibular fracture, the nurse determines that teaching has been successful when the patient says what?
    a. "I can keep my mouth moist by sucking on hard candy."
    b. "I should cut the wires with scissors if I begin to vomit."
    c. "I may use a bulk-forming laxative if my liquid diet causes constipation."
    d. "I should use a moist swab to clean my mouth every time I eat something."

33. *Priority Decision:* Twenty-four hours after a below-the-knee amputation, a patient uses the call system to tell the nurse that his dressing (a compression bandage) has fallen off. What is the first action that the nurse should take?
    a. Apply ice to the site.
    b. Cover the incision with dry gauze.
    c. Reapply the compression dressing.
    d. Elevate the extremity on a couple of pillows.

34. A patient complains of pain in the foot of a leg that was recently amputated. What should the nurse recognize about this pain?
    a. It is caused by swelling at the incision.
    b. It should be treated with ordered analgesics.
    c. It will become worse with the use of a prosthesis.
    d. It can be managed with diversion because it is psychologic.

35. **Priority Decision:** An immediate prosthetic fitting during surgery is used for a patient with a traumatic below-the-knee amputation. During the immediate postoperative period, what is a priority nursing intervention?
    a. Monitor the patient's vital signs.
    b. Assess the incision for hemorrhage.
    c. Elevate the residual limb on pillows.
    d. Have the patient flex and extend the knee every hour.

36. Why does a nurse position a patient with an above-the-knee amputation with a delayed prosthetic fitting prone several times a day?
    a. To prevent flexion contractures
    b. To assess the posterior skin flap
    c. To reduce edema in the residual limb
    d. To relieve pressure on the incision site

37. A patient who had a below-the-knee amputation is to be fitted with a temporary prosthesis. It is most important for the nurse to teach the patient to do what?
    a. Inspect the residual limb daily for irritation.
    b. Apply an elastic shrinker before applying the prosthesis.
    c. Perform range-of-motion (ROM) exercises to the affected leg four times a day.
    d. Apply alcohol to the residual limb every morning and evening to toughen the skin.

38. Which joint surgery is used to arthroscopically remove degenerative tissue in joints?
    a. Osteotomy
    b. Arthrodesis
    c. Debridement
    d. Synovectomy

39. When the nursing student asks the RN what an arthroplasty is, what is the best description the RN can give the student?
    a. Surgical fusion of a joint to relieve pain
    b. Correction of bone deformity by removal of a wedge or slice of bone
    c. Reconstruction or replacement of a joint to relieve pain and correct deformity
    d. Used in rheumatoid arthritis to remove the tissue involved in joint destruction

40. A 65-year-old patient has undergone a right total hip arthroplasty with a cemented prosthesis for treatment of severe osteoarthritis of the hip. What is included in the activity the nurse anticipates for the patient on the patient's first or second postoperative day?
    a. Transfer from the bed to the chair twice a day only
    b. Turning from the back to the unaffected side q2hr only
    c. Crutch walking with non–weight bearing on the operative leg
    d. Ambulation and weight bearing on the right leg with a walker

41. When positioning the patient after a total hip arthroplasty with a posterior approach, it is important that the nurse maintain the affected extremity in what position?
    a. Adduction and flexion
    b. Abduction and extension
    c. Abduction and internal rotation
    d. Adduction and external rotation

42. Following a knee arthroplasty, a patient has a continuous passive motion machine for the affected joint. The nurse explains to the patient that this device is used for what purpose?
    a. To relieve edema and pain at the incision site
    b. To promote early joint mobility and increase knee flexion
    c. To prevent venous stasis and the formation of a deep venous thrombosis
    d. To improve arterial circulation to the affected extremity to promote healing

43. *Priority Decision:* A patient with severe ulnar deviation of the hands undergoes an arthroplasty with reconstruction and replacement of finger joints. Postoperatively, what is it most important for the nurse to do?
    a. Position the fingers lower than the elbow.
    b. Perform neurovascular assessments of the fingers q2-4hr.
    c. Encourage the patient to gently flex, extend, abduct, and adduct the fingers q4hr.
    d. Remind the patient that function of the hands is more important than their cosmetic appearance.

44. *Priority Decision:* Following change-of-shift handoff, which patient should the nurse assess first?
    a. A 58-year-old male experiencing phantom pain and requesting analgesic
    b. A 72-year-old male being transferred to a skilled nursing unit following repair of a hip fracture
    c. A 25-year-old female in left leg skeletal traction asking for the weights to be lifted for a few minutes
    d. A 68-year-old male with a new lower leg cast complaining that the cast is too tight and he cannot feel his toes

---

CASE STUDY

Fracture

Patient Profile

H.A., a 30-year-old telephone lineman, was seen in the emergency department after falling from a pole. His right lower extremity was splinted with a cardboard splint and a large, bulky dressing.

Subjective Data

- Complains of severe pain in the right leg
- Expresses concern about notifying his wife about the accident and his whereabouts
- Asks how long he will be off work

Objective Data

- Open oblique fracture of the anterolateral aspect of the tibia
- Obvious deformity, marked swelling, and ecchymosis in region of injury
- To be treated with closed reduction and a cast

Discussion Questions

Using a separate sheet of paper, answer the following questions:

1. Was the immobilization of the fracture at the scene of the accident appropriate?
2. What is the appropriate nursing neurovascular assessment of the injured extremity?
3. *Priority Decision:* What are the priority therapeutic and nursing interventions to prevent infection?
4. What specific nursing actions should the nurse implement to alleviate H.A.'s pain?
5. How would the nurse answer H.A.'s question about time off from work based on the stages of fracture healing?
6. *Delegation Decision:* What care can be delegated to unlicensed assistive personnel (UAP)?
7. How should the nurse notify H.A.'s wife about her husband's accident?
8. *Priority Decision:* Based on the assessment data presented, what are the priority nursing diagnoses? Are there any collaborative problems?

1. A patient with chronic osteomyelitis has been hospitalized for a surgical debridement procedure. What does the nurse explain to the patient as the rationale for the surgical treatment?
   a. Removal of the infection prevents the need for bone and skin grafting.
   b. Formation of scar tissue has led to a protected area of bacterial growth.
   c. The process of depositing new bone blocks the vascular supply to the bone.
   d. Antibiotics are not effective against microorganisms that cause chronic osteomyelitis.

2. A patient with osteomyelitis has a nursing diagnosis of risk for injury. What is an appropriate nursing intervention for this patient?
   a. Use careful and appropriate disposal of soiled dressings.
   b. Gently handle the involved extremity during movement.
   c. Measure the circumference of the affected extremity daily.
   d. Provide range-of-motion (ROM) exercise q4hr to the involved extremity.

3. A patient who experienced an open fracture of the humerus 2 weeks ago is having increased pain at the fracture site. To identify a possible causative agent of osteomyelitis at the site, what should the nurse expect testing to include?
   a. X-rays
   b. CT scan
   c. Bone biopsy
   d. WBC count and erythrocyte sedimentation rate (ESR)

4. Following 2 weeks of IV antibiotic therapy, a patient with acute osteomyelitis of the tibia is prepared for discharge from the hospital. The nurse determines that additional instruction is needed when the patient makes which statement?
   a. "I will need to continue antibiotic therapy for 4 to 6 weeks."
   b. "I shouldn't bear weight on my affected leg until healing is complete."
   c. "I can use a heating pad on my lower leg for comfort and to promote healing." *— avoid heat, it spreads infection*
   d. "I should notify the health care provider if the pain in my leg becomes worse."

5. During a follow-up visit to a patient with acute osteomyelitis treated with IV antibiotics, the home health nurse is told by the patient's wife that she can hardly get the patient to eat because his mouth is so sore. In assessing the patient's mouth, what should the nurse expect to find?
   a. A dry, cracked tongue with a central furrow
   b. White, curdlike membranous lesions of the mucosa
   c. Ulcers of the mouth and lips surrounded by a reddened base
   d. Single or clustered vesicles on the tongue and buccal mucosa

6. Which type of bone tumor is a benign overgrowth of bone and cartilage and may transform into a malignant form?
   a. Endochroma
   b. Osteoclastoma
   c. Ewing's sarcoma
   d. Osteochondroma

7. Which statement describes osteosarcoma?
   a. High rate of local recurrence
   b. Very malignant and metastasizes early
   c. Arises in cancellous ends of long bones
   d. Develops in the medullary cavity of long bones

8. A 24-year-old patient with a 12-year history of Becker muscular dystrophy is hospitalized with heart failure. What is an appropriate nursing intervention for this patient?
   a. Feed and bathe the patient to avoid exhausting the muscle.
   b. Reposition frequently to avoid skin and respiratory complications.
   c. Provide hand weights for the patient to exercise the upper extremities.
   d. Use orthopedic braces to promote ambulation and prevent muscle wasting.

9. What does radicular pain that radiates down the buttock and below the knee, along the distribution of the sciatic nerve, generally indicate?
   a. Cervical disc herniation
   b. Acute lumbosacral strain
   c. Degenerative disc disease
   d. Herniated intervertebral disc

10. What should the nurse teach the patient recovering from an episode of acute low back pain?
    a. Perform daily exercise as a lifelong routine.
    b. Sit in a chair with the hips higher than the knees.
    c. Avoid occupations in which the use of the body is required.
    d. Sleep on the abdomen or on the back with the legs extended.

11. A laminectomy and spinal fusion are performed on a patient with a herniated lumbar intervertebral disc. During the postoperative period, which finding is of most concern to the nurse?
    a. Paralytic ileus
    b. Urinary incontinence
    c. Greater pain at the graft site than at the lumbar incision site
    d. Leg and arm movement and sensation unchanged from preoperative status

12. *Priority Decision:* Before repositioning the patient on the side after a lumbar laminectomy, what should be the nurse's first action?
    a. Raise the head of the bed 30 degrees.
    b. Have the patient flex the knees and hips.
    c. Place a pillow between the patient's legs.
    d. Have the patient grasp the side rail on the opposite side of the bed.

13. A health care provider diagnoses a patient with a plantar wart. What should the nurse know about this kind of abnormality?
    a. Papilloma growth on the sole of the foot
    b. Thickening of skin on the weight-bearing part of the foot
    c. Local thickening of skin caused by pressure on bony prominences
    d. Tumor on nerve tissue between the third and fourth metatarsal heads

14. The patient has lateral angulation of the large toe toward the second toe. The nurse knows that treatment will include what?
    a. Metatarsal arch support
    b. Trimming with a scalpel after softening
    c. Surgery to remove the bursal sac and bony enlargement
    d. Intraarticular corticosteroids and passive manual stretching

15. In promoting healthy feet, what factor should the nurse recognize is associated with most foot problems?
    a. Poor foot hygiene
    b. Congenital deformities
    c. Improperly fitting shoes
    d. Peripheral vascular disease

16. What are characteristics of Paget's disease (*select all that apply*)?
    a. Results from vitamin D deficiency
    b. Loss of total bone mass and substance
    c. Abnormal remodeling and resorption of bone
    d. Most common in bones of spine, hips, and wrists
    e. Generalized bone decalcification with bone deformity
    f. Replacement of normal marrow with vascular connective tissue

17. Which female patients are at risk for developing osteoporosis (*select all that apply*)?
    a. 60-year-old white aerobics instructor
    b. 55-year-old Asian American cigarette smoker
    c. 62-year-old African American on estrogen therapy
    d. 68-year-old white who is underweight and inactive
    e. 58-year-old Native American who started menopause prematurely

18. Identify methods to specifically prevent osteoporosis in postmenopausal women (*select all that apply*).
    a. Eating more beef
    b. Eating 8 ounces of yogurt daily
    c. Performing weight-bearing exercise
    d. Spending 15 minutes in the sun each day
    e. Taking postmenopausal estrogen replacement

19. A patient is started on alendronate (Fosamax) once weekly for the treatment of osteoporosis. The nurse determines that further instruction about the drug is needed when what is said by the patient?
    a. "I should take the drug with a meal to prevent stomach irritation."
    b. "This drug will prevent further bone loss and increase my bone density."
    c. "I need to sit or stand upright for at least 30 minutes after taking the drug."
    d. "I will still need to take my calcium supplements while taking this new drug."

CASE STUDY
Herniated Intervertebral Disc
Patient Profile
- G.B. is a 38-year-old truck driver who slipped on a wet floor at work and landed on his buttocks.

Subjective Data
- Experienced immediate, severe lower back pain, with pain radiating into his right buttock
- Had worsening of pain in 3 days, with pain radiating down his leg and into his foot
- Experienced tingling of his toes
- Rested at home for 2 weeks without relief
- Smokes a pack of cigarettes a day

Objective Data
- Height: 5 ft, 8 in
- Weight: 253 lb
- Diagnostic studies: MRI revealed a large herniated disc at L4–5 level.

Collaborative Care
- Underwent microdiskectomy at L4–5
- Expected discharge 2 days after surgery

Discussion Questions
Using a separate sheet of paper, answer the following questions:

1. What risk factors for low back pain does G.B. have?
2. What preoperative teaching is indicated for G.B.?
3. What postoperative activity restrictions will G.B. need to follow?
4. What postoperative nursing assessments should be made?
5. *Priority Decision:* What priority needs must be included in the discharge teaching for G.B.?
6. *Priority Decision:* Based on the assessment data presented, what are the priority nursing diagnoses? Are there any collaborative problems?

CHAPTER 65

Nursing Management: Arthritis and Connective Tissue Diseases

1. A 60-year-old woman has pain on motion in her fingers and asks the nurse whether this is just a result of aging. The best response by the nurse should include what information?
   a. Joint pain with functional limitation is a normal change that affects all people to some extent.
   b. Joint pain that develops with age is usually related to previous trauma or infection of the joints.
   c. This is a symptom of a systemic arthritis that eventually affects all joints as the disease progresses.
   d. Changes in the cartilage and bones of joints may cause symptoms of pain and loss of function in some people as they age.

2. Number in sequence from 1 to 6 the pathophysiologic processes that occur in osteoarthritis (OA).
   3 _____ a. Erosion of articular surfaces
   5 _____ b. Incongruity in joint surfaces
   6 _____ c. Reduction in motion
   1 _____ d. Joint cartilage becomes yellow and granular
   4 _____ e. Osteophytes form at joint margins
   2 _____ f. Cartilage becomes softer and less elastic

3. What is most likely to cause the pain experienced in the later stages of OA?
   a. Crepitation   c. Heberden's nodes
   b. Bouchard's nodes   d. Bone surfaces rubbing together

4. To preserve function and the ability to perform activities of daily living (ADLs), what should the nurse teach the patient with OA?
   a. Avoid exercise that involves the affected joints.
   b. Plan and organize task performance to be less stressful to joints.
   c. Maintain normal activities during an acute episode to prevent loss of function.
   d. Use mild analgesics to control symptoms when performing tasks that cause pain.

5. A patient with OA asks the nurse whether he could try glucosamine and chondroitin for control of his symptoms. The best response by the nurse includes what information?
   a. Some patients find these supplements helpful for relieving arthritis pain and improving mobility.
   b. Although these substances may not help, there is no evidence that they can cause any untoward effects.
   c. These supplements are a fad that has not been shown to reduce pain or increase joint mobility in patients with OA.
   d. Only dosages of these supplements available by prescription are high enough to provide any benefit in treatment of OA.

6. A patient taking ibuprofen (Motrin) for treatment of OA has good pain relief but is experiencing increased dyspepsia and nausea with the drug's use. The nurse consults the patient's primary care provider about doing what?
   a. Adding misoprostol (Cytotec) to the patient's drug regimen
   b. Substituting naproxen (Naprosyn) for the ibuprofen (Motrin)
   c. Returning to the use of acetaminophen but at a dose of 5 g/day instead of 4 g/day
   d. Administering the ibuprofen with antacids to decrease the gastrointestinal (GI) irritation

7. Which description is most characteristic of osteoarthritis (OA) when compared to rheumatoid arthritis (RA)?
   a. Not systemic or symmetric   c. Most commonly occurs in women
   b. Rheumatoid factor (RF) positive   d. Morning joint stiffness lasts one to several hours

8. What best describes the manifestations of OA?
   a. Smaller joints are typically affected first.
   b. There is joint stiffness after periods of inactivity.
   c. Joint stiffness is accompanied by fatigue, anorexia, and weight loss.
   d. Pain and immobility may be aggravated by falling barometric pressure.

9. During the physical assessment of the patient with early to moderate RA, what should the nurse expect to find?
   a. Hepatomegaly
   b. Heberden's nodes
   c. Spindle-shaped fingers
   d. Crepitus on joint movement

10. Laboratory findings that the nurse would expect to be present in the patient with RA include
    a. polycythemia.
    b. increased immunoglobulin G (IgG).
    c. decreased white blood cell (WBC) count.
    d. anti-citrullinated protein antibody (ACPA).

11. Which other extraarticular manifestation of RA is most likely to be seen in the patient with rheumatoid nodules?
    a. Lyme disease
    b. Felty syndrome
    c. Sjögren's syndrome
    d. Spondyloarthropathies

12. Which drug that prevents binding of the tumor necrosis factor and inhibits the inflammatory response is used in the management of RA?
    a. Anakinra (Kineret)
    b. Entanercept (Enbrel)
    c. Leflunomide (Arava)
    d. Azathioprine (Imuran)

13. The patient has had RA for some time but has not had success with previous medications. Although there is an increased risk for tuberculosis, which monoclonal antibody is used with methotrexate to best treat symptoms?
    a. Parenteral gold
    b. Certolizumab (Cimzia)
    c. Tocilizumab (Actemra)
    d. Hydroxychloroquine (Paquenil)

14. A 70-year-old patient is being evaluated for symptoms of RA. The nurse recognizes what as the major problem in the management of RA in the older adult?
    a. RA is usually more severe in older adults.
    b. Older patients are not as likely to comply with treatment regimens.
    c. Drug interactions and toxicity are more likely to occur with multidrug therapy.
    d. Laboratory and other diagnostic tests are not effective in identifying RA in older adults.

15. After teaching a patient with RA about the prescribed therapeutic regimen, the nurse determines that further instruction is needed when the patient says what?
    a. "It is important for me to perform my prescribed exercises every day."
    b. "I should perform most of my daily chores in the morning when my energy level is highest."
    c. "An ice pack to a joint for 10 minutes may help to relieve pain and inflammation when I have an acute flare."
    d. "I can use assistive devices such as padded utensils, electric can openers, and elevated toilet seats to protect my joints."

16. A patient recovering from an acute exacerbation of RA tells the nurse that she is too tired to bathe. What should the nurse do for this patient?
    a. Give the patient a bed bath to conserve her energy.
    b. Allow the patient a rest period before showering with the nurse's help.
    c. Tell the patient that she can skip bathing if she will walk in the hall later.
    d. Inform the patient that it is important for her to maintain self-care activities.

17. After teaching a patient with RA to use heat and cold therapy to relieve symptoms, the nurse determines that teaching has been effective when what is said by the patient?
    a. "Heat treatments should not be used if muscle spasms are present."
    b. "Cold applications can be applied for 15 to 20 minutes to relieve joint stiffness."
    c. "I should use heat applications for 20 minutes to relieve the symptoms of an acute flare."
    d. "When my joints are painful, I can use a bag of frozen corn for 10 to 15 minutes to relieve the pain."

18. The nurse teaches the patient with RA that which exercise is one of the most effective methods of aerobic exercise?
    a. Ballet dancing
    b. Casual walking
    c. Aquatic exercises
    d. Low-impact aerobic exercises

19. A patient is seen at the outpatient clinic for a sudden onset of inflammation and severe pain in the great toe. A definitive diagnosis of gouty arthritis is made on the basis of what?
    a. A family history of gout
    b. Elevated urine uric acid levels
    c. Elevated serum uric acid levels
    d. Presence of monosodium urate crystals in synovial fluid

20. During treatment of the patient with an acute attack of gout, the nurse would expect to administer which drug?
    a. Aspirin
    b. Colchicine
    c. Allopurinol (Zyloprim)
    d. Probenecid (Benemid)

21. A patient with gout is treated with drug therapy to prevent future attacks. The nurse teaches the patient that what is most important for the patient to do?
    a. Avoid all foods high in purine, such as organ meats.
    b. Have periodic determination of serum uric acid levels.
    c. Increase the dosage of medication with the onset of an acute attack.
    d. Perform active range of motion (ROM) of all joints that have been affected by gout.

22. What characteristics are common in spondyloarthritides associated with human leukocyte antigen (HLA)–B27?
    a. Symmetric polyarticular arthritis
    b. Absence of extraarticular disease
    c. Presence of rheumatoid factor and autoantibodies
    d. High level of involvement of sacroiliac joints and the axial skeleton

23. An important nursing intervention for the patient with ankylosing spondylitis is to teach the patient to do what?
    a. Wear roomy shoes with good orthotic support.
    b. Sleep on the side with the knees and hips flexed.
    c. Keep the spine slightly flexed while sitting, standing, or walking.
    d. Perform back, neck, and chest stretches and deep-breathing exercises.

24. Which descriptions are related to reactive arthritis (*select all that apply*)?
    a. Methotrexate is a treatment of choice
    b. Symptoms include urethritis and conjunctivitis
    c. Diagnosed by finding of hypersensitive tender points
    d. Increased risk in persons with decreased host resistance
    e. Infection of a joint often caused by hematogenous route
    f. Self-limiting arthritis following GI (enteral) or sexually transmitted infections

25. What is the pathophysiology of systemic lupus erythematosus (SLE) characterized by?
    a. Destruction of nucleic acids and other self-proteins by autoantibodies
    b. Overproduction of collagen that disrupts the functioning of internal organs
    c. Formation of abnormal IgG that attaches to cellular antigens, activating complement
    d. Increased activity of T suppressor cells with B-cell hypoactivity, resulting in an immunodeficiency

26. What is an ominous sign of advanced SLE disease?
    a. Proteinuria from early glomerulonephritis
    b. Anemia from antibodies against blood cells
    c. Dysrhythmias from fibrosis of the atrioventricular node
    d. Cognitive dysfunction from immune complex deposit in the brain

27. A patient with newly diagnosed SLE asks the nurse how the disease will affect her life. What is the best response the nurse can give the patient?
    a. "You can plan to have a near-normal life since SLE rarely causes death."
    b. "It is difficult to tell because the disease is so variable in its severity and progression."
    c. "Life span is shortened somewhat in people with SLE but the disease can be controlled with long-term use of corticosteroids."
    d. "Most people with SLE have alternating periods of remissions and exacerbations with rapid progression to permanent organ damage."

28. During an acute exacerbation, a patient with SLE is treated with corticosteroids. The nurse would expect the corticosteroids to begin to be tapered when which serum laboratory results are evident?
    a. Decreased anti-DNA
    b. Increased complement
    c. Increased red blood cells (RBCs)
    d. Decreased erythrocyte sedimentation rate (ESR)

29. What should the nurse include in the teaching plan for the patient with SLE?
    a. Ways to avoid exposure to sunlight
    b. Increasing dietary protein and carbohydrate intake
    c. The necessity of genetic counseling before planning a family
    d. The use of nonpharmacologic pain interventions instead of analgesics

30. During assessment of the patient with scleroderma, what should the nurse expect to find?
    a. Thickening of the skin of the fingers and hands
    b. Cool, cyanotic fingers with thinning skin over the joints
    c. Swan neck deformity or ulnar drift deformity of the hands
    d. Low back pain, stiffness, and limitation of spine movement

31. When caring for the patient with CREST syndrome (calcinosis, Raynaud's phenomenon, esophageal dysfunction, sclerodactyly, and telangiectasia) associated with scleroderma, what should the nurse teach the patient to do?
    a. Maintain a fluid intake of at least 3000 mL/day.
    b. Avoid exposure to the sun or other ultraviolet light.
    c. Monitor and keep a log of daily blood pressure (BP).
    d. Protect the hands and feet from cold exposure and injury.

32. During the acute phase of dermatomyositis, what is an appropriate patient outcome?
    a. Relates improvement in pain
    b. Does not experience aspiration
    c. Performs active ROM four times daily
    d. Maintains absolute rest of affected joints

33. During assessment of the patient diagnosed with fibromyalgia, what should the nurse expect the patient to report?
    a. Generalized muscle twitching and spasms
    b. Nonrestorative sleep with resulting fatigue
    c. Profound and progressive muscle weakness that limits ADLs
    d. Widespread musculoskeletal pain that is accompanied by inflammation and fever

34. What is one criterion identified by the American College of Rheumatology for a diagnosis of fibromyalgia?
    a. Fiber atrophy found on muscle biopsy
    b. Elimination of all other causes of musculoskeletal pain
    c. The presence of the manifestations of chronic fatigue syndrome
    d. The elicitation of pain on palpation of at least 11 of 18 identified tender points

35. One important nursing intervention for the patient with fibromyalgia is to teach the patient to do what?
    a. Rest the muscles as much as possible to avoid triggering pain.
    b. Plan nighttime sleep and naps to obtain 12 to 14 hours of sleep a day.
    c. Try the use of food supplements such as glucosamine and chondroitin for relief of pain.
    d. Use stress management techniques such as biofeedback, meditation, or cognitive behavioral therapy

36. A patient with debilitating fatigue has been diagnosed with chronic fatigue syndrome. Which criteria are considered the four major criteria that must be present for this diagnosis to be made (*select all that apply*)?
    a. Unexplained muscle pain
    b. Fatigue not due to ongoing exertion
    c. Tender cervical or axillary lymph nodes
    d. Fatigue not substantially alleviated by rest
    e. Headaches of a new type, pattern, or severity
    f. Unexplained, persistent, or relapsing chronic fatigue of new and definite onset
    g. Fatigue resulting in substantial reduction in occupational, educational, social, or personal activities

CASE STUDY
Rheumatoid Arthritis
Patient Profile

N.M. is a 36-year-old overweight white woman who has RA. When her symptoms began to interfere with her daily activities, she sought medical help.

Subjective Data

- Has painful, stiff hands and feet
- Feels tired all of the time
- Reports an intermittent low-grade fever
- Takes naproxen (Aleve) 220 mg twice daily
- Wears a copper bracelet on the advice of a neighbor

Objective Data

- Hands show mild ulnar drift and puffiness
- Temp: 100°F (37.8°C)
- Admitted to the hospital for examination and comprehensive treatment plan
- Methotrexate (Rheumatrex) therapy to be initiated

Discussion Questions

Using a separate sheet of paper, answer the following questions:

1. How should the nurse explain the pathophysiology of rheumatoid arthritis to N.M.?
2. What manifestations does N.M. have that suggest the diagnosis of RA?
3. What diagnostic studies will confirm the diagnosis of RA?
4. What results may be expected from methotrexate therapy? What are the nursing responsibilities related to methotrexate therapy?
5. What are some suggestions that may be offered to N.M. concerning home management and joint protection?
6. How can the nurse help N.M. to recognize ineffective, unproven methods of treatment?
7. What other sources of information regarding arthritis might the nurse suggest to N.M.?
8. *Priority Decision:* Based on the assessment data presented, what are the priority nursing diagnoses? Are there any collaborative problems?

CHAPTER

66

Nursing Management: Critical Care

1. What is an ability that is a primary difference in the skills of a certified critical care nurse compared with nurses certified in medical-surgical nursing?
   a. Diagnose and treat life-threatening diseases
   b. Detect and manage early complications of health problems
   c. Provide intensive psychologic support to the patient and family
   d. Use advanced technology to assess and maintain physiologic function

2. Identify the rationale for the following four patients' admissions to the intensive care unit (ICU) based on the common three reasons why patients are admitted to the ICU.
   _____ a. Patient with diabetic ketoacidosis
   _____ b. Patient with nondisplaced skull fracture who is alert and oriented
   _____ c. Postoperative patient with mitral valve replacement
   _____ d. Comatose patient who had an anaphylactic reaction with cardiopulmonary arrest at home yesterday

   1. Physiologically unstable
   2. Risk for serious complications
   3. Intensive nursing support required

3. What is a nursing intervention that is indicated for the patient in the ICU who has a nursing diagnosis of anxiety *related to* the ICU environment and sensory overload?
   a. Provide flexible visiting schedules for caregivers.
   b. Eliminate unnecessary alarms and overhead paging.
   c. Administer sedatives or psychotropic drugs to promote rest.
   d. Allow the patient to do as many self-care activities as possible.

4. Why should the critical care nurse include caregivers of the patient in the ICU as part of the health care team?
   a. The costs of critical care will affect the entire family.
   b. Caregivers play a valuable role in the patient's recovery.
   c. Caregivers are responsible for making health care decisions for the patient.
   d. Caregivers who are ignored are more likely to question the patient's quality of care.

5. What factor will cause a decrease in cardiac output (CO)?
   a. Decreased afterload
   b. Decreased heart rate (HR)
   c. Increased stroke volume (SV)
   d. Decreased systemic vascular resistance (SVR)

6. The patient with shortness of breath is scheduled for an impedance cardiography to differentiate if the cause is cardiac or pulmonary. How should the nurse best explain this test to the patient?
   a. An invasive method of measuring CO
   b. Electricity is transmitted through the bones in the chest
   c. It will most effective when the patient has generalized edema
   d. Thoracic fluid status is determined by changes in impedance with each heartbeat

7. The patient has experienced an increased preload, which supports an increase in CO. What nursing action contributes to an increased preload?
   a. Diuretic administration
   b. Intropin administration
   c. Increased fluid administration
   d. Calcium channel blocker administration

8. During hemodynamic monitoring, the nurse finds that the patient has a decreased CO with unchanged pulmonary artery wedge pressure (PAWP), HR, and SVR. The nurse identifies that the patient has a decrease in what?
   a. Preload
   b. Afterload
   c. Contractility
   d. Stroke volume

9. Before taking hemodynamic measurements, how must the nurse reference the monitoring equipment?
   a. Confirm that when pressure in the system is zero, the equipment reads zero.
   b. Position the stopcock nearest the transducer level with the phlebostatic axis.
   c. Place the transducer on the left side of the chest at the fourth intercostal space.
   d. Place the patient in a left lateral position with the transducer level with the top surface of the mattress.

10. Which statement is accurate?
    a. A pulmonary artery flow–directed catheter has a balloon at the distal tip that floats into the left atrium.
    b. In the absence of mitral valve impairment, the left ventricular end-diastolic pressure is reflected by the cardiac index.
    c. The pressure obtained when the balloon of the pulmonary artery catheter is inflated reflects the preload of the left ventricle.
    d. When a patient has an arterial catheter placed for arterial blood gas (ABG) sampling, the low pressure alarm must be activated to detect functioning of the line.

11. In preparing the patient for insertion of a pulmonary artery catheter, what should the nurse do?
    a. Place the patient in high Fowler's position.
    b. Obtain an informed consent from the patient.
    c. Perform an Allen test to confirm adequate ulnar artery perfusion.
    d. Ensure that the patient has continuous electrocardiographic (ECG) monitoring.

12. What is a rationale for the use of a pulmonary artery catheter instead of arterial pressure–based CO (APCO) monitoring?
    a. Coagulopathy
    b. Less infection risk
    c. Mechanical tricuspid or pulmonic valve
    d. Needs research for accuracy with more specific illnesses and treatments

13. Which description accurately describes the continuous CO (CCO) method and not the intermittent bolus thermodilution CO (TDCO) method of determining CO?
    a. Room temperature or cold normal saline is injected rapidly.
    b. The TDCO method is easier and faster than the CCO method.
    c. The digital measurements reflect the average CO every 30 to 60 seconds.
    d Systemic vascular resistance (SVR) can be calculated each time CO is measured.

14. A patient in the ICU with hemodynamic monitoring has the following values.
    Blood pressure (BP): 90/68 mm Hg
    HR: 124 bpm
    PAWP: 22 mm Hg
    CO: 3.2 L/min
    Right atrial pressure (central venous pressure [CVP]): 14 mm Hg
    Pulmonary artery pressure: 38/20 mm Hg

    a. Calculate the additional values that can be determined from these findings.
    Mean arterial pressure (MAP) _____
    Pulmonary artery mean pressure (PAMP) _____
    SV _____
    SVR _____

    b. What interpretation can the nurse make about the patient's circulatory status and cardiac function from these values?

15. A patient has central venous oxygen saturation/mixed venous oxygen saturation ($ScvO_2/SvO_2$) of 52%, CO of 4.8 L/min, SpO_2 of 95%, and an unchanged hemoglobin level. What should the nurse assess the patient for?
    a. Dysrhythmias   c. Pulmonary edema
    b. Pain on movement   d. Signs of septic shock

16. The nurse observes a PAWP waveform on the monitor when the balloon of the patient's pulmonary artery catheter is deflated. What should the nurse recognize about this situation?
    a. The patient is at risk for embolism because of occlusion of the catheter with a thrombus.
    b. The patient is developing pulmonary edema that has increased the pulmonary artery pressure.
    c. The patient is at risk for an air embolus because the injected air cannot be withdrawn into the syringe.
    d. The catheter must be immediately repositioned to prevent pulmonary infarction or pulmonary artery rupture.

17. A patient with which disorder would benefit from the use of the intraaortic balloon pump (IABP)?
    a. An insufficient aortic valve
    b. A dissecting thoracic aortic aneurysm
    c. Generalized peripheral vascular disease
    d. Acute myocardial infarction with cardiogenic shock

18. Which statement about the function of the IABP is accurate?
    a. Deflation of the balloon allows the HR to increase.
    b. A primary effect of the IABP is increased systolic blood pressure.
    c. The rapid deflation of the intraaortic balloon causes a decreased preload.
    d. During intraaortic counterpulsation, the balloon is inflated during diastole.

19. What should the nurse do to prevent arterial trauma during the use of the IABP?
    a. Reposition the patient every 2 hours.
    b. Check the site for bleeding every hour.
    c. Prevent hip flexion of the cannulated leg.
    d. Cover the insertion site with an occlusive dressing.

20. A patient who is hemodynamically stable has an order to wean the IABP. How should the nurse accomplish this?
    a. Decrease the augmentation pressure to zero.
    b. Stop the machine since hemodynamic parameters are satisfactory.
    c. Stop the infusion flow through the catheter when weaning is initiated.
    d. Change the pumping ratio from 1:1 to 1:2 or 1:3 until the balloon is removed.

21. What are ventricular assist devices (VADs) designed to do for the patient?
    a. Provide permanent, total circulatory support when the left ventricle fails
    b. Partially or totally support circulation temporarily until a donor heart can be obtained
    c. Support circulation only when patients cannot be weaned from cardiopulmonary bypass
    d. Reverse the effects of circulatory failure in patients with acute myocardial infarction (MI) in cardiogenic shock

22. A comatose patient with a possible cervical spine injury is intubated with a nasal endotracheal (ET) tube. The nurse recognizes that what is a disadvantage of a nasal ET tube in comparison with an oral ET tube?
    a. Requires the placement of a bite block
    b. Is more likely to cause laryngeal trauma
    c. Requires greater respiratory effort in breathing
    d. Requires the placement of an additional airway to keep the trachea open

23. In preparing a patient in the ICU for oral ET intubation, what should the nurse do?
    a. Place the patient supine with the head extended and the neck flexed.
    b. Tell the patient that the tongue must be extruded while the tube is inserted.
    c. Position the patient supine with the head hanging over the edge of the bed to align the mouth and trachea.
    d. Inform the patient that while it will not be possible to talk during insertion of the tube, speech will be possible after it is correctly placed.

24. *Priority Decision:* A patient has an oral ET tube inserted to relieve an upper airway obstruction and to facilitate secretion removal. What is the first responsibility of the nurse immediately following placement of the tube?
    a. Suction the tube to remove secretions.
    b. Place an end tidal CO_2 detector on the ET tube.
    c. Secure the tube to the face with adhesive tape.
    d. Assess for bilateral breath sounds and symmetric chest movement.

25. The nurse uses the minimal occluding volume technique to inflate the cuff on an ET tube to minimize the incidence of what?
    a. Infection
    b. Hypoxemia
    c. Tracheal necrosis
    d. Accidental extubation

26. When suctioning an ET tube, the nurse should use a suction pressure of _____ mm Hg.

27. The nurse suctions the patient's ET tube when the patient has what?
    a. Peripheral wheezes in all lobes
    b. Has not been suctioned for 2 hours
    c. Coarse rhonchi over central airways
    d. A need for stimulation to cough and deep breathe

28. What nursing care is included for the patient with an ET tube?
    a. Check the cuff pressure every hour.
    b. Keep a tracheostomy tray at the bedside.
    c. Hyperoxygenate before and after suctioning.
    d. Reuse the suction catheter at the bedside for 24 hours.

29. *Priority Decision:* While suctioning the ET tube of a spontaneously breathing patient, the nurse notes that the patient develops bradycardia with premature ventricular contractions. What should the nurse do first?
    a. Stop the suctioning and assess the patient for spontaneous respirations.
    b. Attempt to resuction the patient with reduced suction pressure and pass time.
    c. Stop the suctioning and ventilate the patient with slow, small-volume breaths using a bag-valve-mask (BVM) device.
    d. Stop suctioning and ventilate the patient with a BVM device with 100% oxygen until the HR returns to baseline.

30. What precautions should the nurse take during mouth care and repositioning of an oral ET tube to prevent and detect tube dislodgement (*select all that apply*)?
    a. Confirm bilateral breath sounds after care.
    b. Use suction pressures less than 120 mm Hg.
    c. Use water swabs to prevent mucosal drying.
    d. Use humidified inspired gas to help thin secretions.
    e. One staff member holds the tube and one performs care.
    f. Move secretions into larger airways with turning every 2 hours.

31. A patient with an oral ET tube has a nursing diagnosis of risk for aspiration *related to* presence of artificial airway. What are appropriate nursing interventions for this patient (*select all that apply*)?
    a. Assess gag reflex.
    b. Ensure that the cuff is properly inflated.
    c. Suction the patient's mouth frequently.
    d. Keep the ventilator tubing cleared of condensed water.
    e. Raise the head of the bed 30 to 45 degrees unless the patient is unstable.

32. *Priority Decision:* Although his oxygen saturation is above 92%, an orally intubated, mechanically ventilated patient is restless and very anxious. What intervention should be used first to decrease the risk of accidental extubation?
    a. Obtain an order and apply soft wrist restraints.
    b. Remind the patient that he needs the tube inserted to breathe.
    c. Administer sedatives and have a caregiver stay with the patient.
    d. Move the patient to an area close to the nurses' station for closer observation.

33. Which patient's medical diagnosis should the nurse know is most likely to need mechanical ventilation (*select all that apply*)?
    a. Sleep apnea
    b. Cystic fibrosis
    c. Acute kidney failure
    d. Type 2 diabetes mellitus
    e. Acute respiratory distress syndrome (ARDS)

34. What characteristics describe positive pressure ventilators (*select all that apply*)?
    a. Require an artificial airway
    b. Applied to outside of the body
    c. Most similar to physiologic ventilation
    d. Most frequently used with acutely ill patients
    e. Frequently used in the home for neuromuscular or nervous system disorders

35. What is included in the description of positive pressure ventilation (*select all that apply*)?
    a. Peak inspiratory pressure predetermined
    b. Consistent volume delivered with each breath
    c. Increased risk for hyperventilation and hypoventilation
    d. Preset volume of gas delivered with variable pressure based on compliance
    e. Volume delivered varies based on selected pressure and patient lung compliance

36. Which mode of ventilation is used with critically ill patients and allows the patient to self-regulate the rate and depth of spontaneous respirations but may also deliver a preset volume and frequency of breaths?
    a. Assist-control ventilation (ACV)
    b. Pressure support ventilation (PSV)
    c. Pressure-controlled inverse ratio ventilation (PC-IRV)
    d. Synchronized intermittent mandatory ventilation (SIMV)

37. A patient in acute respiratory failure is receiving ACV with a positive end-expiratory pressure (PEEP) of 10 cm H_2O. What sign alerts the nurse to undesirable effects of increased airway and thoracic pressure?
    a. Decreased BP
    b. Decreased PaO_2
    c. Increased crackles
    d. Decreased spontaneous respirations

38. What should the nurse recognize as a factor commonly responsible for sodium and fluid retention in the patient on mechanical ventilation?
    a. Increased release of ADH
    b. Increased release of atrial natriuretic factor
    c. Increased insensible water loss via the airway
    d. Decreased renal perfusion with release of renin

39. ***Delegation Decision:*** The RN caring for a stable patient on mechanical ventilation in a long-term acute care facility plans the interventions listed below. Indicate whether each intervention must be done by the registered nurse (RN) or if it could be delegated to the licensed practical nurse (LPN) or unlicensed assistive personnel (UAP), who would report back to the RN.
    _____ a. Administer routinely scheduled medications.
    _____ b. Administer sedatives, analgesics, and paralytic medications.
    _____ c. Administer enteral nutrition.
    _____ d. Obtain vital signs and measure urine output.
    _____ e. Educate the patient and caregiver about mechanical ventilation and weaning.
    _____ f. Assist the respiratory therapist with repositioning and securing the ET tube.
    _____ g. Auscultate breath sounds and respiratory effort.
    _____ h. Perform passive or assisted range-of-motion (ROM) exercises.
    _____ i. Maintain appropriate cuff inflation on the ET tube.
    _____ j. Provide personal hygiene and skin care.

40. A patient receiving mechanical ventilation is very anxious and agitated and neuromuscular blocking agents are used to promote ventilation. What should the nurse recognize about the care of this patient?
    a. The patient will be too sedated to be aware of the details of care.
    b. Caregivers should be encouraged to provide stimulation and diversion.
    c. The patient should always be addressed and explanations of care given.
    d. Communication will not be possible with the use of neuromuscular blocking agents.

41. While receiving prolonged mechanical ventilation, the patient developed anemia. The patient is also having difficulty being weaned from the ventilator related to a recurrent pneumonia and early fatigue with weaning. What is contributing to the patient's prolonged recovery?
    a. Hypoxemia
    b. Enteral feeding
    c. Inadequate nutrition
    d. Decreased activity level

42. The nurse determines that alveolar hypoventilation is occurring in a patient on a ventilator when what happens?
    a. The patient develops cardiac dysrhythmias.
    b. Auscultation reveals an air leak around the ET tube cuff.
    c. ABG results show a $PaCO_2$ of 32 mm Hg and a pH of 7.47.
    d. The patient tries to breathe faster than the ventilator setting.

43. What plan should the nurse use when weaning a patient from a ventilator?
    a. Decrease the delivered FIO_2 concentration
    b. Intermittent trials of spontaneous ventilation followed by ventilatory support to provide rest
    c. Substitute ventilator support with a manual resuscitation bag if the patient becomes hypoxemic
    d. Implement weaning procedures around the clock until the patient does not experience ventilatory fatigue

44. A patient is to be discharged home with mechanical ventilation. Before discharge, what is most important for the nurse to do for the patient and caregiver?
    a. Teach the caregiver to care for the patient with a home ventilator.
    b. Help the caregiver to plan for placement of the patient in a long-term care facility.
    c. Stress the advantages for the patient in being cared for in the home environment.
    d. Have the caregiver arrange for around-the-clock home health nurses for the first several weeks.

CASE STUDY
Critically Ill Patient
Patient Profile

D.V., age 42, has a history of human immunodeficiency virus (HIV) infection with the development of manifestations of acquired immunodeficiency syndrome (AIDS) 2 years ago. He has been hospitalized and treated twice for *Pneumocystis jiroveci* pneumonia and is now admitted to ICU with suspected cryptococcal meningitis. Intracranial pressure (ICP) monitoring is instituted and an arterial line and flow-directed pulmonary artery catheter are inserted. ET intubation with assist-control mechanical ventilation at 12 breaths/min, 15 cm H_2O PEEP, and FIO_2 of 50% is established. (Note: This patient is very critically ill and requires you to review ICP, septic shock, multiple organ dysfunction syndrome [MODS], and respiratory failure.)

Subjective Data

- Friend relates that D.V. had two generalized tonic-clonic seizures in the 2 hours before admission

Objective Data

- Glasgow Coma Scale (GCS) score: 6
- ICP: 22 mm Hg
- Vital signs: Temp 102.2°F (39°C), HR 80 bpm, RR 26, BP 100/46
- ABGs: PaO_2 65 mm Hg, $PaCO_2$ 32 mm Hg, HCO_3^- 16 mEq/L, pH 7.26
- Other laboratory tests: Glucose 228 mg/dL (12.6 mmol/L), lactate 3 mEq/L (3 mmol/L), white blood cells (WBCs) 18,500/µL
- Hemodynamic monitoring values: CO 6 L/min, PAMP 8 mm Hg, PAWP 15 mm Hg, SVR 530 dynes sec/cm^{-5}, SvO_2 90%, SaO_2 92%
- Skin warm and dry
- Urinary catheter inserted with 30 mL urine return

Discussion Questions

Using a separate sheet of paper, answer the following questions:

1. What are the best indicators to use in D.V.'s case to monitor his hemodynamic status?
2. What effect might the use of PEEP have on D.V.'s ICP?
3. What is D.V.'s MAP? What MAP would be necessary to promote tissue and cerebral perfusion and not increase ICP?
4. What drugs and fluids would be indicated for D.V.'s treatment?
5. How may D.V.'s condition be complicated by gastrointestinal ischemia?
6. Explain the processes that account for the abnormal assessment findings in D.V.
7. ***Priority Decision:*** Based on the assessment data presented, what are the priority nursing diagnoses? Are there any collaborative problems?

67 Nursing Management: Shock, Systemic Inflammatory Response Syndrome, and Multiple Organ Dysfunction Syndrome

1. What is the key factor in describing any type of shock?
   a. Hypoxemia
   b. Hypotension
   c. Vascular collapse
   d. Inadequate tissue perfusion

2. When shock occurs in a patient with pulmonary embolism or abdominal compartment syndrome, what type of shock would that be?
   a. Distributive shock
   b. Obstructive shock
   c. Cardiogenic shock
   d. Hypovolemic shock

3. What physical problems could precipitate hypovolemic shock (*select all that apply*)?
   a. Burns
   b. Ascites
   c. Vaccines
   d. Insect bites
   e. Hemorrhage
   f. Ruptured spleen

4. A 70-year-old patient is malnourished, has a history of type 2 diabetes mellitus, and is admitted from the nursing home with pneumonia. For which kind of shock should the nurse closely monitor this patient?
   a. Septic shock
   b. Neurogenic shock
   c. Cardiogenic shock
   d. Anaphylactic shock

5. Which hemodynamic monitoring description of the identified shock is accurate?
   a. Tachycardia with hypertension is characteristic of neurogenic shock.
   b. In cardiogenic shock the patient will have an increased pulmonary artery wedge pressure (PAWP) and a decreased cardiac output (CO).
   c. Anaphylactic shock is characterized by increased systemic vascular resistance (SVR), decreased CO, and decreased PAWP.
   d. In septic shock, bacterial endotoxins cause vascular changes that result in increased SVR and decreased CO.

6. In the compensatory stage of hypovolemic shock, to what organs does blood flow decrease after the sympathetic nervous system activates the α-adrenergic stimulation (*select all that apply*)?
   a. Skin
   b. Brain
   c. Heart
   d. Kidneys
   e. Gastrointestinal tract

7. As the body continues to try to compensate for hypovolemic shock, there is increased angiotensin II from the activation of the renin-angiotensin-aldosterone system. What physiologic change occurs related to the increased angiotensin II?
   a. Vasodilation
   b. Decreased blood pressure (BP) and CO
   c. Aldosterone release results in sodium and water excretion
   d. Antidiuretic hormone (ADH) release increases water reabsorption

8. The patient is in the compensatory stage of shock. What manifestations indicate this to the nurse (*select all that apply*)?
   a. Pale and cool
   b. Unresponsive
   c. Lower BP than baseline
   d. Moist crackles in the lungs
   e. Hyperactive bowel sounds
   f. Tachypnea and tachycardia

9. The nurse suspects sepsis as a cause of shock when the laboratory test results indicate
   a. hypokalemia.
   b. thrombocytopenia.
   c. decreased hemoglobin.
   d. increased blood urea nitrogen (BUN).

10. Progressive tissue hypoxia leading to anaerobic metabolism and metabolic acidosis is characteristic of the progressive stage of shock. What changes in the heart contribute to this increasing tissue hypoxia?
    a. Arterial constriction causes decreased perfusion.
    b. Vasoconstriction decreases blood flow to pulmonary capillaries.
    c. Increased capillary permeability and profound vasoconstriction cause increased hydrostatic pressure.
    d. Decreased perfusion occurs, leading to dysrhythmias, decreased CO, and decreased oxygen delivery to cells.

11. A patient with severe trauma has been treated for hypovolemic shock. The nurse recognizes that the patient is in the irreversible stage of shock when what is included in assessment findings?
    a. A lactic acidosis with a pH of 7.32
    b. Marked hypotension and refractory hypoxemia
    c. Unresponsiveness that responds only to painful stimuli
    d. Profound vasoconstriction with absent peripheral pulses

12. ***Priority Decision:*** A patient with acute pancreatitis is experiencing hypovolemic shock. Which initial orders for the patient will the nurse implement first?
    a. Start 1000 mL of normal saline at 500 mL/hr.
    b. Obtain blood cultures before starting IV antibiotics.
    c. Draw blood for hematology and coagulation factors.
    d. Administer high-flow oxygen (100%) with a non-rebreather mask.

13. What abnormal finding should the nurse expect to find in early compensatory shock?
    a. Metabolic acidosis
    b. Increased serum sodium
    c. Decreased blood glucose
    d. Increased serum potassium

14. In late irreversible shock in a patient with massive thermal burns, what should the nurse expect the patient's laboratory results to reveal?
    a. Respiratory alkalosis
    b. Decreased potassium
    c. Increased blood glucose
    d. Increased ammonia (NH_3) levels

15. A patient with hypovolemic shock is receiving lactated Ringer's solution for fluid replacement therapy. During this therapy, which laboratory result is most important for the nurse to monitor?
    a. Serum pH
    b. Serum sodium
    c. Serum potassium
    d. Hemoglobin (Hgb) and hematocrit (Hct)

16. The nurse determines that a large amount of crystalloid fluids administered to a patient in septic shock is effective when hemodynamic monitoring reveals what?
    a. CO of 2.6 L/min
    b. CVP of 15 mm Hg
    c. PAWP of 4 mm Hg
    d. Heart rate (HR) of 106 bpm

17. When caring for a patient in cardiogenic shock, the nurse recognizes that the metabolic demands of turning and moving the patient exceed the oxygen supply when what change is revealed in hemodynamic monitoring?
    a. SvO_2 from 62% to 54%
    b. CO from 4.2 L/min to 4.8 L/min
    c. Stroke volume (SV) from 52 to 68 mL/beat
    d. SVR from 1300 dyne/sec/cm^5 to 1120 dyne/sec/cm^5

18. During administration of IV norepinephrine (Levophed), what should the nurse assess the patient for?
    a. Hypotension
    b. Marked diuresis
    c. Metabolic alkalosis
    d. Decreased tissue perfusion

19. When administering any vasoactive drug during the treatment of shock, the nurse should know that what is the goal of the therapy?
    a. Increasing urine output to 50 mL/hr
    b. Constriction of vessels to maintain BP
    c. Maintaining a MAP of at least 60 mm Hg
    d. Dilating vessels to improve tissue perfusion

20. Identify two medical therapies that are specific to each of the following types of shock.

Type of Shock	Medical Therapies
Cardiogenic	
Hypovolemic	
Septic	
Anaphylactic	

21. Identify four drugs and their actions that are used in the treatment of cardiogenic shock but not generally used for other types of shock.

Drug	Action

22. *Priority Decision:* What is the priority nursing responsibility in the prevention of shock?
    a. Frequently monitoring all patients' vital signs
    b. Using aseptic technique for all invasive procedures
    c. Being aware of the potential for shock in all patients at risk
    d. Teaching patients health promotion activities to prevent shock

23. Which indicators of tissue perfusion should be monitored in critically ill patients by the nurse (*select all that apply*)?
    a. Skin
    b. Urine output
    c. Level of consciousness
    d. Activities of daily living
    e. Vital signs, including pulse oximetry
    f. Peripheral pulses with capillary refill

24. A patient in the progressive stage of shock has rapid, deep respirations. The nurse determines that the patient's hyperventilation is compensating for a metabolic acidosis when the patient's arterial blood gas (ABG) results include which results?
    a. pH 7.42, PaO_2 80 mm Hg
    b. pH 7.48, PaO_2 69 mm Hg
    c. pH 7.38, $PaCO_2$ 30 mm Hg
    d. pH 7.32, $PaCO_2$ 48 mm Hg

25. Which interventions should be used for anaphylactic shock (*select all that apply*)?
    a. Antibiotics
    b. Vasodilator
    c. Antihistamine
    d. Oxygen supplementation
    e. Colloid volume expansion
    f. Crystalloid volume expansion

26. A patient in shock has a nursing diagnosis of fear *related to* severity of condition and perceived threat of death as manifested by verbalization of anxiety about condition and fear of death. What is an appropriate nursing intervention for the patient?
    a. Administer antianxiety agents.
    b. Allow caregivers to visit as much as possible.
    c. Call a member of the clergy to visit the patient.
    d. Inform the patient of the current plan of care and its rationale.

27. Which statement describing systemic inflammatory response syndrome (SIRS) and/or multiple organ dysfunction syndrome (MODS) is accurate?
    a. MODS may occur independently from SIRS.
    b. All patients with septic shock develop MODS.
    c. The GI system is often the first to show evidence of dysfunction in SIRS and MODS.
    d. A common initial mediator that causes endothelial damage leading to SIRS and MODS is endotoxin.

28. What mechanism that can trigger SIRS is related to myocardial infarction or pancreatitis?
    a. Endotoxin release
    b. Abscess formation
    c. Global perfusion deficits
    d. Ischemic or necrotic tissue

29. What types of injuries cause a mechanical tissue trauma that can trigger SIRS (*select all that apply*)?
    a. Burns
    b. Fungi
    c. Viruses
    d. Crush injuries
    e. Surgical procedures

30. Which intervention may prevent GI bacterial and endotoxin translocation in a critically ill patient with SIRS?
    a. Early enteral feedings
    b. Surgical removal of necrotic tissue
    c. Aggressive multiple antibiotic therapy
    d. Strict aseptic technique in all procedures

31. **Priority Decision:** A patient with a gunshot wound to the abdomen is being treated for hypovolemic and septic shock. To monitor the patient for early organ damage associated with MODS, what is most important for the nurse to assess?
    a. Urine output
    b. Breath sounds
    c. Peripheral circulation
    d. Central venous pressure

32. Which patient manifestations confirm the development of MODS?
    a. Upper GI bleeding, Glasgow Coma Scale (GCS) score of 7, and Hct of 25%
    b. Elevated serum bilirubin, serum creatinine of 3.8 mg/dL, and platelet count of 15,000/μL
    c. Urine output of 30 mL/hr, BUN of 45 mg/dL, and white blood cell (WBC) count of 1120/μL
    d. Respiratory rate of 45, $PaCO_2$ of 60 mm Hg, and chest x-ray with bilateral diffuse patchy infiltrates

---

CASE STUDY

Septic Shock

Patient Profile

A.M. is an 81-year-old man who was brought to the emergency department via an ambulance from a local nursing home. He was found by the nurses on their 6:00 AM rounds to be very confused, restless, and hypotensive.

Past Health History

A.M. is a type 1 diabetic with a history of prostate cancer, myocardial infarction, and heart failure. He has been a resident of the nursing home for 3 years. He has had an indwelling urinary catheter in place for 5 days because of difficulty voiding. Until today, A.M. has been very oriented and cooperative. His current medications are metoprolol (Lopressor), lisinopril (Zestril), hydrochlorothiazide (HydroDiuril), isosorbide (Isordil), and insulin.

Subjective Data

- Denies any pain or discomfort (but patient is confused and this information may be unreliable)

Objective Data

- Neurologic: Lethargic, confused to place and time, easily aroused, does not follow commands; moves all extremities in response to stimuli
- Cardiovascular: BP 80/60; HR 112 bpm and regular; Temp 103°F (40°C) axillary; heart sounds normal without murmurs or S_3, S_4; peripheral pulses weak and thready
- Skin: Warm, dry, flushed
- Respiratory: RR 34 and shallow; breath sounds audible in all lobes with crackles bilaterally in the bases
- GI/GU: Abdomen soft with hypoactive bowel sounds; urinary catheter in place draining scant, purulent urine

Collaborative Care

In the emergency department, two 16-gauge IVs were inserted and 700 mL of normal saline was given over the first hour. The patient was placed on 40% oxygen via face mask. The urinary catheter was removed and cultured and blood cultures were drawn at two intervals. A new urinary catheter was inserted. The patient was started on IV antibiotics and transferred to the intensive care unit (ICU) with the diagnosis of septic shock resulting from gram-negative sepsis.

- In the ICU, a pulmonary catheter was inserted in addition to an arterial line.
- ABG results: pH 7.25, PaO_2 60 mm Hg, $PaCO_2$ 28 mm Hg, HCO_3^- 12 mEq/L, SaO_2 82%
- Hemodynamic pressures taken were right atrial pressure (CVP), pulmonary artery mean pressure (PAMP), PAWP, CO, and SVR

Laboratory Tests

WBC: 21,000/μL
Na^+: 133 mEq/L
K^+: 4.5 mEq/L
Cl^-: 96 mEq/L
Glucose: 230 mg/dL
Creatinine: 1.7 mg/dL
Hgb: 12 g/dL; Hct: 36%

A.M.'s BP continued to drop despite several liters of crystalloids. In addition to more fluid administration, dopamine (Intropin) was started and titrated up as needed to try to maintain the patient's BP. Despite all efforts, including intubation and mechanical ventilation, A.M. died on the sixth hospital day. Cause of death was MODS caused by gram-negative sepsis.

Discussion Questions

Using a separate sheet of paper, answer the following questions:

1. What risk factors for septic shock were present in A.M.?
2. What preventive measures could have been taken by the nursing home staff in regard to A.M.?
3. What are the major pathophysiologic changes associated with sepsis?
4. Discuss the mechanism for hypotension in the patient with septic shock.
5. Explain the physiologic reasons for the following assessment findings in this patient and any nursing interventions that can improve the patient's condition.

Assessment Finding	Physiologic Basis	Nursing Intervention
Decreased level of consciousness		
Warm, dry, and flushed skin		
Tachycardia		
Tachypnea		
Fever		
Decreased SVR		
Increased CO		
Oliguria		
Hyperglycemia		

6. What are the overall goals for this patient on admission?
7. Why was a pulmonary artery catheter indicated for A.M.?
8. Analyze the results of the ABGs.
9. Describe the changes in the hemodynamic pressure that would be expected as A.M.'s condition worsened.
10. Explain the rationale for fluid therapy and the use of Intropin (dopamine).
11. *Priority Decision:* Based on the assessment data provided, what are the priority nursing diagnoses? What collaborative problems are present?

Nursing Management: Respiratory Failure and Acute Respiratory Distress Syndrome

1. When explaining respiratory failure to the patient's family, what should the nurse use as an accurate description?
   a. The absence of ventilation
   b. Any episode in which part of the airway is obstructed
   c. Inadequate gas exchange to meet the metabolic needs of the body
   d. An episode of acute hypoxemia caused by a pulmonary dysfunction

2. Which descriptions are characteristic of hypoxemic respiratory failure (*select all that apply*)?
   a. Referred to as ventilatory failure
   b. Primary problem is inadequate O_2 transfer
   c. Risk of inadequate O_2 saturation of hemoglobin exists
   d. Body is unable to compensate for acidemia of increased $PaCO_2$
   e. Most often caused by ventilation-perfusion (V/Q) mismatch and shunt
   f. Exists when PaO_2 is 60 mm Hg or less, even when O_2 is administered at 60%

3. When teaching the patient about what was happening when experiencing an intrapulmonary shunt, which explanation is accurate?
   a. This occurs when an obstruction impairs the flow of blood to the ventilated areas of the lung.
   b. This occurs when blood passes through an anatomic channel in the heart and bypasses the lungs.
   c. This occurs when blood flows through the capillaries in the lungs without participating in gas exchange.
   d. Gas exchange across the alveolar capillary interface is compromised by thickened or damaged alveolar membranes.

4. When the V/Q lung scan result returns with a mismatch ratio that is greater than 1, which condition should be suspected?
   a. Pain
   b. Atelectasis
   c. Pulmonary embolus
   d. Ventricular septal defect

5. Which physiologic mechanism of hypoxemia occurs with pulmonary fibrosis?
   a. Anatomic shunt
   b. Diffusion limitation
   c. Intrapulmonary shunt
   d. V/Q mismatch ratio of less than 1

6. Which patient with the following manifestations is most likely to develop hypercapnic respiratory failure?
   a. Rapid, deep respirations in response to pneumonia
   b. Slow, shallow respirations as a result of sedative overdose
   c. Large airway resistance as a result of severe bronchospasm
   d. Poorly ventilated areas of the lung caused by pulmonary edema

7. Which arterial blood gas (ABG) results would most likely indicate acute respiratory failure in a patient with chronic lung disease?
   a. PaO_2 52 mm Hg, $PaCO_2$ 56 mm Hg, pH 7.4
   b. PaO_2 46 mm Hg, $PaCO_2$ 52 mm Hg, pH 7.36
   c. PaO_2 48 mm Hg, $PaCO_2$ 54 mm Hg, pH 7.38
   d. PaO_2 50 mm Hg, $PaCO_2$ 54 mm Hg, pH 7.28

8. The patient is being admitted to the intensive care unit (ICU) with hypercapnic respiratory failure. Which manifestations should the nurse expect to assess in the patient (*select all that apply*)?
   a. Cyanosis
   b. Metabolic acidosis
   c. Morning headache
   d. Respiratory acidosis
   e. Use of tripod position
   f. Rapid, shallow respirations

9. Which assessment finding should cause the nurse to suspect the early onset of hypoxemia?
   a. Restlessness
   b. Hypotension
   c. Central cyanosis
   d. Cardiac dysrhythmias

10. Which changes of aging contribute to the increased risk for respiratory failure in older adults (*select all that apply*)?
    a. Alveolar dilation
    b. Increased delirium
    c. Changes in vital signs
    d. Increased infection risk
    e. Decreased respiratory muscle strength
    f. Diminished elastic recoil within the airways

11. The nurse assesses that a patient in respiratory distress is developing respiratory fatigue and the risk of respiratory arrest when the patient displays which behavior?
    a. Cannot breathe unless he is sitting upright
    b. Uses the abdominal muscles during expiration
    c. Has an increased inspiratory-expiratory (I/E) ratio
    d. Has a change in respiratory rate from rapid to slow

12. A patient has a PaO_2 of 50 mm Hg and a $PaCO_2$ of 42 mm Hg because of an intrapulmonary shunt. Which therapy is the patient most likely to respond best to?
    a. Positive pressure ventilation
    b. Oxygen administration at a FIO_2 of 100%
    c. Administration of O_2 per nasal cannula at 1 to 3 L/min
    d. Clearance of airway secretions with coughing and suctioning

13. A patient with a massive hemothorax and pneumothorax has absent breath sounds in the right lung. To promote improved V/Q matching, how should the nurse position the patient?
    a. On the left side
    b. On the right side
    c. In a reclining chair bed
    d. Supine with the head of the bed elevated

14. A patient in hypercapnic respiratory failure has a nursing diagnosis of ineffective airway clearance *related to* increasing exhaustion. What is an appropriate nursing intervention for this patient?
    a. Inserting an oral airway
    b. Performing augmented coughing
    c. Teaching the patient huff coughing
    d. Teaching the patient slow pursed lip breathing

15. The patient with a history of heart failure and acute respiratory failure has thick secretions that she is having difficulty coughing up. Which intervention would best help to mobilize her secretions?
    a. Administer more IV fluid
    b. Perform postural drainage
    c. Provide O_2 by aerosol mask
    d. Suction airways nasopharyngeally

16. *Priority Decision:* After endotracheal intubation and mechanical ventilation have been started, a patient in respiratory failure becomes very agitated and is breathing asynchronously with the ventilator. What is it most important for the nurse to do first?
    a. Evaluate the patient's pain level, ABGs, and electrolyte values
    b. Sedate the patient to unconsciousness to eliminate patient awareness
    c. Administer the PRN vecuronium (Norcuron) to promote synchronous ventilations
    d. Slow the rate of ventilations provided by the ventilator to allow for spontaneous breathing by the patient

17. What is the primary reason that hemodynamic monitoring is instituted in severe respiratory failure?
    a. To detect V/Q mismatches
    b. To continuously measure the arterial BP
    c. To evaluate oxygenation and ventilation status
    d. To evaluate cardiac status and blood flow to tissues

18. Patients with acute respiratory failure will have drug therapy to meet their individual needs. Which drugs will meet the goal of reducing pulmonary congestion (*select all that apply*)?
    a. Morphine
    b. Furosemide (Lasix)
    c. Nitroglycerin (Tridil)
    d. Albuterol (Ventolin)
    e. Ceftriaxone (Rocephin)
    f. Methylprednisolone (Solu-Medrol)

19. In caring for a patient in acute respiratory failure, the nurse recognizes that noninvasive positive pressure ventilation (NIPPV) may be indicated for which patient?
    a. Is comatose and has high oxygen requirements
    b. Has copious secretions that require frequent suctioning
    c. Responds to hourly bronchodilator nebulization treatments
    d. Is alert and cooperative but has increasing respiratory exhaustion

20. The patient progressed from acute lung injury to acute respiratory distress syndrome (ARDS). He is on the ventilator and receiving propofol (Diprivan) for sedation and fentanyl (Sublimaze) to decrease anxiety, agitation, and pain in order to decrease his work of breathing, O_2 consumption, carbon dioxide production, and risk of injury. What intervention is recommended in caring for this patient?
    a. A sedation holiday
    b. Monitoring for hypermetabolism
    c. Keeping his legs still to avoid dislodging the airway
    d. Repositioning him every 4 hours to decrease agitation

21. Although ARDS may result from direct lung injury or indirect lung injury as a result of systemic inflammatory response syndrome (SIRS), the nurse is aware that ARDS is most likely to occur in the patient with a host insult resulting from
    a. sepsis.
    b. oxygen toxicity.
    c. prolonged hypotension.
    d. cardiopulmonary bypass.

22. What are the primary pathophysiologic changes that occur in the injury or exudative phase of ARDS (*select all that apply*)?
    a. Atelectasis
    b. Shortness of breath
    c. Interstitial and alveolar edema
    d. Hyaline membranes line the alveoli
    e. Influx of neutrophils, monocytes, and lymphocytes

23. In patients with ARDS who survive the acute phase of lung injury, what manifestations are seen when they progress to the fibrotic phase?
    a. Chronic pulmonary edema and atelectasis
    b. Resolution of edema and healing of lung tissue
    c. Continued hypoxemia because of diffusion limitation
    d. Increased lung compliance caused by the breakdown of fibrotic tissue

24. In caring for the patient with ARDS, what is the most characteristic sign the nurse would expect the patient to exhibit?
    a. Refractory hypoxemia
    b. Bronchial breath sounds
    c. Progressive hypercapnia
    d. Increased pulmonary artery wedge pressure (PAWP)

25. The nurse suspects the early stage of ARDS in any seriously ill patient who manifests what?
    a. Develops respiratory acidosis
    b. Has diffuse crackles and rhonchi
    c. Exhibits dyspnea and restlessness
    d. Has a decreased PaO_2 and an increased $PaCO_2$

26. A patient with ARDS has a nursing diagnosis of risk for infection. To detect the presence of infections commonly associated with ARDS, what should the nurse monitor?
    a. Gastric aspirate for pH and blood
    b. Quality, quantity, and consistency of sputum
    c. Subcutaneous emphysema of the face, neck, and chest
    d. Mucous membranes of the oral cavity for open lesions

27. The best patient response to treatment of ARDS occurs when initial management includes what?
    a. Treatment of the underlying condition
    b. Administration of prophylactic antibiotics
    c. Treatment with diuretics and mild fluid restriction
    d. Endotracheal intubation and mechanical ventilation

28. When mechanical ventilation is used for the patient with ARDS, what is the rationale for applying positive end-expiratory pressure (PEEP)?
    a. Prevent alveolar collapse and open up collapsed alveoli
    b. Permit smaller tidal volumes with permissive hypercapnia
    c. Promote complete emptying of the lungs during exhalation
    d. Permit extracorporeal oxygenation and carbon dioxide removal outside the body

29. The nurse suspects that a patient with PEEP is experiencing negative effects of this ventilatory maneuver when which of the following is assessed?
    a. Increasing PaO_2
    b. Decreasing blood pressure
    c. Decreasing heart rate (HR)
    d. Increasing central venous pressure (CVP)

30. Prone positioning is considered for a patient with ARDS who has not responded to other measures to increase PaO_2. The nurse knows that this strategy will
    a. increase the mobilization of pulmonary secretions.
    b. decrease the workload of the diaphragm and intercostal muscles.
    c. promote opening of atelectatic alveoli in the upper portion of the lung.
    d. promote perfusion of nonatelectatic alveoli in the anterior portion of the lung.

CASE STUDY

Acute Respiratory Failure

Patient Profile

P.C. is a 75-year-old married woman with severe oxygen- and corticosteroid-dependent chronic obstructive pulmonary disease (COPD). She is admitted to the medical ICU in acute respiratory failure with pneumonia.

Subjective Data

• Complains of increasing shortness of breath and difficulty breathing with minimal exertion

Objective Data

• ABGs on 2 L O_2/min: pH 7.3, $PaCO_2$ 55 mm Hg, PaO_2 60 mm Hg, SaO_2 84%
• Awake, alert, and oriented
• Sitting in tripod position and using pursed lip breathing

Collaborative Care

• O_2 at 2 L/min per NIPPV
• Albuterol (Ventolin, Proventil) nebulization every hour PRN
• IV aminophylline
• IV antibiotics
• IV corticosteroids

Discussion Questions

Using a separate sheet of paper, answer the following questions:

1. What type of respiratory failure is P.C. primarily experiencing? Briefly describe how this situation illustrates the concept of acute chronic respiratory failure.
2. What factors contributed to the development of respiratory failure in P.C.?
3. What are the pathophysiologic effects and clinical manifestations of P.C.'s respiratory failure?
4. How do the tripod position and pursed lip breathing contribute to respiratory function?
5. What is NIPPV? When is it contraindicated?
6. What other nursing interventions will assist P.C. in recovery?
7. *Priority Decision:* Which of the treatments instituted for P.C. is the most important in returning her to her usual level of respiratory function?
8. What discharge teaching should be started?
9. *Priority Decision:* Based on the assessment data presented, what are the priority nursing diagnoses? Are there any collaborative problems?

69

Nursing Management: Emergency, Terrorism, and Disaster Nursing

1. *Priority Decision:* Triage the following patient situations that may be present in an emergency department (ED) as 1, 2, 3, 4, or 5 on the Emergency Severity Index.

_____ a. A 6-year-old child with a temperature of 103.2°F (39.6°C)

_____ b. A 22-year-old woman with asthma in acute respiratory distress

_____ c. An infant who has been vomiting for 2 days

_____ d. A 50-year-old man with low back pain and spasms

_____ e. A 32-year-old woman who is unconscious following an automobile accident

_____ f. A 40-year-old woman with rhinitis and a cough

_____ g. A 58-year-old man with midsternal chest pain

_____ h. A 16-year-old teenager with an angulated forearm following a sports injury

2. When a nurse is performing a primary survey in the ED, what is she assessing?
   a. Whether the resources of the ED are adequate to treat the patient
   b. The acuity of the patient's condition to determine priority of care
   c. Whether the patient is responsive enough to provide needed information
   d. The status of airway, breathing, circulation, disability, and exposure/environmental control

3. *Priority Decision:* During the primary survey the nurse identified asymmetric chest wall movement in the patient. What intervention should the nurse do first?
   a. Check a central pulse.
   b. Stabilize the cervical spine.
   c. Apply direct pressure to the wound.
   d. Administer bag-mask ventilation with 100% oxygen.

4. During the secondary survey of a trauma patient in the ED, why is it important that the nurse obtain details of the incident?
   a. The mechanism of injury can indicate specific injuries.
   b. Important facts may be forgotten when needed later for legal actions.
   c. Alcohol use associated with many accidents can affect treatment of injuries.
   d. Many types of accidents or trauma must be reported to government agencies.

5. What nursing intervention is performed during the "E" step of the secondary survey?
   a. Obtain full set of vital signs.
   b. Remove the patient's clothing and assess.
   c. Elicit history and head-to-toe assessment.
   d. Assess mental status and capillary refill for signs of shock.

6. When is the placement of a nasogastric tube contraindicated during emergency care?
   a. Inhalation injury
   b. Head or facial trauma
   c. Intraabdominal bleed
   d. Cervical spine fracture

7. In assessing the emergency patient's health history, what information is obtained with the use of the mnemonic AMPLE?
   a. Anatomy of injuries, mucous membranes, peripheral edema, leukocytosis, eczema location
   b. Approximate weight, motor function, palpable swelling, labored breathing, edema severity
   c. Allergies, medications, past health history, last meal, and events/environment leading to the illness or injury
   d. Abdominal sounds, memory loss, people exposed to, last medication, earliest availability of past medical records

8. A 65-year-old trauma patient has open wounds and the nurse questions the patient about her tetanus immunization status. When should tetanus immunoglobulin be administered to the patient?
   a. Had three doses of tetanus toxoid as a child
   b. Has had a dose of tetanus toxoid in the past 10 years
   c. Is unsure of the history of tetanus toxoid vaccinations
   d. Has not had a dose of tetanus toxoid in the past 3 years

9. In which situation would therapeutic hypothermia be instituted in the ED?
   a. 48-year-old male found unconscious by neighbors; on ED arrival, he is moaning and moving all extremities
   b. 62-year-old man defibrillated by emergency medical technicians (EMTs); on ED arrival, he is not responsive although his heart rhythm and blood pressure (BP) are stable
   c. 30-year-old female who suffered heat exhaustion following a marathon; on ED arrival, she is hypotensive and extremely diaphoretic with a temperature of 102.6°F (39.2°C)
   d. 38-year-old female found face down in her bathtub; she has a history of seizures; on ED arrival, she is responsive to pain only and she was intubated by paramedics with evidence of pulmonary edema; her pulse oximetry is 91%

10. Following a death in the ED of a 36-year-old man from a massive head injury, what would be appropriate for the nurse to do?
    a. Ask the family members to consider donating their loved one's organs.
    b. Notify an organ procurement agency that a death has occurred that could result in organ donation.
    c. Explain to the family what a generous act it would be to donate the patient's organs to another patient who needs them.
    d. Ask the family to check the patient's driver's license to determine whether he had designated approval of donation of his organs in case of death.

11. What heat-related emergency would the healthy athlete with inadequate fluid intake be most likely to experience after exercise?
    a. Heatstroke
    b. Heat attack
    c. Heat cramps
    d. Heat exhaustion

12. What describes heat exhaustion (*select all that apply*)?
    a. Volume and electrolyte depletion
    b. High risk of mortality and morbidity
    c. Treated with rapid cooling methods
    d. Rectal temperature of 99.6°F to 104°F (37.5°C to 40°C)
    e. Causes mild confusion, headache, and dilation of pupils

13. What should the nurse do during rewarming of a patient's toes that have suffered deep frostbite?
    a. Apply sterile dressings to blisters.
    b. Place the feet in a cool water bath.
    c. Ensure that analgesics are administered.
    d. Massage the digits to increase circulation.

14. *Priority Decision:* A patient is brought to the ED following a skiing accident after which he was not found for several hours. He is rigid and has slowed respiratory and heart rates. What should the nurse do during the primary assessment of the patient?
    a. Initiate active core rewarming interventions.
    b. Monitor the core temperature via the axillary route.
    c. Manage and maintain ABCs (airway, breathing, circulation).
    d. Expose the patient to check for areas of frostbite and other injuries.

15. A homeless man is brought to the ED in severe hypothermia with a temperature of 85°F (29.4°C). What should the nurse expect to find on initial assessment?
    a. Shivering and lethargy
    b. Fixed and dilated pupils
    c. Respirations of 6 to 8 per minute
    d. BP obtainable only by Doppler

16. What condition occurs with saltwater near-drowning but not with freshwater near-drowning?
    a. Destruction of surfactant
    b. Noncardiogenic pulmonary edema
    c. Water leaks from alveoli to capillary bed and circulation
    d. Fluid is drawn into the alveoli from the pulmonary capillaries

17. *Priority Decision:* What is the priority of management of the near-drowning patient?
    a. Correction of hypoxia
    b. Correction of acidosis
    c. Maintenance of fluid balance
    d. Prevention of cerebral edema

18. The ascending paralysis caused by exposure to the wood tick or dog tick may cause respiratory arrest unless what happens?
    a. The tick is removed.
    b. Antibiotics are administered.
    c. An antidote for the neurotoxin is administered.
    d. Hemodialysis is instituted to remove the neurotoxin.

19. A 68-year-old patient was bitten by the neighbor's dog 8 hours ago. What treatment should the nurse plan to provide for the patient?
    a. Report the bite to the police.
    b. Give rabies prophylaxis now.
    c. Administer IV antibiotics prophylactically.
    d. Dress the wound to prevent exposure to neurotoxins.

20. The patient is admitted with severe acidosis from trying to commit suicide by ingesting aspirin. What should be used to treat this patient?
    a. Milk
    b. Cathartics
    c. Hemodialysis
    d. Whole bowel irrigation

21. For which of the following ingested poisons may gastric lavage be considered (*select all that apply*)?
    a. Bleach
    b. Aspirin
    c. Drain cleaner
    d. Iron supplements
    e. Amitriptyline (Elavil)

22. *Priority Decision:* A patient is admitted to the ED with nausea, vomiting, and right upper quadrant pain. The patient's family brought an empty container of acetaminophen that was found near him. A large oral gastric tube is inserted. What does the nurse prepare to administer first?
    a. Cathartics
    b. Ipecac syrup
    c. Gastric lavage
    d. Activated charcoal

23. Which biologic agent of terrorism is a bacterial neurotoxin that causes paralysis and respiratory failure, with death occurring within 24 hours of exposure?
    a. Sarin
    b. Botulism
    c. Smallpox
    d. Tularemia

24. Which agent of terrorism does not have an established treatment for those exposed to it?
    a. Plague
    b. Anthrax
    c. Tularemia
    d. Hemorrhagic fever

25. Which biologic agents of terrorism can be protected against with a vaccine (*select all that apply*)?
    a. Plague
    b. Anthrax
    c. Botulism
    d. Smallpox
    e. Tularemia
    f. Hemorrhagic fever

26. When a patient is admitted with hemorrhagic fever, what nursing treatment should be provided?
    a. Parenteral analgesics
    b. Supportive treatment
    c. Warfarin administration
    d. Care of the rodent or mosquito bite

27. As a member of a volunteer disaster medical assistance team (DMAT), what would the nurse be expected to do?
    a. Triage casualties of a tornado that hit the local community.
    b. Assist with implementing the hospital's emergency response plan.
    c. Train citizens of communities how to respond to mass casualty incidents.
    d. Deploy to local or other communities with disasters to provide medical assistance.

CASE STUDY

Heatstroke

Patient Profile

M.M., age 72, was taking a short break from nailing new shingles on his roof during the summer when he lost consciousness, fell off of the roof, and collapsed in his yard. Accompanied by his wife, he was brought by ambulance to the ED.

Subjective Data

- Wife states that M.M. has been working all week on the roof, even though he has not felt well for the last day or two

Objective Data

- Vital signs: Temp 106.6°F (41.4°C), HR 124 bpm and weak and thready, RR 36 and shallow, BP 82/40
- Skin hot, dry, and pale

Discussion Questions

Using a separate sheet of paper, answer the following questions:

1. What factors in M.M.'s history place him at risk for heatstroke?
2. What laboratory tests would the nurse anticipate to be ordered and what alterations in these tests would be indications of heatstroke?
3. How would cooling for M.M. be carried out?
4. What supportive treatment is indicated for M.M.?
5. What should M.M.'s wife be told about M.M.'s condition?
6. *Priority Decision:* Based on the assessment data presented, what are the priority nursing diagnoses? Are there any collaborative problems?

CHAPTER 1

Answer Key

1. a, b, d, f, g, i
2. a, b, d. Certification usually requires an examination to verify a certain knowledge base and experience in the specialty area to develop the expertise. Certification is a voluntary process that provides recognition of one's expertise.
3. d. The Joint Commission establishes National Patient Safety Goals (NPSG) and evidence-based solutions are provided to prevent persistent safety problems. Nurses are vital to promoting this culture of safety. Rapidly expanding technology and knowledge are increasing the complexity of the health care system. With the aging population there will be more patients with chronic illnesses. The QSEN project identified six core competencies for nursing education to include in the curriculum to enable graduates to be ready for practice.
4. QSEN's six competencies are (1) Patient-centered care, (2) Teamwork and collaboration, (3) Evidence-based practice, (4) Quality improvement, (5) Safety, and (6) Informatics.
5. In order:
   6 Make recommendations for practice or generate data
   1 Ask a clinical question
   3 Critically analyze the evidence
   2 Find and collect the evidence
   5 Evaluate the outcomes in the clinical setting
   0 Create a spirit of inquiry
   4 Use evidence, clinical expertise, and patient preferences to determine care
6. b. The C part of the PICOT format stands for Comparison. "Restraint" is the Intervention. "During a seizure" is the Time period. "Adult seizure patients" is the Patient/ population.
   "Protecting them from injury" is the Outcome.
7. d. Evidence-based clinical practice guidelines are developed from summaries of research results and reflect the best known state of practice at the time. Use of these guidelines leads to more positive outcomes of care and would be best to use in planning care or programs.
8. d, e, f. Only standardized terminologies describe and organize nursing practice that includes patient responses, nursing interventions, and patient outcomes.
9. d. The use of a standardized electronic health record for each person is being promoted primarily to provide all health care providers ready access to patient information to coordinate care and to prevent duplication of information and erratic delivery of care.
10. a, e. The nurse informaticist designs, builds, implements, evaluates, and maintains computer systems used for health care. The studies done by nurse informaticists develop ways to avoid errors. Nurses are trained by informaticists to use computer systems but not all nursing actions. All nurses use the accessing of information and communication aspects of technology.
11. a. 2; b. 3; c. 4; d. 1; e. 2; f. 5; g. 3; h. 2; i. 5; j. 4

12. b, e, f. Collaborative problems are potential or actual complications of disease or treatment. As stated, fatigue, constipation, and excess fluid volume are not complications of disease or treatment.
13. Many answers may be correct. Examples include the following:
    a. Turn the patient every 2 hours using the following schedule: L side → back → R side → L side → back. Inspect and document all at-risk areas for blanching and erythema at each position change.
    b. Provide 8 oz of fluids every 2 hours (even hours) while the patient is awake (the patient prefers cold liquids). Assist the patient in choosing five fresh fruits or vegetables from the menu each day.
14. d. The mistake was made during assessment when the nurse did not ask why the patient had not taken her medication regularly and the appropriate etiology for the nursing diagnosis was not validated.
15. b, d, f, g, h. Right task, right circumstance, right person, right direction and communication, and right supervision and evaluation.
16. a, c, d, f, g. These actions or interventions require judgment and clinical decision making; therefore they should be performed by an RN.
17. 3 A plan that directs an entire health care team
    1 Used as guides for routine nursing care
    1, 2 Used in nursing education to teach the nursing process and care planning
    3 A description of patient care required at specific times during treatment
    1 Should be personalized and specific to each patient
    2 A visual diagram representing relationships between patient problems, interventions, and data
    3 Used for high-volume and highly predictable case types
18. c, e. Hands are to be washed with soap and water or gel before and after each patient. SBAR is suggested to improve the effectiveness of communication among caregivers. Restraints are not suggested as part of the National Patient Safety Goals (NPSG), although evaluating fall risk and taking action to reduce fall risk are included. All medications may not be administered if there is interaction between them. The physician would be notified before administering any questionable medications. The "time-out" is not for the nurse's fatigue but to ensure that the correct patient procedure and site are verified before surgical procedures. To prevent health care–related pressure ulcers, NPSG suggest assessing patients at risk initially on admission and on a regular basis throughout their care. To improve the accuracy of patient identification, it is suggested that two identifiers are used whenever a patient is identified, including for but not limited to medication administration.
19. a, c, d, e. Only regulatory agencies are not quality of care measures, although they do affect patient safety, which is another quality of care measure that affects payment for care.

CHAPTER 2

Answer Key

1. b. The determinants of health are factors that influence the health of individuals and groups. Today the major determinant of health is behavior. Although the other factors could influence this patient's health, the smoking behavior is the most important causative factor in this situation.
2. a. Rural setting; b. Low income; c. Gender; d. Age
3. a, b, e, f. Health literacy is the patient's ability to obtain, process, and understand basic health information needed to make appropriate decisions. Age, language, and education may interfere with the patient's ability to read, comprehend, and analyze information to make health care decisions. Place may be associated with limited health literacy because rural populations tend to be older and have lower literacy rates. The accepted health behaviors are affected by the areas in which people grow up, work, and live. Gender, race, and ethnicity are not associated with health literacy.
4. a, b, c. Values, culture, and ethnicity provide the nurse with information to help plan care for the patient that ensures that cultural histories, experiences, and traditions are valued. Stereotyping, acculturation, and ethnocentricity all presuppose information about the individual because of his or her culture or ethnicity without assessing the individual.
5. d. Culture is dynamic and ever changing, may not be shared by all members of the same cultural group, is adapted to specific conditions such as environmental factors, and is learned through oral and written histories as well as socialization.
6. a. Cultural skill is the ability to complete a cultural assessment by collecting cultural data.
7. Examples may include any instances of the following and others:

Cultural Factor	Effect on Nursing Care	Health Care Team
Time orientation	Patients may be late for appointments, skip appointments entirely, or delay seeing a health care provider because social events are more important to them.	Health care providers may be late to work or in providing time-sensitive care.
Economic factors	Lack of health insurance, limited financial resources, or undocumented immigrant status may deter patients from using the health care system.	The health care worker may not be able to afford new uniform items or transportation to work.
Nutrition	Ethnic foods may be high in sodium and fat or low in calcium and protein. If dietary changes required by health problems are not made within the context of the patient's normal diet, chances are high that the patient will not make the changes.	Ethnic foods may not be available in the cafeteria, so the health care provider must bring food for meals.
Personal space	Personal space zones are a strong cultural trait.	A patient may move closer to the nurse, causing a feeling of discomfort for the nurse, or if the nurse increases the personal space, the patient might be offended.
Beliefs and practices	Religious beliefs or practices, faith in folk medicine, or negative experiences with culturally insensitive health care may delay or prevent patients from seeking health care.	Health care workers may need to practice certain behaviors while at work (i.e., fasting during Ramadan, not caring for patients having abortions, not eating milk and meat together).

8. a. As a follower of Islam, pork or pork-derived products are prohibited (this is also true for strict followers of Judaism). Strict relationships between men and women are also characteristic of Islam. The Amish seldom purchase health insurance. Artificial contraception and abortion are prohibited in Catholicism. For Jehovah's Witness, the administration of blood or blood products is prohibited.
9. b. Traditional Native American rituals may include healing ceremonies used in addition to conventional therapy to promote a balance of physical, spiritual, and emotional wholeness believed to be necessary for wellness. These rituals may or may not be part of formal religious beliefs and may positively alter the progression of physical illnesses.
10. a. Empacho causes pain and cramping from food balls forming in the stomach or intestinal tract. Susto is a culture-bound syndrome also known as "fright sickness." Ghost sickness for Native Americans causes nightmares, weakness and a sense of suffocation. Bilis brought on by strong anger causes headaches, stomach disturbances, and loss of consciousness.
11. b. In some cultural groups, especially Asian, Hispanic, and Native American, there is an emphasis on interdependence rather than independence. The nurse should be aware that in other cultures, decisions for the patient may be made by other family members or may be made collectively by the patient and his or her family. All of the other options reflect an insensitive assumption that the patient should make an autonomous decision.
12. c. In the Arabic culture, male and female roles are strictly observed. A woman should not be touched by a man other than her husband, nor should she be alone with another man. An Arabic woman would be very uncomfortable being cared for by a male nurse or would be put in the position of having to refuse the care.
13. b, d, e. From eTable 2-1. With antipsychotics use is more frequent and dose is higher. Tricyclic antidepressants show faster response but more side effects in African Americans. Antihypertensives are not responded to as well as they are by European Americans. There is no difference in the effect of analgesics or benzodiazepines.

14. c. Hispanics or Latino individuals may not return the nurse's direct gaze because of their respect for authority.

15. b, d

16. a, c. Using standardized evidence-based care guidelines guides care based on the patient's outcomes. Using cultural competency guidelines guides the nurse in practice. Using a family member as the interpreter is not recommended because of the possibility of misunderstandings as well as potential privacy issues. Completing the health history rapidly may not allow patients from other cultures than the nurse to explain themselves well enough. Racial cultural differences cannot be assumed. The individual patient must be assessed to determine the differences to be included in the care.

CHAPTER 3

Answer Key

1.

Subjective	Objective
Short of breath, pain in chest upon breathing, coughing makes head hurt, aches all over	Respiratory rate of 28 bpm, coughing yellow sputum, skin hot and moist, temperature 102.2°F (39°C)

2. d. The focused assessment is used to evaluate the status of previously identified problems and monitor for signs of new problems. In this case, the chest must be assessed related to the shortness of breath, chest pain with breathing, increased respiratory rate, yellow sputum, increased temperature, and elevated white blood cell count. If the patient's headache and achiness are not reduced after the cough and temperature have been treated, further nursing and medical assessments will be done.

3. Examples: Many answers could be correct. It is helpful to preface the question with the reason it is being asked.
   a. "Many patients taking drugs for hypertension have problems with sexual function. Have you experienced any problems?"
   b. "Alcohol may interact dangerously with drugs you receive or it may cause withdrawal problems in the hospital. Can you describe your recent alcohol intake?"
   c. "It is important to contact and treat others who might have the same infection you do. Would you tell me with whom you have been sexually intimate in the last 6 weeks?"
   d. "Today medications are so expensive that some people must choose between eating and taking their medications. Are you able to get and take all of the medications prescribed for you?"

4. d. Data are required regarding the immediate problem but gathering additional information can be delayed. The patient should not receive pain medication before pertinent information related to allergies or the nature of the problem is obtained. Questions that require brief answers do not elicit adequate information for a health profile.

5. c. When a patient describes a feeling, the nurse should ask about the factors surrounding the situation to clarify the etiology of the problem. An incorrect nursing diagnosis may be made if the statement is taken literally and its meaning is not explored with the patient. A sense of "being tired and unable to function" does not necessarily indicate a need for rest or sleep and there is no way to know that treatment will relieve the problem.

6. There may be many correct answers. Examples include the following:

   a. "Can you tell me how you are feeling?"
   b. "Describe your relationship with your spouse."
   c. "Can you describe your experience with this illness?"
   d. "What is your usual activity during the day?"

7. c, d, e. Severity, palliative, and radiation are not addressed. The timing, quality, and precipitating factors are described.

8. a. 1; b. 10; c. 10; d. 8; e. 4; f. 4, 6; g. 2, 3; h. 6; i. 6; j. 6; k. 7; l. 5; m. 3, 9; n. 2; o. 4; p. 12; q. 11; r. 2; s. 10; t. 13

9. d. Abnormal lung sounds are usually associated with chronic bronchitis and their absence is a negative finding. Chest pain is a positive finding and radiation is not expected for all chest pain. Elevated blood pressure in hypertension is a positive finding and pupils that are equal and react to light and accommodation are normal findings.

10. a. 2; b. 4; c. 3; d. 2; e. 1; f. 4; g. 1; h. 2

11. d. The usual sequence of physical assessment techniques is inspection, palpation, percussion, and auscultation. However, because palpation and percussion can alter bowel sounds, in abdominal assessment the sequence should be inspection, auscultation, percussion, and palpation.

12. b. A nurse should use the same efficient sequence in each examination to avoid forgetting a procedure, a step in the sequence, or a body part. However, a specific method is not required. Patient safety, comfort, and privacy are considerations but are not the priorities. The nursing history data should be collected in an interview to avoid prolonging the examination.

13. b, c, e. Older adults may have decreased vision and hearing so providing a quiet environment free from distractions will make the assessment easier than having the distraction of the TV.

14. b, c. These are situations in which an initial and thorough baseline assessment needs to be completed. Options a. and e. would require focused assessments; option d. would require an emergency assessment.

15. a, b, e. The watch is used to assess pulses, the stethoscope is used to hear pulses and heart sounds, and the blood pressure cuff is used to assess blood pressure. The ophthalmoscope is used to assess the retina and the percussion hammer is used to assess reflexes.

16. c. Subjective data or symptoms are obtained by interview during the nursing history. These data can be described only by the patient or caregiver. Objective data or signs are data that are obtained on physical examination. Comprehensive data are obtained from a detailed health history and physical examination of one or more body systems.

17. a, d, e. The general survey is considered a scanning procedure that includes mental state, behavior, speech, body movements, body features, obvious physical signs, and nutritional status. The physical examination includes auscultation and percussion of lung sounds and bowel tones, palpation of temperature and pulses, auscultation of pulses and heart sounds, and inspection of mobility. If there are obvious physical signs or abnormal sounds, a focused assessment will be done to assess the specific problems.

CHAPTER 4

Answer Key

1. a. Maintenance of health. b. Management of illness. c. Appropriate selection and use of treatment options. d. Prevention of disease.

2. In your own words, the answer should be something like this: Use every opportunity (interaction [e.g., administering medications]) to assess patients for educational needs, to provide the teaching needed, and to reinforce the teaching that has already occurred. The time for patient teaching is limited and every opportunity needs to be used efficiently.

3. a, b, e. Learning is acquiring a skill or knowledge and may occur from experience rather than teaching. Planned teaching using a variety of methods may increase learning and teaching that is planned helps to make learning more efficient. Teaching may occur as an incidental experience without prior planning. One hopes that the learner's behavior will change as a result of teaching. However, it is the choice of the learner to either change behavior or not.

4. a. 1, 2; b. 1, 2, 4, 6; c. 2, 4; d. 5; e. 2, 6; f. 5; g. 3

5. c. This patient is in the precontemplation stage of behavior change; he is not considering a change, nor is he ready to learn. During this stage the best intervention by the nurse is to describe the benefits of change and the risks of not changing. The consequences of not changing should not be presented as threats but rather as a disadvantage of the current behavior. Describing what is involved in behavior change and setting priorities are recommended for later stages of change.

6. a. Example: A sudden episode (acute) in which the heart muscle (myocardium) is damaged from a lack of blood supply (infarction)
   b. Example: The intravenous (IV) injection of a dye to visually record (gram) the kidneys (pyelo)
   c. Example: Damage (pathy) to the retina (retino) of the eye as a complication of diabetes

7. b. An empathetic approach to teaching requires that the nurse provide positive feedback and try to understand the patient's world. The other options are important but are not directly related to empathy.

8.

Barrier	Strategy
Lack of time	Set learning priorities with the patient and use every encounter. Let the patient know how much time you have for each session.
Your feeling as a teacher	Prepare ahead of time. Use available written materials. Respect the patient's response to the health problem.
Patient circumstances	Know your resources. Anticipate each contact with your patient and use it to teach throughout the day. Provide the patient with written materials and contact numbers if clarification is needed. Provide access to resources that the patient or caregiver may need.

9. c. Because the patient's father died of a myocardial infarction at a young age, the nurse needs to assess how his anxiety may affect his ability to learn about his treatment and follow-up care. There is no information about the learner characteristics or sociocultural characteristics, although these areas would also need to be assessed.

10. b. To promote self-efficacy it is important that the person is successful in new endeavors to strengthen the belief in his or her ability to manage a situation. To avoid early failure the nurse should work with the patient to present simple concepts related to knowledge and skills the person already has. Motivation and relevancy are important factors in adult learning but are more often a result of self-efficacy, not a method of promoting it.

11.

Patient Characteristic	Teaching Intervention
Impaired hearing	Use supplementary illustrations and written materials. Provide audiotapes or audiovisual presentations with headphones that block environmental noise and promote auditory function.
Patient refuses to see a need for a change in health behaviors	Support the patient during this time and do not argue about the need for a change in health behaviors. Wait until the patient is ready to learn before beginning teaching.
Drowsiness caused by use of sedatives	Evaluate the medication schedule and change it, if possible, to increase alertness. If sedation is the objective of the medication, consider teaching family members or other caregivers.
Presence of pain	Provide only brief explanations and wait until the pain has been controlled to present more detailed instruction.
Uncertain of reading ability	Be sure that educational materials are written at fifth-grade or lower reading level. Use audiovisual materials with simple, layperson language.
Visual learning style	Provide a variety of written educational materials. Refer the patient to appropriate Internet resources for information.
Primary language is not English	Use translators and translation software programs. Obtain patient teaching materials in the patient's primary language.

12. b. The nursing diagnosis should specify the exact nature of the knowledge deficit so that the objectives, strategies, implementation, and evaluation relate to the identified problem. The problem is deficient knowledge and a nursing diagnosis stating that the knowledge deficit is related to a lack of interest is in error. The statement "risk for cardiac dysrhythmias" is a collaborative problem rather than a nursing diagnosis.

13. Example: The patient will identify foods that are high in potassium from a given list of common foods by the time of discharge.

14. a, c, d. DVDs or videos and printed materials can be left with the patient, then discussed or "taught back" later to be sure that all goals are met. Role play and lecture-discussion may take more time than is available to meet the goals.

15. a, b. In role playing patients need to examine attitudes and behaviors that they may not be comfortable with if they are not mature enough. Demonstration is best used for teaching motor skills. Lecture-discussion is used in teaching basic information. Audiovisual strategies are easily combined with other teaching strategies.

16. c. If audiovisual and written materials do not help the patient to meet the learning goals, they are a waste of time and expense. The nurse should ensure that these materials are accurate and appropriate for each patient. Audiovisual materials are often supplementary materials that are used either before or after other presentation of information and do not need to include all of the information the patient needs to learn to be of value. Patients with auditory and visual limitations may find these materials useful because they can adjust the volume and size of the images.

17. a, e. When using the Internet as a teaching strategy, the nurse will assist the patient or caregiver in accessing trustworthy sites. The nurse personally cannot evaluate all sites that a patient or caregiver uses. The Internet is a valuable source of health information but it is also unregulated and much information is unreliable or inaccurate. As a result, both nurses and patients should learn to evaluate sources and identify accurate information. Reliable sources include universities, government health agencies, and reputable health care organizations.

18.

Learning Goal	Evaluation Technique
The patient will demonstrate to the nurse the preparation and administration of a subcutaneous insulin injection to himself with correct technique before discharge.	Direct observation
Before discharge, the patient will identify five serious side effects of Coumadin that should be reported to the doctor.	Ask a direct question or use a written measurement tool (ask the patient to write down the serious side effects that need to be reported to the doctor)
The patient's wife will select the foods highest in potassium for each meal from the hospital menu with 80% accuracy.	Direct observation with observation of verbal and nonverbal cues
The patient will verbalize "no shortness of breath" when ambulating unassisted with the walker each of three times a day.	Direct observation with observation of verbal and nonverbal cues
The patient's caregiver will state that they are ready to change the patient's dressing today.	Talk with a member of the patient's family

19. b. A statement that documents what the patient does as a result of teaching indicates whether the learning objective has been met and provides the best documentation of patient instruction. "Understand" is not a measurable behavior and does not validate that learning has occurred.

20. d, f. Baby boomers grew up sitting quietly in rows at school with the teacher lecturing or watching a movie and then discussing the information. They are used to learning with these methods although some individuals may be comfortable with the other methods as well.

21. a, b, c, d, e. Adult children who are caregivers have lost their parents as they knew them before the illness. Possible stressors in her life include changing roles within the family, lack of respite from caregiving responsibilities, conflict with her brother related to decisions about caregiving, financial depletion of resources as a result of her inability to work, and social isolation and loss of friends from an inability to have time for herself.

22. c. Adjusting to rather than opposing the patient's resistance as well as expressing empathy and reinforcing the positive outcome of attending therapy previously will encourage her to continue therapy. The other options are argumentative and confrontational, focus on the negative rather than the patient's strengths, and do not help the patient to recognize the "gap" between where she is and where she hopes to be.

CHAPTER 5

Answer Key

1. b, c, e, f. The diabetes mellitus and residual right-sided weakness from the cerebrovascular accident (CVA) contribute to the residual disability and permanent impairments. The diabetes requires long-term management and both problems contribute to nonreversible pathologic changes.

2.

Chronic Condition	Task
Diabetes mellitus	Prevent and manage crisis, carry out prescribed regimens, adjust to changes in the course of the disease, control symptoms
Visual impairment	Prevent social isolation, attempt to normalize interactions with others
Heart disease	Carry out prescribed regimens, control symptoms, prevent and manage a crisis
Hearing impairment	Prevent social isolation, attempt to normalize interactions with others
Alzheimer's disease	Prevent and manage crisis, reorder time, adjust to changes in the course of the disease, attempt to normalize interactions with others, control symptoms
Arthritis	Control symptoms, carry out prescribed regimens, reorder time, adjust to changes in the course of the disease, prevent social isolation
Orthopedic impairment	Reorder time, prevent and manage crisis, prevent social isolation

3. a. secondary
   b. primary
4. c. Coronary artery disease is the leading cause of death in the United States.
5. d. The trajectory defines a life-threatening situation as a crisis. Increasing disability is described as downward. A gradual return to an acceptable way of life is a comeback.
6. a, b, d, e. Ageism is a negative attitude based on age.
7. There may be other correct responses but examples include the following:
   a. Decreased intestinal villae, decreased digestive enzyme production and secretion, decreased dentine and gingival retraction, decreased taste threshold for salt and sugar
   b. Decreased force of cardiac contraction, decreased cardiac muscle mass, increased fat and collagen
   c. Decreased skeletal muscle mass; decreased joint flexion; stiffening of tendons and ligaments; decreased cortical and trabecular bone; changes in eyes and ears that impair vision, hearing, and balance; slowed response/reaction time
   d. Decreased bladder smooth muscle and elastic tissue, decreased sphincter control
   e. Decreased ciliary action, decreased respiratory muscle strength, decreased elastic recoil, decreased cough force
   f. Decreased muscle and subcutaneous fat, collagen stiffening, decreased sebaceous gland activity, decreased sensory receptors, decreased tissue fluid, increased capillary fragility
   g. Decreased vessel elastin and smooth muscle, increased arterial rigidity
   h. Decreased blood flow to colon, decreased intestinal motility, decreased sensation to defecate, decreased muscle mass
8. d. Age-associated memory impairment is characterized by a memory lapse or benign forgetfulness that is not the same as a decline in cognitive functioning. Forgetting a name, date, or recent event is not serious but the other examples indicate abnormal functioning.
9.

S	Sadness (mood)
C	Cholesterol (high)
A	Albumin (low)
L	Loss (or gain of weight)
E	Eating problems
S	Shopping (and food preparation problems)

10. d. Older adults with an ethnic identity often have disproportionately low incomes and might not be able to afford Medicare deductibles or medications to treat health problems. Although they often live in older urban neighborhoods with extended families, they are not isolated. Ethnic diets have adequate nutrition but health could be impaired if money is not available for food.
11. c. This statement indicates that this patient does not understand the importance of having the test every week and that the test results will determine ongoing dosing. The other three statements indicate that the patient is thinking about ways to get into town weekly.
12. Any three of the following are appropriate: unplanned weight loss (≥10 lb in the last year), weakness, poor endurance and energy, slowness and low activity.

13. a. Psychologic abuse, psychologic neglect, physical neglect, and perhaps violation of personal rights
    b. Perform a very careful medical history and screening for mistreatment; interview the mother alone; use an assessment tool designed specifically for elder mistreatment; specifically assess for dehydration, malnutrition, pressure ulcers, and poor personal hygiene; evaluate explanations about physical findings that are not consistent with what is seen or contradictory statements made by the daughter and the mother
    c. Caregiver role strain
    d. Community caregiver support group, formal support system for respite care, adult day care
14. Possible factors that accelerate placement decisions are deteriorating cognition, incontinence, or a major health event.
    a. Rapid patient deterioration
    b. Caregiver exhaustion
    c. Alteration in or loss of family support system
15. c. During an initial contact with an older adult, the nurse should perform a comprehensive nursing assessment that includes a history using a functional health pattern format, physical assessment, assessment of activities of daily living (ADLs) and instrumental activities of daily living (IADLs), mental status evaluation, and a social-environmental assessment. If available, a comprehensive interdisciplinary geriatric assessment may then be done to maintain and enhance the functional abilities of the older adult. The older adult and the caregiver should be interviewed separately and the older adult should identify his or her own needs.
16. a. The results of mental status evaluation often determine whether the patient is able to manage independent living, a major issue in older adulthood. Other elements of comprehensive assessment could determine eligibility for special problems, determination of frailty, and total service and placement needs.
17. c. Exercise for all older adults is important to prevent deconditioning and subsequent functional decline from many different causes. Walkers and canes may improve mobility but can also decrease mobility if they are too difficult for the patient to use. Nutrition is important for muscles but muscle strength is primarily dependent on use. Risk appraisals are usually performed for specific health problems.
18. Any of the following eight nursing interventions listed in Table 5-13: (1) Evaluate cognitive function and ensure ability to self-administer medication, (2) Attempt to reduce medication use that is not essential, (3) Screen all medication use, (4) Assess alcohol use, (5) Encourage the use of written or medication-reminder systems, (6) Encourage the use of one pharmacy, (7) Work with health care providers and pharmacists to establish routine drug profiles on all older adult patients, (8) Advocate with drug companies for low-income prescription support services.
19. a, b, c. These actions are alternatives to restraints that may help to reduce falls and keep the patient safe. A jacket vest and a seat belt are forms of restraint and require an order and frequent reassessment and order renewal.
20. a, b, c, d, e. Any of these actions will promote health.
21. b. Long-term acute care provides acute care for an average length of greater than 25 days. Acute rehabilitation is a post-acute level of care with therapies for returning the patient to the best level of functioning as possible. Intermediate care facilities provide convalescent care. Transitional subacute care facilities are used for 5 to 21 days.

CHAPTER 6

Answer Key

1. a. The natural products category uses dietary supplements and herbs. The other categories do not.

2. b, c, d. Mind-body medicine includes communication with the Creator or prayer, self-directed focusing or meditation, and learned control of physiologic body responses or biofeedback. The use of hands to realign energy flow or healing touch is part of the other CAM practices, in this case an energy therapy. The soft tissue manipulation or massage and spinal manipulation or chiropractic therapy are included in the category of manipulative and body-based methods.

3. d. Ayurveda from India is a whole medical system that views disease as an imbalance between the person's life force and basic metabolic condition. Acupuncture is part of Traditional Chinese Medicine and uses fine needles to manipulate energy channels. The principle of "like cures like" is used in homeopathy. Acupressure uses finger and hand pressure at energy meridians to improve energy flow.

4. c. The integrative health care model focuses on the mind-body-spirit connections with the individual responsible for care that uses natural, less invasive modalities and is less costly. The conventional health care model is directed by the health care provider and focuses on treatment of symptoms with medications and surgery.

5. d. CAM therapy practices vary by culture and time. CAM therapy incorporates the physical, emotional, mental, and spiritual realms of the patient. The increase of CAM therapies is due in part to increased chronic disease and stress-related disorders. Research and education related to CAM therapies are supported by the National Center for Complementary and Alternative Medicine (NCCAM) of the National Institutes of Health (NIH).

6. b. Complementary and alternative therapies are harmonious with the values of nursing, which include a view of humans as holistic beings, an emphasis on healing and partnership relationships with patients, and a focus on health promotion and illness prevention.

7. a. The basic concept of disease in Traditional Chinese Medicine is that the opposing phenomena of yin and yang are out of balance and this imbalance alters the movement of the vital energy of the body, known as Qi, that influences physiologic functions of the body. Acupoints are holes in the Qi meridians where the flow of Qi can be influenced but not released. Naturopathy is based on promotion of health rather than symptom management and focuses on enhancing the body's natural healing response using individualized interventions. Harmony with nature is necessary for health in Native American beliefs and spiritualism and mysticism are frequently a part of Hispanic health care.

8. b, d. Acupuncture is used to regulate the flow of Qi with the insertion of needles at acupoints, areas where needles may be inserted to unblock obstruction of energy and reestablish the flow of Qi. It can relieve nausea and vomiting postoperatively, with pregnancy, or related to chemotherapy. Counterirritation and inflammation are not consistent with the theory of Qi and although electrical stimulation may be applied to the needles in electroacupuncture, this procedure releases neuropeptides within the central nervous system.

9. b. If the nurse knows enough acupressure to suggest its use to a patient, it is appropriate to use with the patient's permission.

The PRN medication for postoperative pain is not usually appropriate for a headache, nor would biofeedback training be appropriate for this situation. Simply reassuring the patient that the headache will go away is not helpful.

10. c. Massage therapy is one of the body-based methods commonly used by nurses for many different effects. As part of nursing care, nurses can use specific massage techniques that are not as comprehensive as those of massage therapists. It would be quite appropriate for the nurse to massage the patient's back. The other options are inappropriate at this time.

11. a. Journaling may be very helpful for this patient who has difficulty verbalizing her fears and concerns. Yoga is a helpful general stress management but is not specific to this problem. The nurse cannot prescribe herbal therapy or provide chiropractic care.

12. a. Because of a lack of governmental control for clinical testing of herbs or standardization of ingredient concentration or acceptable levels of contamination of pesticides, solvents, bacteria, and heavy metals, the safety and efficacy of herbal preparations are based on the manufacturer's standards. As such, the reputation and history of the manufacturer are the major criteria for purchasing herbs. Herbs indeed can be toxic and are contraindicated or should be used with caution in certain people.

13. b. To serve as a resource for patients regarding complementary and alternative therapies, nurses must first develop their own knowledge base. To teach patients about their use, monitor for adverse effects and interactions with conventional therapies, and assist patients to use the therapies knowledgeably and safely, nurses themselves must be informed.

14. a. Encourage the patient to seek the guidance of the physician regarding the safety and efficacy of using the herbal therapy rather than the medical therapy. See the answer to Question 15 for further clarification.

15. a, b, c, f. Professional nurses should be knowledgeable about the various complementary and alternative therapies, assess their use in patients, and promote their safety. Suggesting specific herbs is "prescribing" and is outside the scope of nursing. Advice against use of all herbs related to side effects is not appropriate.

16. b. Feverfew is used to prevent migraine headaches. Valerian is used for insomnia and anxiety. Echinacea and zinc are used to prevent and treat upper respiratory infections. Soy and black cohosh have been used for menopausal symptom relief.

17. b. Ginger may be used with monitoring to treat nausea and vomiting related to pregnancy. Aloe is an effective laxative and is also used for skin lesions. Cranberry juice is used to prevent urinary tract infections. Evening primrose is used for eczema and skin irritation.

18. a. Melatonin decreases the time needed to fall asleep. Depression may be relieved by St. John's wort, although it may have many side effects. The dietary supplements red yeast rice and soy and the herb garlic may help to lower cholesterol. Saw palmetto has been used for benign prostatic hyperplasia but current research shows that it has little or no benefit.

19. a. Kava may be used to relieve anxiety but the U.S. Food and Drug Administration has issued a warning of severe liver damage, so patients with liver problems or those taking other medications that affect the liver must avoid kava. Ginseng is used to improve mental performance, enhance the immune system, and lower blood glucose in healthy adults. It may also affect blood pressure. Although not proven effective, milk thistle has been used for liver disease and does not

affect anxiety. Although not proven effective, ginkgo biloba has been used in the early stage of Alzheimer's disease.

CHAPTER 7

Answer Key

1. b. When individuals do not become stressed with a situation or an event, it is because the event is not perceived by them as a demand that is being made on them or as a threat to their well-being. Perceptions of stressors have great variability and, for whatever reasons, this patient does not perceive this diagnosis as stressful.

2. a. 1; b. 1; c. 3; d. 3; e. 1; f. 2

3. Resilience, hardiness, attitude, and optimism. Other factors that could have been selected are age, health status, personality characteristics, prior experience with stress, nutritional status, sleep status, and genetic background. These are all factors that are internal to the individual and may affect the response to stress.

4. See chart below.

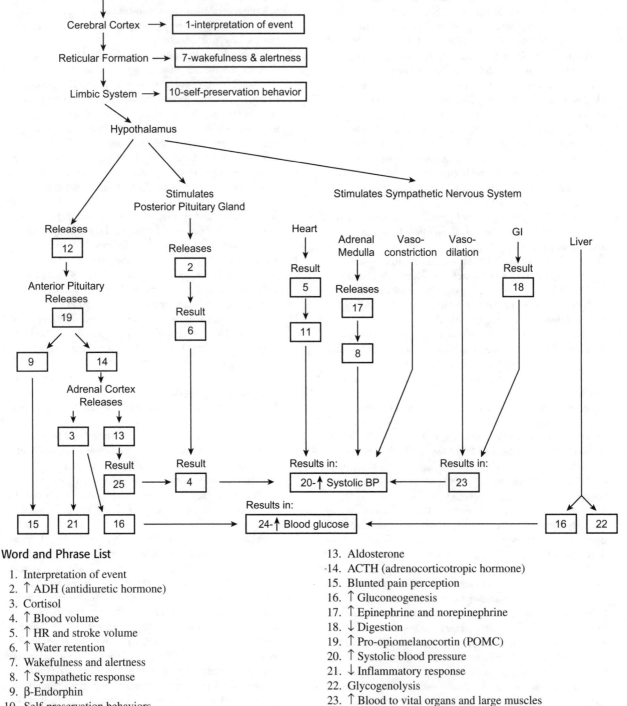

Word and Phrase List

1. Interpretation of event
2. ↑ ADH (antidiuretic hormone)
3. Cortisol
4. ↑ Blood volume
5. ↑ HR and stroke volume
6. ↑ Water retention
7. Wakefulness and alertness
8. ↑ Sympathetic response
9. β-Endorphin
10. Self-preservation behaviors
11. ↑ Cardiac output
12. Corticotropin-releasing hormone
13. Aldosterone
14. ACTH (adrenocorticotropic hormone)
15. Blunted pain perception
16. ↑ Gluconeogenesis
17. ↑ Epinephrine and norepinephrine
18. ↓ Digestion
19. ↑ Pro-opiomelanocortin (POMC)
20. ↑ Systolic blood pressure
21. ↓ Inflammatory response
22. Glycogenolysis
23. ↑ Blood to vital organs and large muscles
24. ↑ Blood glucose
25. ↑ Na and H_2O reabsorption

5. **Objective Manifestations**
   a. Increased heart rate
   b. Increased blood pressure
   c. Cool, clammy skin
   d. Decreased bowel sounds
   e. Hyperglycemia
   f. Decreased lymphocytes
   g. Decreased eosinophils
   h. Decreased urinary output
   Subjective Findings
   a. Anxiety, fear
   b. Decreased perception of pain
   c. Verbalization of stress
   d. Wakefulness, restlessness
6. b. One of the many physiologic changes that occur as a result of prolonged, increased stress is immunosuppression, which may exacerbate or increase the risk of progression of immune-based diseases, including asthma. The other options are not valid explanations for the worsening asthma.
7. a. N; b. N; c. P; d. P; e. P
8. a, d, e. The other answers are problem-focused coping mechanisms.
9. a. Because it is almost impossible to maintain muscle tension while breathing slowly and deeply, relaxation breathing is a component of all relaxation therapies. Progressive muscle relaxation and meditation first require relaxed breathing and although soft music can decrease stress, it should be used with other therapies.
10. a. Peptic ulcer disease is one of several disorders with a known stress component. Although many patients have stress related to a health problem, stress-relieving interventions are always indicated for patients with diseases in which stress contributes to the problem.
11. a, c, e. Humor, journaling, and relaxation activities are realistic strategies that can be used during hospitalization by a patient with an acute episode of a chronic disease. Exercise or a cleansing diet would not be appropriate for an exacerbation of Crohn's disease.

Case Study

1. **Physiologic:** Fever, pain, anemia, inflammatory disease itself
   Psychologic: No income, no insurance, duration and chronicity of the disease, frequent hospital admissions, lack of social support systems
   Effects: Prolonged healing of illness, progression of the inflammatory disease. Cardiovascular, respiratory, and immune system involvement can also occur.
2. Her refusal to seek support from boyfriend
   Her depression, weakness
   Her experience with the illness and hospitalizations
   Her lack of financial resources
3. Increased weight, hemoglobin and hematocrit levels, strength
   Decreased body temperature, number of stools
4. One approach might be using a hospital stress-rating scale to clarify the patient's perception of the situation. The nurse and the patient might not rate the stressors as being the same in intensity. Specific questions may include the following:

"What is the most stressful thing to you about being in the hospital?"
"Can you tell me what having this illness means to you?"
5. Reduce additional stressors, such as sleep deprivation, environmental stimuli.
   Set short-term outcomes to achieve success.
   Provide pain relief, measures for comfort, rest.
   Provide stress-reducing interventions, such as relaxation and guided imagery.
6. **Nursing diagnoses:**
   • Ineffective coping *related to* inadequate resources as manifested by crying, depression
   • Stress overload *related to* excessive amounts of demands
   • Ineffective role performance *related to* lack of employment
   • Acute pain *related to* inflammatory process
   • Risk for impaired skin integrity *related to* frequent stools and emaciation
   • Imbalanced nutrition: less than body requirements *related to* nausea and frequent watery stools
   • Risk for deficient fluid volume *related to* frequent watery stools and low-grade fever
   Collaborative problems:
   Potential complications: fluid-electrolyte imbalances, intestinal obstruction, fistula-fissure-abscess
7. Acute pain, a physiologic need that takes priority over other physiologic and psychosocial problems

CHAPTER 8

Answer Key

1. c. Lack of sleep does not cause medical and psychiatric disorders, although people with these diagnoses may have fragmented sleep. Most adults need 7 to 8 hours of sleep per day. In 2011, 87% of Americans reported sleep problems.
2. b, c, e, f. Manifestations of insomnia include difficulty falling asleep, frequent awakenings, prolonged nighttime awakening or awakening too early and not being able to fall back to sleep, and feeling unrefreshed on awakening and having daytime sleepiness and difficulty concentrating.
3. d. Parasomnias are unusual and often undesirable behaviors that occur while falling asleep, transitioning between sleep stages, or arousing from sleep. Cataplexy is brief and sudden loss of skeletal muscle tone and is experienced with narcolepsy episodes. Hypopnea is shallow respirations and sleep apnea is the cessation of spontaneous respirations for longer than 10 seconds.
4. c. The nervous system controls the cyclic changes of wake and sleep through a complex arrangement of structures with key nuclei in the brainstem, hypothalamus, and thalamus. Melatonin is an endogenous hormone that increases sleep efficiency and is released in the evening. The light-dark cycles influence our circadian rhythms and neuropeptides influence wake behavior. These all play a role in the sleep/wake cycle and are components of the nervous system.
5. a. 4; b. 3; c. 2, 3; d. 3; e. 4; f. 1; g. 2; h. 1; i. 2; j. 3

6. Any three of these can contribute to insomnia:
   - Consumption of stimulants (caffeine, nicotine, methamphetamine) close to bedtime
   - Side effect of medications (antidepressants, antihypertensives, corticosteroids, psychostimulants, analgesics)
   - Drinking alcohol or using over-the-counter medications as a sleep aid
   - Long naps in the afternoon
   - Sleeping in late
   - Exercise near bedtime
   - Jet lag
   - Nightmares
   - Stressful life event
   - Medical conditions or psychiatric illnesses
   - Irregular sleep/wake schedules
   - Worry about getting enough sleep

7. a, b, e, f, g, h, i, k

8. b. Cognitive-behavioral therapies are effective therapies for insomnia and should be tried first. These include relaxation training, guided imagery, education about good sleep hygiene, and regular exercise several hours before bedtime. The other therapies are used to treat insomnia, with benzodiazepine-receptor-like agents being the first choice for drug therapy. Many patients will try over-the-counter medications such as diphenhydramine (Benadryl) but tolerance develops rapidly. Complementary and alternative therapies such as melatonin have been found to be useful to help individuals to fall asleep but they are not first-line therapy.

9. b. It is not recommended that a person lie in bed awake. Alcohol should not be consumed within 6 hours of bedtime. The other statements represent strategies that may help the individual go to sleep. Exercise is good but not within 6 hours of bedtime; a light snack may help to relax the person.

10. b. Hot chocolate has 5 mg of caffeine. A Hershey's bar has 10 mg of caffeine, Dannon coffee yogurt has 45 mg of caffeine, and Ben & Jerry's nonfat coffee fudge frozen yogurt contains 85 mg of caffeine.

11. a. Reducing the light and noise levels in the ICU can help to promote opportunities for sleep. Having the TV on at all times will only add to the noise level. Analgesics given for actual pain may help a patient to sleep or rest but they may also alter sleep. The alarms should not be silenced except for short periods to address why they were alarming. Silencing alarms to prevent them from making noise puts the patient at risk because the nurse may not be alerted to patient changes on the monitor or problems with the infusion device.

12. a. Desipramine and protriptyline are both tricyclic antidepressants used to treat cataplexy and methylphenidate is an amphetamine.

13. Any of these responses would be appropriate:
   - Start to get in harmony with the Moscow time zone several days before you travel.
   - Be sure to expose yourself to daytime daylight, which will assist with synchronizing your body's clock to environmental time.
   - Melatonin has been shown to be an effective sleep aid to help synchronize the body's rhythm.
   - Resynchronization of the body's clock will occur at a rate of 1 hr/day if the patient travels eastward.

14. a. 4; b. 7; c. 6; d. 5; e. 2; f. 1; g. 8; h. 3. Obstructive sleep apnea has the risk factors listed. Airflow obstruction occurs because of narrowing of the air passages with relaxation of muscle tone during sleep or when the tongue and soft palate fall backward and partially or completely obstruct the pharynx. With apnea lasting 10 to 90 seconds, hypoxemia and hypercapnia occur. The startle response causes a brief arousal, so the tongue and soft palate move forward and the airway opens. This cycle occurs 200 to 400 times during 6 to 8 hours of sleep.

15. c. CPAP is continuous positive airway pressure and is the treatment of choice for more serious sleep apnea. Bilevel positive airway pressure (BiPAP) is the therapy that delivers a high inspiratory pressure and a low expiratory pressure to prevent airway collapse. CPAP is not well tolerated and compliance is low. Compliance may be improved by involving the patient in the selection of the device and mask, showing the CPAP before therapy begins, and teaching troubleshooting to reduce anxiety. An oral appliance is used to prevent airway occlusion from the relaxed mandible and tongue.

16. d. The most common complications in the immediate postoperative period are airway obstruction and hemorrhage. The patient may experience a sore throat, foul-smelling breath, and snoring during the recovery but they will resolve. Infection is a potential complication of any surgery but is not common with this procedure. Loss of voice and electrolyte imbalance generally are not complications of this procedure.

17. d. Assess the patient to determine what the problem is and then offer sleep hygiene instruction and collaborate with the physician to improve the patient's sleep behavior. Disturbed sleep is not a normal result of aging and people need about the same amount of sleep throughout their life span. Over-the-counter and prescription sleep aids need to be used very cautiously in older adults and patient response must be monitored closely.

18. Any three of these would be correct:
   - Nurse is too sleepy to be fully awake at work
   - Nurse is too alert to sleep soundly the next day
   - Increased morbidity and mortality related to cardiovascular problems
   - Mood disorders are higher
   - Fatigue could result in errors and accidents, as perceptual skills, judgment, and decision-making abilities may be diminished

19. a, b, c, d, e. All of these measures can be used to help a nurse who works rotating shifts to get adequate sleep.

CHAPTER 9

Answer Key

1. c. Because the patient's self-report is the most valid means of pain assessment, patients who have decreased cognitive function, such as those who are comatose, have dementia, or are mentally disabled, might not be able to report pain. In these cases, nonverbal information and behaviors are necessary considerations in pain assessment.

2. c. Administering the smallest prescribed analgesic dose when given a choice is not consistent with current pain management guidelines and leads to undertreatment of pain and inadequate pain control. Without reassessing the

pain within 30 minutes of the IV analgesic the nurse is unsure how well the previous dose of medication worked for the patient to determine the current dose needed. Unnecessary suffering, impaired recovery from acute illness, increased morbidity as a result of respiratory dysfunction, increased heart rate and cardiac workload, and other physical dysfunction can occur.

3. a. Physiologic—the anatomic and physical determinants of pain
   b. Affective—the emotional response to pain
   c. Cognitive—the beliefs, attitudes, and meanings attributed to pain
   d. Behavioral—observable actions that express or control pain
   e. Sociocultural—age and gender, family and caregiver influence, and culture that influences the pain experience

4. a. Although a peripheral nerve is one cell that carries an impulse directly from the periphery to the dorsal horn of the spinal cord with no synapses, transmission of the impulse can be interrupted by drugs known as membrane stabilizers or sodium-channel inhibitors, such as local anesthetics and some antiseizure drugs. The nerve fiber produces neurotransmitters only at synapses, not during transmission of the action potential.

5. a. The right neck and flank are common areas of referred pain from liver damage and examination of the liver should be considered when pain occurs without other findings in these areas. Other common referred areas are midscapular and left arm for cardiac pain, inner legs for bladder pain, and shoulders for gallbladder pain.

6. b. It is known that the brain is necessary for pain perception but because it is not clearly understood where in the brain pain is perceived, pain may be perceived even in a comatose patient who may not respond behaviorally to noxious stimuli. Any noxious stimulus should be treated as potentially painful.

7. a. 3; b. 4; c. 2; d. 1

8. a. 2, 7/9; b. 2, 7; c. 2, 6; d. 1, 3; e. 1, 5; f. 2, 8; g. 1, 4

9. c. Several antidepressants affect the modulatory systems by inhibiting the reuptake of serotonin and norepinephrine in descending modulatory fibers, thereby increasing their availability to inhibit afferent transmission of pain impulses. Although chronic pain is often accompanied by anxiety and depression, the antidepressants that affect the physiologic process of pain modulation are used for pain control whether depression is present or not.

10. a. Damage to peripheral or cranial nerves causes neuropathic pain that is not well controlled by opioid analgesics alone and often includes the adjuvant use of tricyclic antidepressants or antiseizure drugs to help inhibit pain transmission. Salicylates and NSAIDs are not effective for the intensity of neuropathic pain.

11. a. Onset: About 4 hours ago
    b. Duration and pattern of the pain: Continuously for about 4 hours. Similar episodes in the past month but lasted only 2 hours.
    c. Location: Right upper quadrant
    d. Intensity: Severe, 10 on a scale of 0 to 10
    e. Quality: Severe cramping, radiates to back
    f. Associated symptoms: Nausea
    g. Management strategies: Pain better walking bent forward, more intense lying in bed

12. a. Follow the principles of pain assessment.
    b. Use a holistic approach to pain management.
    c. Every patient deserves adequate pain management.
    d. Base treatment on the patient's goals.
    e. Use both drug and nondrug therapies.
    f. When appropriate, use a multimodal approach to analgesic therapy.
    g. Address pain using an interdisciplinary approach.
    h. Evaluate the effectiveness of all therapies to ensure that they are meeting the patient's goals.
    i. Prevent or manage medication side effects.
    j. Incorporate patient and caregiver teaching throughout assessment and teaching.

13. a. Analgesics should be scheduled around the clock for patients with constant pain to prevent pain from escalating and becoming difficult to relieve. If pain control is not adequate, the analgesic dose may be increased or an adjunctive drug may be added to the treatment plan.

14. a. As cancer pain increases, stronger drugs are added to the regimen. This patient is using a nonsteroidal antiinflammatory drug (NSAID) and an antidepressant. A stronger preparation would be an opioid but because an NSAID is already being used, a combination NSAID/opioid is not indicated. An appropriate stronger drug would be an oral opioid, in this case oral oxycodone, and this still leaves stronger drugs for expected increasing pain. Propoxyphene is not recommended in analgesic guidelines because of its limited efficacy and toxicities.

15. c. Although tolerance to many of the side effects of opioids (nausea, sedation, respiratory depression, pruritus) develops within days, tolerance to opioid-induced constipation does not occur. A bowel regimen that includes a gentle-stimulant laxative and a stool softener should be started at the beginning of opioid therapy and continue for as long as the drug is taken.

16. d. Use of a basal dose may increase the risk of serious respiratory events in opioid-naive patients and those at risk for respiratory difficulties (older age, existing pulmonary disease, etc.). Overdose is not expected, as the dosages are calculated and the PCA pump is programmed to prevent this. Nausea and itching are common side effects but not related to a basal dose of analgesic. A lack of pain control would not be expected with or without a basal dose. The nurse would be assessing the patient and notify the physician if a lack of pain control occurs but, again, this is not related to receiving a basal dose of analgesic via PCA pump.

17. b, d, e, f. Distraction is effective in the perception stage. Epidural opioids are effective in the transmission stage.

18. a, b, c, d, e, f. The major complications of epidural analgesia are catheter displacement and migration, accidental infusions of neurotoxic agents, and infection. These actions will help to reduce those risks.

19. b. When a patient wants to be stoic about pain, it is important that he or she understand that pain itself can have harmful physiologic effects and that failure to report pain and participate in its control can result in severe unrelieved pain. No evidence that indicates fear of taking the medication is present in this situation.

20. a. Duragesic is frequently used for chronic pain in patients who are not opiate-naive. Oramorph SR given buccally will have the same absorption as morphine, so it would not be expected to be more effective than oral morphine.

Hydrocodone is used for acute and short-term pain, not chronic pain. Intranasal butorphanol (Stadol) is used for acute headaches and recurrent, not chronic pain. The route used will depend on the swallowing ability of the patient.

Case Study

1. Assess the location, quality, and specific pattern of the pain. Also assess R.D.'s prior medication use, experience with opioids, and any addictions.
2. Affective: Worried about worsening of disease, afraid of opioids
   Behavioral: Posturing, slow gait, stays in bed with severe pain
   Cognitive: Uses emptying mind to block pain
3. The symptoms that R.D. has in the mornings are related to withdrawal because of physical dependence and the long interval during the night when the opioid is not used. An adjuvant drug should be added to his regimen and it and the Percocet should be taken around the clock. If the pain is not controlled with this measure, a stronger, sustained-release opioid such as MS Contin should be substituted for the Percocet.
4. Teach R.D. to evaluate the dose required to control his pain and the range and frequency of his dose.
5. Explain that tolerance and physical dependence are expected with long-term opiate use and should not be confused with addiction. Addiction is a psychologic condition characterized by a drive to obtain and compulsively take substances other than for their prescribed therapeutic value and despite risk of harm.
6. There are several physical techniques that could be used, depending on the location of R.D.'s pain, including dermal stimulation, such as massage and pressure. Additional cognitive-behavioral therapies, such as distraction or relaxation (imagery, meditation), could be taught. R.D. has a potential for using cognitive-behavioral therapies successfully because he can already mentally block the pain somewhat.
7. **Nursing diagnoses:**
   - Chronic pain *related to* ineffective pain management
   - Anxiety *related to* effects of disease process and inadequate relief from pain-relief measures
   - Activity intolerance *related to* pain, fatigue
   Collaborative problems:
   Potential complications: drug-induced constipation, respiratory depression, negative nitrogen balance, opioid toxicity

CHAPTER 10

Answer Key

1. a, c, d, f, g, i. Table 10-1 lists the goals of palliative care. Overall, goals of palliative care are to prevent and relieve suffering and to improve the quality of life for the patient.
2. a. The family may not understand what hospice care is and may need information. Some cultures and ethnic groups may underuse hospice care because of a lack of awareness of the services offered, a desire to continue with potentially curative therapies, and concerns about a lack of minority hospice workers.
3. a. Patient must desire services and agree in writing that only hospice care can be used to treat the terminal illness (palliative care)
   b. Patient must meet eligibility, which is less than 6 months to live, certified initially by two physicians

4. **Respiratory**
   a. Cheyne-Stokes respiration
   b. Death rattle (inability to cough and clear secretions)
   c. Increased, then slowing, respiratory rate
   (Also: irregular breathing, terminal gasping)
   Skin
   a. Mottling on hands, feet, and legs that progresses to the torso
   b. Cold, clammy skin
   c. Cyanosis on nose, nail beds, and knees
   (Also: waxlike skin when very near death)
   Gastrointestinal
   a. Slowing of the gastrointestinal tract with accumulation of gas and abdominal distention
   b. Loss of sphincter control with incontinence
   c. Bowel movement before imminent death or at time of death
   Musculoskeletal
   a. Loss of muscle tone with sagging jaw
   b. Difficulty speaking
   c. Difficulty swallowing
   (Also: loss of ability to move or maintain body position, loss of gag reflex)
5. b. Hearing is often the last sense to disappear with declining consciousness and conversations can distress patients even when they appear unresponsive. Conversation around unresponsive patients should never be other than that which one would maintain if the patients were alert.
6. a. Coma
   b. Absent brainstem reflexes
   c. Apnea
7. b. Bargaining is demonstrated by "if-then" grief behavior that is described by Kübler-Ross. Kübler-Ross's stage of depression is seen when the person says "yes me, and I am sad." Prolonged grief disorder is seen when there is a dysfunctional reaction to loss and the individual is unable to move forward after the death of a loved one. In the Grief Wheel model, the new normal stage is when the grief is resolved but the normal state, because of the loss, is not the same as before.
8. a. Spiritual distress may surface when an individual is faced with a terminal illness and it is characterized by verbalization of inner conflicts about beliefs and questioning the meaning of one's own existence. Individuals in spiritual distress may be able to resolve the problem and die peacefully with effective grief work but referral to spiritual leaders should be the patient's choice.
9. a. Natural death acts in each state have their own requirements. Allow natural death is the new term being used for the Do Not Resuscitate order. Advance care planning is the process of having patients and their families think through their values and goals for treatment and document those wishes as advance directives.
10. b. Palliative care is aimed at symptom management rather than curative treatment for diseases that no longer respond to treatment and is focused on caring interventions rather than curative treatments. "Palliative care" and "hospice" are frequently used interchangeably.
11. d. There currently are no clinical practice guidelines to relieve the shortness of breath and air hunger that often occur at the end of life. The principle of beneficence would encourage any of the options to be tried, based on knowing that whatever gives the patient the most relief should be used.

12. d. In assisting patients with dying, end-of-life care promotes the grieving process, which involves saying goodbye. Physical care is very important for physical comfort but assessment should be limited to essential data related to the patient's symptoms. Analgesics should be administered for pain but patients who are sedated cannot participate in the grieving process.

13. a, b, c, d, e, f. Teaching, along with support and encouragement, can decrease some of the anxiety. Teaching about pain relief, the dying process, and the care provided will help the patient and family know what to expect. Allowing the patient to make decisions will help to decrease feelings of powerlessness and hopelessness. The nurse who is the target of anger needs to not react to this anger on a personal level.

14. d. Using the open-ended statement to seek information related to the patient's and family's perspective and expectations will best guide the plan of care for this patient. This will open the discussion about palliative or hospice care and preferences for end-of-life care.

Case Study

1. Additional assessment data should include S.J.'s and her husband's reasons for not discussing her illness and impending death with their children, an assessment of their spiritual needs, what decisions (if any) they have made about where and how S.J. prefers to die, and what resources they have used or could use to assist them through the dying process. In addition, assessment and evaluation of their coping skills are necessary. A functional assessment of S.J.'s activities of daily living (ADLs) should also be made.

2. Maladaptive or dysfunctional grief is demonstrated in this family. S.J. appears to have some degree of acceptance of her impending death but feels rejected by her children. The children may be experiencing fear, guilt, anger, powerlessness, and other emotions that they cope with by withdrawing from the family. S.J.'s husband is also feeling guilt about wishing that the ordeal would be over. Healthy grieving is blocked in this family because communication has not occurred.

3. Pain patterns should be assessed and dosages and frequencies of medication increased to provide pain relief that is acceptable to S.J. without unnecessary sedation. Complementary and alternative therapies to enhance the effect of pain medication should be instituted. As opioids are increased, constipation and abdominal distention could become a problem and stool softeners may be needed. Although S.J. is underweight, patients tend to take in less food and fluid as death approaches and maintaining food and fluid intake is not a high priority. Because S.J. spends most of her time in bed and is very thin, measures to prevent skin breakdown are essential. Oxygen therapy should be considered as a measure to relieve her shortness of breath.

4. Arrange for family meetings to discuss S.J.'s condition and her feelings and those of the family. The hospice nurse or a grief counselor can help all members of the family to express and acknowledge their feelings of anger, fear, or guilt. S.J. and the family need to know that the grief reaction is normal and they should be taught what to expect and how each individual's needs can be met as S.J.'s death approaches.

5. A multidisciplinary team of nurses, health care providers, pharmacists, dietitians, nursing assistants, social workers, clergy, and volunteers is available to this family to provide care and support to the patient and family through hospice care.

6. **Nursing diagnoses:**
   - Compromised family coping *related to* inadequate coping mechanisms
   - Dysfunctional grieving *related to* blocked communication and guilt
   - Chronic pain *related to* ineffective pain management
   - Risk for impaired skin integrity *related to* immobility and emaciation
   - Risk for constipation *related to* decreased oral intake and effects of drugs
   - Ineffective breathing pattern *related to* weakness
   - Impaired physical mobility *related to* pain

CHAPTER 11

Answer Key

1. d. Substance abuse negatively affects psychologic, physiologic, and/or social functioning of an individual. The compulsive need for pleasure is psychologic dependence. Behavior to maintain addiction is addictive behavior. Absence of a substance causing withdrawal symptoms is physical dependence.

2. b. Tolerance is described. Relapse is when the person returns to substance use after a period of abstinence. Abstinence is avoidance of substance use. Withdrawal is the response that occurs after abrupt cessation of a substance.

3. a. Ask; b. Advise; c. Assess; d. Assist; e. Arrange

4. d. Nurses have a professional responsibility to help individuals stop smoking. The advice and motivation of health care professionals can be very helpful to the individual. Nurses should encourage and provide information to patients and work with physicians to identify ways to assist patients with quitting.

5. **Nicotine**
   a. Chronic obstructive pulmonary disease (COPD)
   b. Cancers: lung, mouth, larynx, esophagus, stomach, bladder, pancreas
   Others: coronary artery disease, peripheral artery disease, peptic ulcer disease, gastroesophageal reflux disease (GERD) (see Table 11-2)
   Alcohol
   a. Dementia
   b. Cirrhosis
   Others: peripheral neuropathy, increased risk for several cancers, anemia, coronary artery disease (CAD), hypertension, GERD (see Table 11-7)
   Cocaine and amphetamines
   a. Cardiac dysrhythmias
   b. Psychosis
   Others: nasal sores, myocardial infarction (MI), stroke (see Table 11-2)
   Opioids
   a. Gastric ulcer
   b. Glomerulonephritis
   Other: sexual dysfunction (see Table 11-2)
   Cannabis
   a. Bronchitis, chronic sinusitis
   b. Memory impairment
   Other: impaired immune system, reproductive dysfunction (see Table 11-2)

6. b, c, f. Cocaine and amphetamines cause nasal damage when snorted, sexual arousal, and tachycardia and

hypertension. Drowsiness and constricted pupils are seen with sedative-hypnotics and opioids. There is anorexia with cocaine, not increased appetite.

7. a. Opioids produce these physiologic responses. Although alcohol intake can cause euphoria, drowsiness, and slurred speech, the abuser of alcohol develops tolerance and does not usually have these manifestations. Effects of chronic alcohol abuse include impairment of all body systems (see Table 11-7). Cannabis produces euphoria, sedation, and hallucinations. Depressants may cause slurred speech and drowsiness but not euphoria or decreased respirations unless there is an overdose.

8. a. Seizures may be experienced with phenobarbital or a long-acting benzodiazepine. Tremors, chills, sweating, nausea, and cramps are seen with opioid withdrawal. Hallucinogens are least likely to have withdrawal symptoms. Suicidal thoughts and violence are more likely to occur in patients withdrawing from stimulants.

9. d. Nicotine replacement contains the same nicotine as that in tobacco but with slower absorption. The nicotine will help to prevent withdrawal symptoms because its use is reduced gradually. While the addiction is treated, the carcinogens and gases associated with tobacco smoke are eliminated.

10. a. 2; b. 3; c. 4; d. 1; e. 3; f. 4; g. 3

11. a. Headache is a common symptom of caffeine withdrawal and often occurs in heavy caffeine users who are NPO for diagnostic tests and surgery.

12. b, c, f. Seizures, gross tremors, visual and auditory hallucinations, and alcohol withdrawal delirium are the four major withdrawal syndrome manifestations. Apathy and depression occur in withdrawal from stimulants. Cardiovascular collapse is seen in sedative-hypnotic withdrawal.

13. c. Open-ended questions indicating that substance use is normal or at least understandable are helpful in eliciting information from patients who are reluctant to disclose substance use.

14. b. Smoking is the single most preventable cause of death and most smokers start smoking by age 16. If smoking in preadolescents and adolescents could be prevented, it is unlikely that these individuals would start smoking at a later age. Health problems associated with smoking and future use of other addictive substances would be significantly reduced.

15. a. Naloxone (Narcan) is given when opioids are the cause of central nervous system (CNS) depression.
    b. Flumazenil (Romazicon) is given when benzodiazepines are the cause of CNS depression.

16. a. The knowledge of when the patient last had alcohol intake will help the nurse to anticipate the onset of withdrawal symptoms. In patients with alcohol tolerance, the amount of alcohol and the blood alcohol concentration do not reflect impairment as consistently as in the nondrinker. The type of alcohol ingested is not important because in the body it is all alcohol.

17. c. An extreme autonomic nervous system response may be life threatening and requires immediate intervention. A quiet room is recommended but it should be well lighted to prevent misinterpretation of the environment and visual hallucinations. Cessation of alcohol intake causes low blood alcohol levels leading to withdrawal symptoms and fluids should be administered carefully to prevent dysrhythmias.

Patients should not be restrained if at all possible because injury and exhaustion can occur as patients struggle against restraint.

18. d. Alcohol-induced central nervous system (CNS) depression can lead to respiratory and circulatory failure in an alcoholic patient. Vital signs are monitored closely because of the increased risk of infection from malnutrition. Emergency magnesium would not be expected, although an emergency dose of thiamine may have been given before surgery. Pain medication requirements may be increased if the patient is cross-tolerant to opiates.

19. a. Because Wernicke's encephalopathy resulting from a thiamine deficiency is a possibility with chronic alcoholism, IV thiamine is often administered to intoxicated patients to prevent the development of Korsakoff's psychosis. Thiamine should be given before any glucose solutions are administered because glucose can precipitate Wernicke's encephalopathy. Benzodiazepines may be used for sedation and to minimize withdrawal symptoms but would not be given before thiamine, and haloperidol could be used if hallucinations occur.

20. d. The "five Rs" are used for individuals who are unwilling to quit tobacco use. The "five As" are used for individuals who want to quit tobacco use. Although cost, cough, cleanliness, and the use of Chantix as well as deduce, describe, decide, and deadline may be ways to assist this patient, these are not recommendations or clinical practice guidelines.

21. d. Older adult patients have the highest use of OTC and prescription drugs, and simultaneous use of these drugs with alcohol is a major problem. Illegal drug use is minimal in older patients except in long-term addicts.

Case Study

1. Because there is a tendency among substance abusers to take a variety of drugs simultaneously or in a sequence to obtain specific effects, as shown by this patient's history, he should be assessed for his pattern of abuse. Regular alcohol use in addition to other drug use or the common use of cocaine in combination with heroin or phencyclidine hydrochloride could cause withdrawal symptoms and additional manifestations that would complicate his condition and direct his care. Information about all of the drugs he uses, including both over-the-counter (OTC) and prescription drugs, is necessary to avoid withdrawal syndromes, acute intoxication, overdose, or drug interactions that might be life threatening.

2. The nurse should be aware that common behaviors that are likely to influence history taking from this patient include manipulation, denial, avoidance, underreporting or minimizing substance abuse, giving inaccurate information, and inaccurate self-reporting. To obtain reliable information about his drug abuse patterns, the nurse should first explain that information about his drug use is essential in the monitoring for and prevention of serious effects of the drugs while he already is very ill. Providing a need for the information and explaining how the information will be used may facilitate more honest responses by the patient. The nurse should question him without judgment about his pattern of abuse with open-ended questions such as "How much or how often do you use alcohol?" or "Can you describe how you use cocaine with other drugs?"

3. Physical effects of drug use that provide clues to drug abuse include collapsed and scarred veins used to inject drugs, nasal septum and mucosa damage, brown or black sputum production, and wound abscesses and cellulitis.

4. Continuous monitoring of this patient's vital signs, cardiac activity, level of consciousness, respiratory status, temperature, fluid and electrolyte balance, liver function, and renal function is necessary. Complications of cocaine toxicity that may occur and can be detected by monitoring include myocardial ischemia or infarction, heart failure, cardiopulmonary arrest, rhabdomyolysis with acute renal failure, stroke, respiratory distress or arrest, seizures, agitated delirium and hallucinations, electrolyte imbalances, and fever. In severe intoxication the patient may progress rapidly through stages of stimulation and depression, which may result in death. His use of cocaine with alcohol also increases his risk of liver injury and sudden death.

5. Assessment for neurologic, cardiovascular, and respiratory problems as described above is a critical nursing intervention in the patient with cocaine toxicity. In addition, the nurse should institute seizure precautions, provide airway management, keep open IV lines, administer medications aggressively as prescribed, and use cardiac life-support measures as indicated. Nursing interventions that are indicated for his anxiety, nervousness, and irritability include explaining procedures using short, simple, clear statements in a calm manner; providing a safe, secure environment; decreasing environmental stimuli; reinforcing reality orientation; and encouraging participation in relaxation exercises if possible.

6. Engaging an individual who is addicted to cocaine in treatment is difficult because of the intense craving for the drug and a strong denial that cocaine is addicting or that the individual cannot control it. Motivational interviewing is indicated in even this initial encounter with this patient. The nurse should help him to increase his awareness of risks and problems related to his current behavior and create doubt about the use of substances. Asking him what he thinks could happen if the behavior continues, pointing out the physical symptoms he is experiencing, and offering factual information about the risks of substance abuse are indicated. Often the only motivation for a patient with a cocaine addiction to enter a treatment program is family threats, loss of job or professional license, legal action, or major health consequences. A treatment program is indicated to provide him with new skills and an ability to deal with his addictive behavior.

7. **Nursing diagnoses:**
   - Ineffective health maintenance
   - Risk-prone health behavior
   - Impaired memory
   - Ineffective denial
   - Ineffective coping

   Collaborative problems:
   Potential complications: cardiopulmonary arrest, seizures, sudden death, cerebrovascular accident, acute renal failure

CHAPTER 12

Answer Key

1.

Clinical Manifestation	Chemical Mediators	Physiologic Change
Fever	Interleukin-1 (IL-1) released from mononuclear phagocytic cells and prostaglandin E_2 (PGE_2) synthesis	Increases the hypothalamic thermostatic set point
Redness	Histamine, kinins, prostaglandins	Vasodilation and hyperemia
Edema	Histamine, kinins, prostaglandins	Increased capillary permeability and fluid shift to tissues
Leukocytosis	Release of chemotactic factors at site of injury	Increased release of neutrophils and monocytes from bone marrow

2. d. *A shift to the left* is the term used to describe the presence of immature, banded neutrophils in the blood in response to an increased demand for neutrophils during tissue injury. Monocytes are increased in leukocytosis but are mature cells.

3. c. Chemotaxis involves the release of chemicals at the site of tissue injury that attract neutrophils and monocytes to the site of injury. The attraction is chemotaxis and when monocytes move from the blood into tissue, they are transformed into macrophages. The complement system is a pathway of chemical processes that results in cellular lysis, vasodilation, and increased capillary permeability causing the slowing of blood flow at the area.

4. d. The processes that are stimulated by the activation of the complement system include enhanced phagocytosis, increased vascular permeability, chemotaxis, and cellular lysis. Prostaglandins and leukotrienes are released by damaged cells and body temperature is increased by the action of prostaglandins and interleukins. All chemical mediators of inflammation increase the inflammatory response and, as a result, increase pain.

5. c. The nurse will encourage Rest to prevent further injury. Ice or cold compresses will be applied to decrease swelling with vasoconstriction. Compression will help to reduce edema and stop bleeding if it is occurring. Elevation will help to decrease edema and pain. The other options are not correct.

6. b. The injurious agent of chronic inflammation persists or repeatedly injures tissue. It lasts for weeks, months, or years. Infective endocarditis is a subacute inflammation that lasts for weeks or months. Neutrophils are the predominant cell type in acute inflammation. Lymphocytes and macrophages are the predominant cell types at chronic inflammation sites.

7. a. Labile cells of the skin, lymphoid organs, bone marrow, and mucous membranes divide constantly and regenerate rapidly following injury. Stable cells, such as those in bone, liver, pancreas, and kidney, regenerate only if they are injured and permanent cells found in neurons and cardiac muscle are not expected to regenerate when damaged.

8. a. 1; b. 10; c. 2; d. 4; e. 8; f. 6; g. 7; h. 9; i. 3; j. 5

9. c. The process of healing by secondary intention is essentially the same as primary healing. With the greater defect and gaping wound edges of an open wound, healing and granulation take place from the edges inward and from the bottom of the wound up, resulting in more granulation tissue and a much larger scar. In primary healing the edges of the wound may be sutured. Tertiary healing involves delayed suturing of two layers of granulation tissue together and may require debridement of necrotic tissue.

10. b. Adhesion is a band of scar tissue that forms between organs. It may occur in the abdominal cavity and cause intestinal obstruction. Infection could be seen with undernutrition or necrotic tissue but would not cause these symptoms. Contractures shorten the muscle or scar tissue but would not contribute to abdominal symptoms. Evisceration of an abdominal wound would occur sooner after surgery when the wound edges separate and the intestines protrude through the wound.

11. d. A fistula is an abnormal passage between organs or between a hollow organ and skin that will leak fluid or pus until it is healed. In this situation there may be a fistula between the vagina and rectum. The student nurse did not describe dehiscence, hemorrhage, or keloid scar formation.

12. c. Vitamin C aids healing with capillary synthesis and collagen production by fibroblasts. Fats provide synthesis of fatty acids and triglycerides used for cellular membranes. Protein corrects negative nitrogen balance from increased metabolism and contributes synthesis of immune factors, blood cells, fibroblasts, and collagen. Vitamin A aids in epithelialization, increasing collagen synthesis and tensile strength of the healing wound.

13. d. The B-complex vitamins are necessary coenzymes for many metabolic reactions, including protein, fat, and carbohydrate metabolism. Carbohydrates provide metabolic energy for inflammation and are protein sparing. Fluid is needed to replace that used in exudates as well as the extra fluid used for the increased metabolic rate required for healing.

14. d. A yellow wound would have creamy ivory to yellow-green exudate with soft necrotic tissue. A red wound will be a clean pink wound, possibly with serosanguineous drainage. A black wound would have adherent gray necrotic tissue.

15. b. A yellow wound would be treated with absorptive dressings. A red wound would be treated with a hydrocolloid dressing or a telfa dressing with antibiotic ointment to keep the wound moist and encourage granulation. A dry, sterile dressing would be used for a closed wound. A black wound would be treated with autolytic debridement or negative pressure wound therapy.

16. c. For the negative pressure therapy to work, a vacuum is created between the device and the wound so that the excess fluid, bacteria, and debris are removed from the wound. The wound is cleaned weekly or when the dressing is replaced. A hyperbaric oxygen therapy chamber is not used with a wound vac device. Nutrition must be maintained, as protein and electrolytes may be removed from the wound.

17. d. Hand washing is the most important factor in preventing infection transmission and is recommended before and after the use of gloves by the Centers for Disease Control and Prevention for all types of isolation precautions in health care facilities.

18. c. The immobility, mental deterioration, and possible neurologic disorder of the comatose patient present the greatest risk for tissue damage related to pressure. His Braden score is 9, which puts him at very high risk. Although obesity, hyperglycemia, advanced age, mental deterioration, malnutrition, and incontinence contribute to development of pressure ulcers, the risk is not as high with any of the other patients.

19. c. Relief of pressure on tissues is critical to prevention and treatment of pressure ulcers. Although pressure-reduction devices may relieve some pressure and lift sheets and trapeze bars prevent skin shear, they are no substitute for frequent repositioning of the patient. Massage is contraindicated if there is the presence of acute inflammation or possibly damaged blood vessels or fragile skin.

20. d. Stage IV pressure ulcers are full-thickness tissue loss with muscle, tendon, or bone exposed. Stage I pressure ulcers are intact skin with nonblanchable localized redness. Stage II pressure ulcers have a shallow open area with a red-pink wound bed. Stage III pressure ulcers exhibit full-thickness tissue loss without bone, tendon, or muscle exposure with possible tunneling into the tissue.

21. c. Stage III is full-thickness tissue loss; subcutaneous fat may be visible but bone, tendon, and muscle are not exposed. Option a. describes a Stage IV pressure ulcer, option b. describes a Stage II pressure ulcer, and option d. describes a Stage I pressure ulcer.

22. d, e. Measuring the size of the wound and repositioning do not require judgment, patient teaching, or evaluation of care. The other interventions listed relate to assessment, judgment, and teaching, all of which are responsibilities of the RN. However, the LPN can reinforce teaching by the RN.

Case Study

1. Pain, redness of leg, edema of leg, fever, elevated WBC

2. Purulent, which means that this is a yellow wound.

3. This is likely to be a venous ulcer because it is located medially above the ankle, is shallow with an irregular shape, is extremely painful, is infected, and is accompanied by edema. Venous ulcers occur distally because circulation may be compromised, as commonly seen in diabetic patients. (See eTable 12-1.)

4. The WBC count is increased, indicating a pronounced leukocytosis that would be seen in acute inflammation. Neutrophils are normally 50% to 70% of the WBCs and hers are increased to 80%, indicating an early response of neutrophils to tissue damage. She also has a "shift to the left" in that she has 12% bands. (Normally only 0% to

8% of the neutrophils in the blood are immature, banded-nucleus.) All of these findings are consistent with an acute inflammatory process.

5. History of diabetes, with possible circulatory impairment to lower extremities and altered blood glucose levels; increased weight; inadequate nutrients (e.g., vitamin C, protein, carbohydrates, zinc) for healing possible because of confinement to bed; has no one to help with meals; and the presence of infection in the wound

6. Acetaminophen acts on the heat-regulating center in the hypothalamus, resulting in peripheral dilation and heat loss. Mild to moderate fevers (up to 103°F [39.4° C]) are not usually harmful and may benefit defense mechanisms. Antipyretics are often prescribed only to control higher temperatures. To prevent acute swings in temperature and cycles of chilling and perspiring, antipyretics should be given regularly at 2- to 4-hour intervals as ordered.

7. The wound should be kept moist with frequent cleansing with high-quality tap water to remove nonviable tissue. Moist gauze, hydrocolloids, alginates, and/or hydrogel dressings will keep the wound moist and help with debridement, which would be the best choice in this infected wound.

8. Hand washing—Before application of clean gloves and immediately after gloves are removed
Clean gloves—When in contact with infectious material, such as dressings or linens with exudate
Biohazard disposal—Of dressings, gloves

9. **Nursing diagnoses:**
   - Acute pain *related to* inflammation of left leg
   - Impaired skin integrity *related to* wound left ankle
   - Hyperthermia *related to* inflammatory process and infection
   - Risk for deficient fluid volume *related to* an increased metabolic rate
   - Risk for imbalanced nutrition: less than body requirements *related to* decreased intake of essential nutrients and diabetes mellitus
   - Impaired physical mobility *related to* pain of left leg
   Collaborative problems:
   Potential complications: septicemia, hyperglycemia

CHAPTER 13

Answer Key

1. c. The phenotype is the observable characteristics of the individual. An allele is one of two or more alternative forms of a gene on a particular locus. Genomics is the study of all of a person's genes (the genome), including interactions of these genes with each other and the person's environment. Chromosomes are compact structures containing DNA and proteins that are present in nearly all cells of the body.

2. c. Genotype is the genetic identity of an individual without outward characteristics. A gene is the basic unit of heredity at a specific locus on a chromosome. Transmission of a disease from parent to child is termed hereditary. The pedigree is the family tree that contains the genetic characteristics and disorders of that particular family.

3. c, e. The age of disease diagnosis as well as the age and cause of death of three generations of the biological relatives will be most helpful for making lifestyle changes, if necessary, and family planning. Cholecystitis, prostate cancer, and kidney stones are not known to be genetically linked.

4. a. An error during meiosis causes an abnormal number of chromosomes. In Down syndrome there are three copies of chromosome 21. There can also be a copy of a chromosome missing. Translocation occurs when genetic material is exchanged between two chromosomes in a cell, such as in chronic myelocytic leukemia.

5.

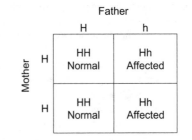

a. 50%
b. 50%

6. a, b, e. Genetic testing may raise psychologic and emotional issues if someone is identified with a positive result or as a carrier of a disease. A woman with a positive *BRCA1* or *BRCA2* genetic test may have a bilateral mastectomy to prevent breast cancer. Privacy issues also arise with genetic testing. Genetic testing can be used to provide the risk of a genetic condition only if both parents are tested. Newborn screening for phenylketonuria is done in all states. It may also be completed for congenital hypothyroidism and cystic fibrosis.

7. 25%. With autosomal recessive diseases, the pedigree will show 25% having the disease, 25% not having the disease, and 50% being carriers whether the offspring are male or female.

8. a. When both parents are tested, genetic testing can provide information about the couple's risk of having a child with a genetic condition by identifying changes in the genes tested. Not all diseases are genetically identified or familial disorders. Genetic testing kits are available but a genetic counselor will help them to understand the purpose of the testing, the pros and cons of having testing, and the emotional and medical impact of the test results.

9. a. Because Huntington's disease is an autosomal dominant disease and her father has it, she has a 50% chance of getting it. A positive result of genetic testing will mean that she will get the disease. There are no carriers of Huntington's disease and changing her lifestyle will not affect the disease diagnosis.

10. d. Multifactorial conditions are caused by a combination of genetic and environmental factors. In diabetes, several genes have been identified that increase the likelihood of getting diabetes. Single gene disorders result from a single gene mutation, for example, sickle cell disease. Chromosome disorders are caused by structural changes within chromosomes or an excess or deficiency of the genes in that locus. People are born with these disorders. Acquired genetic disorders occur when there is an error in replication or damage to DNA from toxins at some time in the person's life.

11. a. Trastuzumab is effective only for women whose breast cancer tumors have genes that overproduce the protein HER2. Testing for *BRCA* genes is used to identify women at risk for developing breast cancer. The stage of cancer is not relevant to whether this drug should be used.

12. a. Pharmacogenetic testing can assist the health care provider in prescribing the appropriate dosage of warfarin. Giving bivalirudin IV would be done only in the hospital. Clopidogrel and aspirin will not give the level of anticoagulant effect that warfarin does, as they are only platelet inhibitors and do not block clotting factors. Enoxoparin injections can be given at home but the patient is less likely to continue the therapy because of the injections and the added expense of the medication.

13. b. Yearly colonoscopies are done to monitor the polyp growth and remove polyps. A colectomy may be considered to prevent cancer. Changing the diet will not affect the growth of polyps that develop in the colon and potentially become cancerous. Gene therapy is still considered experimental therapy. If he has children, they will need to have genetic testing.

14. b. Because gene therapy is risky, it is currently studied only in research settings with diseases that have no cure. Gene therapy may inactivate or "knock out" a mutated malfunctioning gene. A new gene inserted into the body usually does not function without using a carrier molecule called a vector to deliver it to the target cells. It will replace a mutated gene with a healthy copy of a gene.

15. b. The hematopoietic stem cells are adult stem cells. The red blood cells are returned to the donor so that he or she does not become anemic. Although bone marrow aspirations and transplants may be done for recipients, stem cells are now usually obtained from the blood via large-bore intravenous needles.

Case Study

1. The nurse will provide accurate information pertaining to genetics and the genetic disease. This information should be tailored to the patient based on culture, religion, knowledge level, literacy, and preferred language. The nurse will identify and assess inheritance patterns and explain them to the patient and family through the use of family pedigrees (see Fig. 13-4 and Fig. 13-5) and the Punnett square (see Fig. 13-9). Maintain the patient's confidentiality and respect the patient's values and beliefs because genetic information may have major health and social implications. The nurse will also be an advocate for the patient and her family by facilitating access to genetics resources, such as a genetic clinical nurse or genetic counselor.

2. Duchenne muscular dystrophy (MD) is an X-linked recessive genetic disorder.

3. D.L. will not develop MD, as it is present at birth but usually does not become clinically apparent until age 3. Few individuals with MD live into adulthood. She is too old to develop MD now.

4. Because MD is X-linked recessive genetic disorder, if she carries the gene, each son will have a 50% chance of having the disease and each daughter will have a 50% chance of being a carrier of the gene.

5. This is an ethical concern. As with all medical information, this information should not be misused and the nurse should protect the privacy of the patient. The nurse should tell her about the Genetic Information Nondiscrimination Act (GINA), which protects her from discrimination by employers and health insurance companies.

CHAPTER 14

Answer Key

1. c. Innate immunity is present at birth and its primary role is first-line defense against pathogens. Innate immunity is not antigen specific so it can respond within minutes to an invading microorganism without prior exposure to that organism.

2. a, c, d. Passive acquired immunity is received from the injection of gamma globulin, provides immediate immunity, and may last for several weeks or months. Immunization with an antigen and the need for boosters contribute to active acquired immunity. Maternal immunoglobulins in the neonate provide temporary passive innate immunity.

3. a. Both B and T lymphocytes must be sensitized by a processed antigen to activate the immune response. Processing involves the taking up of an antigen by macrophages, expression of the antigen on the macrophage cell membrane, and presentation to the lymphocytes. Antigens do not need to be proteins and a few antigens may combine with larger molecules that are antigenic.

4. d. T cytotoxic cells directly attack antigens on the cell membrane of foreign pathogens and release cytolytic substances that destroy pathogens. Dendritic cells primarily capture antigens at sites of contact with the external environment and then transport the antigen to a T cell with specificity for the antigen. Natural killer cells are involved in cell-mediated immunity but are not considered T lymphocytes. CD4 cells (T helper cells) are involved in the regulation of cell-mediated immunity and humoral antibody response.

5. c. Interferon produces an antiviral effect in cells by reacting with viruses and inducing the formation of an antiviral protein that prevents new viruses from becoming assembled. Most cytokines are immunomodulatory and do not directly affect antigens, and cytokines such as interleukins may stimulate activation of immune cells.

6. b. Production of immunoglobulins (or antibodies) by B lymphocytes differentiated into plasma cells is the essential component in humoral immunity. Tumor surveillance and the production of cytokines are functions of T lymphocytes in cellular immunity and B lymphocytes do not directly attack antigens.

7. b. B lymphocytes activated in the bone marrow by the presentation of an antigen differentiate into many plasma cells that secrete immunoglobulins and only a few memory cells that retain recognition of the antigen as foreign. Helper cells are T lymphocytes and natural killer cells are large, granular lymphocytes that are neither B nor T lymphocytes. The spleen filters foreign substances from the blood. The thymus differentiates T lymphocytes. The bursa of Fabricius is found in birds, not humans.

8. d. IgM immunoglobulin is predominant in the primary immune response and produces antibodies against ABO blood antigens.

9. a, d. IgA is passed to the neonate in the colostrum and IgG crosses the placenta for fetal protection.

10. a, b. Immunoglobulin E (IgE) assists in parasitic infections and causes allergic reactions. IgA protects body surfaces and mucous membranes. IgD assists in B-lymphocyte differentiation and is present on the lymphocyte surface. IgG is predominant in the secondary immune response.

11. a, c, d. Functions of cell-mediated immunity include fungal infections, rejection of foreign tissue, contact hypersensitivity reactions, immunity against pathogens that survive inside cells, and destruction of cancer cells and tuberculosis. Transfusion reactions are from humoral immunity.

12. d. Aging has a pronounced effect on the thymus, which decreases in size and activity, leading to a decline in T cells and cell-mediated immunity. T-cell reduction is responsible for decreased tumor surveillance, resulting in an increase in cancer. B-cell activity also declines with advancing age but the bone marrow is relatively unaffected by increasing age. Circulating autoantibodies increase and are a factor in autoimmune diseases.

13. c. When sensitized T lymphocytes attack antigens or release cytokines that attract macrophages and cause tissue damage, a type IV or delayed hypersensitivity reaction is occurring with transplant rejections as well as contact dermatitis, some drug sensitivity reactions, and hypersensitivity reactions to bacterial fungal and viral infections.

14. a, b, c, d, e, g. These are the anaphylactic or atopic responses that can be seen with a type I or IgE-mediated hypersensitivity reaction to specific allergens. Contact dermatitis is seen with a type IV or delayed hypersensitivity reaction. Transfusion reactions and Goodpasture syndrome are seen with a type II or cytotoxic hypersensitivity reaction.

15. c. With rheumatoid arthritis and acute glomerulonephritis, type III or immune-complex mediated hypersensitivity reaction is seen when the antigens combined with IgG and IgM are too small to be removed by the mononuclear phagocytic system and are deposited in tissue, which activates the complement system.

16. d. The best drugs for allergic rhinitis are antihistamines. However, of those listed, minor sympathomimetic/decongestant drugs are used primarily for allergic rhinitis. Nasal corticosteroids may be used for seasonal allergic rhinitis; oral corticosteroids are used briefly if the patient is incapacitated. Immunotherapy is used when the allergen cannot be avoided and after it is found that drug therapy is not effective. Antipruritic drugs are topical and used to relieve itching.

17. a, f. Wheezing and a feeling of impending doom can both occur with anaphylaxis. Other common physiologic systemic anaphylactic responses are hypotension; rapid, weak pulse; dilated pupils; and edema and itching at the injection site. An arm rash would be more likely with a simple allergic reaction.

18. a. 2; b. 4; c. 1; d. 6; e. 5; f. 3; g. 7; h, 8. Airway is always first and oxygen will help with the dyspnea. Knowing that the patient has hypotension leads to placing the patient recumbent with elevated legs. Knowing that the patient has a bee sting, the stinger will be removed next. Then an IV is started. Anticipation of intubation with severe respiratory distress is also needed after the initial interventions.Having diphenhydramine and nebulized albuterol as well as methylprednisolone IV available is important, as they may be needed.

19. c. Allergic individuals have elevated levels of IgE that react with allergens to produce symptoms. Immunotherapy involves injecting allergen extracts that will stimulate increased IgG that combines more readily with allergens without releasing histamine. The goal is to keep the "blocking" level of IgG high.

20. d. This describes a type IV allergic contact dermatitis that is caused by chemicals used in the manufacturing process of latex gloves. A type I allergic reaction that is a response to the natural rubber latex proteins occurs within minutes of contact with the proteins and may manifest with reactions ranging from skin redness to full-blown anaphylactic shock. Powder-free gloves will avoid respiratory exposure to latex proteins but nonlatex gloves are more helpful. Avoidance of oil-based hand creams when wearing gloves can also help to prevent latex allergic reactions.

21. b. Multiple chemical sensitivities are commonly seen with scented products, paint fumes, petroleum products, smoke, pesticides, plastics, and synthetic products and occur in Gulf War veterans. Symptoms vary but include headache, sore throat, breathing problems, nausea as well as pain, skin rash, gastrointestinal (GI) problems, confusion, difficulty concentrating, memory problems, and mood changes. Diagnosis is made based on the patient's health history, as there is no test to diagnose it.

22. c, d. Autoimmune causative factors are genetic susceptibility and initiation of autoreactivity by a trigger. Females and older patients are more likely to develop autoimmune diseases. A viral infection may be a trigger but medications and hormones may also be triggers.

23. c. Plasmapheresis is the removal of plasma from the blood and in autoimmune disorders is used to remove pathogenic substances found in plasma, such as autoantibodies, antigen-antibody complexes, and inflammatory mediators. Circulating blood cells are not affected by plasmapheresis, nor are blood cells added.

24. d. A crossmatch mixes recipient serum with donor lymphocytes. A positive crossmatch shows that the recipient has cytotoxic antibodies to the donor and this organ cannot be transplanted without hyperacute rejection occurring. A negative crossmatch indicates that it is safe to do the transplant.

25. c. Drug-induced immunosuppression with antineoplastic agents and corticosteroids is the most common cause of secondary immunodeficiency. Chronic stress and AIDS, not HIV, may cause secondary immunodeficiency but they are not the most common causes. Primary immunodeficiency is caused by common variable hypogammaglobulinemia.

26. d, e, f. Acute transplant rejection occurs when the recipient's T cytotoxic lymphocytes attack the foreign organ. Long-term immunosuppressants help to combat it and it is usually reversible with additional immunosuppression. Treatment of chronic rejection is supportive and irreversible with infiltration of the organ with B and T lymphocytes. Hyperacute rejection occurs when the recipient has antibodies against the donor's human leukocyte antigen (HLA), is most common with kidney transplants, and results in the organ needing to be removed.

27. b. Chronic rejection of a kidney transplant manifests as fibrosis and glomerulopathy (seen with proteinuria, edema, and renal failure), occurs over months or years, and is irreversible. Acute rejection occurs in the first 6 months after transplant. Hyperacute rejection occurs minutes to hours after transplantation and is rare. "Delayed rejection" is not a term used with transplantation.

28. d. Standard immunotherapy involves the use of three different immunosuppressants that act in different ways:

a calcineurin inhibitor (cyclosporine, tacrolimus), a corticosteroid, and the antimetabolite mycophenolate mofetil. Although cyclosporine is still used, tacrolimus is the most frequently prescribed calcineurin inhibitor. Azathioprine (Imuran) is similar to mycophenolate mofetil and they cannot be taken together.

29. c. Graft-versus-host (GVH) disease is occurring as the graft is rejecting the host tissue, which usually manifests in a pruritic or painful skin rash; in the GI tract with diarrhea, severe abdominal pain, GI bleeding, and malabsorption; or in the liver with mild jaundice and elevated liver enzymes. GVH disease is more effectively prevented with immunosuppressive agents than treated.

Case Study

1. The comprehensive assessment should include past health history of respiratory problems and any allergies, medication use and response, family history of allergies, food intolerances, GI problems, activity intolerance symptoms, presence of pets, and altered home or work environment. The eyes, ears, nose, and throat should be assessed for drainage and discomfort. The lung sounds should also be assessed.

2. IgE is the immunoglobulin involved in most allergic reactions. Chemical mediators that would be active in the patient's allergic rhinitis include histamine, serotonin, leukotrienes, prostaglandins, eosinophil chemotactic factor of anaphylaxis (ECF-A), kinins, bradykinin, and complement anaphylatoxins.

3. The procedure would involve either the scratch test or the prick test technique to identify specific allergens. Intradermal allergy testing is not used unless other methods do not result in conclusive reactions. An allergy blood test for IgE antibodies to specific allergens may be used if the patient cannot tolerate the many needle sticks or scratches needed for the skin test, has a skin disorder, or cannot stop using antihistamines or corticosteroids before skin testing. The patient must have been taught not to take antihistamines or corticosteroids for a few days before the test to achieve a positive result. A positive result is manifested by a local wheal-and-flare reaction that occurs within minutes after insertion of the extract and may last for 8 to 12 hours.

4. Precautions to prevent or treat severe allergic reactions are important:
   - Never leave the patient alone during the testing period.
   - Always have the following available:
     ○ Emergency equipment (oral airway, laryngoscope, endotracheal tubes, oxygen, tourniquet, IV therapy equipment, cardiac monitor with defibrillator
     ○ Essential drugs (epinephrine, antihistamines, corticosteroids, vasopressors)
   - Severe local reactions should be treated with removal of the extract and application of antiinflammatory topical cream to the site.

5. Antihistamines relieve allergic symptoms by competing with histamine for H_1 histamine receptors and thus block the effect of histamine. The action of most antihistamines is not very effective against histamine-induced bronchoconstriction. This patient should be taught to take antihistamines on a regular basis because he has perennial allergic rhinitis that is not limited to contact with seasonal allergens. He also must be cautioned about the common

side effects of antihistamines: drowsiness and impaired coordination, dry mouth, GI upset, urinary retention, blurred vision, and dizziness.

6. Household dust is controlled with air conditioners and air filtration systems in the home as well as daily damp dusting and frequent vacuuming with high-filtration vacuum bags.

7. Advantages of using sublingual immunotherapy include a lower risk of severe adverse reactions and being able to do it at home. However, sublingual immunotherapy is considered investigational, as the Food and Drug Administration (FDA) considers this an "off-label" use, and is not covered by most insurance plans.

8. Precautions with subcutaneous immunotherapy are as follows.
   - Always having the following available:
     ○ Health care provider
     ○ Emergency equipment (oral airway, laryngoscope, endotracheal tubes, oxygen, tourniquet, IV therapy equipment, cardiac monitor with defibrillator)
     ○ Emergency drugs (epinephrine, antihistamines, corticosteroids, vasopressors)
   - Administer the extract in an extremity away from a joint so that a tourniquet can be applied for a severe reaction.
   - Always aspirate for blood before injection of the allergen extract.
   - Assess for systemic reactions manifested by pruritus, urticaria, sneezing, laryngeal edema, and hypotension.
   - Observe the patient for systemic reactions for 20 minutes following the injection.

9. **Nursing diagnoses:**
   - Ineffective health maintenance *related to* insufficient knowledge of medications and methods of decreasing exposure to allergens
   - Risk for injury *related to* effects of antihistamines, skin testing, and immunotherapy
   Collaborative problems:
   Potential complication: anaphylaxis

CHAPTER 15

Answer Key

1. a, b, c, e. Infectious agents, such as the human immunodeficiency virus (HIV) and hantavirus, have evolved to affect humans through closer association with animals as human populations push into wild animal habitats. The transfer of infectious agents from animals to humans has also resulted in West Nile virus and avian flu. Bacterial infections have also become untreatable as the result of genetic and biochemical changes stimulated by unnecessary or inadequate exposure to antibiotics. The increased number of immunosuppressed and chronically ill people also increase the emergence of untreatable infections.

2. Methicillin-resistant *Staphylococcus aureus* (MRSA); vancomycin-resistant enterococci (VRE); penicillin-resistant *Streptococcus pneumoniae* (PRSP).

3. d, e. Hand washing and the use of alcohol-based sanitizers and personal protective equipment (e.g., gloves) will prevent health care–associated infections (HAIs). Although the other interventions will not hurt a patient and they are good practice, they will not prevent HAIs.

4. b. Contact precautions are used with standard precautions when microorganisms can be transmitted by direct patient contact.

5. a. A mask will be worn even 3 feet from the patient to avoid droplet transmission. The gown and gloves will be used as with standard precautions, when working closely with the patient and there is a risk of contamination.

6. b. Infection in older adults often has atypical presentations, cognitive and behavioral changes occurring before fever, pain, or altered laboratory values. Fatigue and ICU psychosis (if the patient is in the ICU) could be occurring but these are not as dangerous for the patient as infection can be. Cognitive and behavioral changes are not typical manifestations of medication allergy.

7. d. One of the most important factors in the development of antibiotic-resistant strains of organisms has been inappropriate use of antibiotics. Following directions regarding timing and completion of antibiotics will not allow antibiotic-resistant bacteria to develop. Antibiotics are not effective against viruses, which cause colds and flu. Not completing the antibiotic may allow the hardiest bacteria to survive and multiply and the potential development of an antibiotic-resistant infection.

8. a. women; b. vascular access; c. first 2 to 6 months of infection; d. HIV-infected mothers using no therapy; e. needle-stick exposure to HIV-infected blood

9. a. 3; b. 5; c. 1; d. 6; e. 2; f. 7; g. 4

10.
Drug	Mechanism of Action
Entry inhibitors	Inhibit entry into cell (step 2 from Question 9)
Reverse transcriptase inhibitors	Inhibit conversion of viral RNA to single-stranded viral DNA with the assistance of the enzyme reverse transcriptase (step 3 from Question 9)
Integrase inhibitors	Viral DNA is spliced into cell genome using the enzyme integrase (step 5 from Question 9)
Protease inhibitors	Inhibit cutting of the long strands of viral RNA in the presence of the enzyme protease (step 7 from Question 9)

11. a. Activated CD4$^+$ T cells are an ideal target for HIV because these cells are attracted to the site of concentrated HIV in the lymph nodes, where they become infected through viral contact with CD4 receptors. CD4$^+$ T cells normally are a major component of the immune system and their infection renders the immune system ineffective against HIV and other agents. The virus does not affect natural killer cells and B lymphocytes are functional early in the disease, as evidenced by positive antibody titers against HIV. Monocytes do ingest infected cells and may become sites of HIV replication and spread the virus to other tissue but this does not make the immune response ineffective.

12. b. The symptoms of acute HIV infection occur 2 to 4 weeks after initial infection and last for 1 to 2 weeks. The CD4$^+$ T-cell counts fall temporarily but quickly return to baseline levels. Burkitt's lymphoma and *Pneumocystis jiroveci* pneumonia are two of the opportunistic diseases that can occur in acquired immunodeficiency syndrome (AIDS). Persistent fevers and drenching night sweats occur in the symptomatic infection stage.

13. d. Cytomegalovirus retinitis could be an opportunistic viral infection that occurs when AIDS is diagnosed. Flu-like symptoms occur in the acute HIV infection stage. CD4$^+$ T cells drop to 200–500/μL and oral hairy leukoplakia are seen in the symptomatic infection stage of HIV.

14. d. Organisms that are nonvirulent or that cause limited or localized diseases in an immunocompetent person can cause severe, debilitating, and life-threatening infections in persons with impaired immune function.

15. c. *Pneumocystis jiroveci* infection is characterized by pneumonia with a dry, nonproductive cough. *Cryptococcus* infection may cause fungal meningitis. Non-Hodgkin's lymphoma is diagnosed by lymph node biopsy. Cytomegalovirus infection is characterized by viral retinitis, stomatitis, esophagitis, gastritis, or colitis.

16. a. Hyperpigmented lesions of skin, lungs, and GI tract are seen in Kaposi sarcoma. *Candida albicans* is a common yeast infection of the mouth, esophagus, GI tract, or vagina. Herpes simplex type 1 infection has oral and mucocutaneous vesicular and ulcerative lesions. Varicella-zoster virus infection or shingles is a maculopapular, pruritic rash and is treated with acyclovir.

17. b. Because there is a median delay of several weeks after infection before antibodies can be detected, testing during this "window" may result in false-negative results. Risky behaviors that may expose a person to HIV should be discussed and possible scheduling for repeated testing done. Positive results on initial testing will be verified by additional testing. Identification of sexual partners and prevention practices are important but do not relate immediately to the testing situation.

18. c. Although the "rapid" test is highly reliable and results are available in about 20 minutes, if results are positive from any testing, blood will be drawn for more specific enzyme immunosorbent assay (EIA) or Western blot testing and another visit will be necessary to obtain the results of the additional testing. CD4$^+$ T-cell counts are not used for screening but rather are used to monitor the progression of HIV infection and new assay tests measure resistance of the virus to antiviral drugs.

19. b. The use of potent combination antiretroviral therapy limits the potential for development of resistance to antiretroviral medications, the major factor that limits the ability of antiretroviral drugs to inhibit virus replication and delay disease progression. The drugs selected should be ones with which the patient has not been previously treated and that are not cross-resistant with antiretroviral agents previously used by the patient.

20. c. Guidelines for initiating antiretroviral therapy (ART) are being updated continuously because of the development of alternative drugs and problems with long-term side effects and compliance with regimens. In the past, ART was always recommended at the time of HIV infection diagnosis but today new guidelines suggest that treatment can be delayed until higher levels of immunosuppression are observed. Whenever treatment is started, an important

consideration is the patient's readiness to initiate ART because adherence to drug regimens is a critical component of the therapy.

21. b. An undetectable viral load in the blood does not mean that the virus is gone; it is still present in lymph nodes and other organs. Transmission is still possible and use of protective measures must be continued.

22. c. Pneumococcal pneumonia, influenza, and hepatitis A and B vaccines should be given as early as possible in HIV infection while there is still immunologic function. Isoniazid (INH) is used for 9 to 12 months only if a patient has reactive purified protein derivative (PPD) >5 mm, has had high-risk exposure, or has prior untreated positive PPD. Trimethoprim/sulfamethoxazole (TMP/SMX) is initiated when CD4+ T-cell count is <200/μL or when there is a history of *Pneumocystis jiroveci* pneumonia (PCP) and varicella-zoster immune globulin (VZIG) is indicated only after significant exposure to chickenpox or shingles in patients with no history of disease or a negative varicella-zoster virus (VZV) antibody test. Prophylaxis for other opportunistic diseases is noted in eTable 15-2.

23. d. After a patient has positive HIV antibody testing and is in acute disease, the overriding goal is to keep the viral load as low as possible and to maintain a functioning immune system. The nurse should provide teaching regarding ways to enhance immune function to prevent the onset of opportunistic diseases in addition to teaching about the spectrum of the infection, options for care, signs and symptoms to watch for, ways to prevent HIV spread, and ways to adhere to treatment regimens.

24. **Sexual Intercourse**
   - Abstain from sexual activity
   - Noncontact sexual activities (outercourse)
   - Use of male or female condoms during sexual activity

   Drug Use
   - Abstain from drug use
   - Do not share equipment
   - Use alternative routes to injecting
   - Do not have sexual intercourse while under the influence of drugs

   Perinatal Transmission
   - Use family planning to avoid pregnancy
   - Use antiretroviral therapy to reduce the risk of transmission

25. a. All of the nursing interventions are appropriate for a patient with impaired memory but the priority is the safety of the patient when cognitive and behavioral problems impair the ability to maintain a safe environment.

Case Study

1. Posttest counseling should include the following:
   - Provide resources for medical and emotional support, with immediate assistance.
   - Evaluate suicide risk.
   - Determine the need to test others who have had risky contact with the patient.
   - Discuss retesting to verify results.
   - Discuss risk reduction.
   - Encourage optimism: treatment options are available, health habits can improve immune function, the patient can visit HIV-infected people, the patient is

infected with HIV but does not have AIDS. Empower the patient to identify needs, direct care, and seek services.

2. Vague symptoms of fatigue, headaches, lymphadenopathy, and night sweats are characteristic of asymptomatic infection. CD4+ T-cell counts are usually >500/μL in asymptomatic infection. This patient experienced what could have been acute infection only 2 weeks ago and it is unlikely that he would be at a later stage than asymptomatic infection.

3. Additional testing at this visit should include the following:
   - Complete blood count (CBC) with differential
   - Another CD4+ T-cell count
   - Viral load assessment (bDNA or PCR)
   - Hepatitis B and/or hepatitis C serology
   - Purified protein derivative (PPD) skin test by Mantoux method
   - Liver function tests
   - Phenotype assay to determine medications to use for the patient
   - Genotype assay to detect drug-resistant viral mutations

4. Pneumococcal, influenza, and hepatitis A and B vaccines should be given. INH should be given if PPD is >0.5 mm reactive or, if the patient has had high-risk exposure, nutritional support and education should be provided. Varicella-zoster immune globulin (VZIG) should be given if the patient is exposed to chickenpox or shingles with no past disease.

5. The drug therapy is not curative but has resulted in dramatic improvements in many HIV-infected patients by maintaining immune function and decreasing viral load. It is critical to take the drug combination specifically as prescribed to prevent the development of resistance by the virus. If the drugs cannot be taken for any reason, the health care provider or nurse practitioner should be notified. There are many side effects of the drugs, some of which can be controlled and are not serious but some of which can prevent use of the drugs. It is important to report any changes in the patient's condition or symptoms that develop. The patient will be closely monitored and viral loads will be assessed 2 to 4 weeks after therapy is started and periodically after that.

6. Genotype and phenotype testing can be done to test for resistance to antiretroviral drugs. The genotype assay detects drug-resistant viral mutations that are present in the reverse transcriptase and protease genes. The phenotype assay measures the growth of the virus in various concentrations of antiretroviral drugs (similar to bacteria-antibiotic sensitivity tests).

7. **Nursing diagnoses:**
   - Anxiety
   - Fear
   - Ineffective denial
   - Anticipatory grieving
   - Deficient knowledge
   - Fatigue
   - Risk-prone health behavior

   Collaborative problems:

   Potential complications: opportunistic infections, opportunistic malignancies, myelosuppression

CHAPTER 16

Answer Key

1. a. Lung cancer is the leading cause of cancer deaths in the United States for both women and men and smoking cessation is one of the most important cancer prevention behaviors. Approximately one half of cancer-related deaths in the U.S. are related to tobacco use, unhealthy diet, physical inactivity, and obesity. Cancers of the reproductive organs are the second leading cause of cancer deaths.

2. d. Malignant cells proliferate indiscriminately and continuously and also lose the characteristic of contact inhibition, growing on top of and in between normal cells. Cancer cells usually do not proliferate at a faster rate than normal cells, nor can cell cycles be skipped in proliferation. However, malignant proliferation is continuous, unlike normal cells.

3. a. Cancer cells become more fetal and embryonic (undifferentiated) in appearance and function and some produce new proteins, such as carcinoembryonic antigen (CEA) and α-fetoprotein (AFP), on cell membranes that reflect a return to more immature functioning. The other options are unrelated to CEA and AFP.

4. d. The major difference between malignant and benign cells is the ability of malignant tumor cells to invade and metastasize. Benign tumors can cause death by expansion into normal tissues and organs. Benign tumors are more often encapsulated and often grow at the same rate as malignant tumors.

5. d. Alkylating agents are used to treat Hodgkin's lymphoma and are carcinogens associated with initiation of acute myelogenous leukemia. Working with radiation would lead to a higher incidence of bone cancer. Epstein-Barr virus is seen in vitro with Burkitt's lymphoma. Intense tanning or exposure to ultraviolet radiation is associated with skin cancers.

6. a. Mutations in the *p53* tumor suppressor gene have been found in many cancers, including bladder, breast, colorectal, esophageal, liver, lung, and ovarian cancers. *APC* gene mutations increase a person's risk for familiar adenomatous polyposis, which is a precursor for colorectal cancer. *BRCA1* and *BRCA2* mutations increase the risk for breast and ovarian cancer.

7. a, c, d. Promoting factors such as obesity and tobacco smoke promote cancer in the promotion stage of cancer development. Eliminating risk factors can reduce the chance of cancer development as the activity of promoters is reversible in this stage. Increased growth, invasion, and metastasis are seen in the progressive stage.

8. b. Carcinoma in situ has the histologic features except invasion. Evasion of the immune system by cancer cells by various methods is immunologic escape. Oncogenic factors are capable of causing cellular alterations associated with cancer. Tumor cell surface antigens that stimulate an immune response are tumor-associated antigens.

9. a. Oncogenes are the mutation of protooncogenes, which then induce tumors. Oncogenic viruses cause genetic alterations and mutations that allow the cell to express the abilities and properties it had in fetal development and may lead to cancer. Oncofetal antigens are antigens that are found on the surface and inside the cancer cells. They are an expression of the cells usually associated with embryonic or fetal periods of

life and may be used as tumor markers to monitor treatment. Tumor angiogenesis factor is the substance within tumors that promotes blood vessel development.

10. d. Meningeal sarcoma is from the embryonal mesoderm, is located in the meninges, and is malignant. A meningioma has the same tissue of origin and anatomic site but it is benign. Meningitis is inflammation or infection of the meninges. Meningocele is a hernia cyst filled with cerebrospinal fluid.

11. c. The breast cancer origination gives it the anatomic classification of a carcinoma. Grade II has moderate abnormal cells with moderate differentiation. $T_1N_1M_0$ represents a small tumor with only minimal regional spread to the lymph nodes and no metastasis. Sarcomas originate from embryonal mesoderm or connective tissue, muscle, bone, and fat. Leukemias and lymphomas originate from the hematopoietic system. The other histologic grading and TNM classifications do not represent this patient's tumor.

12. b. Healthy men and women should have a colonoscopy every 10 years, an annual fecal occult blood test, or a barium enema every 5 years. These frequencies may change depending on the results. Annual PSA and digital rectal exams screen for prostate problems, although the decision to test is made by the patient with his health care provider.

13. b. Although other tests may be used in diagnosing the presence and extent of cancer, biopsy is the only method by which cells can be definitely determined to be malignant.

14. a. A simple mastectomy can be done to prevent breast cancer in women with high risk and can be used to control, cure, or provide palliative care for breasts with cancerous tumors. A mastectomy would not be used for biopsy or otherwise to establish a diagnosis of cancer.

15. a. 4; b. 1; c. 3; d. 2; e. 3; f. 2; g. 1; h. 2. Mammoplasty is done for rehabilitation post mastectomy. A bowel resection and debulking procedure to enhance radiation therapy are done to cure or control cancer. Cordotomy for pain control and colostomy to bypass bowel obstruction are done for palliation. Supportive care includes insertion of a feeding tube, placement of a central venous catheter, and surgical fixation of bones at risk for pathologic fracture.

16. b. Neuroblastomas are cured with chemotherapy. A positive response of cancer cells to chemotherapy is most likely in solid or hematopoietic tumors that arise from tissue that has a rapid rate of cellular proliferation and new tumors with cells that are rapidly dividing. A state of optimum health and a positive attitude of the patient will also promote the success of chemotherapy.

17. a. Nitrosureas are cell cycle phase–nonspecific, break the DNA helix, and cross the blood-brain barrier. Antimetabolites are cell cycle phase–specific drugs that mimic essential cellular metabolites to interfere with DNA synthesis. Mitotic inhibitors are cell cycle phase–specific drugs that arrest mitosis. Antitumor antibiotics bind with DNA to block RNA production.

18. b. One of the major concerns with the IV administration of vesicant chemotherapeutic agents is infiltration or extravasation of drugs into tissue surrounding the infusion site. When infiltrated into the skin, vesicants cause pain, severe local breakdown, and necrosis. Specific measures to ensure adequate dilution, patency, and early detection of extravasation and treatment are important.

19. a. Intravesical regional chemotherapy is administered into the bladder via a urinary catheter. Leukemia is treated with IV chemotherapy. Osteogenic sarcoma is treated with intraarterial chemotherapy via vessels supplying the tumor. Metastasis to the brain is treated with intraventricular or intrathecal chemotherapy via an Ommaya reservoir or lumbar punctures.

20. d. Intraperitoneal regional chemotherapeutic administration is used to treat metastasis from a primary colorectal cancer. Intrathecal administration is used with the spinal cord or the brain. Intraarterial administration is used to deliver chemotherapy to tumors via specific vessels. IV administration is used for systemic administration.

21. b. Patients should always be taught what to expect during a course of chemotherapy, including side effects and expected outcome. Side effects of chemotherapy are serious but it is important that patients be informed about what measures can be taken to help them to cope with the side effects of therapy. Hair loss related to chemotherapy is usually reversible and wigs, scarves, or turbans can be used during and following chemotherapy until the hair grows back.

22. c. Tissue that is actively proliferating, such as GI mucosa, esophageal and oropharyngeal mucosa, and bone marrow, exhibits early acute responses to radiation therapy. Radiation ionization breaks chemical bonds in DNA, which renders cells incapable of surviving mitosis. This loss of proliferative capacity yields cellular death at the time of division for both normal cells and cancer cells but cancer cells are more likely to be dividing because of the loss of control of cellular division. Cartilage, bone, kidney, and nervous tissues that proliferate slowly manifest subacute or late responses.

23. d. Avoiding sources of excessive heat and cold will prevent damage to the skin. Only nonmedicated, nonperfumed lotions or creams (e.g., calendula ointment, aloe gel, Aquaphor) are recommended for dry skin. The area should be exposed to air if possible. Gentle cleansing, thorough rinsing, and patting the treatment area dry are recommended.

24. b. Brachytherapy is the implantation or insertion of radioactive materials directly into the tumor or in proximity to the tumor and may be curative. The patient is a source of radiation and in addition to implementing the principles of time, distance, and shielding, film badges should be worn by caregivers to monitor the amount of radiation exposure. Computerized dosimetry and simulation are used in external radiation therapy.

25. a. Walking programs scheduled during the time of day when the patient feels better are a way for patients to keep active without overtaxing themselves and help to combat the depression caused by inactivity. Ignoring the fatigue or overstressing the body can make symptoms worse and the patient should rest before activity and as necessary.

26. b. Alkylating chemotherapeutic agents and high-dose radiation are most likely to cause secondary malignancies as a late effect of treatment. The other conditions are not known to be late effects of radiation or chemotherapy.

27. c. Biologic therapies are normal components of the immune system and are used therapeutically to restore, augment, or modulate host immune system mechanisms. They have direct antitumor effects or other biologic effects to assist in immune activity against cancer cells. Virtually all biologic therapies may cause a flu-like syndrome. The other options are not correct.

28. c. The nadir is the point of the lowest blood counts after chemotherapy is started and it is the time when the patient is most at risk for infection. Because infection is the most common cause of morbidity and death in cancer patients, identification of risk and interventions to protect the patient are of the highest priority. The other problems will be treated but they are not the priority.

29. c. An allogenic hematopoietic stem cell or bone marrow transplant is one in which peripheral stems cells or bone marrow from an HLA-matched donor is infused into a patient who has received high doses of chemotherapy, with or without radiation, to eradicate cancerous cells. In an autologous bone marrow transplant, the patient's own bone marrow is removed before therapy to destroy the bone marrow. The marrow is treated to remove cancer cells and may be infused shortly after conditioning treatment or frozen and stored for later use. With either source, the new bone marrow will take several weeks to produce new blood cells and protective isolation is necessary during this time.

30. a. Hyperkalemia and hyperuricemia are characteristic of tumor lysis syndrome, which is the result of rapid destruction of large numbers of tumor cells. Signs include hyperuricemia that causes acute kidney injury, hyperkalemia, hyperphosphatemia, and hypocalcemia. To prevent renal failure and other problems, the primary treatment includes increasing urine production using hydration therapy and decreasing uric acid concentrations using allopurinol (Zyloprim).

31. d. The priority in pain management is to obtain a comprehensive history of the patient's pain. This will determine the medications most useful for this patient's pain to enable giving the dose that relieves the pain with the fewest side effects. Teaching the patient about the lack of tolerance and addiction associated with effective cancer pain management will also be important for this patient's pain management.

32. a, b, d. Feeling in control, having a strong support system, and the potential of cure or control of the cancer will have a positive effect on coping with the diagnosis. The other options will make coping more difficult for the patient. (See Table 16-19.)

Case Study

1. Chemotherapy-induced bone marrow suppression is probably the most relevant factor in the patient's decreased WBC and neutrophil count. Inadequate protein intake would also contribute to impaired recovery of normal blood cells.

2. A temperature of 99.4°F (37.4°C) in an immunosuppressed patient is a significant finding for infection. He also has warm skin, with some degree of dehydration. His risk of infection is high, with a WBC count of 3200/μL and neutrophils of 500/μL. The risk for infection increases when neutrophils are <1000/μl.

3. Assess for sore throat, chest pain, persistent cough, urinary symptoms, skin lesions, rectal pain, or confusion. Also note the catheter site for chemotherapy as a possible source of infection.

4. His nausea, vomiting, and anorexia as well as any other side effects of chemotherapy may contribute to his negative

attitude. Negative attitude may also be promoted by lack of social support, an inability to cope with stress, an inability to express his feelings and concerns, the lack of control he may be feeling, a past negative experience with cancer in a friend, and lack of information about expected results of treatment.

5. **Nursing measures:**
   - Use antiemetic protocols to control treatment-related nausea and vomiting.
   - Offer small, frequent feedings of bland, high-calorie, high-protein foods (e.g., milk shake, eggnog, cottage cheese) in a pleasant environment.
   - Provide or encourage frequent oral care.
   - Use relaxation techniques and distraction when the patient is nauseated.
   - Offer any fluids or foods that the patient can tolerate and that may be appealing to him.
   - Avoid nagging or being judgmental about food intake.
   - Keep a food diary to track daily calories and fluids.

6. Metastasis can occur when cancer cells detach from the primary tumor to invade tissue surrounding the tumor. Via tumor angiogenesis, hematogenous metastasis can occur through the vascular circulation.

7. There is a lesser incidence of lung cancer in African American women than men but a high morbidity. Less cancer is seen with avoidance of exposure to carcinogens (e.g., limited alcohol use, no tobacco use, limited sun exposure), regular physical activity, maintaining a normal body weight, reducing fat consumption, increasing fruit and vegetable consumption, and regular physical examinations. There are no specific screening tests for lung cancer but the seven warning signs of cancer include change in bowel or bladder habits, a sore that does not heal, unusual bleeding or discharge from any body orifice, thickening or a lump in the breast or elsewhere, indigestion or difficulty swallowing, obvious change in a wart or mole, and nagging cough or hoarseness. The routine screenings that are done to detect cancer include colorectal screening, breast self-examination, clinical breast examination, mammogram, and Papanicolaou (Pap) tests.

8. **Teaching measures:**
   - Hand washing with antibacterial soap for staff, patient, and visitors
   - Do not scratch skin or use a razor with a blade
   - Careful sterile technique in caring for IV catheter site
   - Avoidance of visitors with infection
   - Wear shoes to prevent cuts
   - Use a soft toothbrush to prevent cuts in the mouth
   - Report any manifestations of infection

9. **Nursing diagnoses:**
   - Hopelessness *related to* uncertainty about outcomes and insufficient knowledge about cancer and treatment
   - Imbalanced nutrition: Less than body requirements *related to* decreased oral intake, increased metabolic demands of cancer
   - Deficient fluid volume *related to* decreased oral fluid intake
   - Risk for infection *related to* immunosuppression

   Collaborative problems:
   Potential complications: septicemia, negative nitrogen balance, myelosuppression

CHAPTER 17

Answer Key

1. 1000
2. $90 \text{ kg} \times 60\% = 54$
3. a, d, e. Third spacing is when fluid moves into spaces that normally have little or no fluid. A cell surrounded by hypoosmolar fluid will swell and burst as water moves into the cell. A cell surrounded by hyperosmolar fluid will shrink and die as water moves out of the cell.
4. a. 3; b. 6; c. 7; d. 4; e. 5; f. 1; g. 2
5. $2 \times 147 + 126/18 = 301$. The patient's serum osmolality is increased.
6. c, e. At the arterial end of the capillary, capillary hydrostatic pressure exceeds plasma oncotic pressure and fluid moves into the interstitial space.
7.

Event or Factor	Direction of Fluid Shift	Mechanism of Fluid Movement Involved
Burns	1	b
Dehydration	2	c
Fluid overload	3, 4	d
Hyponatremia	4	a
Low serum albumin	1	e
Administration of 10% glucose	1	a
Application of elastic bandages	4	c

8. a. Serum osmolality increases as a large amount of sodium is absorbed.

   b. Intake of these foods stimulates antidiuretic hormone (ADH) release from the posterior pituitary, which increases water reabsorption from the kidney, lowering the sodium concentration but increasing vascular volume and hydrostatic pressure, perhaps causing fluid shift into interstitial spaces.

9. d. Aldosterone is secreted by the adrenal cortex in response to a decrease in plasma volume (loss of water), serum sodium, or renal perfusion. It is also secreted in response to an increase in serum potassium.

10. b. A decrease in renin and aldosterone and an increase in antidiuretic hormone (ADH) and atrial natriuretic peptide (ANP) lead to decreased sodium reabsorption and increased water retention by the kidney, both of which lead to hyponatremia. Skin changes lead to increased insensible water loss and plasma oncotic pressure is more often decreased because of lack of protein intake.

11. a, b, c, d, e. All of these are important in assessing fluid balance in a postoperative patient. These assessments will provide data about potential fluid volume abnormalities.

12. d. A major cause of hypernatremia is a water deficit, which can occur in those with a decreased sensitivity to thirst, the major protection against hyperosmolality. All other conditions lead to hyponatremia.

13. d. As water shifts into and out of cells in response to the osmolality of the blood, the cells that are most sensitive to shrinking or swelling are those of the brain, resulting in neurologic symptoms.

14. a. 8; b. 4; c. 6; d. 1; e. 7; f. 2; g. 9; h. 3; i. 6, 10; j. 6; k. 1; l. 5; m. 1, 4, 10; n. 3, 6, 8, 9; o. 4, 2, 6, 10

15. d. Because of the osmotic pressure of sodium, water will be excreted with the sodium lost with the diuretic. A change in the relative concentration of sodium will not be seen but an isotonic fluid loss will occur.

16. c. Potassium maintains normal cardiac rhythm, transmission and conduction of nerve impulses, and contraction of muscles. Cardiac cells demonstrate the most clinically significant changes with potassium imbalances because of changes in cardiac conduction. Although paralysis may occur with severe potassium imbalances, cardiac changes are seen earlier and much more commonly.

17. b. In metabolic acidosis, hydrogen ions in the blood are taken into the cell in exchange for potassium ions as a means of buffering excess acids. This results in an increase in serum potassium until the kidneys have time to excrete the excess potassium.

18. d. Chvostek's sign is a contraction of facial muscles in response to a tap over the facial nerve. This indicates the neuromuscular irritability of low calcium levels and IV calcium is the treatment used to prevent laryngeal spasms and respiratory arrest. Calcitonin is indicated for treatment of high calcium levels and loop diuretics may be used to decrease calcium levels. Oral vitamin D supplements are part of the treatment for hypocalcemia but not for impending tetany.

19. c. Kidneys are the major route of phosphate excretion, a function that is impaired in renal failure. A reciprocal relationship exists between phosphorus and calcium and high serum phosphate levels of kidney failure cause low calcium concentration in the serum.

20. c. 7.35 to 7.45; 20 to 1. The other answers are incorrect.

21. a, b, c. Shifts of H^+ in and out of the cell are characteristics of the cellular buffer system. Free basic radical dissociation is characteristic of the protein buffer system.

22. a, b, d. Free acid radical dissociation is characteristic of the protein buffer system. Chloride shifting in and out of red blood cells is characteristic of the hemoglobin buffer system.

23. c. The amount of carbon dioxide in the blood directly relates to carbonic acid concentration and subsequently hydrogen ion concentration. The carbon dioxide combines with water in the blood to form carbonic acid and in cases in which carbon dioxide is retained in the blood, acidosis occurs.

24. a. 3; b. 4; c. 2; d. 1. Respiratory acid-base imbalances are associated with excesses or deficits of carbonic acid. Metabolic acid-base imbalances are associated with excesses or deficits of bicarbonate.

25. d. Shifting of bicarbonate for Cl^- may buffer acute respiratory alkalosis. The kidney conserves bicarbonate and excretes hydrogen to compensate for respiratory acidosis. Kussmaul respirations occur with metabolic acidosis to compensate.

26. a. 1; b. 1; c. 1; d. 3; e. 2; f. 2; g. 4; h. 3; i. 4

27. b. Calculation of the anion gap by subtracting the serum chloride and bicarbonate levels from the serum sodium level should normally be 10 to 14 mmol/L. The anion gap is increased in metabolic acidosis associated with acid gain (e.g., diabetic acidosis) but remains normal in metabolic acidosis caused by bicarbonate loss (e.g., diarrhea).

28. a. 1. pH >7.45 indicates alkalosis.
    2. $PaCO_2$ is low, indicating respiratory alkalosis.
    3. HCO_3^- is normal.
    4. Respiratory alkalosis matches the pH.
    5. Although uncommon, if the HCO_3^- were decreased, compensation would be present.
    Interpretation: Respiratory alkalosis
    b. 1. pH <7.35 indicates acidosis.
    2. $PaCO_2$ is low, indicating respiratory alkalosis.
    3. HCO_3^- is low, indicating metabolic acidosis.
    4. Metabolic acidosis matches the pH.
    5. The $PaCO_2$ does not match the acidic pH but is in the opposite direction, which indicates that the lungs are attempting to compensate for the metabolic acidosis.
    Interpretation: Metabolic acidosis; partially compensated
    c. 1. pH <7.35 indicates acidosis.
    2. $PaCO_2$ is high, indicating respiratory acidosis.
    3. HCO_3^- is normal.
    4. Respiratory acidosis matches the pH.
    5. Normal HCO_3^- is found until the kidneys have time to retain bicarbonate.
    Interpretation: Respiratory acidosis
    d. 1. pH >7.45 indicates alkalosis.
    2. $PaCO_2$ is high, indicating respiratory acidosis.
    3. HCO_3^- is high, indicating metabolic alkalosis.
    4. Metabolic alkalosis matches the pH.
    5. The $PaCO_2$ does not match the alkalotic pH but is in the opposite direction, indicating that the lungs are attempting to compensate for the alkalosis.
    Interpretation: Metabolic alkalosis; partially compensated
    e. 1. pH is within normal range but toward alkalosis.
    2. $PaCO_2$ is high, indicating respiratory acidosis.
    3. HCO_3^- is high, indicating metabolic alkalosis.
    4. Because the body will not overcompensate, the metabolic alkalosis is a closer match with the pH.
    5. The high $PaCO_2$ indicates the ability of the lungs to compensate for the metabolic alkalosis.
    Interpretation: Compensated or chronic metabolic alkalosis indicated by the high $PaCO_2$ and a pH within normal range
    f. 1. pH is within normal range but toward acidosis.
    2. $PaCO_2$ is high, indicating respiratory acidosis.
    3. HCO_3^- is high, indicating metabolic alkalosis.
    4. Because the body will not overcompensate, the respiratory acidosis is a closer match with the pH.
    5. The high HCO_3^- indicates the ability of the kidneys to compensate for the respiratory acidosis.
    Interpretation: compensated respiratory acidosis as reflected by high HCO_3^- and pH in normal range

29. a. Fluids such as 5% dextrose in water (D_5W) allow water to move from the extracellular fluid to the intracellular fluid. Although D_5W is physiologically isotonic, the dextrose is rapidly metabolized, leaving free water to shift into cells.

30. c. An isotonic solution does not change the osmolality of the blood and does not cause fluid shifts between the extracellular fluid and intracellular fluid. In the case of extracellular fluid loss, an isotonic solution, such as lactated Ringer's solution, is ideal because it stays in the extracellular compartment. A hypertonic solution would pull fluid from the cells into the extracellular compartment, resulting in cellular fluid loss and possible vascular overload.

31. d. The greatest risk with CVAD is systemic infection. Dressings that are loose should be changed immediately to reduce this risk.

32. a. 3; b. 7; c. 4; d. 8; e. 2; f. 5; g. 6; h. 1. The first nursing action to be completed after a CVAD is inserted and before it is used is to ensure proper placement with a chest x-ray. Assessments, flushing, dressing changes, and cap changes are completed according to facility policies but hand hygiene must be completed before manipulating the CVAD to prevent infection. Strict sterile technique is used with dressing and cap changes as well as having the patient turn his or her face away from the insertion site to avoid contamination.

33. a. Catheters tunneled to the distal end of the superior vena cava or the right atrium are vascular access devices inserted into central veins, which decrease the incidence of extravasation, provide for rapid dilution of chemotherapy, and reduce the need for venipunctures. Most right atrial catheters, except for a Groshong catheter, need to be flushed with heparin to prevent clotting in the tubing. Regional chemotherapy administration delivers the drug directly to the tumor and is the only administration route that can decrease the systemic effects of the drugs.

34. b. With a low magnesium level there is an increased risk for hypokalemia and hypocalcemia as well as altered sodium-potassium pump and altered carbohydrate and protein metabolism. Hypokalemia could lead to dysrhythmias and severe muscle weakness. The sodium and phosphate levels are also not within normal limits. However, the implications are not as life-threatening. The calcium level is normal.

Case Study

1. Status: Fluid volume deficit
   Physical assessment: Decreased skin turgor; dry mucous membranes; weak pulses, low blood pressure; confusion
   Laboratory findings: Elevated blood urea nitrogen (BUN); elevated hematocrit
   Status: Hypokalemia
   Physical assessment: Weakness, confusion; irregular heart rhythm, tachycardia
   Laboratory findings: Potassium 2.5 mEq/L
   Etiology: Diuretic therapy

2. Electrocardiographic (ECG) changes are associated with hypokalemia and metabolic alkalosis.

3. Metabolic alkalosis: pH 7.52 with increased base bicarbonate (34 mEq/L)
   Etiology: Diuretic-induced hypokalemia is the primary factor.
   Compensation: Not complete because the pH is out of normal range but increased $PaCO_2$ and slow and shallow respirations indicate the attempt by the lungs to increase carbon dioxide to compensate for excess bicarbonate.

4. P.B. has less fluid reserve because older adults have less total body fluid; older adults also have decreased thirst sensation.

5. Aldosterone would be secreted in response to low fluid volume (decreased plasma volume). P.B.'s low blood pressure and extracellular fluid deficit would stimulate secretion of aldosterone to increase sodium and water retention.

6. **General care:** Encourage and assist with oral fluid intake
   Provide skin care with assessment, changes in position, no soap

Assessments:
- Vital signs q4hr
- Intake and output; daily weights
- Cardiac monitoring until electrolytes and acid-base normal
- Type and rate of IV fluid and electrolyte replacement
- Lung sounds for signs of fluid overload in cardiac-compromised patient
- Daily serum electrolyte and blood gas levels

7. **Nursing diagnoses:**
- Deficient fluid volume *related to* excessive extracellular fluid (ECF) loss or decreased fluid intake
- Ineffective health maintenance *related to* lack of knowledge of drugs and preventive measures
- Risk for injury *related to* confusion, muscle weakness
- Risk for impaired skin integrity *related to* dehydration

Collaborative problems:
Potential complications: dysrhythmias, hypovolemic shock, hypoxemia

CHAPTER 18

Answer Key

1. d, e. Gastroscopy is for the purpose of diagnosis. Rhinoplasty is done for a cosmetic improvement. A tracheotomy is palliative.

2. a. Ambulatory surgery is usually less expensive and more convenient, generally involving fewer laboratory tests, fewer preoperative and postoperative medications, less psychologic stress, and less susceptibility to hospital-acquired infections. However, the nurse is still responsible for assessing, supporting, and teaching the patient who is undergoing surgery, regardless of where the surgery is performed.

3. a. Excessive anxiety and stress can affect surgical recovery and the nurse's role in psychologically preparing the patient for surgery is to assess for potential stressors that could negatively affect surgery. Specific fears should be identified and addressed by the nurse by listening and by explaining planned postoperative care. Falsely reassuring the patient, ignoring her behavior, and telling her not to be anxious are not therapeutic.

4. a, b, d, f. Valerian may cause excess sedation. Astragalus may increase blood pressure before and during surgery.

5. c. Risk factors for latex allergies include a history of hay fever and allergies to foods such as avocados, kiwi, bananas, potatoes, peaches, and apricots. When a patient identifies such allergies, the patient should be further questioned about exposure to latex and specific reactions to allergens. A history of any allergic responsiveness increases the risk for hypersensitivity reactions to drugs used during anesthesia but the hay fever and fruit allergies are specifically related to latex allergy. After identifying the allergic reaction, the anesthesia care provider (ACP) should be notified, the allergy alert wristband should be applied, and the note in the record will include the allergies and reactions as well as the nursing actions related to the allergies.

6. d. BUN, serum creatinine, and electrolytes are used to assess renal function and should be evaluated before surgery. Other tests are often evaluated in the presence of diabetes, bleeding tendencies, and respiratory or heart disease.

7. a. Obesity, as well as spinal, chest, and airway deformities, may compromise respiratory function during and after surgery. Dehydration may require preoperative fluid therapy and an enlarged liver may indicate hepatic dysfunction that will increase perioperative risk related to glucose control, coagulation, and drug interactions. Weak peripheral pulses may reflect circulatory problems that could affect healing.

8. a, b, e. Procedural information includes what will or should be done for surgical preparation, including what to bring and what to wear to the surgery center, length and type of food and fluid restrictions, physical preparation required, pain control, need for coughing and deep breathing (if appropriate), and procedures done before and during surgery (such as vital signs, IV lines, and how anesthesia is administered). The other options are sensory and process information (see Table 18-6).

9. a. The health care provider is ultimately responsible for obtaining informed consent. However, the nurse may be responsible for obtaining and witnessing the patient's signature on the consent form. The nurse may be a patient advocate during the signing of the consent form, verifying that consent is voluntary and that the patient understands the implications of consent, but the primary legal action by the nurse is witnessing the patient's signature.

10. a. The nurse should notify the health care provider because the patient needs further explanation of the planned surgery.
    b. Sufficient comprehension

11. a. The preoperative fasting recommendations of the American Society of Anesthesiology indicate that clear liquids may be taken up to 2 hours before surgery for healthy patients undergoing elective procedures. There is evidence that longer fasting is not necessary.

12. b. Preoperative checklists are a tool used to ensure that the many preparations and precautions performed before surgery have been completed and documented. Patient identification, instructions to the family, and administration of preoperative medications are often documented on the checklist, which ensures that no details are omitted.

13. c. One of the major reasons that older adults need increased time preoperatively is the presence of impaired vision and hearing that slows understanding of preoperative instructions and preparation for surgery. Thought processes and cognitive abilities may also be impaired in some older adults. The older adult's decreased adaptation to stress because of physiologic changes may increase surgical risks and overwhelming surgery-related losses may result in ineffective coping that is not directly related to time needed for preoperative preparation. The involvement of caregivers in preoperative activities may be appropriate for patients of all ages.

14. d. This finding may indicate an infection. The surgeon will probably postpone the surgery until the cause of the elevated WBC count has been found.

15. a, b, c, d, e. All of these are actions that are needed to ensure that the patient is ready for surgery. In addition, the nurse should verify that the identification band and allergy band (if applicable) are on; the patient is not wearing any cosmetics; nail polish has been removed; valuables have been removed and secured; and prosthetics, such as eyeglasses, have been removed and secured.

Case Study

1. Family: children with cystic fibrosis who require extra care and expense and concern that the wife will not be able to manage without him; fear of cancer and the unknown; anemia: contributes to fatigue and ability to cope

2. Three criteria for informed consent:
   - Adequate disclosure of the diagnosis; the nature and purpose of the proposed treatment; risks and consequences of the proposed treatment; the availability, benefits, and risks of alternative treatments; and the prognosis if treatment is not instituted.
   - Sufficient comprehension of the information is provided.
   - Voluntary consent is given without persuasion or coercion.

3. Outpatient instructions: When to arrive and the time of the surgery, how and where to register, what to wear and bring, the need for a responsible adult for transportation home after the procedure
   General preoperative instruction: Information related to preoperative routines and preparation, such as food and fluid restrictions; approximate length of surgery; postoperative recovery

4. Smoking history increases the risk for postoperative respiratory complications; the longer the patient can stop smoking before surgery, the less the risk will be Mild obesity may contribute to problems with clearance of respiratory secretions and complete expansion of the lungs. The patient should have preoperative instruction about deep-breathing and coughing techniques. Fear of a diagnosis of cancer can alter adaptation and recovery. The nurse can help to minimize this risk by providing specific information about the experience and through supportive listening.

5. **Nursing diagnoses:**
   - Fear *related to* possible diagnosis of cancer
   - Interrupted family processes *related to* shift in family roles
   - Ineffective health maintenance *related to* tobacco use

   Collaborative problems:

   Potential complications: hemorrhage, laryngospasm/ bronchospasm, pneumonia, pneumothorax

CHAPTER 19

Answer Key

1. b. Although all of the factors listed are important to the safety and well-being of the patient, the first consideration in the physical environment of the surgical suite is prevention of transmission of infection to the patient.

2. b. Persons in street clothes or attire other than surgical scrub clothing can interact with personnel of the surgical suite in unrestricted areas, such as the holding area, nursing station, control desk, or locker rooms. Only authorized personnel wearing surgical attire and hair covering are allowed in semirestricted areas, such as corridors, and masks must be worn in restricted areas, such as operating rooms and clean core and scrub sink areas.

3. a, c, e. The circulating nurse documents intraoperative care, checks mechanical and electrical equipment, and monitors blood and other fluid loss and urine output.

4. a. The protection of the patient from injury in the operating room environment is maintained by the circulating nurse by ensuring functioning equipment, preventing falls and injury during transport and transfer, monitoring asepsis, and providing supportive care for the anesthetized patient.

5. d. The Universal Protocol supported by The Joint Commission (TJC) is used to prevent wrong site, wrong procedure, and wrong surgery in view of a high rate of

these problems nationally. It involves pausing just before the procedure starts to verify patient identity, surgical site, and surgical procedure.

6. a. The mask covering the face is not considered sterile and if in contact with sterile gloved hands, it contaminates the gloves. The gown at chest level and to 2 inches above the elbows is considered sterile, as is the drape placed at the surgical area.

7. c. Musculoskeletal deformities can be a risk factor for positioning injuries and require special padding and support on the operating table. Skin lesions and break in sterile technique are risk factors for infection and electrical or mechanical equipment failure may lead to other types of injury.

8. d. The Perioperative Nursing Data Set includes outcome statements that reflect standards and recommended practices of perioperative nursing. Outcomes related to physiologic responses include those of physiologic function, such as respiratory function; perioperative safety includes the patient's freedom from any type of injury; and behavioral responses include knowledge and actions of the patient and family, including the consistency of the patient's care with the perioperative plan and the patient's right to privacy.

9. d, e. Nitrous oxide is a weak gaseous anesthetic. Propofol (Diprivan) is a nonbarbiturate hypnotic that has a rapid onset and may be used for induction. Isoflurane (Forane) is a volatile liquid inhalation agent.

10. b. The volatile liquid inhalation agents have very little residual analgesia and patients experience early onset of pain when the agents are discontinued. These agents are associated with a low incidence of nausea and vomiting. Prolonged respiratory depression is not common because of their rapid elimination. Hypothermia is not related to use of these agents but they may precipitate malignant hyperthermia in conjunction with neuromuscular blocking agents.

11. a. Midazolam (Versed) is a rapid, short-acting, sedative-hypnotic benzodiazepine that is used to prevent recall of events under anesthesia because of its amnestic properties.

12.

Drug	Use	Nursing Implication
Ketamine (Ketalar)	Maintenance anesthesia	Monitor for cardiopulmonary depression, early pain, and nausea and vomiting
Fentanyl (Sublimaze)	Dissociative anesthesia with analgesia and amnesia	Monitor for agitation, hallucinations, and nightmares
Desflurane (Suprane)	Induction and maintenance of anesthesia	Promote early analgesia—assess for nausea and vomiting, monitor respiratory status
Succinylcholine (Anectine)	Produce deep muscle relaxation	Monitor respiratory muscle movement, airway patency, and temperature

13. d. MAC refers to sedation that is similar to general anesthesia using sedative, anxiolytic, and/or analgesic medications. It can be administered by an ACP. The patient must be assessed and the physiologic problems that may develop must be managed because of the high risk of complications resulting in clinical emergencies.

14. a. 3; b. 5; c. 1; d. 4; e. 2

15. d. Moderate sedation uses sedative, anxiolytic, and/or analgesic medications. Inhalation agents are not used. It is not expected to induce levels of sedation that would impair a patient's ability to protect the airway.

16. b. During epidural and spinal anesthesia, a sympathetic nervous system blockade may occur that results in hypotension, bradycardia, and nausea and vomiting. A spinal headache may occur after, not during, spinal anesthesia and loss of consciousness and seizures are indicative of IV absorption overdose. Upward extension of the effect of the anesthesia results in inadequate respiratory excursion and apnea.

17. b. Although malignant hyperthermia can result in cardiac arrest and death, if the patient is known or suspected to be at risk for the disorder, appropriate precautions taken by the ACP can provide for safe anesthesia for the patient. Because preventive measures are possible if the risk is known, it is critical that preoperative assessment include a careful family history of surgical events. Dantrolene (Dantrium) is given as a treatment for malignant hyperthermia, not as a preventive measure. The cooling blanket would have no effect.

Case Study

1. Ensure that enough help is available to transfer the patient from the stretcher to the OR table. Position the patient carefully to prevent injury. Apply safety straps. Place electrocardiogram (ECG) leads, blood pressure (BP) cuff, and pulse oximetry. Check the IV to verify insertion and patency. Ensure that the grounding pad is placed correctly. Complete the patient safety checklist. Implement the Universal Protocol: take a surgical timeout with the surgical team members to verify patient name, birth date, and operative procedure and location and to compare the hospital ID number on the patient ID band with the chart. Aseptic technique must be maintained by all surgical team members. A fire risk assessment may also be completed.

2. The patient position should allow for operative site accessibility. Place in correct musculoskeletal alignment. Be sure that no undue pressure is occurring to bony prominences, nerves, earlobes, and eyes. Be sure that there can be adequate thoracic wall movement. Prevent any pressure or occlusion of veins and arteries. Secure the patient's extremities and provide adequate padding. Respect patient modesty. Respect the patient's specific aches and pains or deformities.

3. T.M. should be monitored for hypotension, bradycardia, nausea and vomiting, respiratory difficulties, and apnea.

4. Monitor the effect of anesthetic agents and adjuncts closely. Ensure clear communication and verify patient understanding. Closely monitor the patient's skin, especially where tape, electrodes, and pads have been applied. Position the older patient carefully with close attention to patient alignment and joint support. Consider using warming

devices and monitor closely if these are used. Assess the postoperative recovery from the anesthetic agents before the patient is transferred out of the postanesthesia care unit (PACU).

5. **Nursing diagnoses:**
   - Risk for infection
   - Risk for impaired skin integrity
   - Risk for injury
   - Risk for hypothermia

CHAPTER 20

Answer Key

1. a. Although some surgical procedures and drug administration require more intensive postanesthesia care, how fast and through which levels of care patients are moved depend on the condition of the patient. A physiologically unstable outpatient may stay an extended time in Phase I, whereas a patient requiring hospitalization but who is stable and recovering may well be transferred quickly to an inpatient unit.

2. c. Physiologic status of the patient is always prioritized with regard to airway, breathing, and circulation, and respiratory adequacy is the first assessment priority of the patient on admission to the PACU from the operating room. Following assessment of respiratory function, cardiovascular, neurologic, and renal function should be assessed as well as the surgical site.

3. c. The admission of the patient to the PACU is a joint effort between the ACP, who is responsible for supervising the postanesthesia recovery of the patient, and the PACU nurse, who provides care during anesthesia recovery. The ACP gives a verbal report that presents the details of the surgical and anesthetic course, preoperative conditions influencing the surgical and anesthetic outcome, and PACU treatment plans to ensure patient safety and continuity of care.

4. b. Even before patients awaken from anesthesia, their sense of hearing returns and all activities should be explained by the nurse from the time of admission to the PACU to assist in orientation and decrease confusion.

5. b. ECG monitoring is performed on patients to assess initial cardiovascular problems during anesthesia recovery. Fluid and electrolyte status is an indication of renal function and determinations of arterial blood gases and direct arterial blood pressure monitoring are used only in special cardiovascular or respiratory problems.

6. a. Hypoxemia occurs with atelectasis and aspiration as well as pulmonary edema, pulmonary embolism, and bronchospasm. Hypercapnia is caused by decreased removal of CO_2 from the respiratory system that could occur with airway obstruction or hypoventilation. Hypoventilation may occur with depression of central respiratory drive, poor respiratory muscle tone due to disease or anesthesia, mechanical restriction, or pain. Airway obstruction could occur with the tongue blocking the airway, restrained thick secretions, laryngospasm, or laryngeal edema.

7. d. An unconscious or semiconscious patient should be placed in a lateral position to protect the airway from obstruction by the tongue. Deep breathing and elevation of the head of the bed are implemented to facilitate gas exchange when the patient is responsive. Oxygen administration is often used but the patient must first have a patent airway.

8. c. Incisional pain is often the greatest deterrent to patient participation in effective ventilation and ambulation and adequate and regular analgesic medications should be provided to encourage these activities. Controlled breathing may help the patient to manage pain but does not promote coughing and deep breathing. Explanations and use of an incentive spirometer help to gain patient participation but are more effective if pain is controlled.

9. c. Hypotension with normal pulse and skin assessment is typical of residual vasodilating effects of anesthesia and requires continued observation. An oxygen saturation of 88% indicates hypoxemia, whereas a narrowing pulse pressure accompanies hypoperfusion. A urinary output >30 mL/hr is desirable and indicates normal renal function.

10. a. The most common cause of emergence delirium is hypoxemia and initial assessment should evaluate respiratory function. When hypoxemia is ruled out, other causes, such as a distended bladder, pain, and fluid and electrolyte disturbances, should be considered. Delayed awakening may result from neurologic injury and cardiac dysrhythmias most often result from specific respiratory, electrolyte, or cardiac problems.

11. a. During hypothermia, oxygen demand is increased and metabolic processes slow down. Oxygen therapy is used to treat the increased demand for oxygen. Antidysrhythmics and vasodilating drugs would be used only if the hypothermia caused symptomatic cardiac dysrhythmias and vasoconstriction. Sedatives and analgesics are not indicated for hypothermia.

12. c. On initial assessment in PACU the airway, breathing, and circulation (ABC) status is assessed using a standardized tool that usually includes consciousness, respiration, oxygen saturation, circulation, and activity. Increased or decreased respiratory rate, hypertension, and a SaO_2 below 90% indicate inadequate oxygenation that will be treated or managed in the PACU before discharging the patient to the next phase.

13. b, d, e, f. These problems are improved with ambulation. Other collaborative problems could be potential complications: urinary retention, atelectasis, and pneumonia.

14. c. The stress response causes fluid retention during the first 1 to 3 days postoperatively and fluid overload is possible during this time. Fluid retention results from secretion and release of antidiuretic hormone (ADH) and adrenocorticotropic hormone (ACTH) by the pituitary and activation of the renin-angiotensin-aldosterone system (RAAS). ACTH stimulates the adrenal cortex to secrete cortisol and aldosterone. The RAAS increases aldosterone release, which also increases fluid retention. Aldosterone causes renal potassium loss with possible hypokalemia and blood coagulation is enhanced by cortisol.

15. c. Slow progression to ambulation by slowly changing the patient's position will help to prevent syncope. Monitoring vital signs after walking will not prevent or treat syncope. Monitor the patient's pulse and blood pressure (BP) before, during, and after position changes. Elevate the patient's head, then slowly have the patient dangle, then stand by the bed to help determine if the patient is safe for walking. Eating will not have an effect on syncope. Deep breathing and coughing will not decrease syncope, although it will prevent respiratory complications.

16. c, e. The nasogastric tube and gastrointestinal tube drain gastric contents. The T-tube drains bile, the Hemovac drains blood from a surgical site, and the indwelling catheter drains urine from the bladder.

17. d. Bile is drained by a T-tube, urine is drained by an indwelling urinary catheter, and gastric contents are drained by a nasogastric tube or a gastrointestinal tube.

18. a. 2; b. 5; c. 4; d. 1; e. 3. The nurse must be aware of drains, if used, and the type of surgery to help predict the expected drainage. Dressings over surgical sites are initially removed by the surgeon unless otherwise specified and should not be changed, although reinforcing the dressing is appropriate. Some drainage is expected for most surgical wounds and the drainage should be evaluated and recorded to establish a baseline for continuing assessment. The surgeon should be notified of excessive drainage. Dressings will then be changed as ordered with assessment for infection being done as well.

19. d. During the first 24 to 48 postoperative hours, temperature elevations to 100.4°F (38°C) are a result of the inflammatory response to surgical stress. Dehydration and lung congestion or atelectasis in the first 2 days will cause a temperature elevation above 100.4°F (38°C). Wound infections usually do not become evident until 3 to 5 days postoperatively and manifest with temperatures above 100°F (37.8°C).

20. d. Before administering all analgesic medications, the nurse should first assess the nature and intensity of the patient's pain to determine if the pain is expected, prior doses of the medication have been effective, and any undesirable side effects are occurring. The administration of PRN analgesic medication is based on the nursing assessment. If possible, pain medication should be in effect during painful activities but activities may be scheduled around medication administration.

21. c. All postoperative patients need discharge instructions regarding what to expect and what self-care can be assumed during recovery. Diet, activities, follow-up care, symptoms to report, and instructions about medications are individualized to the patient.

Case Study

1. Priority nursing actions for this patient are orienting as the patient recovers from the sedating medication, promoting voiding, and providing oral fluids and intake.

2. Syncope is possible because of the effects of the drug and instrumentation of the bladder. The patient should be slowly progressed to ambulation by elevating the head of the bed, then dangling the legs, and then standing at the side of the bed before attempting ambulation.

3. Inability to void is the most likely problem. The patient could also have respiratory depression or unstable vital signs because of the effects of the drugs or have complications such as bladder bleeding.

4. The nurse can determine this by using standard discharge criteria for PACUs—stable vital signs, oxygen saturation >90%, awake and oriented, no excessive bleeding or drainage, and no respiratory depression—in addition to the specific criteria ordered for this patient.

5. In an outpatient setting, the patient also needs to be alert and ambulatory with the ability to provide self-care near the level of preoperative functioning. Postoperative pain, nausea, and vomiting must be controlled and the patient must be accompanied by an adult to drive her home. No opioids should have been given for 30 minutes before discharge.

6. **Nursing diagnoses:**
   - Impaired urinary elimination *related to* bladder irritation
   - Acute pain *related to* bladder irritation
   - Risk for infection *related to* incomplete bladder emptying
   - Risk for injury *related to* sedation

   Collaborative problems:
   Potential complications: hemorrhage, infection

CHAPTER 21

Answer Key

1. a. lens; b. pupil; c. cornea; d. anterior chamber; e. iris; f. posterior chamber; g. ciliary body; h. retina; i. choroid; j. sclera; k. vitreous cavity; l. optic nerve; m. optic disc

2. d. The zonule connects the lens to the ciliary body. The cornea is a transparent external structure that is responsible for the majority of light refraction needed for clear vision. Aqueous humor fills the anterior and posterior chambers of the anterior cavity of the eye.

3. c. The lens bends light rays so they fall on the retina. Aqueous humor is produced from capillary blood in the ciliary body. Rods are the photoreceptor cells stimulated in dim lighting.

4. c. The junction of the eyelids is the medial and lateral canthi. The optic disc is the point where the optic nerve leaves the eyeball. The puncta drain the tears to the lacrimal canals.

5. c. The pupil is the opening of the iris, the cones are photoreceptors sensitive to color in bright light, and the canal of Schlemm is the drainage path for aqueous humor.

6.

Eye Function	Cranial Nerve
Eyelid movement	CN VII (facial)
Pupil constriction	CN III (oculomotor)
Pupil dilation	CN V (trigeminal)
Visual acuity	CN II (optic)

7.

Assessment Finding	Cause
Floaters	Liquefaction and detachment of vitreous
Ectropion	Loss of orbital fat
Pinguecula	Chronic exposure to ultraviolet (UV) light or other environmental irritants
Arcus senilis	Cholesterol deposits in the peripheral cornea
Yellowish sclera	Deposition of lipids
Dry, irritated eyes	Decreased tear secretion
Decreased pupil size	Increased rigidity of iris
Changes in color percept	Decreased cones

8. a. The use of corticosteroids has been associated with the development of cataracts and glaucoma. Use of oral hypoglycemic agents alerts the nurse to the presence of diabetes and risk for diabetic retinopathy. Antihistamine and decongestant drugs may cause eye dryness. β-Adrenergic blocking agents may cause additive effects in patients with glaucoma for whom these medications may be prescribed.

9.

Functional Health Pattern	Risk Factor or Response to Visual Problem
Health perception–health management	UV light exposure; age-related eye problems; improper contact lens care; family history of ocular problems; diseases affecting the eye; allergies causing eye problems
Nutritional-metabolic	Deficiencies of zinc or vitamins C and E
Elimination	Constipation and straining to defecate increases intraocular pressure
Activity-exercise	Work and leisure activities that increase eye strain; lack of protective eyewear during sports; visual difficulties with activities
Sleep-rest	Lack of sleep
Cognitive-perceptual	Presence of eye pain; unable to read
Self-perception–self-concept	Decreased self-concept and self-image; loss of independence
Role-relationship	Loss of roles and responsibilities; occupational eye injuries
Sexuality-reproductive	Eye medications that may cause fetal abnormalities; change in sexual activity related to self-image; use of erectile dysfunction drugs in males
Coping–stress tolerance	Grief related to loss of vision; emotional stress
Value-belief	Values and beliefs that limit treatment decisions

10. With the right eye, the patient standing at 20 feet from a Snellen chart can read to the 40-foot line on the chart with two or fewer errors; with the left eye, the patient can read only to the 50-foot line on the chart. This patient can read at 20 feet what a person with normal vision can read at 40 and 50 feet.

11. d. PERRLA means pupils equal (in size), round, and react to light (pupil constricts when light shines into same eye and also constricts in the opposite eye) and accommodation (pupils constrict with focus on near object). Nystagmus on far lateral gaze is normal but is not part of the assessment of pupil function.

12.

Assessment Data	Assessment Technique
Peripheral vision field	Confrontation test
Extraocular muscle functions	Cardinal field of gaze
Near visual acuity	Jaeger chart
Visual acuity	Snellen chart
Intraocular pressure	Tono-Pen

13. b. A normal yellowish hue to the normally white sclera is found in dark-pigmented persons and in older adults. Infants and some older adults may exhibit a normal blue cast to the sclera because of thin sclera. Iris color does not affect the color of the sclera and infections of the eye may cause dilation of small blood vessels in the normally clear bulbar conjunctiva, reddening the sclera and conjunctiva.

14. b. Fluorescein is a dye that is used topically to identify corneal irregularities; irregularities stain a bright green on application of the dye. A tonometer is used to measure intraocular pressure. Light from either a penlight or an ophthalmoscope often is not able to illuminate corneal injuries.

15. a, c. Ptosis is drooping of the upper lid. Blepharitis is redness, swelling, and crusting along the lid margins. Strabismus is seen with extraocular muscle assessment. Anisocoria is pupils that are unequal. See Table 21-5. The pinna is the outer part of the ear.

16. c. Photophobia (light intolerance) is seen with inflammation or infection of the cornea or anterior uveal tract. Anisocoria is seen with central nervous system disorders, although some people normally have a slight difference in pupil size. Stabismus is seen with overaction or underaction of one or more extraocular muscles.

17. c. A break in the retina anywhere in the eye is abnormal and indicates a potential loss of vision. Depression of the center of the optic disc and blurring of the optic disc at the nasal border are normal findings. Pieces of liquefied vitreous are "floaters" and are a normal finding in older adults and others.

18. b. Although fluorescein dye can be used topically to identify corneal lesions, in angiography the dye is injected intravenously and outlines the vasculature of the retina, locating areas of retinopathy. Intraocular pressure is measured indirectly with a tonometer and a keratometry is measurement of the corneal curvature.

19. d. The receptor organ for hearing is the cochlea. It contains the organ of Corti, whose tiny hair cells respond to stimulation according to pitch. The ossicular chain moves and transmits sound waves to the oval window.

20. c. The eustachian tube equalizes air pressure between the middle ear and the throat. The other options have nothing to do with the eustachian tube. The vestibulocochlear nerve (CN VIII) transmits sound stimuli to the brain. The tympanic membrane sets the bones (ossicles) in motion. The semicircular canals are the organ of balance.

21. a, c, f. Increased hair growth occurs but this does not cause hearing loss. The vestibular apparatus is less effective. There is a decrease in blood supply, which decreases cochlear efficiency.

22. d. Presbycusis is a sensorineural hearing loss that occurs with aging and is associated with decreased ability to hear high-pitched sounds. Tinnitus is present in some, but not all, cases of presbycusis. A sensation of fullness in the ears is related to a blocked eustachian tube and difficulty understanding the meaning of words is associated with a central hearing loss occurring with problems arising from the cochlea to the cerebral cortex.

23.

Question	Significance
Do you have a history of childhood ear infections or ruptured eardrums?	Childhood middle ear infections with perforations and scarring of the eardrum lead to conductive hearing impairments in adulthood.
Do you use any over-the-counter (OTC) or prescription medications on a regular basis?	Many medications are ototoxic, causing damage to the auditory nerve. OTC agents such as aspirin and nonsteroidal antiinflammatory drugs (NSAIDs) are potentially ototoxic, as are prescription diuretics, antibiotics, and chemotherapeutic drugs.
Have you ever been treated for a head injury?	A head injury can damage areas of the brain to which auditory and vestibular stimuli are transmitted, with a resultant loss of hearing or balance.
Is there a history of hearing loss in your parents?	Some congenital hearing disorders are hereditary and the age of onset of presbycusis also follows a familial pattern.
Have you been exposed to excessive noise levels in your work or recreational activities?	It is well documented that exposure to loud noises causes damage to the auditory organs and hearing loss. Noise exposure earlier in life also can result in increased hearing loss with age.
Has the amount of scial activities you are involved in changed?	Persons with hearing loss may withdraw from social relationships because of difficulty with communication. A hearing loss often leaves the patient feeling isolated and cut off from valued relationships.

24. a. The tympanic retraction indicates negative pressure in the middle ear. The lack of landmarks and a bulging eardrum describe acute otitis media. Straightening the ear canal by pulling the auricle downward and backward describes otoscope use for children; for adults the auricle is pulled upward and backward to insert the otoscope.

25. a, d, f. Positive Rinne test, Weber lateralization to the good ear, and inner ear or nerve pathway pathology indicate sensorineural hearing loss. Negative Rinne test, Weber lateralization to impaired ear, and external or middle ear pathology indicate conductive hearing loss.

26. b. Hearing is most sensitive between 500 and 4000 Hz and a 10-dB loss is not significant at 8000 Hz. A 40- to 45-dB loss in the frequency between 4000 and 8000 Hz will cause difficulty in distinguishing high-pitched consonants. A hearing aid is rarely recommended for a hearing loss of less than 26 dB, and problems in everyday communication situations occur only when the thresholds are 25 dB or higher.

27. b. Irrigation of the external ear with cold or warm water causes a disturbance in the endolymph that normally results in nystagmus directed opposite the side of instillation. The absence of nystagmus indicates that peripheral or central vestibular functions are impaired. An improvement in hearing would occur only if an obstruction of the ear canal was present, which would not be an indication for caloric testing. Severe pain upon irrigation would not be related to vestibular function.

28.

Functional Health Pattern	Risk Factor for or Response to Hearing Problem
Health perception–health management	Gradual or sudden hearing loss, use of protective earwear for high noise environments or with swimming
Nutritional-metabolic	Alcohol, sodium and dietary supplements used; changes in symptoms with food eaten; ear pain with chewing, grinding of the teeth
Elimination	Constipation and straining may increase intracranial pressure
Activity-exercise	Changes in activity related to hearing or equilibrium problems
Sleep-rest	Tinnitus disturbs sleep; snoring may be caused by swelling in nasopharynx, which impairs eustachian tube function and causes the sensation of ear fullness or pain
Cognitive-perceptual	Pain and relief methods; inability to pay attention or hear and follow directions
Self-perception–self-concept	Effect on personal life, feelings about self, embarrassing social situations
Role-relationship	Strained family life, work, and social relationships; dangerous situations with vertigo or dizziness
Sexuality-reproductive	Interference with establishing or maintaining a satisfactory sexual relationship
Coping–stress tolerance	Denial is common with hearing problems
Value-belief	Values and beliefs that limit treatment options

CHAPTER 22

Answer Key

1. a, d, e. Myopic people may have abnormally long eyeballs, not abnormally short ones, which occurs in hyperopia. Unequal corneal curvature results in astigmatism.
2. d. Absence of crystalline lens is aphakia. Astigmatism is corrected with a cylinder lens. People with myopia have abnormally long eyeballs.
3. a. A light shined at an angle over the cornea will illuminate a contact lens and fluorescein should not have to be used. Cotton balls should not be placed on the cornea and simply tensing the outer canthus will not dislodge the lens.
4. a, d, e. Refractive errors are the most common visual problem and treatment may include nonsurgical corrections such as corrective glasses and contact lenses. Surgical therapy includes LASIK, PRK, LASEK, and intraocular lens implants.
5. d. A person who is legally blind may have some usable vision that will benefit from vision enhancement techniques. A person with total blindness has no light perception and no usable vision and a person with functional blindness has the loss of usable vision but some light perception. As only 4% of blindness occurs suddenly from injuries, the grieving is probably already in process. Dependency on others from visual impairment is individual and cannot be assumed.
6. a. Address the patient, not others with the patient, in normal conversational tones.
   b. Face the patient and make eye contact.
   c. Introduce self when approaching the patient and let the patient know when you are leaving.
   d. Orient to sounds, activities, and physical surroundings.
   e. Use sighted-guide technique to ambulate and orient patient.
   (Other options: Do not move objects positioned by the patient without the knowledge and consent of the patient; ask the patient what help is needed and how to provide it.)
7. c. Emergency management of foreign bodies in the eye includes covering and shielding the eye, with no attempt to treat the injury, until an ophthalmologist can evaluate the injury. Irrigations are performed as emergency management in chemical exposure. Pressure should never be applied because it might further injure the eye.
8. b. Epidemic keratoconjunctivitis is an ocular adenoviral disease. Sebaceous glands do not exist on the cornea.
9. a. Blepharitis is inflammation of the eyelid. Hordeolum is an infection of the sebaceous glands in the lid margin. Conjunctivitis is infection or inflammation of the conjunctiva.
10. d. All infections of the conjunctiva or cornea are transmittable and frequent, thorough hand washing is essential to prevent spread from one eye to the other or to other persons. Artificial tears are not normally used in external eye infections. Photophobia is not experienced by all patients with eye infections and cold compresses are indicated for some infections.

11. a, b, f. There are also headaches, reddened and swollen conjunctiva, and corneal edema. Eyelid edema, reddened sclera, and bleeding conjunctiva do not occur with endophthalmitis.

12. d. Although cataracts do become worse with time, surgical extraction is considered an elective procedure and is usually performed when the patient decides that he or she wants or needs to see better for his or her lifestyle. There are no known measures to prevent cataract development or progression. Surgical extraction is safe but the patient will still need glasses for near vision and for any residual refractive error of the implanted lens.

13. c. The lens opacity of cataracts causes a decrease in vision, abnormal color perception, and glare. Blurred vision, halos around lights, and eye pain are characteristic of glaucoma. Light flashes, floaters, and "cobwebs" or "hairnets" in the field of vision followed by a painless, sudden loss of vision are characteristic of detached retina.

14. a. Assessment of the visual acuity in the patient's unoperated eye enables the nurse to determine how visually compromised the patient may be while the operative eye is patched and healing and to plan for assistance until vision improves. The patch on the operative eye is usually removed within 24 hours and although vision in the eye may be good, it is not unusual for visual acuity to be reduced immediately after surgery. Activities that are thought to increase intraocular pressure, such as bending, coughing, and Valsalva maneuver, are restricted postoperatively.

15. a, d. Vitrectomy is an intraocular procedure but it may be used with sclera buckling. Pneumatic retinopexy is an intraocular procedure that may be used with photocoagulation or cryotherapy. Penetrating keratoplasty is used for corneal scars or opacities and removes the cornea.

16. a. Postoperatively the patient must position the head so that the bubble is in contact with the retinal break and may have to maintain this position for up to 16 hours a day for 5 days. The patient may go home within a few hours of surgery or may remain in the hospital for several days. No matter what the type of repair, reattachment is successful in 90% of retinal detachments. Postoperative pain is expected and is treated with analgesics.

17. b. The patient with AMD can benefit from low-vision aids despite increasing loss of vision and it is important to promote a positive outlook by not giving patients the impression that "nothing can be done" for them. Laser treatment may help a few patients with choroidal neovascularization and photodynamic therapy is indicated for a small percentage of patients with wet AMD but there is no treatment for the increasing deposit of extracellular debris in the retina.

18. c. Verteporfin, the dye used with photodynamic therapy to destroy abnormal blood vessels, is a photosensitizing drug that can be activated by exposure to sunlight or other high-intensity light. Patients must cover all of their skin to avoid thermal burns when exposed to sunlight. Blind spots occur with laser photocoagulation used for dry AMD. Head movements and position are not of concern following this procedure.

19. c. Because glaucoma develops slowly and without symptoms, it is important that intraocular pressure be evaluated every 2 to 4 years in persons between the ages of 40 and 64 and every 1 to 2 years in those over 65 years old. More frequent measurement of intraocular pressure should be done in a patient with a family history of glaucoma, African American patients, and a patient with diabetes or cardiovascular disease. The disease is chronic but vision impairment is preventable in most cases with treatment.

20. a, d, f. The other answers are associated with primary angle-closure glaucoma (PACG).

21. a, c, e, f. The other answers are associated with primary open-angle glaucoma (POAG).

22.

Drug	Rationale for Use
Betaxolol	An adrenergic blocking agent that decreases aqueous humor production
Dipivefrin	An adrenergic agonist that decreases the production of aqueous humor and enhances outflow facility
Carbachol	A cholinergic agent that stimulates iris sphincter contraction, leading to miosis and opening of the trabecular network, increasing aqueous outflow
Acetazolamide	A carbonic anhydrase inhibitor that decreases aqueous humor production

23. b. Patients receiving ototoxic drugs should be monitored for tinnitus, hearing loss, and vertigo to prevent further damage caused by the drugs. Ears should not be cleaned with anything but a washcloth and finger and ear protection should be used in any environment with noise levels above 90 dB. Exposure to the rubella virus during the first 16 weeks of pregnancy may cause fetal deafness and the vaccine should never be given during pregnancy.

24. a. 5; b. 4; c. 3; d. 6; e. 1; f. 2

25. Advanced age; use of three potentially ototoxic drugs (aspirin, quinidine, and furosemide)

26. d. Antibiotic eardrops for external otitis should be applied without touching the auricle to avoid contaminating the dropper and the solution and the patient should hold the ear upward for several minutes to allow the drops to run down the canal. The drops may be placed onto an ear wick that is placed in the canal but it remains in the ear throughout the course of treatment. The use of lubricating eardrops followed by irrigation is performed for impacted cerumen. "Swimmer's ear" is best prevented by avoiding swimming in contaminated waters; prophylactic antibiotics are not used.

27. c, e. Antibiotics are used to treat acute otitis media. Both acute and chronic otitis media occur in the middle ear. A cholesteatoma may destroy structures in the middle ear or invade the dura of the brain.

28. a. Otosclerosis is an autosomal dominant hereditary disease that causes fixation of the footplate of the stapes, leading to conductive hearing loss. Tuning fork testing

in conductive hearing loss would result in a negative Rinne test and lateralization to the poor ear or the ear with greater hearing loss upon Weber testing. During a stapedectomy, the patient often reports an immediate improvement in hearing but the hearing level decreases temporarily postoperatively.

29. b. Stimulation of the labyrinth intraoperatively may cause postoperative dizziness, increasing the risk for falls. Nystagmus on lateral gaze may result from perilymph disturbances but does not constitute a risk for injury. A tympanic graft is not performed in a stapedectomy, nor is postoperative tinnitus common.

30. a, c, d. Vertigo, tinnitus, and sensorineural hearing loss are the triad of symptoms that occur with inner ear problems.

31. b. Nursing care should minimize vertigo by keeping the patient in a quiet, dark environment. Movement aggravates the whirling and roaring sensations and the patient should be moved only for essential care. Fluorescent lights or television flickering may also increase vertigo and should be avoided. Side rails should be raised when the patient is in bed but padding is not indicated.

32. c. The benign acoustic neuroma can compress the facial nerve and arteries in the internal auditory canal and may expand into the cranium but if removed when small, hearing and vestibular function can be preserved. During surgery for a tumor that has expanded into the cranium, preservation of hearing and the facial nerve is reduced.

33. b, c, e, f. The remaining answers are characteristics of sensorineural hearing loss.

34. a, c, e. The remaining answers are characteristics of conductive hearing loss.

35. c. Initial adjustment to a hearing aid should include voices and household sounds and experimenting with volume in a quiet environment. The next recommended exposure is small parties; the outdoors; and, finally, uncontrolled areas, such as shopping areas.

Case Study

1. Her race, her family history of glaucoma, and her increasing age place her at a high risk for glaucoma. Glaucoma is the leading cause of blindness among African Americans and in older persons, 1 in 10 African Americans has glaucoma. African Americans in every age category should have examinations more often than persons without risk factors because of the increased incidence and more aggressive course of glaucoma in these individuals. Glaucoma may have no symptoms until visual impairment occurs, resulting from increased intraocular ischemic pressure on the retina and optic nerve.

2. Appropriate hand washing and aseptic technique should be used to administer the eyedrops. To prevent systemic absorption of the drug this patient should use punctal occlusion, as she already uses one β-adrenergic blocker (metoprolol) for her hypertension and systemic absorption of the betaxolol could cause additive effects.

3. The antihistamine comes into question because of its anticholinergic effects. It is allowed because A.G. has

open-angle glaucoma (OAG) with no abnormal angle on gonioscopy. In angle-closure glaucoma, the drug is contraindicated because anticholinergic effects of the antihistamine would dilate the pupil, obstructing an already narrowed angle.

4. No, because glaucoma is a chronic disease with no cure. It can be controlled with medication and some surgical interventions but it cannot be cured.

5. Alternatives to topical therapy for primary open-angle glaucoma (POAG) include a trabeculoplasty that opens outflow channels in the trabecular meshwork; a trabeculectomy, in which part of the iris and trabecular meshwork are removed; or cyclocryotherapy, in which parts of the ciliary body are destroyed, decreasing production of aqueous humor.

6. Optic disc cupping with the disc becoming wider, deeper, and paler occurs with progression of glaucoma. Visual complaints with increasing damage include increasing peripheral visual-field loss with eventual tunnel vision and loss of sight.

7. **Nursing diagnoses:**
   • Anxiety *related to* potential permanent visual impairment
   • Ineffective health maintenance *related to* lack of routine assessments for glaucoma
   • Ineffective self-health management *related to* lack of knowledge about disease, treatment, administration of eyedrops, follow-up recommendations
   Collaborative problems:
   Potential complications: increased intraocular pressure, blindness

CHAPTER 23

Answer Key

1. a. hair shaft; b. stratum corneum; c. stratum germinativum; d. melanocyte; e. sebaceous gland; f. eccrine sweat gland; g. apocrine sweat gland; h. blood vessels; i. nerves; j. hair follicle; k. arrector pili muscle; l. connective tissue; m. adipose tissue; n. subcutaneous tissue; o. dermis; p. epidermis

2. c. In older adults the dermis loses volume and has fewer blood vessels, which contributes to decreased extracellular water. Some older people do not drink enough fluids and this can also contribute to dry skin. In older adults there are also decreased surface lipids and apocrine and sebaceous gland activity. Increased bruising from capillary fragility does not contribute to dry skin.

3. d. A careful medication history is important because many medications cause dermatologic side effects and patients also use many over-the-counter preparations to treat skin problems. Freckles are common in childhood and are not related to skin disease. Communicable childhood illnesses are not directly related to skin problems, although varicella viruses may affect the skin in adulthood. Patterns of weight gain and loss are not significant but the presence of obesity may cause skin problems in overlapping skin areas.

4.

Functional Health Pattern	Risk Factor for or Patient Response to Skin Problem
Health perception–health management	Poor skin hygiene; excessive or unprotected sun exposure; family history of alopecia, ichthyosis, psoriasis; history of skin cancer
Nutritional-metabolic	Decreased intake of vitamins A, D, E, or C; malnutrition; food allergies; obesity
Elimination	Incontinence; fluid imbalances
Activity-exercise	Exposure to carcinogens or chemical irritants
Sleep-rest	Itching that interferes with sleep
Cognitive-perceptual	Pain; decreased perception of heat, cold, and touch
Self-perception–self-concept	Feelings of rejection, prejudice, loss of self-esteem, and decreased body image
Role-relationship	Exposure to irritants and allergens; altered relationships with others
Sexuality-reproductive	Changes in sexual intimacy because of appearance, pain
Coping–stress tolerance	Skin problems exacerbated by stress
Value-belief	High social value placed on appearance and skin condition with tanning, use of cosmetics

5. d. It is necessary for the patient to be completely undressed for an examination of the skin. Gowns should be provided and exposure minimized as the skin is inspected generally first, followed by a lesion-specific examination. Skin temperature is best assessed with the back of the hand and turgor is best assessed with the skin over the sternum.

6. b. Discolored lesions that are caused by intradermal or subcutaneous bleeding do not blanch with pressure, whereas those caused by inflammation and dilated blood vessels will blanch and refill after palpation. Varicosities are engorged, dilated veins that may empty with pressure applied along the vein.

7. a. vesicles; b. discrete, localized to the chest and abdomen. c. color, size, and configuration

8. d. An excoriation is a focal loss of epidermis; it does not involve the dermis and, as such, does not scar with healing. Ulcers do penetrate into and through the dermis and scarring does occur with these deeper lesions. Epidermal and dermal thinning is atrophy of the skin but does not involve a break in skin integrity. Both excoriations and ulcers have a break in skin integrity and may develop crusts or scabs over the lesions.

9. b. A shave biopsy is done for superficial lesions that can be scraped with a razor blade, removing the full thickness of the stratum corneum. An excisional biopsy is done when the entire removal of a lesion is desired. Punch biopsies are done with larger nodules to examine for pathology, as are incisional biopsies.

10. a. A culture can be performed to distinguish among fungal, bacterial, and viral infections. A Tzanck test is specific for herpesvirus infections, potassium hydroxide slides are specific for fungal infections, and immunofluorescent studies are specific for infections that cause abnormal antibody proteins.

11. b. Telangiectasia looks like small, superficial, dilated blood vessels. A small circumscribed, flat discoloration describes a macule. A benign tumor of blood or lymph vessels describes an angioma. Tiny purple spots resulting from tiny hemorrhages describes petechiae.

12. b. Scales are excess dead epidermal cells. A pustule is a circumscribed collection of leukocytes and free fluid. Comedo is associated with acne vulgaris.

13. b. Intertrigo is dermatitis in the folds of her skin. Thickening of the skin is lichenification. Loss of color in diffuse areas of skin is vitiligo. A firm plaque caused by fluid in the dermis is a wheal.

CHAPTER 24

Answer Key

1. a, e, f. Vitamin A, not vitamin C, is critical in maintaining and repairing the structure of epithelial cells. Exposure to UVB rays, not UVA rays, is believed to be the most important factor in the development of skin cancer. Sunscreen, not topical hydrocortisone, can block the photosensitivity caused by various drugs.

2. b, c, d. Actinic and firm lesions are actinic keratosis and squamous cell carcinoma. Squamous cell carcinoma frequently occurs in previously damaged skin.

3. b. Actinic keratosis is an irregularly shaped, flat, slightly erythematous papule with indistinct borders and an overlying hard keratotic scale or horn. Malignant melanoma tumors arise in melanocytes. Malignant melanoma is the deadliest skin cancer and has an increased risk in people with dysplastic nevus syndrome. Squamous cell carcinoma is a malignant neoplasm of keratinizing epidermal cells.

4. a. Basal cell carcinoma is noduloulcerative with pearly borders. Malignant melanoma tumors arise in melanocytes. Malignant melanoma is the deadliest skin cancer and has an increased risk in people with dysplastic nevus syndrome. Squamous cell carcinoma is a malignant neoplasm of keratinizing epidermal cells.

5. d. Dysplastic nevus syndrome involves atypical moles with irregular borders and various shades of color.

6. **A**symmetry: one half unlike the other half; **B**order: irregular and poorly circumscribed; **C**olor: varied within lesion; **D**iameter: larger than 6 mm; **E**volving: look and appearance is changing

7. b. Thirty years ago, when the patient was a teenager, radiation therapy was used to treat cystic acne with the result that many of these patients now have developed basal cell carcinoma. For a person with dark skin, radiation therapy is a higher risk factor for skin cancer than exposure to the sun or other irritants.

8. b, c. In the early stages, surgical excision with a margin of normal skin is the initial treatment for malignant melanoma. Mohs' surgery can also be used to treat malignant melanoma. Radiation may be used after excision for malignant melanoma, depending on staging of the disease. Topical nitrogen mustard may be used for treatment of cutaneous T-cell lymphoma.

9. a. chronic disease; b. obesity; c. recent antibiotic therapy; d. recent corticosteroid therapy

10. d. A plantar wart is caused by human papillomavirus (HPV). A furuncle is a deep skin infection with staphylococci around the hair follicle. A carbuncle is multiple, interconnecting furuncles. Erysipelas is superficial cellulitis primarily involving the dermis.

11. b. Seborrheic keratoses are irregularly round or oval shaped and are often verrucous papules or plaques. Candidiasis is a white patchy yeast infection. Cellulitis is a deep inflammation of subcutaneous tissue. Psoriasis is an excessive turnover of epithelial cells.

12. a. In scabies mites penetrate the skin and deposits eggs. An allergic reaction can result from the presence of eggs, feces, and mite parts. Impetigo involves vesiculopustular lesions that develop a thick, honey-colored crust surrounded by erythema. Folliculitis is a small pustule at the hair follicle opening with minimal erythema. Pediculosis is lice.

13. c, e, f. Patients who are immunocompromised are at an increased risk for candidiasis (a fungal infection), herpes simplex 1 (caused by a virus), and Kaposi sarcoma (vascular lesions on the skin, mucous membranes, and viscera with wide range of presentation). The other options are not at increased risk with immunosuppression. Acne is caused by inflammation of sebaceous glands. Lentigo (also called "liver spots" or "age spots") is caused by an increased number of normal melanocytes in the basal layer of epidermis. Herpes zoster, which is caused by an activation of the varicella-zoster virus, is a group of vesicles and pustules resembling chickenpox located in a linear distribution along a dermatome.

14. b. Urticaria is inflammation and edema in the upper dermis, most commonly caused by histamine released during an antibody-allergen reaction. The best treatment for all types of allergic dermatitis is avoidance of the allergen. Sunlight and warmth would increase the edema and inflammation. Antihistamines may be used for an acute outbreak but not to prevent the dermatitis. Topical benzene hexachloride is used to treat pediculosis.

15. a. Pediculosis (head lice and body lice) causes very small, red, noninflammatory lesions that progress to papular wheal-like lesions and cause severe itching. Lice live on the body as nits (tiny white eggs) that are firmly attached to hair shafts on the head and body. Burrows, especially in interdigital webs, are found with scabies.

16. c. A lotion is a suspension of insoluble powders in water, which has cooling and drying properties, useful when itching is present. Creams and ointments have an oil and water base that lubricates and protects skin whereas a paste is a mixture of powder and ointment.

17. d. Psoralen is absorbed by the lens of the eye and eyewear that blocks 100% of UV light must be used for 24 hours after taking the medication. Because UVA penetrates glass, the eyewear must also be worn indoors when near a bright window. Psoralen does not affect the accommodative ability of the eye.

18.

Medication	Nursing Instruction
Topical antibiotics	Clean skin; no occlusive dressings
Topical corticosteroids	Diagnosis of the lesion first; thin layers; massage at prescribed frequency
Systemic antihistamines	Advise of side effects and risks associated with driving or operating heavy machinery
Topical fluorouracil	Avoid sunlight; causes photosensitivity; warn patient that it will cause painful, eroded dermatitis before healing

19. a. 4; b. 1, 2, 3, 5; c. 1, 3; d. 2, 3, 6; e. 2, 3, 6

20. a. Dressings used to treat pruritic lesions should be cool to cause vasoconstriction and to have an antiinflammatory effect. Water is most commonly used and it does not need to be sterile. Acetic acid solutions are bacteriocidal and are used to treat skin infections.

21. b. Tepid or warm solutions should be used when the purpose is debridement and saline is a common debridement solution. Baths are appropriate for debridement but sodium bicarbonate and oatmeal are used for pruritus.

22.

Intervention	Rationale
Cool environment	Vasoconstriction
Topical menthol, camphor, or phenol	Decreased inflammation and blood flow, numbing of itch receptor
Soaks and baths	Vasoconstriction and stopping itch sensation

23. b. Defining characteristics for body image problems include verbalization of self-disgust and reluctance to look at lesions, as evidenced in this patient. Social isolation is indicated only if there is evidence of decreased social activities and of anxiety by verbalization of anxiety or frustration. Ineffective self-health management is indicated by evidence of a lack of self-care or understanding of the disease process.

24. a. Lichenification is thickening of the skin caused by chronic scratching or rubbing and can be prevented by controlling itching. It is not an infection, nor is it contagious, as the other options indicate.

25. a. Improvement of body image is the most common reason for undergoing cosmetic surgery; appearance is an important part of confidence and self-assurance. Acne scars, pigmentation problems, and wrinkling can be treated with cosmetic surgery but the surgery does not prevent the skin changes associated with aging.

26. d. A facelift is used for preauricular lesions and redundant soft tissue reduction. Liposuction is used for obesity with subcutaneous fat accumulation.
27. a. Skin flaps as grafts include moving skin and subcutaneous tissue to another part of the body and are used to cover wounds with poor vascular beds, add padding, and cover wounds over cartilage and bone. Both types of free grafts include just skin and soft tissue extension involves placement of an expander under the skin, which stretches the skin over time to provide extra skin to cover the desired area.
28. b. The appearance of candidiasis on the skin shows diffuse papular erythematous rash with pinpoint satellites around the affected area. Height and weight could show if the patient is obese but it would be better to ask if the areas affected are moist. The chemotherapy could contribute to candidiasis but it does not matter if the chemotherapy treatments are finished. Culture and sensitivity of the area may be ordered by the physician at the patient's appointment.
29. a, d, e, f. Glucocorticoid excess can cause acne and decreased subcutaneous fat over the extremities. Diabetes mellitus can cause erythematous plaques of the shins and both the corticosteroids and diabetes can impair or delay wound healing. Increased sweating is seen with hyperthyroidism and coarse, brittle hair is seen with hypothyroidism.

Case Study

1. The nurse would assess the size and depth of the injury, what the knife was being used for before the patient cut himself, and whether the patient had problems like this in the past.
2. W.B. should have cleansed the wound with soap and water and sought medical care for cleaning and suturing. A sterile dressing should have been applied and the arm should have been elevated to reduce edema.
3. *Staphylococcus aureus* and streptococcus are the usual etiologies of this type of infection.
4. Systemic antibiotics will be necessary and warm, moist packs or dressings should be used to help localize the infection. Hospitalization will be necessary if it becomes severe.
5. If treatment is not initiated and maintained, gangrene of the extremity and possible septicemia could occur.
6. **Nursing diagnoses:**
   - Impaired skin integrity *related to* trauma
   - Acute pain *related to* inflammatory process
   - Hyperthermia related to inflammatory process
   - Readiness for enhanced coping *related to* self-care post injury
   - Deficient knowledge *related to* self-care post injury
   Collaborative problems:
   Potential complications: gangrene, septicemia

CHAPTER 25

Answer Key

1. b. An electrical injury causes tissue damage from intense heat generated by the electrical current passing through tissue, including muscle contractions that can fracture long bones and vertebrae. Myoglobin is released into the circulation when massive muscle damage occurs. The electric shock even can cause cardiac standstill or dysrhythmias as well as delayed dysrhythmias during the first 24 hours after injury.

2. d, e. With chemical burns, removing the chemical from the skin is important. Lavaging the skin for 20 minutes to 2 hours post exposure may be needed. Alkali tends to adhere to skin and causes prolonged damage with protein hydrolysis and liquefaction. Metabolic asphyxiation is from the inhalation of carbon monoxide or hydrogen cyanide. Metabolic acidosis is most common in electrical burns, as is the "iceberg effect" of tissue injury below the skin.
3. a. Dry, waxy white, leathery, or hard skin is characteristic of full-thickness burns in the emergent phase and it may turn brown and dry in the acute phase. Deep partial-thickness burns in the emergent phase are red and shiny and have blisters. Edema may not be as extensive in full-thickness burns because of thrombosed vessels.
4. a. $3\frac{1}{2} + 1 + 6\frac{1}{2} + 2 + 1\frac{1}{2} + 3\frac{1}{2} = 18\%$ TBSA
   b. $4\frac{1}{2} + 9 + 4\frac{1}{2} + 4\frac{1}{2} = 22\frac{1}{2}\%$ TBSA
   c. No, because edema and inflammation obscure the demarcation of zones of injury.
5. a. 2; b. 4; c. 3; d. 1. The first intervention in emergency management of a burn injury is to remove the burn source and stop the burning process. Airway maintenance would be second, then establishing IV access, followed by assessing for other injuries.
6. b. The emergent phase is usually 24 to 72 hours after the time the burn occurred and focuses on fluid resuscitation. The acute phase is after the emergent phase and may last weeks to months after the burn occurred but begins when the extracellular fluid is mobilized and diuresis occurs. There is no postacute phase. The rehabilitative phase begins weeks to months after the injury, when the wounds have healed and the patient participates in self-care.
7. a. With increased capillary permeability, water, sodium, and plasma proteins leave the plasma and move into the interstitial spaces, decreasing serum sodium and albumin. Serum potassium is elevated because injured cells and hemolyzed red blood cells (RBCs) release potassium from cells. An elevated hematocrit is caused by water loss into the interstitium, creating a hemoconcentration.
8. a. Although all of the selections add to the hypovolemia that occurs in the emergent burn phase, the initial and most pronounced effect is caused by fluid shifts out of the blood vessels as a result of increased capillary permeability.
9. c. Burn injury causes widespread impairment of the immune system, with impaired WBC functioning, bone marrow depression, and a decrease in circulating immunoglobulins, which allows microorganisms to grow.
10. b. Shivering often occurs in a patient with a burn as a result of chilling that is caused by heat loss, anxiety, or pain. Severe pain is not common in full-thickness burns, nor is unconsciousness unless other factors are present. Fever is a sign of infection in later burn phases.
11. d. In circumferential burns, circulation to the extremities can be severely impaired and pulses should be monitored closely for signs of obstruction by edema. Swelling of the arms would be expected but it becomes dangerous when it occludes blood vessels. Pain and eschar are also expected.
12. c. Patients with major injuries involving burns to the face and neck require intubation within 1 to 2 hours after burn injury to prevent the need for emergency tracheostomy, which is done if symptoms of upper respiratory obstruction occur. Carbon monoxide poisoning is treated with 100% oxygen and eschar constriction of the chest is treated with an escharotomy.

13. To calculate fluid replacement, the patient's weight in pounds must be converted to kilograms: 132 lb = 60 kg.
    a. lactated Ringer's solution; 4 mL × 60 × 40 = 9600 mL
    b. 4800 mL between 10:15 PM and 5:30 AM; 2400 mL between 5:30 AM and 1:30 PM; 2400 mL between 1:30 PM and 9:30 PM
    c. 720–1200 mL (0.3–0.5 mL/kg/%/TBSA or 0.3 or 0.5 mL × 60 × 40)
    d. urine output (0.5 to 1 mL/kg/hr = 30–50 mL/hr) and vital signs (systolic BP 90, HR <120 bpm, RR 16–20).

14. b. When the patient's wounds are exposed with the open method, the staff must wear caps, masks, gowns, and gloves. Sterile water is not necessary in the debridement tank and topical antiinfective agents should be applied with sterile gloves. If some dressings are used with the open method, they are removed and wounds are washed with clean gloves.

15. a. Morphine is the drug of choice for pain control and during the emergent phase it should be administered IV because GI function is impaired and IM injections will not be absorbed adequately.

16. b. The patient with large burns often develops paralytic ileus within a few hours and a nasogastric tube is inserted and connected to low, intermittent suction. After GI function returns, feeding tubes may be used for nutritional supplementation and H_2 histamine blockers may be used to prevent Curling's ulcers. Free water is not given to drink because of the potential for water intoxication.

17. c. Patients with ear burns are not allowed to use pillows because of the danger of the burned ear sticking to the pillowcase and patients with neck burns are not allowed to use pillows because contractures of the neck can occur.

18. b, c, e. There is a hypermetabolic state proportional to the size of the burn, which increases the core temperature. Massive catabolism can occur and lead to malnutrition and delayed healing without adequate calorie and protein supplementation. The electrolyte imbalance has more effect on the fluid resuscitation than the nutritional needs.

19. c. At the end of the emergent phase, fluid mobilization moves potassium back into the cells and sodium returns to the vascular space, causing hypokalemia and hypernatremia. As diuresis in the acute phase continues, sodium will be lost in the urine and potassium will continue to be low unless it is replaced. Excessive fluid replacement with 5% dextrose in water without potassium supplementation can cause hyponatremia with hypokalemia. Prolonged hydrotherapy and free oral water intake can cause a decrease in both sodium and potassium.

20. b. The limited ROM in this situation is related to the patient's inability or reluctance to exercise the joints because of pain and the appropriate intervention is to help control the pain so that exercises can be performed. The patient is probably never without some pain and although exercises and enlisting the help of the physical therapist are important, neither of these interventions addresses the cause.

21. a. Early signs of sepsis include an elevated temperature and increased pulse and respiratory rate accompanied by decreased blood pressure and, later, decreased urine output and perhaps paralytic ileus. A burn wound may become locally infected without causing sepsis.

22.

Body System	Complication
Neurologic	Confusion or delirium
Gastrointestinal	Curling's ulcer
Endocrine	Hyperglycemia

23. a. cultured epithelial autograft. b. eschar (or necrotic tissue); autograft. c. aspirating the fluid with a tuberculosis syringe, performed by individuals instructed in this skill.

24. a. Midazolam is useful when patients' anticipation of the pain experience increases their pain because it causes a short-term memory loss and, if given before a dressing change, the patient will not recall the event. A dosage range of morphine is useful, as is patient-controlled analgesia, but seldom will these doses effectively relieve the discomfort of dressing changes. Buprenorphine is an opioid agonist/antagonist and cannot be used with other opioids.

25. a. Pressure garments help to keep scars flat and prevent elevation and enlargement above the original burn injury area. Lotions and splinting are used to prevent contractures. Avoidance of sunlight is necessary for at least 3 months to prevent hyperpigmentation and sunburn injury to healed burn areas.

26. c. There is tremendous psychologic impact with a burn injury. Open communication with caregivers, close friends, and the burn team about fears regarding loss of life as she once knew it, loss of function, temporary or permanent deformity and disfigurement, return to routine life, financial burdens, rehabilitation, and her future are all essential. Simply convincing her to have the wound cared for ignores her psychologic, emotional, and perhaps spiritual needs.

27. a. 3; b. 2; c. 1; d. 4. Face and neck burns are frequently associated with airway inhalation. Therefore this patient requires airway assessment (priority = ABCs). Severe pain would be the next priority (high physiologic need). The patient returning from the PACU will need to be seen soon to assess vital signs, level of consciousness, IV fluids, and wounds. However, at the current time the transport personnel should be with her. The 18-year-old is not at risk related to ABCs and it will probably take a few minutes to talk with him about why he doesn't want to go for the dressing change.

Case Study

1. Discharge planning should be initiated soon after admission, when D.K. is stabilized. Resuming a functional role in society and accomplishing functional and cosmetic reconstruction are the end goals toward which all care is directed. The nurse should coordinate the discharge process with the whole health care team involved with D.K.'s care: the health care provider, physical and occupational therapists, dietitian, home care nurses, and counselors.

2. D.K will continue to need a high-calorie, high-protein diet but not to the same extent as during the acute phase. She should be taught about her diet as well as to monitor for unwanted weight gain and reduce calories as indicated. She may also have a functional disability in feeding herself and may need padded utensils or special assistive devices.

3. D.K. will need to continue the splinting and exercise routine diligently until healing is complete, probably for at least a year.

4. It should be emphasized that exercise and performance of activities of daily living will decrease the tightness and limitation of movement. Set achievable short-term

goals with D.K. that can be measured or have her identify a few activities she wants most to do that are realistic and work toward success with those. D.K. is receiving a secondary gain from her husband in her dependence and regression and the nurse should help her husband to see the importance of her reestablishing independence and enlist his help in coaching the patient with exercises.

5. The staff should provide information and expected outcomes related to the healing of her injuries to both D.K. and her husband. Encourage both D.K. and her husband to participate in D.K.'s care and have them identify how care can be managed at home. Let them know that it is possible to maintain contact with hospital personnel after discharge to answer questions and provide support. A visiting nurse may also be ordered to assist them in adapting to the burn care at home.

6. D.K. and her family may experience a wide range of emotional responses—fear, anxiety, anger, guilt, and depression—and D.K. may be very concerned about her children's reactions to the appearance of her injuries. Encourage D.K.'s expression of negative feelings and fears while still hospitalized. Arranging for short visits by her children while she is still hospitalized and while the visits can be controlled would be helpful. Preparation of the family can also be enhanced by helping all family members to become aware of routines and activities that will need to be continued during rehabilitation.

7. The procedures for dressing changes and graft care should be formally demonstrated to D.K. and her husband with time for them to practice and return the demonstrations. It is most likely that the husband will need be involved because D.K. will be unable to manage applying dressings to her hands. Referral to home care nurses is essential for follow-up and evaluation when the patient is discharged to ensure that rehabilitation is continuing.

8. **Nursing diagnoses:**
   - Grieving *related to* impact of injury on appearance, relationships, and lifestyle
   - Anxiety *related to* appearance
   - Interrupted family processes *related to* altered health status of family member
   - Self-care deficit *related to* inability or unwillingness to participate in self-care
   - Ineffective self-health management *related to* insufficient knowledge of wound care and follow-up care
   - Situational low self-esteem *related to* effects of burn on appearance, increased dependence on others, and disruption of lifestyle and role responsibilities
   - Risk for disuse syndrome *related to* effects of immobility

   Collaborative problems:

   Potential complications: skin graft rejection, infection, contractures

CHAPTER 26

Answer Key

1. a. 9; b. 6; c. 7; d. 8; e. 5; f. 1; g. 12; h. 3; i. 2; j. 13; k. 4; l. 10; m. 11

2. b, e. This patient is older and short of breath. To obtain the most information, auscultate the posterior to avoid breast tissue and start at the base because of her respiratory difficulty and the chance that she will tire easily. Important sounds may be missed if the other strategies are used first.

3. b. Surfactant is a lipoprotein that lowers the surface tension in the alveoli. It reduces the pressure needed to inflate the alveoli and decreases the tendency of the alveoli to collapse. The other options do not maintain inflation of the alveoli. The carina is the point of bifurcation of the trachea into the right and left bronchi. Empyema is a collection of pus in the thoracic cavity. The thoracic cage is formed by the ribs and protects the thoracic organs.

4. c. Alveolar sacs are terminal structures of the respiratory tract where gas exchange takes place. The visceral pleura lines the lungs and forms a closed, double-walled sac with the parietal pleura. Turbinates warm and moisturize inhaled air. The 150 mL of air is dead space in the trachea and bronchi.

5. b. The epiglottis is a small flap closing over the larynx during swallowing. The trachea separates the larynx and the bronchi. The turbinates warm and moisturize inhaled air. The parietal pleura is a membrane that lines the chest cavity.

6. a. Normal findings in arterial blood gases (ABGs) in the older adult include a small decrease in PaO_2 and SaO_2 but normal pH and $PaCO_2$. No interventions are necessary for these findings. Usual PaO_2 levels are expected in patients 60 years of age or younger.

7. d. Normal venous blood gas values reflect the normal uptake of oxygen from arterial blood and the release of carbon dioxide from cells into the blood, resulting in a much lower PaO_2 and an increased $PaCO_2$. The pH is also decreased in mixed venous blood gases because of the higher $PvCO_2$. Normal mixed venous blood gases also have much lower PvO_2 and SvO_2 than ABGs. Mixed venous blood gases are used when patients are hemodynamically unstable to evaluate the amount of oxygen delivered to the tissue and the amount of oxygen consumed by the tissues.

8. c. Pulse oximetry is inaccurate if the probe is loose, if there is low perfusion, or when skin color is dark. Before other measures are taken, the nurse should check the probe site. If the probe is intact at the site and perfusion is adequate, an ABG analysis will be ordered by the health care provider to verify accuracy and oxygen may be administered, depending on the patient's condition and the assessment of respiratory and cardiac status.

9. c. Poor peripheral perfusion that occurs with hypovolemia or other types of conditions that cause peripheral vasoconstriction will cause inaccurate pulse oximetry and ABGs may need to be used to monitor oxygenation status and ventilation status in these patients. Pulse oximetry would not be affected by fever or anesthesia and is a method of monitoring arterial oxygen saturation in patients who are receiving oxygen therapy.

10. d. The respiratory rate, pulse rate, and blood pressure will all increase with decreased oxygenation when compared to the patient's own normal results. The position of the oximeter should also be assessed. The oxygenation status with a stress test would not assist the nurse in caring for the patient now. Hyperkalemia is not occurring and will not directly affect oxygenation initially. The SpO_2 compared with normal values will not be helpful in this older patient or in a patient with respiratory disease, as the patient's expected normal will not be the same as standard normal values.

11. d. An SpO_2 of 88% and a PaO_2 of 55 mm Hg indicate inadequate oxygenation and are the criteria for prescription of continuous oxygen therapy (see Table 26-3). These values may be adequate for patients with chronic hypoxemia if no cardiac problems occur but will affect the patients' activity tolerance.

12. c. A combination of excess CO_2 and H_2O results in carbonic acid, which lowers the pH of cerebrospinal fluid and stimulates an increase in the respiratory rate. Peripheral chemoreceptors in the carotid and aortic bodies also respond to increases in $PaCO_2$ to stimulate the respiratory center. Excess CO_2 does not increase the amount of hydrogen ions available in the body but does combine with the hydrogen of water to form an acid.

13. c. Ciliary action impaired by smoking and increased mucus production may be caused by the irritants in tobacco smoke, leading to impairment of the mucociliary clearance system.

Smoking does not directly affect filtration of air, the cough reflex, or reflex bronchoconstriction but it does impair the respiratory defense mechanism provided by alveolar macrophages.

14. a, b. Decreased functional cilia and decreased force of cough from declining muscle strength cause decreased secretion clearance. The other options contribute to other age-related changes. Decreased compliance contributes to barrel chest appearance. Early small airway closure contributes to decreased PaO_2. Decreased immunoglobulin A (IgA) decreases the resistance to infection.

15.

Functional Health Pattern	Risk Factor for or Response to Respiratory Problem
Health perception–health management	Smoking history; gradual change in health status; family history of lung disease; sputum production; no immunizations for influenza or pneumococcal pneumonia received; travel to developing countries
Nutritional-metabolic	Decreased fluid intake; anorexia and rapid weight loss; obesity
Elimination	Constipation; incontinence
Activity-exercise	Decreased exercise tolerance; dyspnea on rest or exertion; sedentary habits
Sleep-rest	Sleep apnea; awakening with dyspnea, wheezing, or cough; night sweats
Cognitive-perceptual	Decreased cognitive function with restlessness, irritability; chest pain or pain with breathing
Self-perception–self-concept	Inability to maintain lifestyle; altered self-esteem
Role-relationship	Loss of roles at work or home; exposure to respiratory toxins at work
Sexuality-reproductive	Sexual activity altered by respiratory symptoms
Coping–stress tolerance	Dyspnea-anxiety-dyspnea cycle; poor coping with stress of chronic respiratory problems
Value-belief	Noncompliance with treatment plan; conflict with values

16. c. Dullness and hyperresonance are found in the lungs using percussion, not the other assessment techniques.

17. c, d, e. Palpation identifies tracheal deviation, limited chest expansion, and increased tactile fremitus. Stridor is identified with auscultation. Finger clubbing and accessory muscle use are identified with inspection.

18. c. To assess the extent and symmetry of chest movement, the nurse places the hands over the lower anterior chest wall along the costal margin and moves them inward until the thumbs meet at the midline and then asks the patient to breathe deeply and observes the movement of the thumbs away from each other. The palms are placed against the chest wall to assess tactile fremitus. To determine the tracheal position, the nurse places the index fingers on either side of the trachea just above the suprasternal notch and gently presses backward.

19. b. An increased AP diameter is characteristic of a barrel chest, in which the AP diameter is about equal to the side-to-side diameter. Normally the AP diameter should be one third to one half the side-to-side diameter. A prominent protrusion of the sternum is the pectus carinatum and diminished movement of the two sides of the chest indicates decreased chest excursion. Lack of lung expansion caused by kyphosis of the spine results in shallow breathing with decreased chest expansion.

20. d. Bronchovesicular breath sounds are normal breath sounds when they are heard anteriorly over the mainstem bronchi on either side of the sternum and posteriorly between the scapulae. If they are heard in the peripheral lung fields, they are considered abnormal breath sounds. Adventitious lung sounds are extra abnormal sounds that include crackles, rhonchi, wheezes, and pleural friction rubs. See Table 26-7 for descriptions of these sounds.

21. a. 7; b. 6; c. 5; d. 8; e. 1; f. 2; g. 4; h. 3

22. d. A 10-mm red indurated injection site could be a positive result for a nurse as an employee in a high-risk setting. Because antibody production in response to infection with the TB bacillus may not be sufficient to produce a reaction to TB skin testing immediately after infection, two-step testing is recommended for individuals likely to be tested often, such as health care providers. An initial negative skin test should be repeated in 1 to 3 weeks and if the second test is negative, the individual can be considered uninfected. All other answers indicate a negative response to skin testing.

23. c. Samples for ABGs must be iced to keep the gases dissolved in the blood (unless the specimen is to be analyzed in <1 minute) and taken directly to the lab. The syringe used to obtain the specimen is rinsed with heparin before the specimen is taken and pressure is applied to the arterial puncture site for 5 minutes after obtaining the specimen. Changes in oxygen therapy or interventions should be avoided for 20 minutes before the specimen is drawn because these changes might alter blood gas values.

24. a. A pulmonary angiogram involves the injection of an iodine-based radiopaque dye and iodine or shellfish allergies should be assessed before injection. A bronchoscopy requires NPO status for 6 to 12 hours before the test and invasive tests (e.g., bronchoscopy, mediastinoscopy, biopsies) require informed consent that the physician should obtain from the patient. Nuclear scans use radioactive materials for diagnosis but the amounts are very small and no radiation precautions are indicated for the patient.

25. a. 6; b. 1; c. 7; d. 2; e. 5; f. 4; g. 3. The nurse will gather the supplies as soon as the order to do a thoracentesis is given. Hopefully the family will have some time to discuss this before they are instructed to leave the room, unless it is an emergency. The patient is positioned and instructed not to talk or cough to avoid damage to the lung. Observing for hypoxia is done to keep the physician informed. Breath sounds in all lobes are verified to be sure that there was no damage to the lung. This is done before sending the sample to the lab if there is no one else who can send the sample to the lab.

26. a. The greatest chance for a pneumothorax occurs with a thoracentesis because of the possibility of lung tissue injury during this procedure. Ventilation-perfusion scans and positron emission tomography (PET) scans involve injections but no manipulation of the respiratory tract is involved. Pulmonary function tests are noninvasive.

27. d. A pulmonary angiogram outlines the pulmonary vasculature and is useful to diagnose obstructions or pathologic conditions of the pulmonary vessels, such as a pulmonary embolus. The tissue changes of TB and cancer of the lung may be diagnosed by chest x-ray or computed tomography (CT), magnetic resonance imaging (MRI), or PET scans. Airway obstruction is most often diagnosed with pulmonary function testing.

28. a. 3; b. 7; c. 2; d. 4; e. 5; f. 6; g. 1; h. 8

CHAPTER 27

Answer Key

1. a. Direct pressure on the entire soft lower portion of the nose against the nasal septum for 10 to 15 minutes is indicated for epistaxis. In addition, have the patient upright and leaning forward to prevent swallowing blood.

2. d. All of the assessments are appropriate but the most important is the patient's oxygen status. After the posterior nasopharynx is packed, some patients, especially older adults, experience a decrease in PaO_2 and an increase in $PaCO_2$ because of impaired respiration and the nurse should monitor the patient's respiratory rate and rhythm and SpO_2.

3. b. The most important factor in managing allergic rhinitis is identification and avoidance of triggers of the allergic reactions. Immunotherapy may be indicated if specific allergens are identified and cannot be avoided. Drug therapy is an alternative to avoidance of the allergens but long-term use of decongestants can cause rebound nasal congestion.

4. d. Dyspnea and severe sinus pain as well as tender swollen glands, severe ear pain, or significantly worsening symptoms in a patient who has a viral upper respiratory infection (URI) indicate lower respiratory involvement and a possible secondary bacterial infection. Bacterial infections are indications for antibiotic therapy but unless symptoms of complications are present, injudicious administration of antibiotics may produce resistant organisms. Low-grade elevated temperature, cough, sore throat, myalgia, and purulent nasal drainage at the end of a cold are common symptoms of viral rhinitis and influenza.

5. a. The injected trivalent inactivated influenza vaccine is recommended for individuals 6 months of age and older and those at increased risk for influenza-related complications, such as people with chronic medical conditions or those who are immunocompromised, residents of long-term care facilities, health care workers, and providers of care to at-risk persons. The live attenuated influenza vaccine is given intranasally and is recommended for all healthy people between the ages of 2 and 49 but not for those at increased risk of complications or health care providers. The immunity will not protect for several years, as new strains of influenza may develop each year. Antiviral agents will help to reduce the duration and severity of influenza in those at high risk but immunization is the best control.

6. c. Although inadequately treated β-hemolytic streptococcal infections may lead to rheumatic heart disease or glomerulonephritis, antibiotic treatment is not recommended until strep infections are definitely diagnosed with culture or antigen tests. The manifestations of viral and bacterial infections are similar and appearance is not diagnostic except when the white irregular patches on the oropharynx suggest that candidiasis is present.

7. a, b, c. With partial airway obstruction, choking, stridor, use of accessory muscles, suprasternal and intercostals retraction, flaring nostrils, wheezing, restlessness, tachycardia, cyanosis, and change in level of consciousness may occur. Partial airway obstruction may progress to complete obstruction without prompt assessment and treatment.

8. c. With a tracheostomy (versus an endotracheal [ET] tube), patient comfort is increased because there is no tube in the mouth. Because the tube is more secure, mobility is improved. The ET tube is more easily inserted in an emergency situation. It is preferable to perform a tracheostomy in the operating room because it requires careful dissection but it can be performed with local anesthetic in the intensive care unit (ICU) or in an emergency. With a cuff, tracheal pressure necrosis is as much a risk with a tracheostomy tube as with an ET tube and infection is also as likely to occur because the defenses of the upper airway are bypassed.

9. e, f. The fenestrated tracheostomy tube has openings on the outer cannula to allow air to pass over the vocal cords to allow speaking. If the steps of using the fenestrated tracheostomy tube are not completed in the correct order, severe respiratory distress may result. The cuff of the tracheostomy tube with a foam-filled cuff passively fills with air and does require pressure monitoring, although cuff integrity must be assessed daily. The speaking tracheostomy tube has two tubes attached. One tube allows air to pass over the vocal cords to enable the person to speak with the cuff inflated.

10. b. An inner cannula is a second tubing that fits inside the outer tracheostomy tube. Disposable inner cannulas are frequently used but nondisposable ones can be removed and cleaned of mucus that has accumulated on the inside of the tube. Many tracheostomy tubes do not have inner cannulas because when humidification is adequate, accumulation of mucus should not occur.

11. d, e, f. Changing the tracheostomy tapes or the tube too soon will be irritating to the trachea and could contribute to dislodgement of the tracheostomy tube. Suctioning should be done when increased secretions are evident in the tube to prevent the patient from severe coughing, which could cause tube dislodgement. Tracheostomy care is done every 8 hours. Keeping the patient in a semi-Fowler position will not prevent dislodgement. Keeping an extra tube at the bedside will speed reinsertion if the tracheostomy tube is dislodged but it will not prevent dislodgement.

12. a, b, c. LPNs may determine the need for suctioning, suction the tracheostomy, and determine whether the patient has improved after the suctioning when caring for stable patients. They also may perform tracheostomy care using sterile technique. The patient's swallowing ability is assessed by a speech therapist, videofluoroscopy, or fiberoptic endoscopic evaluations. The RN will teach the patient about home tracheostomy care.

13. b. Cuff pressure should be monitored every 8 hours to ensure that an air leak around the cuff does not occur and that the pressure is not too high to allow adequate tracheal capillary perfusion. Respiratory therapists in some institutions will record the cuff pressure but the nurse must be able to assess cuff pressure and identify if there is a problem maintaining cuff pressure. Tracheostomy tubes are not usually changed sooner than 7 days after a tracheotomy. Mouth care should be performed a minimum of every 8 hours and more often as needed to remove dried secretions. ABGs are not routinely assessed with tracheostomy tube placement unless symptoms of respiratory distress continue.

14. a. If a tracheostomy tube is dislodged, the nurse should immediately attempt to replace the tube by grasping the retention sutures (if available) and spreading the opening. The obturator is inserted in the replacement tube, water-soluble lubricant is applied to the tip, and the tube is inserted in the stoma at a 45-degree angle to the neck. The obturator is immediately removed to provide an airway. If the tube cannot be reinserted, the health care provider should be notified and the patient should be assessed for the level of respiratory distress, positioned in semi-Fowler position, and ventilated with a manual resuscitation bag (MRB) only if necessary until assistance arrives.

15. b. The primary risk factors associated with head and neck cancers are heavy tobacco and alcohol use and family history. Chronic infections are not known to be risk factors, although cancers in patients younger than age 50 have been associated with human papillomavirus (HPV) infection. Oral cancer may cause a change in the fit of dentures but denture use is not a risk factor for oral cancer.

16. a. If laryngeal tumors are small, radiation is the treatment of choice because it can be curative and can preserve voice quality. Surgical procedures are used if radiation treatment is not successful or if larger or advanced lesions are present.

17. a. With removal of the larynx, the patient will not be able to communicate verbally and it is important to arrange with the patient a method of communication before surgery so that postoperative communication can take place. Dry mouth and stomatitis result from radiation therapy. Vigorous coughing is not encouraged immediately postoperatively and information related to community resources is usually introduced during the postoperative period.

18. a. Following a radical neck dissection, drainage tubes are often used to prevent fluid accumulation in the wound as well as possible pressure on the trachea. The patient has placement of a nasogastric tube to suction immediately after surgery, which will later be used to administer tube feedings until swallowing can be accomplished. A tracheostomy tube is in place but mechanical ventilation is usually not indicated.

19. c. A supraglottic laryngectomy involves removal of the epiglottis and false vocal cords and the removal of the epiglottis allows food to enter the trachea. Supraglottic swallowing protects the trachea from aspiration by taking a deep breath, putting the food or fluid in the mouth, swallowing while holding the breath, coughing immediately after swallowing to remove the food from the top of the vocal cord, swallowing again, then breathing. Super-supraglottic swallowing requires performance of the Valsalva maneuver before placing food in the mouth and swallowing. See Table 27-9.

20. b. Suctioning of the tracheostomy with the use of a mirror is a self-care activity taught to the patient before discharge. Voice rehabilitation is usually managed by a speech therapist or speech pathologist but the nurse should discuss the various types of voice rehabilitation and the advantages and disadvantages of each option. The laryngectomy stoma should be covered with a shield during showering and covered with light scarves or fabric when aspiration of foreign materials is likely.

21. b. Transesophageal puncture provides the most normal voice reproduction but requires a surgical fistula made between the esophagus and the trachea and possibly a valve prosthesis. Esophageal speech involves trapping air in the esophagus and releasing it to form sound but only 10% of patients can develop fluent speech with this method. The electrolarynx, whether placed in the mouth or held to the neck, allows speech that has a metallic or robotic sound.

Case Study

1. Clear drainage in the nose after facial trauma may be cerebrospinal fluid (CSF) that is leaking from the central nervous system following fractures of the face. Testing at the bedside or in the laboratory with strips that indicate glucose can differentiate CSF from mucus.

2. The vascularity of the face may cause excessive edema following facial trauma and surgery to repair fractures may need to be delayed until the edema subsides.

3. Airway can be maintained best by keeping F.N. in an upright position and controlling edema of the upper airway. After surgery, cold compresses and head elevation may help to decrease edema, reduce dyspnea, and minimize discomfort. F.N. may have PO fluids when awake and cold fluids will help to decrease the swelling. Activity restriction to prevent bleeding and injury include no nose blowing, swimming, heavy lifting, strenuous exercise, or large facial movements.

4. Respiratory status—rate, depth, and rhythm—should be assessed frequently to note respiratory distress. Vital signs should be taken and observation of the surgical site for hemorrhage and edema should also be done often.

5. F.N. needs to be taught how to clean the nose and nares with cotton swabs and water or hydrogen peroxide and to apply water-soluble jelly to the nares; to continue using the external plastic splint as ordered; to report any continued drainage of serosanguineous fluid from the nose after 24 hours or any fresh bleeding; and to not use aspirin or aspirin-containing products for pain relief. F.N. should also be educated about symptoms of postoperative infection. Activity restriction to prevent bleeding and injury will be decreased as the rhinoplasty heals.

6. **Nursing diagnoses:**
   - Disturbed body image *related to* postoperative edema and changed facial appearance
   - Acute pain *related to* incisional edema
   - Risk for ineffective breathing pattern *related to* presence of packing and nasal edema

   Collaborative problems:
   Potential complications: nasal hemorrhage, nasal hematoma, infection

CHAPTER 28

Answer Key

1. a, c, e. Microorganisms that cause pneumonia reach the lungs by aspiration from the nasopharynx or oropharynx, inhalation of microbes in the air, and hematogenous spread from infections elsewhere in the body. The other causes of infection do not contribute to pneumonia.

2. c. Pneumonia that has its onset in the community is usually caused by different microorganisms than pneumonia that develops related to hospitalization and treatment can be empiric—based on observations and experience without knowing the exact causative organism. Frequently a causative organism cannot be identified from cultures and treatment is based on experience.

3. b. People at risk for opportunistic pneumonia include those with altered immune responses. *Pneumocystis jiroveci* rarely causes pneumonia in healthy individuals but is the most common cause of pneumonia in persons with HIV disease. Cytomegalovirus (CMV) occurs in people with an impaired immune response. Medical care-associated pneumonia is frequently caused by *Pseudomonas aeruginosa, Escherichia coli, Klebsiella,* and *Acinetobacter* species. Community-acquired pneumonia is most commonly caused by *Streptococcus pneumonia.*

4. a, b, f. Community-acquired pneumonia (CAP) and medical care–associated pneumonia (MCAP) are both associated with *Klebsiella, Staphylococcus aureus,* and *Streptococcus pneumonia. Haemophilus influenzae* and *Mycoplasma pneumonia* are only associated with CAP. *Pseudomonas aeruginosa* is only associated with MCAP.

5. a. 4; b. 3; c. 1; d. 2. With most pneumonia-causing organisms the inflammatory response sends increased blood flow and neutrophils to engulf the offending organisms. The alveoli are filled with extra fluid from increased blood flow and capillary permeability from surrounding vessels, which leads to hypoxia. Mucus production is increased and can further obstruct airflow. With bacterial pneumonia the alveoli fill with fluid and debris. Macrophages lyse and process the debris so that normal gas exchange returns.

6. a. Confusion possibly related to hypoxia may be the only finding in older adults. Although CAP is most commonly caused by *Staphylococcus aureus* pneumonia and is associated with an acute onset with fever, chills, productive cough with purulent or bloody sputum, and pleuritic chest pain, the older patient may not have classic symptoms. Other causes of pneumonia have a more gradual onset with dry, hacking cough; headache; and sore throat. A recent loss of consciousness or altered consciousness is common in those pneumonias associated with aspiration, such as anaerobic bacterial pneumonias.

7. d. Prompt treatment of pneumonia with appropriate antibiotics is important in treating bacterial and mycoplasma pneumonia and antibiotics are often administered on the basis of the history, physical examination, and a chest x-ray indicating a typical pattern characteristic of a particular organism without further testing. Sputum and blood cultures take 24 to 72 hours for results and microorganisms often cannot be identified with either Gram stains or cultures. Whether the pneumonia is community acquired or medical-care associated is more significant than the severity of symptoms.

8. c. A sputum specimen for Gram stain and culture should be done before initiating antibiotic therapy and while waiting for the antibiotic to be delivered from the pharmacy in a hospitalized patient with suspected pneumonia and then antibiotics should be started without delay. If the sputum specimen cannot be obtained rapidly, the chest x-ray will be done to assess the typical pattern characteristic of the infecting organism. Blood cell tests will not be altered significantly by delaying the tests until after the first dose of antibiotics.

9.

Clinical Situation	Nursing Intervention
Patient with altered consciousness	Position to side, protect airway
Patient with a feeding tube	Check placement of the tube before feeding, residual feeding; keep head of bed up after feedings or continuously with continuous feedings
Patient with local anesthetic to throat	Check gag reflex before feeding or offering fluids
Patient with difficulty swallowing	Cut food in small bites, encourage thorough chewing, and provide soft foods that are easier to swallow than liquids

10. a. Oxygen saturation obtained by pulse oximetry should be between 90% and 100%. An SpO_2 lower than 90% indicates hypoxemia and impaired gas exchange. Crackles, purulent sputum, and fever are all manifestations of pneumonia, but do not necessarily relate to impaired gas exchange.

11. b. Clear lung sounds indicate that the airways are clear. SpO_2 of 90% to 100% indicates appropriate gas exchange. Tolerating walking in the hallway also indicates appropriate gas exchange, not improved airway clearance. Deep breaths are necessary to move mucus from distal airways but this is not an outcome.

12. b. A second dose of the pneumococcal vaccine should be provided to all persons 65 years of age or older who have not received the vaccine within 5 years and were younger than 65 years of age at the time of vaccination. Influenza vaccine should be taken each year by those older than 65 years of age. Antibiotic therapy is not appropriate for all upper respiratory infections unless secondary bacterial infections develop.

13. b. Drug-resistant strains of TB have developed because TB patients' compliance with drug therapy has been poor and there has been general decreased vigilance in monitoring and follow-up of TB treatment. TB can be diagnosed effectively with sputum cultures. Antitubercular drugs are almost exclusively used for TB infections. The incidence of TB is at epidemic proportions in patients with HIV but this does not account for drug-resistant strains of TB.

14. b. A patient with class 3 TB has clinically active disease and airborne infection isolation is required for active disease until the patient is noninfectious, indicated by negative sputum smears. Cardiac monitoring and observation will need to be done with the patient in isolation. The nurse will administer the antitubercular drugs after the patient is in isolation. There should be no need for suction or extra linens after the TB patient is receiving drug therapy.

15. b. TB usually develops insidiously with fatigue, malaise, anorexia, low-grade fevers, and night sweats. Pleuritic pain,

flu-like symptoms, and a productive cough may occur with an acute sudden presentation but dyspnea and hemoptysis are late symptoms.

16. a, b, c, f. For the first 2 months, a four-drug regimen consists of isoniazid (INH), rifampin (Rifadin), pyrazinamide (PZA), and ethambutol (Myambutol). Rifabutin (Mycobutin) and levofloxacin (Levaquin) may be used if the patient develops toxicity to the primary drugs. Rifabutin (Mycobutin) may be used as first-line treatment for patients receiving medications that interact with rifampin.

17. d. Notification of the public health department is required. If drug compliance is questionable, follow-up of patients can be made by directly observed therapy by a public health nurse or a responsible family member. A patient who cannot remember to take the medication usually will not remember to come to the clinic daily or will find it too inconvenient. Additional teaching or support from others is not usually effective for this type of patient.

18. b. Although all of the precautions identified in this question are appropriate in decreasing the risk of occupational lung diseases, using masks and effective ventilation systems to reduce exposure is the most efficient and affects the greatest number of employees.

19. a, b, d, e. Smoking by women is taking a great toll, as reflected by the increasing incidence and deaths from lung cancer in women, who develop lung cancer at a younger age than men. Nonsmoking women are at greater risk of developing lung cancer. The incidence of small cell carcinoma is higher in women than in men. Men still have a worse prognosis than women from lung cancer.

20. d. The use of radiology, computed tomography (CT), and sputum cytology has been shown to detect lung cancer at earlier stages. Low-dose spiral CT scanning has been shown to decrease lung cancer mortality compared with those who had chest x-rays. To be considered for screening for lung cancer, patients must be 55 to 74 years old, current smokers with at least a 30 pack-year smoking history or former smokers who quit within the past 15 years, have no history of lung cancer, and not be on home oxygen A patient who has a smoking history always has an increased risk for lung cancer compared with an individual who has never smoked but the risk decreases as the period of nonsmoking increases.

21. c. Although chest x-rays, lung tomograms, CT scans, MRI, and positron emission tomography (PET) can identify tumors and masses, a definitive diagnosis of a lung cancer requires identification of malignant cells in either sputum specimens or biopsies.

22. a. 3; b. 6; c. 8; d. 7; e. 1; f. 9; g. 5; h. 2; i. 4

23. b. Before making any judgments about the patient's statement, it is important to explore what meaning he or she finds in the pain. It may be that the patient feels it is deserved punishment for smoking but further information needs to be obtained from the patient. Immediate referral to a counselor negates the nurse's responsibility in helping the patient and there is no indication that the patient is not dealing effectively with his or her feelings.

24. d. Spontaneous pneumothorax is seen from the rupture of small blebs on the apex of the lung in patients with lung disease or smoking, as well as in tall, thin males with a family history of or a previous spontaneous pneumothorax. Tension pneumothorax occurs with mechanical ventilation and with blocked chest tubes. Iatrogenic pneumothorax occurs due to the laceration or puncture of the lung during medical procedures. Traumatic pneumothorax can occur with penetrating or blunt chest trauma.

25. b. A tension pneumothorax causes many of the same manifestations as other types of pneumothoraces but severe respiratory distress from collapse of the entire lung with movement of the mediastinal structures and trachea to the unaffected side is present in a tension pneumothorax. Percussion dullness on the injured site indicates the presence of blood or fluid and decreased movement and diminished breath sounds are characteristic of a pneumothorax. Muffled and distant heart sounds indicate a cardiac tamponade.

26. d. Flail chest may occur when two or more ribs are fractured, causing an unstable segment. The chest wall cannot provide the support for ventilation and the injured segment will move paradoxically to the stable portion of the chest (in on expiration; out on inspiration). Hypotension occurs with a number of conditions that impair cardiac function, and chest pain occurs with a single fractured rib and will be of high priority with flail chest. Absent breath sounds occur following pneumothorax or hemothorax.

27. A. Suction control chamber or dry suction regulator; B. water-seal chamber; C. air leak monitor; D. collection chamber; E. suction monitor bellows

28.

Chamber	Function
Water-seal	This chamber contains 2 cm of water, which acts as a one-way valve. Incoming air enters from the collection chamber and bubbles up through the water. The water prevents backflow of the air into the patient from the system
Suction control	This chamber supplies suction to the chest drainage. The water suction type system contains a column of water with the top end vented to the atmosphere to control the amount of suction, with bubbles to indicate it is working. The amount of suction applied is controlled by the amount of water in the chamber (usually −20 cm), not by the wall suction applied to it. The dry suction device contains no water and uses a regulator to dial the desired negative pressure.
Collection	This chamber receives fluid and air from the pleural or mediastinal space. Nurses keep track of the amount of drainage and can mark the container for easy measuring.
Suction monitor bellows	The dry model has the suction monitor bellows, which expands to show that the suction is operating, as this model does not make the bubbling noise made by the models that control the suction with water.

29. b. The water-seal chamber should bubble intermittently as air leaves the lung with exhalation in a spontaneously breathing patient. Continuous bubbling indicates a leak. The water in the suction control chamber will bubble continuously and the fluid in the water-seal chamber fluctuates with the patient's breathing. Water in the suction control chamber, and perhaps in the water-seal chamber, evaporates and may need to be replaced periodically.

30. c. If chest tubes are to be milked or stripped, this procedure should be done only by the professional nurse. This procedure is no longer recommended, as it may dangerously increase pleural pressure, but there is no indication to milk the tubes when there is no bloody drainage, as in a pneumothorax. The UAP can loop the chest tubing on the bed to promote drainage and patients should be reminded to cough and deep breathe at least every 2 hours to aid in lung reexpansion. Securing the drainage container in an upright position is also a necessary activity that can be completed by UAP.

31. b. Decortication is the stripping of a thick fibrous membrane. A lobectomy is the removal of one lung lobe. A thoracotomy is the incision into the thorax. A wedge resection is used to remove a small lesion.

32. d. During video-assisted thoracic surgery (VATS), a video scope is inserted into the thorax to assess, diagnose, and treat intrathoracic injuries. A pneumonectomy is the removal of a lung. A wedge resection is the removal of a lung segment. Lung volume–reduction surgery is the removal of lung tissue by excising multiple wedges.

33. d. A thoracotomy incision is large and involves cutting into bone, muscle, and cartilage, resulting in significant postoperative pain. The patient has difficulty deep breathing and coughing because of the pain and analgesics should be provided before attempting these activities. Water intake is important to liquefy secretions but is not indicated in this case, nor should a patient with chest trauma or surgery be placed in Trendelenburg position, because it increases intrathoracic pressure.

34. a. 8; b. 7; c. 2; d. 3; e. 6; f. 1; g. 9; h. 4; i. 5

35. a. All of the activities are correct but the first thing to do is to raise the head of the bed to promote respiration in the patient who is dyspneic. The health care provider would not be called until the nurse has assessment data relating to vital signs, pulse oximetry, and any other patient complaints.

36. b. A spiral (helical) CT scan is the most frequently used test to diagnose pulmonary emboli because it allows illumination of all anatomic structures and produces a 3-D picture. If a patient cannot have contrast media, a ventilation-perfusion scan is done. Although pulmonary angiography is most sensitive, it is invasive, expensive, and carries more risk for complications. Chest x-rays do not detect pulmonary emboli until necrosis or abscesses occur.

37. a. Chronic obstructive pulmonary disease (COPD) causes pulmonary capillary and alveolar damage. Sarcoidosis is a granulomatous disease. Pulmonary fibrosis stiffens the pulmonary vasculature and pulmonary embolism obstructs pulmonary blood flow.

38. b. High pressure in the pulmonary arteries increases the workload of the right ventricle and eventually causes right ventricular hypertrophy and dilation, known as cor pulmonale. Eventually, decreased left ventricular output may occur because of decreased return to the left atrium but it is not the primary effect of pulmonary hypertension. Alveolar interstitial edema is pulmonary edema associated with left ventricular failure. Pulmonary hypertension does not cause systemic hypertension.

39. d. If possible, the primary management of cor pulmonale is treatment of the underlying pulmonary problem that caused the heart problem. Low-flow oxygen therapy will help to prevent hypoxemia and hypercapnia, which cause pulmonary vasoconstriction.

40. c. Acute rejection may occur as early as 5 to 7 days after surgery and is manifested by low-grade fever, fatigue, and oxygen desaturation with exertion. Complete remission of symptoms can be accomplished with bolus corticosteroids. Cytomegalovirus and other infections can be fatal but usually occur weeks after surgery and manifest with symptoms of pneumonia. Obliterative bronchiolitis is a late complication of lung transplantation, reflecting chronic rejection.

Case Study

1. Low-flow oxygen; calcium channel blocking agents (nifedipine [Adalat], diltiazem [Cardizem]); phosphodiesterase (type 5) enzyme inhibitors (sildenafil [Revatio]); parenteral vasodilators (epoprostenol [Flolan], adenosine [Adenocard]); inhaled vasodilators (iloprost [Ventavis], treprostinil [Tyvaso]); endothelin receptor antagonists (bosentan [Tracleer], ambrisentan [Letairis]); diuretics; and anticoagulants.

2. Yes, because her medical treatment has failed, she has worsening right-sided heart failure, and she potentially can be treated with either a lung or a heart-lung transplant. She meets additional criteria of being less than 60 years old and a nonsmoker.

3. A heart-lung transplant is indicated for T.S. because she has heart damage from the pulmonary hypertension, although there is evidence that even a single-lung transplantation can markedly correct pulmonary hypertension and the resultant cor pulmonale.

4. T.S. needs preoperative teaching to help her to cope with the postoperative regimen, which includes the following:
   * Strict adherence to immunosuppressive drugs
   * Continuous monitoring and reporting of manifestations of infection
   * Self-care activities and accurately identifying when to call the transplant team
   * Rehabilitation program
   * Financial resources for the procedure, drugs, and follow-up care
   * Social and emotional support system because she is a single mother

5. Vital sign and cardiac monitoring, oxygen administration, positioning T.S. in high-Fowler position, sequential compression stockings, medication administration, and consultation with a chaplain, social worker, or psychologist for counseling related to recent divorce and care of children while in the hospital and postoperatively.

CHAPTER 29

Answer Key

1. d. Respiratory infections are one of the most common precipitating factors of an acute asthma attack. Sensitivity to food and drugs may also precipitate attacks and exercise-induced asthma occurs after exercise, especially in cold, dry air. Psychologic factors may interact with the asthmatic response to worsen the disease but it is not a psychosomatic disease.

2. b. Diminished or absent breath sounds may indicate a significant decrease in air movement resulting from exhaustion and an inability to generate enough muscle force to ventilate and is an ominous sign. The other symptoms are expected in an asthma attack.

3. c. Early in an asthma attack, an increased respiratory rate and hyperventilation create a respiratory alkalosis with increased pH and decreased $PaCO_2$, accompanied by hypoxemia. As the attack progresses, pH shifts to normal, then decreases, with arterial blood gases (ABGs) that reflect respiratory acidosis with hypoxemia. During the attack, high-flow oxygen should be provided. Breathing in a paper bag, although used to treat some types of hyperventilation, would increase the hypoxemia.

4.

Agent	Role or Relationship to Asthma
Salicylates	Associated with the asthma triad—people with nasal polyps, asthma, and sensitivity to salicylates and nonsteroidal antiinflammatory drugs (NSAIDs)
α-Adrenergic blockers	Contraindicated in patients with asthma because they prevent bronchodilation
Beer and wine	Contain sulfites that are common triggers of asthma

5. b. Peak expiratory flow rates (PEFR) are normally up to 600 L/min and in status asthmaticus may be as low as 100 to 150 L/min. An SaO_2 of 85% and a FEV_1 of 85% of predicted are typical of mild to moderate asthma. A flattened diaphragm may be present in the patient with long-standing asthma but does not reflect current bronchoconstriction.

6. d. The albuterol nebulizer will rapidly cause bronchodilation and be easier to use in an emergency situation than an inhaler. It will be used every 20 minutes to 4 hours as needed. The ipratropium inhaler could be used if the patient does not tolerate the short-acting β_2-adrenergic agonists (SABA) but its onset is slower than albuterol. Inhaled or oral corticosteroids will be used to decrease the inflammation and provide better symptom control after the emergency situation is over.

7. c, f, g, i. These are the corticosteroids described. Zileuton (Zyflo CR) and montelukast (Singulair) are leukotriene modifiers that interfere with the synthesis or block the action of the leukotriene inflammatory mediators that cause bronchoconstriction. Omalizumab (Xolair) is an anti-IgE, which prevents IgE from attaching to mast cells and prevents the release of chemical mediators. Salmeterol (Serevent) is a long-acting β_2-adrenergic agonist

bronchodilator. Methylxanthine (theophylline) is used when other long-term bronchodilators are not available or affordable.

8. d. Storing the dry powder inhaler (DPI) in the bathroom will expose it to moisture, which could cause clumping of the medication and an altered dose. The other statements show patient understanding.

9. a, f. Salmeterol (Serevent) should not be taken without inhaled corticosteroids. Asthma medications may make gastroesophageal reflux disease (GERD) symptoms worse and GERD medications may make asthma symptoms worse. The rest of the statements show patient understanding.

10. b. The patient in an acute asthma attack is very anxious and fearful. It is important to stay with the patient and interact in a calm, unhurried manner. Helping the patient to breathe with pursed lips will facilitate expiration of trapped air and help the patient to gain control of breathing. Pursed lip breathing also is used with COPD for this same reason.

11. c. A yellow zone reading with the PEFR indicates that the patient's asthma is getting worse and quick-relief medications should be used. The meter is routinely used only each morning before taking medications and does not have to be on hand at all times. The meter measures the ability to empty the lungs and involves blowing through the meter.

12. b. Nonprescription drugs should not be used by patients with asthma because of dangers associated with rebound bronchospasm, interactions with prescribed drugs, and undesirable side effects. All of the other responses are appropriate for the patient with asthma.

13. d. Increased risk of infection, hyperplasia of mucous glands, cancer, and chronic bronchitis are the long-term effects of smoking.

14. a. A; b. C; c. C; d. C; e. C; f. B; g. C; h. B; i. B; j. C; k. A

15. b. Constriction of the pulmonary vessels, leading to pulmonary hypertension, is caused by alveolar hypoxia and the acidosis that results from hypercapnia. Polycythemia is a contributing factor in cor pulmonale because it increases the viscosity of blood and the pressure needed to circulate the blood. Long-term low-flow oxygen therapy dilates pulmonary vessels and is used to treat cor pulmonale. High oxygen administration is not related to cor pulmonale.

16. d. Smoking cessation is one of the most important factors in preventing further damage to the lungs in COPD but prevention of infections that further increase lung damage is also important. The patient is very susceptible to infections and these infections make the disease worse, creating a vicious cycle. Bronchodilators, inhaled corticosteroids, and lung volume–reduction surgery help to control symptoms but these are symptomatic measures.

17. a. A Venturi mask is helpful to administer low, constant O_2 concentrations to patients with COPD and can be set to administer a varied percentage of O_2. The amount of O_2 inhaled via the nasal cannula depends on room air and the patient's breathing pattern. The simple face mask must have a tight seal and may generate heat under the mask. The non-rebreathing mask is more useful for short-term therapy with patients needing high O_2 concentrations.

18. b. The partial rebreathing mask has O_2 flow into the reservoir bag and mask during inhalation.

The O_2-conserving cannula is used for long-term therapy at home versus during hospitalization. The Venturi mask is able to deliver the highest concentrations of O_2. The nasal cannula is the most comfortable and mobile delivery device.

19. c. Oxygen concentrators or extractors continuously supply O_2 concentrated from the air. O_2-conserving units will last for up to 20 hours. Portable liquid O_2 units will hold about 6 to 8 hours of O_2 but because of the expense they are only used for portable and emergency use. Compressed O_2 comes in various tank sizes but generally it requires weekly deliveries of four to five large tanks to meet a 7- to 10-day supply.

20. c. Pursed lip breathing prolongs exhalation and prevents bronchiolar collapse and air trapping. Huff coughing is a technique used to increase coughing patterns to remove secretions. Thoracic breathing is not as effective as diaphragmatic breathing and is the method most naturally used by patients with COPD. Diaphragmatic breathing emphasizes the use of the diaphragm to increase maximum inhalation but it may increase the work of breathing and dyspnea.

21. c. Many postural drainage positions require placement in Trendelenburg position but patients with heart disease, hemoptysis, chest trauma, or severe dyspnea should not be placed in these positions. Postural drainage should be done 1 hour before and 3 hours after meals if possible. Coughing, percussion, and vibration are all performed after the patient has been positioned.

22. b. Eating is an effort for patients with COPD and frequently these patients do not eat because of fatigue, dyspnea, and difficulty holding their breath while swallowing. Foods that require much chewing cause more exhaustion and should be avoided. A low-carbohydrate diet is indicated if the patient has hypercapnia because carbohydrates are metabolized into carbon dioxide. Fluids should be avoided at meals to prevent a full stomach and cold foods seem to give less of a sense of fullness than hot foods.

23. a. Assistance with positioning and activities of daily living (ADL) is within the training of unlicensed assistive personnel (UAP). Teaching, assessing, and planning are all part of the RN's practice.

24. d. Indacaterol (Arcapta Neohaler) is a DPI that is used only for COPD. Roflumilast (Daliresp) is an oral medication used for COPD. Salmeterol (Serevent) is a DPI but it is also used in asthma with inhaled corticosteroids. Ipratropium (Atrovent HFA) is used for COPD but it is delivered via metered-dose inhaler or nebulizer.

25. d. The tripod position with an elevated backrest and supported upper extremities to fix the shoulder girdle maximizes respiratory excursion and an effective breathing pattern. Staying with the patient and encouraging pursed lip breathing also helps. Bronchodilators may help but can also increase nervousness and anxiety; rescue inhalers would be used before routine bronchodilators. Postural drainage is not tolerated by a patient in acute respiratory distress and oxygen is titrated to an effective rate based on ABGs because of the possibility of carbon dioxide narcosis.

26. d. Specific guidelines for sexual activity help to preserve energy and prevent dyspnea and maintenance of sexual activity is important to the healthy psychologic well-being of the patient. Open communication between partners is needed so that the modifications can be made with consideration of both partners.

27. c. Shortness of breath usually increases during exercise but the activity is not being overdone if breathing returns to baseline within 5 minutes after stopping. Bronchodilators can be administered 10 minutes before exercise but should not be administered for at least 5 minutes after activity to allow recovery. Patients are encouraged to walk 15 to 20 minutes per day with gradual increases but actual patterns will depend on patient tolerance. Dyspnea most frequently limits exercise and is a better indication of exercise tolerance than is heart rate in the patient with COPD.

28. b. These results show worsening respiratory function and failure. The results in option a show potential normal results for the patient described. The results in option c show normal ABGs. The results in option d show alkalosis, probably respiratory, but the HCO_3^- results are needed to be sure.

29. b, c, e. Decreasing anxiety, depression, and hospitalizations along with improving exercise capacity are the anticipated effects of pulmonary rehabilitation. The other options may occur but are not predicted.

30. c. Cystic fibrosis (CF) is an autosomal recessive, multisystem disease involving altered transport of sodium and chloride ions in and out of epithelial cells, which affects the lungs, pancreas, and sweat glands. Abnormally thick, abundant secretions from mucous glands lead to a chronic, diffuse, obstructive pulmonary disorder in almost all patients, whereas exocrine pancreatic insufficiency occurs in about 85% to 90% of patients with CF.

31. d. The major objective of therapy in CF is to promote removal of the secretions and performance of postural drainage, vibration, and percussion has been the mainstay of treatment. Aerobic exercise also seems to be effective in clearing the airways and is an important part of treatment. Antibiotics are used for early signs of infection and long courses are necessary but they are not used prophylactically. Bronchodilators have no long-term benefit. Although CF has become a leading indication for heart-lung transplant, this treatment option is not available for most patients.

32. b. The presence of a chronic disease that is present at birth and significantly lowers life span and the many treatments needed by those with CF affects all relationships and development of these patients. Although a lung transplant may be needed, not all CF patients need one. Children of a parent with CF will either be carriers of CF or have the disease. Many men with CF are sterile and women may have difficulty becoming pregnant. Educational and vocational goals may be met in those who maintain treatment programs and health.

33. d. In adults, most forms of bronchiectasis are associated with bacterial infections that damage the bronchial walls. In children, cystic fibrosis is the prominent cause of bronchiectasis. The incidence of bronchiectasis has decreased with the use of measles and pertussis vaccines and better treatment of lower respiratory tract infections.

34. d. Mucus production is increased in bronchiectasis and collects in the dilated, pouched bronchi. A major goal of treatment is to promote drainage and removal of the mucus, primarily through deep breathing, coughing, and postural drainage.

35. d. α$_1$-Antitrypsin (AAT) deficiency is an autosomal recessive disorder that is a genetic risk factor for COPD. AAT occurs in 1 in 1700 to 3500 live births with an onset between ages 20 and 40 years. Although cystic fibrosis occurs in 1 in 3000 white births, legislation requires babies to be screened at birth, so it would have been previously diagnosed. Asthma is a multifactorial genetic disorder.

36. d. Positive expiratory pressure (PEP) is the principle behind the airway clearance devices (ACDs) that mobilize secretions and benefit patients. Vibration, a form of chest physiotherapy, and inhalation therapy are therapies to assist patients with excessive secretions or to increase bronchodilation but they are not principles of ACDs' function.

Case Study

1. Blood pressure; presence of perspiration; PEFR; neck vein distention; triggers; presence of GERD; frequent lung sounds; ABGs as ordered; pulmonary function studies to determine the reversibility of bronchoconstriction (using bronchodilators) after the acute situation; Asthma Control Test; serum IgE level; sputum culture and sensitivity may be done; fractional exhaled nitric oxide (FENO) may be measured.

2. Oxygen therapy needs to be started immediately. The goal is to get E.S.'s oxygen saturation above 90% and to maintain it at or above that level. Although oxygen could be administered using a nasal cannula or face mask, it is important to ensure that E.S. is receiving the oxygen supplement. Her SpO$_2$ or PaO$_2$ needs to be monitored closely. Also, the nurse must assess whether the patient with a nasal cannula or face mask device keeps it on (some patients complain that the face mask is suffocating them).

3. E.S. is using accessory muscles and has audible wheezing, a respiratory rate >30, and a heart rate >120. Her responses to questions are very short (one- to three-word sentences). She is sitting upright and is extremely anxious and restless. Her breath sounds are not audible in the bases of her lungs and her oxygen saturation is <90%. These are all manifestations of a severe asthma attack. Other observations that might be evident during severe attacks are agitation, PEF rate <150 mL, neck vein distention, and a pulsus paradoxus of 40 mm Hg. Patients with life-threatening asthma are usually too dyspneic to speak and are perspiring profusely. They may be drowsy and the ABGs will reveal further deterioration (lower PaO$_2$, lower O$_2$ saturation, rising PaCO$_2$, and pH that is acidotic). Breath sounds may become very difficult to hear and wheezing may no longer be present (very little airflow). These patients become bradycardic and may require airway intubation, mechanical ventilation, and admission to the ICU.

4. SABA stimulate the β$_2$-adrenergic receptors in the bronchioles, producing bronchodilation (relieve bronchospasm) as well as increased mucociliary clearance. The SABA medications will be given by nebulizer repetitively. Often a SABA plus the anticholinergic agent ipratropium (Atrovent) is given in severe asthma attacks and provides partial relief but it has a slower onset of action.

Inhaled corticosteroids are the second classification of medications given in severe attacks. They can be administered orally or IV. Corticosteroids are antiinflammatory agents that reduce bronchial hyperresponsiveness, block the late phase reaction, and inhibit migration of inflammatory cells.

5. Patients experiencing a severe asthma attack are extremely anxious and may not be able to follow the direction of health care providers. Nurses can decrease a patient's sense of panic by providing a calm, quiet, reassuring attitude. Position the patient for comfort (usually sitting upright), stay with the patient, and be available to provide comfort. Gain eye contact with the patient and in a firm and calm voice coach the patient to use pursed lip breathing and abdominal breathing (technique called "talking down"). This helps the patient to remain calm and improves ventilation (maintains a positive airway pressure, slows down the respiratory rate, and encourages deeper breaths).

6. PEFR is measured by the peak expiratory flow rate meter, which correlates with forced expiratory volume in 1 second (FEV$_1$) and is helpful to diagnose and manage asthma. Since there are no standardized PEFR reference values, spirometry is preferred. PEFR can be useful to monitor the asthma patient's response to treatments.

7. Teaching of the written asthma action plan that prescribes a step increase in medications during an acute phase should include medication use and response to medication; avoidance of triggers; a diary with medication use, the presence of wheezing or coughing, PEFR measurement, the drug's side effects, and the activity level; balanced nutrition; physical exercise within the patient's tolerance, possibly with pretreatment; interrupted sleep means poorly controlled asthma; and relaxation therapies. Teaching is done with both patient and family or caregiver.

8. **Nursing diagnoses:**
   - Ineffective airway clearance *related to* bronchospasm and fatigue
   - Anxiety *related to* difficulty breathing and fear
   - Deficient knowledge *related to* lack of information and education about asthma
   - Ineffective health maintenance *related to* lack of primary health care provider

   Collaborative problems:
   Potential complications: severe acute asthma, life-threatening asthma

CHAPTER 30

Answer Key

1. a, b, c, f. These characteristics are evident with neutrophils. Platelets arise from megakaryocytes and are stored in the spleen. Eosinophils are increased in individuals with allergies and make up 2% to 4% of WBCs.

2. c. Increased reticulocytes, or immature RBCs, indicate an increased rate of erythropoiesis or stimulation of erythrocyte (RBC) production by the bone marrow. Basophils release granules that increase allergic and inflammatory responses and are stimulated by granulocyte colony-stimulating factor. Monocytes may become tissue macrophages. Lymphocytes are primarily responsible for the immune response.

3. a, c, d. Basophils, eosinophils, and neutrophils are the granulocytic leukocytes. Lymphocytes are the agranular leukocytes that form the basis of the cellular and humoral immune responses. Monocytes are agranulocytes that are potent phagocytic cells.

4. a. Lymphedema is the obstruction of lymph flow that results in accumulation of lymph fluid for the patient in the right arm following a right-sided breast mastectomy. The other options are not hematologic problems that would cause extreme swelling.

5. a, b, e. Although all of the listed nutrients are helpful, iron, folic acid, and cobalamin (vitamin B_{12}) are essential for erythropoiesis.

6. a. 4; b. 1; c. 3; d. 2

7. a. Protein C and protein S are examples of anticoagulants that are involved in the lysis of clots. Fibrinolysis is also achieved by thrombin-activating conversion of plasminogen to plasmin, which attacks fibrin or fibrinogen and splits it into smaller elements known as fibrin split products (FSPs) or fibrin degradation products (FDPs).

8. a, b, e. The abdominal organs that are primarily involved in hematologic function are the liver, spleen, and lymph nodes. The liver filters the blood, produces procoagulants, and stores iron. The spleen removes old and defective erythrocytes and filters iron for reuse. The lymph nodes filter pathogens and foreign particles from lymphatic circulation.

9. b. During fibrinolysis by plasmin, the fibrin clot is split into smaller molecules known as FSPs or FDPs. Increased FSPs impair platelet aggregation, reduce prothrombin, and prevent fibrin stabilization and lead to bleeding.

10. c. As a person ages the partial thromboplastin time (PTT) is normally decreased, so an abnormally high PTT of 60 seconds is an indication that bleeding could readily occur. Platelets are unaffected by aging and 150,000/µL is a normal count. Serum iron levels are decreased and the erythrocyte sedimentation rate (ESR) is significantly increased with aging, as are reflected in these values.

11. a, b, d. The myeloblast is a committed hematopoietic cell found in the bone marrow from which granulocytes develop. A disorder in which myeloblasts are overproduced would result in increased basophils, eosinophils, and neutrophils.

12. a. The parietal cells of the stomach secrete intrinsic factor, a substance necessary for the absorption of cobalamin (vitamin B_{12}), and if all or part of the stomach is removed, the lack of intrinsic factor can lead to impaired RBC production and pernicious anemia. Recurring infections indicate decreased WBCs and immune response and corticosteroid therapy may cause a neutrophilia and lymphopenia. Oral contraceptive use is strongly associated with changes in blood coagulation.

13.

Functional Health Pattern	Risk Factor for or Response to Hematologic Problem
Health perception–health management	Ethnic background; family history of hematologic disorders; alcohol, illicit drug, and cigarette use
Nutritional-metabolic	Weight; history of anorexia, nausea, vomiting, or oral discomfort; deficiencies of iron, vitamin B_{12}, and folic acid; GI bleeding; petechiae or bruising of the skin; fever; lymph node swelling
Elimination	Frankly bloody or dark, tarry stools; dark or bloody urine
Activity-exercise	Fatigue and weakness; change in ability to perform normal activities of daily living
Sleep-rest	Fatigue unrelieved by sleep
Cognitive-perceptual	Pain, especially in joints or bones; paresthesias, numbness, or tingling; changes in hearing, vision, taste, or mental status
Self-perception–self-concept	Altered self-perception because of lymph node enlargement or skin changes
Role-relationship	Home or work exposure to radiation or chemicals; military history; change in role or responsibility
Sexuality-reproductive	Menstrual history and characteristics of bleeding; intrapartum or postpartum bleeding problems; impotence
Coping–stress tolerance	Lack of support to meet daily needs; methods of coping with stress
Value-belief	Values conflict with treatment, especially blood product or bone marrow transplants

14. a. Superficial lymph nodes are evaluated by light palpation but they are not normally palpable. It may be normal to find small (<1.0 cm), mobile, firm, nontender nodes. Deep lymph nodes are detected radiographically.

15. b. Petechiae are small, flat, red, or reddish-brown pinpoint microhemorrhages that occur on the skin when platelet levels are low. When petechiae are numerous, they group, causing reddish bruises known as purpura. Sternal tenderness is associated with leukemias. Jaundice occurs when anemias are of a hemolytic origin, resulting in accumulation of bile pigments from RBCs. Enlarged, tender lymph nodes are associated with infection or cancer.

16. b. A smooth, shiny, reddened tongue is an indication of iron-deficiency anemia or pernicious anemia that would be reflected by a decreased hemoglobin level. The decreased neutrophils would be indicative of neutropenia. The increased WBC count could be indicative of an infection and the increased RBC count of polycythemia.

17. c. Any platelet count <150,000/μL is considered thrombocytopenia and could place the patient at risk for bleeding, necessitating special consideration in nursing care. Chemotherapy may cause bone marrow suppression and a depletion of all blood cells. The other factors are all within normal range.

18.

Laboratory Finding	Possible Etiology
Serum iron 40 mcg/dL (7 μmol/L)	Iron-deficiency anemia
ESR 30 mm/hr	Inflammatory conditions of any kind
Increased band neutrophils	Infection, usually acute
Activated partial thromboplastin time 60 sec	Heparin therapy
Indirect bilirubin 2.0 mg/dL (34 μmol/L)	Hemolysis of RBCs
Bence Jones protein in urine	Multiple myeloma

19. b. A patient with type O Rh$^+$ blood has no A or B antigens on the RBC but does have anti-A and anti-B antibodies in the blood and has an Rh antigen. Type AB Rh$^-$ blood has both A and B antigens on the RBC but no Rh antigen and no anti-A or anti-B antibodies. If the type AB Rh$^-$ blood is given to the patient with type O Rh$^+$ blood, the antibodies in the patient's blood will react with the antigens in the donor blood, causing hemolysis of the donor cells. There will be no Rh reaction because the donor blood has no Rh antigen.

20. a. A contrast CT scan involves the use of an iodine-based dye that could cause a reaction if the patient is sensitive to iodine. Metal implants or internal appliances and claustrophobia should be determined before magnetic resonance imaging (MRI). Prior blood transfusions are not a factor in this diagnostic test.

21. c. The aspiration of bone marrow content is done with local anesthesia at the site of the puncture but the aspiration causes a suction pain that is quite painful but very brief. There generally is no residual pain following the test.

22. d. Lymph node biopsy is usually done to determine whether malignant cells are present in lymph nodes and can be used to diagnose lymphomas as well as metastatic spread from any malignant tumor in the body. Leukemias may infiltrate lymph nodes but biopsy of the nodes is more commonly used to detect any type of neoplastic cells.

23. c. Pancytopenia is decreased RBCs, WBCs, and platelets. Hemolysis is RBC destruction. Leukopenia is WBC <4000/μL. Thrombocytosis is increased platelets and thrombocytopenia is decreased platelets.

24. b, c. Bone marrow and lymph node biopsies are preferred methods to obtain the sample for gene analysis. If a large number of abnormal cells are circulating in the blood, peripheral blood may be used. The other options will not provide the desired information.

CHAPTER 31

Answer Key

1.

Type or Cause of Anemia	Etiology	Morphology
Malaria	3	4
Thalassemia	1	6
Acute trauma	2	4
Aplastic anemia	1	4
Pernicious anemia	1	5
Sickle cell anemia	3	4
Anemia of gastritis	2	4
Anemia of leukemia	1	4
Iron-deficiency anemia	1	6
Anemia of renal failure	1	4
Glucose-6-phosphate dehydrogenase (G6PD)	3	4
Anemia associated with prosthetic heart valve	3	4

2. b. The patient's hemoglobin (Hgb) level indicates a moderate anemia and at this severity additional findings usually include dyspnea and fatigue. Pallor, smooth tongue, and sensitivity to cold usually manifest in severe anemia when the Hgb level is below 6 g/dL (60 g/L).

3. c. In the older adult, confusion, ataxia, and fatigue are common manifestations of anemia and place the patient at risk for injury. Nursing interventions should include safety precautions to prevent falls and injury when these symptoms are present. The nurse, not the patient's family, is responsible for the patient and although a quiet room may promote rest, it is not as important as protection of the patient.

4. d. Dyspnea at rest indicates that the patient is making an effort to provide adequate amounts of oxygen to the tissues. If oxygen needs are not met, angina, myocardial infarction, heart failure, and pulmonary and systemic congestion can occur. The other manifestations are present in severe anemia but they do not reflect hypoxemia, a priority problem.

5. b. Aplastic anemia has a decrease of all blood cell types and hypocellular bone marrow. Thalassemia is characterized by inadequate production of normal hemoglobin and decreased erythrocyte production. Megaloblastic anemias (cobalamin deficiency and folic acid deficiency anemias) are caused by impaired DNA synthesis, which results in the presence of large red blood cells (RBCs). Anemia of chronic disease occurs with chronic inflammation, autoimmune and infectious disorders, heart failure, malignancies, or bleeding episodes. It manifests with underproduction of RBCs and shortened RBC survival.

6. c, d, f. Iron-deficiency anemia is the most common type of anemia and occurs with chronic blood loss or malabsorption in the duodenum so it may occur with duodenal removal. The other options are associated with cobalamin deficiency.

7. d. Folic acid deficiency megaloblastic anemia is related to dietary deficiency as seen in anorexia and with the use of oral contraceptives and antiseizure medications. The other anemias are unrelated to this patient's history.

8.

Finding	Explanation
Reticulocyte counts are increased in chronic blood loss but decreased in cobalamin (vitamin B$_{12}$) deficiency.	The hypoxia resulting from loss of RBCs in chronic blood loss stimulates the kidney to release erythropoietin, stimulating production of RBCs and reticulocytes. However, in pernicious anemia, normal reticulocytes are not produced because of the lack of cobalamin.
Bilirubin levels are increased in sickle cell anemia but are normal in acute blood loss.	Sickle cell anemia is a hemolytic anemia involving an accelerated RBC breakdown, leading to increased serum bilirubin levels, whereas acute blood loss results in loss of the RBC and the bile pigments from the body.
Mean corpuscular volume (MCV) is increased in folic acid deficiency but decreased in iron-deficiency anemia.	The MCV is a determination of the relative size of an RBC and macrocytic anemias, such as folic acid deficiency and cobalamin deficiency, are characterized by the production of large, immature RBCs that would reflect an increased MCV. In iron-deficiency anemia, the MCV is low because of the lack of Hgb in the cells.

9. a. Constipation is a common side effect of oral iron supplementation and increased fluids and fiber should be consumed to prevent this effect. Because iron can be bound in the gastrointestinal (GI) tract by food, it should be taken before meals unless gastric side effects of the supplements necessitate its ingestion with food. Black stools are an expected result of oral iron preparations. Taking iron with ascorbic acid or orange juice enhances absorption of the iron but enteric-coated iron often is ineffective because of unpredictable release of the iron in areas of the GI tract where it can be absorbed.

10. b. Pernicious anemia is a type of cobalamin (vitamin B$_{12}$) deficiency that results when parietal cells in the stomach fail to secrete enough intrinsic factor to absorb ingested cobalamin. Folic acid deficiency may contribute to folic acid deficiency anemia, not pernicious anemia. Extrinsic factor may be a factor in some cobalamin deficiencies but not in pernicious anemia. Lack of cobalamin intake can cause cobalamin deficiency but not pernicious anemia. Increasing cobalamin intake cannot improve pernicious anemia without intrinsic factor to aid its absorption.

11. c. Neurologic manifestations of weakness, paresthesias of the feet and hands, and impaired thought processes are characteristic of cobalamin deficiency and pernicious anemia. Hepatomegaly and jaundice often occur with hemolytic anemia and the patient with cobalamin deficiency often has achlorhydria or decreased stomach acidity and would not experience effects of gastric hyperacidity.

12. a. Without cobalamin replacement individuals with pernicious anemia will die in 1 to 3 years but the disease can be controlled with cobalamin supplements for life. Hematologic manifestations can be completely reversed with therapy but long-standing neuromuscular complications might not be reversed. Because pernicious anemia results from an inability to absorb cobalamin, dietary intake of the vitamin is not a treatment option, nor is a bone marrow transplant.

13. d. Because red meats are the primary dietary sources of cobalamin, a strict vegetarian is most at risk for cobalamin deficiency anemia. Meats are also an important source of iron and folic acid but whole grains, legumes, and green leafy vegetables also supply these nutrients. Thalassemia is not related to dietary deficiencies.

14. a, c, e. Aplastic anemia may cause an inflamed, painful tongue. The thrombocytopenia may contribute to blood-filled bullae in the mouth and gingival bleeding. The leukopenia may lead to stomatitis and oral ulcers and infections. MCV will be normal or slightly increased. Ferritin and coagulation factors are not affected in aplastic anemia.

15. b. Hemorrhage from thrombocytopenia and infection from neutropenia are the greatest risks for the patient with aplastic anemia. The patient will experience fatigue from anemia but bleeding and infection are the major causes of death in aplastic anemia.

16. a, d, e. With rapid blood loss, hypovolemic shock may occur. Clinical manifestations will be more reliable, as they reflect the body's attempt to meet oxygen requirements. As the percentage of blood loss increases, clinical manifestations worsen. Blood transfusions will first be used, then iron, vitamin B$_{12}$, and folic acid supplements may be used.

17. b. Because RBCs are abnormal in sickle cell anemia, the mean RBC survival time is 10 to 15 days (rather than the normal 120 days) because of accelerated RBC breakdown by the spleen, not in the blood vessels. Antibody reactions with RBCs may be seen in other types of hemolytic anemias but are not present in sickle cell anemia.

18. b. During a sickle cell crisis, the sickling cells clog small capillaries and the resulting hemostasis promotes a self-perpetuating cycle of local hypoxia, deoxygenation of more erythrocytes, and more sickling. Administration of oxygen may help to control further sickling but additional oxygen does not reach areas of local hypoxia caused by occluded vessels.

19. d. Because pain usually accompanies a sickle cell crisis and may last for 4 to 6 days, pain control is an important part of treatment. Rest is indicated to reduce metabolic needs and fluids and electrolytes are administered to reduce blood viscosity and maintain renal function. Although thrombosis does occur in capillaries, elastic stockings that primarily affect venous circulation are not indicated; anticoagulants are used instead.

20. d. The patient with sickle cell disease is particularly prone to upper respiratory infection and infection can precipitate a sickle cell crisis. Patients should seek medical attention quickly to counteract upper respiratory infections because

pneumonia is the most common infection of patients with sickle cell disease. Fluids should be increased to decrease blood viscosity, which may precipitate a crisis, and moderate activity is permitted. Dehydration in hot weather may precipitate a sickling episode but humid weather alone will not do so.

21. a, c, d. Immune thrombocytopenic purpura (ITP) is characterized by increased platelet destruction by the spleen. Thrombotic thrombocytopenic purpura (TTP) has decreased platelets and RBCs with enhanced agglutination of the platelets. Platelet deficiencies lead to superficial site bleeding. ITP is the most common acquired thrombocytopenia. Petechiae, not ecchymosis, is a common manifestation of thrombocytopenia.

22. b. The symptoms describe hemochromatosis, which is treated with iron chelating agents to remove accumulated iron via the kidneys.

23. b. Thrombus and embolization are the major complications of polycythemia vera because of increased hypervolemia and hyperviscosity. Active or passive leg exercises and ambulation should be implemented to prevent thrombus formation. Hydration therapy is important to decrease blood viscosity. However, because the patient already has hypervolemia, a careful balance of intake and output must be maintained and fluids are not increased injudiciously.

24. b. Corticosteroids are used in initial treatment of ITP because they suppress the phagocytic response of splenic macrophages, decreasing platelet destruction. They also depress autoimmune antibody formation and reduce capillary fragility and bleeding time. All of the other therapies may be used but only in patients who are unresponsive to corticosteroid therapy.

25. c. The major complication of thrombocytopenia is hemorrhage and it may occur in any area of the body. Cerebral hemorrhage may be fatal and evaluation of mental status for central nervous system (CNS) alterations to identify CNS bleeding is very important. Fever is not a common finding in thrombocytopenia. Protection from injury to prevent bleeding is an important nursing intervention but strict bed rest is not indicated. Oral care is performed very gently with minimum friction and soft swabs.

26. Any five of these are appropriate: Discontinue heparin administration and expect a direct or indirect thrombin inhibitor to be ordered. Monitor for signs and symptoms of bleeding (check IV sites, wounds, any secretions). Monitor ordered coagulation studies. Avoid injections. Use an electric razor. Protect the patient from trauma. Administer ordered blood products. Instruct the patient and caregiver to avoid aspirin and other anticoagulants. Instruct the patient to avoid high-contact activities (many sports).

27. d. A prolonged partial thromboplastin time (PTT) occurs when there is a deficiency of clotting factors, such as factor VIII associated with hemophilia A. Factor IX is deficient in hemophilia B and prolonged bleeding time and decreased platelet counts are associated with platelet deficiencies.

28. c. Although whole blood and fresh frozen plasma contain the clotting factors that are deficient in hemophilia, specific factor concentrates have been developed that are more pure and safer in preventing infection transmission. Thromboplastin is factor III and is not deficient in patients with hemophilia.

29. b. During an acute bleeding episode in a joint, it is important to rest the involved joint totally and slow bleeding with application of ice. Drugs that decrease platelet aggregation, such as aspirin or nonsteroidal antiinflammatory drugs (NSAIDs), should not be used for pain. As soon as bleeding stops, mobilization of the affected area is encouraged with range-of-motion (ROM) exercises and physical therapy.

30. d. This description is characteristic of von Willebrand disease with prolonged bleeding time occurring because of defective platelets, which does not occur with either type of hemophilia. Although inherited thrombocytopenia is believed to be autosomal dominant, the number of platelets is decreased.

31. a. 5; b. 8; c. 3; d. 6; e. 2; f. 7; g. 1; h. 4

32. a. Yes, as the WBC count is below 4000/µL.
    b. The neutrophil count is $2300 \times 40\% = 920/\mu L$.
    c. Yes, as the neutrophil count is less than 1000/µL.
    d. Yes, the patient is at moderate risk of infection with opportunistic pathogens and nonpathogenic organisms from normal body flora.

33. a. An elevated temperature is of most significance in recognizing the presence of an infection in the neutropenic patient because there is no leukocytic response to injury. When the WBC count is depressed, the normal phagocytic mechanisms of infection are impaired and the classic signs of inflammation may not occur. Cultures are indicated if the temperature is elevated but are not used to monitor for infection.

34. d. Despite its seeming simplicity, hand washing before, during, and after care of the patient with neutropenia is the major method to prevent transmission of harmful pathogens to the patient. IV antibiotics are administered when febrile episodes occur. Some oral antibiotics may be used prophylactically in some neutropenic patients. High-efficiency particulate air (HEPA) filtration and laminar airflow (LAF) rooms may reduce the number of aerosolized pathogens but they are expensive and LAF use is controversial.

35. a. Although myelodysplastic syndromes, like leukemias, are a group of disorders in which hematopoietic stem cells of the bone marrow undergo clonal change and may cause eventual bone marrow failure, the primary difference from leukemias is that myelodysplastic cells have some degree of maturation and the disease progression is slower than in acute leukemias.

36. c. Acute myelogenous leukemia (AML) is seen in 80% of adults with acute leukemia and is characterized by hyperplasia of the bone marrow with uncontrolled proliferation of myeloblasts, the precursors of granulocytes. Acute lymphocytic leukemia (ALL), the other acute leukemia, is most common in children and is characterized by small, immature lymphocytes, primarily of B-cell origin, proliferated in the bone marrow. Fever, bleeding, and central nervous system manifestations are also common with ALL. The other two leukemias are chronic in onset and the maturity of WBCs.

37. a, c, f. Chronic lymphocytic leukemia (CLL) is the most common leukemia in adults. It is a neoplasm of activated B lymphocytes that are mature appearing but functionally inactive. As it progresses, pressure on nerves from enlarged lymph nodes causes pain and paralysis. Mediastinal node enlargement leads to pulmonary symptoms. The other characteristics are related to chronic myelogenous leukemia (CML).

38. c. Almost all leukemias cause some degree of hepatosplenomegaly because of infiltration of these organs as well as the bone marrow, lymph nodes, bones, and central nervous system by excessive WBCs in the blood.

39. c. Whether the donor bone marrow is from a human leukocyte antigen (HLA)-matched donor or taken from the patient during a remission for later use, hematopoietic stem cell transplant always involves the use of chemotherapy and/or total-body radiation to eliminate leukemic cells and the patient's bone marrow stem cells totally before IV infusion of the donor cells. A severe pancytopenic period follows the transplant, during which the patient must be in protective isolation and during which RBC and platelet transfusions may be given.

40. a. NHL; b. HL; c. B; d. NHL; e. B; f. HL; g. HL; h. NHL; i. HL; j. B

41. b. The patient is monitored for infection as leukopenia and thrombocytopenia may develop from the disease or usually as a consequence of treatment. Staging of Hodgkin's disease is important to determine treatment. Multiple myeloma is characterized by proliferation of malignant activated B cells that destroy the bones. The intervention of increasing fluid to manage hypercalcemia is used with multiple myeloma.

42. c. Splenectomy may be indicated for treatment for ITP and when the spleen is removed, platelet counts increase significantly in most patients. In any of the disorders in which the spleen removes excessive blood cells, splenectomy will most often increase peripheral RBC, WBC, and platelet counts.

43. a. Chills and fever are symptoms of an acute hemolytic or febrile transfusion reaction and if these develop, the nurse should stop the transfusion, infuse saline through the IV line, notify the health care provider and blood bank immediately, recheck the ID tags, and monitor vital signs and urine output. The addition of a leukocyte reduction filter may prevent a febrile reaction but is not helpful once the reaction has occurred. Mild and transient allergic reactions indicated by itching and hives might permit restarting the transfusion after treatment with antihistamines.

44. b. Because platelets adhere to the plastic bags, the bag should be gently agitated throughout the transfusion. Platelets do not have A, B, or Rh antibodies and ABO compatibility is not a consideration. Baseline vital signs should be taken before the transfusion is started and the nurse should stay with the patient during the first 15 minutes. Platelets are stored at room temperature and should not be refrigerated.

45. a. Febrile nonhemolytic reaction is the most common transfusion reaction. Allergic reactions occur with sensitivity to foreign plasma proteins and can be treated prophylactically with antihistamines. Acute hemolytic reactions are related to the infusion of ABO-incompatible blood or components with 10 mL or more of RBCs. Massive blood transfusion reactions occur when patients receive more RBCs or blood than the total blood volume.

46. a, c, d. ABO incompatibility, destruction of donor RBCs, and acute kidney injury may occur in an acute hemolytic transfusion reaction. Hypothermia, hypocalcemia, and hyperkalemia are most likely to occur in massive blood transfusion reactions. Epinephrine may be used for severe allergic transfusion reactions and the infusion may be restarted after treatment with antihistamines in mild cases.

47. b, c. All other actions are the responsibility of the RN. The licensed practical nurse may be able to assist with the ID checks (depending on the state and the facility policy).

48. a. 1; b. 3; c. 4; d. 2; e. 5; f. 6; g. 10; h. 9; i. 8; j. 7.

Case Study

1. Traumatized placental and uterine tissues that release tissue factor into circulation, initiating the coagulation cascade.

2. Venipuncture site bleeding; oozing of blood from other sites; respiratory problems, such as tachypnea, hemoptysis, orthopnea, and cyanosis; upper or lower GI bleeding and abdominal pain; hematuria and oliguria; neurologic manifestations such as vision changes, dizziness, headache, and changes in mental status and irritability; musculoskeletal complaints such as bone and joint pain; electrocardiogram changes; and venous distention.

3. Elevated fibrin degradation products (elevated split products); reduced factors V, VIII, X, and XIII; elevated D-dimers (cross-linked fibrin fragments); prolonged prothrombin time and PTT; prolonged activated partial thromboplastin time; prolonged thrombin time; reduced fibrinogen, platelets, antithrombin III (AT III), and proteins C and S.

4. Oxygen and fluid replacement will be administered as needed. In this bleeding patient, therapy is administered on the basis of specific component deficiencies. Platelets are given to correct thrombocytopenia, cryoprecipitate replaces factor VIII and fibrinogen, and fresh frozen plasma replaces all clotting factors except platelets and provides a source of antithrombin. This patient is not manifesting symptoms of thrombosis, so anticoagulation is probably not indicated at this time. Treatment of the underlying condition may include a dilation and curettage or even a hysterectomy, if necessary, to remove the stimulus of DIC.

5. **Nursing diagnoses:**
   * Ineffective tissue perfusion: cardiopulmonary, cerebral, peripheral, and renal *related to* blood loss and thrombosis
   * Decreased cardiac output *related to* fluid volume deficit
   * Risk for impaired tissue integrity *related to* altered coagulation
   * Anxiety or fear *related to* disease process and therapy
   Collaborative problems:
   Potential complications: hemorrhage, thrombosis, hypovolemia and shock, renal failure

CHAPTER 32

Answer Key

1. a. Pulmonic (semilunar) valve; b. tricuspid valve; c. interventricular septum; d. papillary muscle; e. chordae tendineae; f. mitral valve; g. aortic (semilunar) valve

2. a. Aorta; b. superior vena cava; c. right atrium; d. right coronary artery; e. right marginal artery; f. posterior descending artery; g. right ventricle; h. left ventricle; i. left anterior descending artery; j. left marginal artery; k. circumflex artery; l. left atrium; m. left coronary artery; n. pulmonary trunk; o. aorta; p. superior vena cava; q. right atrium; r. small cardiac vein; s. middle cardiac vein; t. right ventricle; u. left ventricle; v. great

cardiac vein; w. coronary sinus; x. posterior vein; y. left atrium; z. pulmonary trunk

3. c, d, f. The left circumflex and left anterior descending arteries branch from the left coronary artery. The left coronary artery and right coronary artery arise from the aorta to supply the atria, ventricles, and interventricular septum.

4. a. 4; b. 7; c. 3; d. 5; e. 8; f. 1; g. 2; h. 6

5. a. P; b. Q; c. R; d. S; e. T; f. U; g. PR interval; h. QRS interval; i. QT interval

6. a. 2; b. 4; c. 2; d. 4; e. 5; f. 3; g. 3; h. 1

7.

Situation	Stroke Volume Factor	Cardiac Output
Valsalva maneuver	Preload, ↓	↓
Venous dilation	Preload, ↓	↓
Hypertension	Afterload, ↑	↓
Administration of epinephrine	Contractility, ↑	↑
Obstruction of pulmonary artery	Preload, ↓	↓
Hemorrhage	Preload, ↓	↓

8. b, d, f. The sympathetic nervous system increases the heart rate, the speed of impulse conduction through the atrioventricular (AV) node, and the force of atrial and ventricular contractions via the β-adrenergic receptors.

9.

Cardiovascular Problem	Physiologic Change
Widened pulse pressure	Loss of vascular distensibility and elastic recoil during systole
Decreased cardiac reserve	Increased collagen and decreased elastin
Increased cardiac dysrhythmias	Decrease in sinoatrial (SA) node cells, conduction cells in the intermodal tracts, the bundle of His, and bundle branches
Decreased response to sympathetic stimulation	Decreased number and function of β-adrenergic receptors
Aortic or mitral valve murmurs	Valvular lipid accumulation and calcification

10. d. Recreational or abused drugs, especially stimulants such as cocaine and methamphetamine, are a growing cause of cardiac dysrhythmias and problems associated with tachycardia and IV injection of abused drugs is a risk factor for inflammatory and infectious conditions of the heart. Although calcium is involved in the contraction of muscles, calcium supplementation is not a significant factor in heart disease, nor is metastatic cancer. Streptococcal, but not viral, pharyngitis is a risk factor for rheumatic heart disease.

11.

Functional Health Pattern	Risk Factor for or Response to Cardiovascular Problem
Health perception–health management	Family history of coronary artery disease, cardiomyopathy, or hypertension; the patient's history of hyperlipidemia, hypertension, smoking, obesity, or sedentary or stressful lifestyle; history of hereditary or familial cardiovascular disease or diabetes mellitus; alcohol use or use of recreational drugs; experience of drug, allergic, or anaphylactic reaction
Nutritional-metabolic	Underweight or obesity; high intake of sodium, fat, and cholesterol
Elimination	Dependent edema; incontinence or constipation; use of diuretics with increased urinary output
Activity-exercise	Lack of aerobic exercise; decreased activity tolerance; symptoms during exercise
Sleep-rest	Attacks of shortness of breath interrupting sleep; use of several pillows to sleep; sleep apnea
Cognitive-perceptual	Vertigo, syncope, language memory problems, or other cognitive changes
Self-perception–self-concept	Loss of self-esteem resulting from fatigue and decreased activity tolerance
Role-relationship	Stress or conflict in roles
Sexuality-reproductive	Change in sexual activity caused by shortness of breath or fatigue; impotence and medications taken for erectile dysfunction; oral contraceptives, hormone therapy for menopause, or medications for breast cancer
Coping–stress tolerance	Depression, high stress, or anxiety; support system; denial, anger, or hostility as coping mechanisms
Value-belief	Diagnosis or treatment conflict with value system

12. d. A palpable vibration of a blood vessel is called a thrill and usually indicates turbulent blood flow through the vessel. A weak, thready pulse has little pressure and is difficult to palpate. A bruit is an abnormal buzzing or humming sound that may be auscultated over diseased blood vessels and a bounding pulse is an extra full, hard pulse that may occur with atherosclerosis or hypervolemia.

13. a. Angle of Louis; b. Aortic area; c. Mitral area (apex) and PMI; d. Tricuspid area; e. Erb's point; f. Pulmonic area

14. a. S_1; b. S_2; c. S_1; d. S_2; e. S_2; f. S_1
15. c, d, f. The cardiac murmurs are produced by turbulent blood flow across diseased heart valves, S_3 is heard with mitral valve regurgitation, and S_4 is heard with aortic stenosis. Arterial bruits are from turbulent peripheral blood flow. Pulsus alternans, seen in heart failure, is a variation in the strength of each pulse when palpated. Pericardial friction rub is the sound heard with pericarditis.
16. c. The bell of the stethoscope will enable better hearing of the low-pitched extra heart sounds. Having the patient lean forward best enables hearing the aortic and pulmonic areas; having the patient on the left side will enhance the mitral area sounds; both of these positions bring the heart closer to the chest wall. Having the patient supine or prone will not improve the auscultation.
17. b. Central cyanosis is evident with a blue tinge in the lips, conjunctiva, or tongue. Finger clubbing results from endocarditis, congenital defects, or prolonged O_2 deficiency. Peripheral cyanosis is evident with blue-tinged extremities or in the nose and ears. Decreased capillary refill may be seen in reduced arterial capillary perfusion or anemia.
18. a. In an exercise nuclear imaging scan, a radioisotope is injected at the maximum heart rate on a bicycle or treadmill and used to evaluate blood flow in different parts of the heart. Insertion of electrodes into the heart chambers via the venous system to record intracardiac electrical activity is an electrophysiology study. Simply monitoring ECG activity during exercise is an exercise stress test and an echocardiogram uses transducers to bounce sound waves off of the heart.
19. d. All actions will be done but in order to perform a transesophageal echocardiogram (TEE), the throat must be numbed. Until sensation returns, as evidenced by the gag reflex, the patient is at risk of aspiration so this action has the highest priority (priority related to airway—ABCs).
20. b. Holter monitoring involves placing electrodes on the chest attached to a recorder that will record ECG rhythm for 24 to 48 hours while the patient engages in normal activities of daily living (ADLs). The recording is later analyzed for cardiac dysrhythmias. Serial ECGs are frequent but not continuous ECGs. The 6-minute walk test measures the distance walked in 6 minutes to determine response to treatments and functional capacity for ADLs. An event monitor or loop recorder is used to record infrequent rhythm disturbances when the patient activates the recording with symptom occurrence.
21. c. An absence of pulses distal to the catheter insertion site indicates that clotting is occluding blood flow to the extremity and is an emergency that requires immediate medical attention. Some swelling and pain at the site are expected but the site is also monitored for bleeding and a pressure dressing and perhaps a sandbag or clamp may be applied. Hives may occur as a result of iodine sensitivity and will require treatment but the priority is the lack of pulses.
22. d. A risk assessment for coronary artery disease (CAD) is determined by comparing the total cholesterol to high-density lipoprotein (HDL) and a ratio can be calculated by dividing the total cholesterol level by the HDL level. The ratio provides more information than either value alone and an increased ratio indicates an increased risk. The female patient has a ratio of 3.56, which is average risk, compared with the male patient's ratio of 6.56, which is increased risk.
23. b, d, e. Increased levels of cardiac tropinin T (cTnT), high-sensitivity C-reactive protein, and lipoprotein-associated phospholipase A_2 are indicators of risk for or evidence of myocardial injury. Increased b-type natriuretic peptide (BNP) is a marker for heart failure and increased CK-creatine kinase (CK)-MM is most commonly associated with skeletal muscle injury.

CHAPTER 33

Answer Key

1.

	Increasing Cardiac Output	Increasing Systemic Vascular Resistance	Mechanisms Causing Increases
β_1-Adrenergic stimulation	X	X	Increased rate and contractility of the heart increases cardiac output (CO). Peripheral artery vasoconstriction. Stimulation of renin production that activates the renin-angiotensin-aldosterone system (RAAS).
α_1-Adrenergic stimulation	X	X	Peripheral arteriole vasoconstriction and increased contractility of the heart
α_2-Adrenergic stimulation		X	Constriction of selected vascular beds
Endothelin release		X	Vasoconstriction
Angiotensin II		X	Arteriole vasoconstriction
Aldosterone release	X		Increased vascular volume
Antidiuretic hormone (ADH) release	X		Increased vascular volume

2. The vasoconstriction caused by the α_1-adrenergic agent raises the BP, stimulating the baroreceptors. The baroreceptors send impulses to the sympathetic vasomotor center in the brainstem, which inhibits the sympathetic nervous system, resulting in a decreased heart rate (HR), decreased force of contraction, and vasodilation.

3. The drug will lower BP because of decreased stroke volume and decreased HR, both of which decrease CO.

4. a, c, d, e. Hypertension progresses with increasing age. It is more prevalent in men up to age 45 and above the age of 64 in women. African Americans have a higher incidence of hypertension than do white Americans. Children and siblings of patients with hypertension should be screened and taught about healthy lifestyles.

5. c. Secondary hypertension has an underlying cause that can often be treated, in contrast to primary or essential hypertension, which has no single known cause. Isolated systolic hypertension occurs when the systolic blood pressure (SBP) is consistently elevated over 140 mm Hg but the diastolic blood pressure (DBP) remains less than 90 mm Hg, which is more prevalent in older adults. The only type of hypertension that does not cause target organ damage is pseudohypertension.

6. a. Hypertension is often asymptomatic, especially if it is mild or moderate, and has been called the "silent killer." The absence of symptoms often leads to noncompliance with medical treatment and a lack of concern about the disease in patients. With severe hypertension, symptoms usually occur and may include a morning occipital headache, fatigability, dizziness, palpitations, angina, and dyspnea.

7. b. Elevated BP causes the entire inner lining of arterioles to become thickened from hyperplasia of connective tissues in the intima and affects coronary circulation, cerebral circulation, peripheral vessels, and renal and retinal blood vessels. The narrowed vessels lead to ischemia and ultimately to damage of these organs.

8. b. The increased systemic vascular resistance (SVR) of hypertension directly increases the workload of the heart and heart failure occurs when the heart can no longer pump effectively against the increased resistance. The heart may be indirectly damaged by atherosclerotic changes in the blood vessels, as are the brain, retina, and kidney.

9.

Laboratory Test Result	Significance
Blood urea nitrogen (BUN): 48 mg/dL (17.1 mmol/L) Creatinine: 4.3 mg/dL (380 mmol/L)	Elevated BUN and creatinine may indicate destruction of glomeruli and tubules of the kidney resulting from hypertension.
Serum K^+: 3.1 mEq/L (3.1 mmol/L)	Serum potassium levels are decreased when hypertension is associated with hyperaldosteronism.
Serum uric acid: 9.2 mg/dL (547 mmol/L)	An increased uric acid level may be caused by diuretics used to treat hypertension.
Fasting blood glucose: 183 mg/dL (10.2 mmol/L)	Fasting glucose levels are elevated when hypertension is associated with glucose intolerance and insulin resistance.
Low-density lipoproteins (LDL): 154 mg/dL (4.0 mmol/L)	An elevated LDL level indicates an increased risk for atherosclerotic changes in the patient with hypertension.

10. a. Dietary modifications to restrict sodium, cholesterol, and saturated fat; maintain intake of potassium, calcium, and magnesium; and promote weight reduction if overweight
    b. Daily moderate-intensity physical activity for at least 30 minutes on most days of the week
    c. Cessation of smoking (if a smoker)
    d. Moderation or cessation of alcohol intake; usually medications and monitor BP at home.
    Also, psychosocial risk factors must be addressed.

11. c. Cardioselective β-adrenergic blockers decrease CO, reduce sympathetic vasoconstrictor tone, and decrease renin secretion by kidneys. Calcium channel blockers reduce BP by causing blocking movement of calcium into cells, which causes vasodilation of arterioles. Spironolactone blocks the effect of aldosterone. Central adrenergic antagonists such as clonidine (Catapres) inhibit sympathetic outflow from the central nervous system (CNS).

12. c. Angiotensin II receptor blockers (ARBs) prevent the action of angiotensin II and produce vasodilation and increased salt and water excretion. Thiazide diuretics decrease extracellular fluid volume by increasing Na^+ and Cl^- excretion with water. Direct vasodilators act directly on smooth muscle of arterioles to cause vasodilation. Angiotensin-converting enzyme (ACE) inhibitors prevent the conversion of angiotensin I to angiotensin II.

13. d. Hydrochlorothiazide is a thiazide diuretic that causes sodium and potassium loss through the kidneys. High-potassium foods should be included in the diet or potassium supplements should be used to prevent hypokalemia. Enalapril and spironolactone may cause hyperkalemia by inhibiting the action of aldosterone and potassium supplements should not be used by patients taking these drugs. As a combined α/β-blocker, labetalol does not affect potassium levels.

14. b. Prazosin is an α-adrenergic blocker that causes dilation of arterioles and veins and causes orthostatic hypotension. The patient may feel dizzy, weak, and faint when assuming an upright position after sitting or lying down and should be

taught to change positions slowly, avoid standing for long periods, do leg exercises to increase venous return, and lie or sit down when dizziness occurs. Direct-acting vasodilators often cause fluid retention; dry mouth occurs with diuretic use, although orthostatic hypotension may occur with hydrochlorothiazide as well; and centrally acting α- and β-blockers may cause bradycardia.

15. c. Sexual dysfunction, which can occur with many of the antihypertensive drugs, including thiazide and potassium-sparing diuretics and β-adrenergic blockers, can be a major reason that a male patient does not adhere to his treatment regimen. It is helpful for the nurse to raise the subject because sexual problems may be easier for the patient to discuss and handle once it has been explained that the drug might be the source of the problem.

16. a, c, e, f. The age-related changes that contribute to hypertension include decreased renal function, increased peripheral vascular resistance, increased collagen and stiffness of the myocardium, and decreased elasticity in large arteries from arteriosclerosis. The baroreceptor reflexes are blunted. The adrenergic receptor sensitivity and renin response are both decreased with aging.

17. a. Centrally acting α-adrenergic blockers may cause severe rebound hypertension if the drugs are abruptly discontinued and patients should be taught about this effect because many are not consistently compliant with drug therapy. Diuretics should be taken early in the day to prevent nocturia and the profound orthostatic hypotension that occurs with first-dose α-adrenergic blockers can be prevented by taking the initial dose at bedtime. Aspirin use may decrease the effectiveness of ACE inhibitors.

18. d. Correct technique in measuring BP includes taking two or more readings at least 1 minute apart. Initially BP measurements should be taken in both arms to detect any differences. If there is a difference, the arm with the higher reading should be used for all subsequent BP readings. The patient may be supine or sitting. The important point is that the arm being used is at the heart level and the cuff needs to fit snugly.

19. b. Unlicensed assistive personnel (UAP) may check postural changes in BP as directed. The licensed practical nurse (LPN) may administer antihypertensive medications to stable patients. The RN must monitor the patient receiving IV enalapril (Vasotec), as he or she is in a hypertensive crisis. The RN must also do the teaching related to home BP monitoring.

20. c. Hypertensive emergency, a type of hypertensive crisis, is a situation that develops over hours or days in which a patient's BP is severely elevated with evidence of acute target organ disease (e.g., cerebrovascular, cardiovascular, renal, or retinal). The neurologic manifestations are often similar to the presentation of a stroke but do not show the focal or lateralizing symptoms of stroke. Hypertensive crises are defined by the degree of organ damage and how rapidly the BP rises, not by specific BP measurements. A hypertensive urgency is a less severe crisis in which a patient's BP becomes severely elevated over days or weeks but there is no evidence of target organ damage.

21. d. Hypertensive crises are treated with IV administration of antihypertensive drugs, including the vasodilators sodium nitroprusside, fenoldopam, and nicardipine; adrenergic blockers such as phentolamine, labetalol, and esmolol;

the ACE inhibitor IV enalaprilat; and the calcium channel blocker clevidipine. Sodium nitroprusside is the most effective parenteral drug for hypertensive emergencies. Drugs that are used specifically for hypertensive emergencies include sodium nitroprusside, nitroglycerin with myocardial infarction, hydralazine with other medications, and oral captopril.

22. a. Initially the treatment goal in hypertensive emergencies is to reduce the mean arterial pressure (MAP) by no more than 20% to 25% in the first hour, with further gradual reduction over the next 24 hours. In this case the MAP is 172, so decreasing it by 25% equals 129. Lowering the BP too far or too fast may cause a stroke, myocardial infarction (MI), visual changes, or renal failure. Only when the patient has an aortic dissection, angina, or signs of MI or an ischemic stroke does the SBP need to be lowered to 100 to 120 mm Hg or less as quickly as possible.

23. d. Hypertensive urgencies are often treated with oral drugs on an outpatient basis but it is important for the patient to be seen by a health care professional within 24 hours to evaluate the effectiveness of the treatment. Hourly urine measurements, titration of IV drugs, and ECG monitoring are indicated for hypertensive emergencies.

Case Study

1. Increasing age, which leads to loss of elasticity in large arteries from atherosclerosis, and more prevalent in women (and in African Americans).

2. High sodium intake from canned foods, sedentary lifestyle, and weight gain.

3. The Dietary Approaches to Stop Hypertension (DASH) eating plan is rich in fresh or frozen fruits and vegetables, fat-free or low-fat milk, whole grains, fish, poultry, beans, seeds, and nuts. In this eating plan there are less salt and sodium, less sweets, less fat, and less red meat than in the typical American diet. Increasing activity and losing weight (if necessary) is encouraged. Increasing calcium, magnesium, potassium, and fiber occurs with the increased fruits and vegetables.

4. Because of K.J.'s low potassium level, a potassium-sparing diuretic, such as spironolactone, amiloride, or triamterine, could be used. If a stronger diuretic were needed, potassium supplementation would be indicated. If an ACE inhibitor were also needed, the diuretic would need to be changed related to additional potassium sparing.

5. The nurse should teach K.J. about regular daily aerobic exercise and weight reduction; avoiding canned food and reading labels for sodium content; the need for stress management indicated by weight gain in response to her husband's death and availability of counseling; the pathology, complications, and management of hypertension; and medications and the potential of orthostatic hypotension.

6. **Nursing diagnoses:**
   - Ineffective health maintenance *related to* increased caloric intake and deficiency of potassium sources
   - Ineffective coping *related to* use of food as coping mechanism
   - Deficient knowledge *related to* lack of knowledge of pathology, complications, and management of hypertension and treatment

   Collaborative problems:
   Potential complications: cerebrovascular accident, MI, renal failure

CHAPTER 34

Answer Key

1. c. The fibrous plaque stage has progressive changes that can be seen by age 30. Collagen covers the fatty streak and forms a fibrous plaque in the artery. The thrombus adheres to the arterial wall in the complicated lesion stage. Rapid onset of coronary artery disease (CAD) with hypercholesterolemia may be related to familial hypercholesterolemia, not a stage of CAD development. The fatty streak stage is the earliest stage of atherosclerosis and can be seen by age 15.

2. b. The etiology of CAD includes atherosclerosis as the major cause. The pathophysiology of atherosclerosis development is related to endothelial chemical injury and inflammation, which can be the result of tobacco use, hyperlipidemia, hypertension, toxins, diabetes mellitus, hyperhomocysteinemia, and infection causing a local inflammatory response in the inner lining of the vessel walls. Partial or total occlusion occurs in the complicated lesion stage. Extra collateral circulation occurs in the presence of chronic ischemia. Therefore it is more likely to occur in an older patient.

3. b. This white woman has one unmodifiable risk factor (age) and two major modifiable risk factors (hypertension and physical inactivity). Her gender risk is as high as a man's because she is over 65 years of age. The white man has one unmodifiable risk factor (gender), one major modifiable risk factor (smoking), and one minor modifiable risk factor (stressful lifestyle). The Asian woman has only one major modifiable risk factor (hyperlipidemia) and Asians in the United States have fewer myocardial infarctions (MIs) than do whites. The African American man has an unmodifiable risk factor related to age and one major modifiable risk factor (obesity).

4. d. CAD is the number-one killer of American women and women have a much higher mortality rate within 1 year following MI than do men. Smoking carries specific problems for women because smoking has been linked to a decrease in estrogen levels and to early menopause and it has been identified as the most powerful contributor to CAD in women under the age of 50. Fewer women than men present with classic manifestations and women delay seeking care longer than men. Recent research indicates that estrogen replacement does not reduce the risk for CAD, even though estrogen lowers low-density lipoprotein (LDL) and raises high-density lipoprotein (HDL) cholesterol.

5. b, c, e. LDLs contain more cholesterol than the other lipoproteins, have an attraction for arterial walls, and correlate most closely with increased incidence of atherosclerosis and CAD. HDLs increase with exercise and carry lipids away from arteries to the liver for metabolism. A high HDL level is associated with a lower risk of CAD.

6. b. Elevated fasting triglyceride levels are associated with cardiovascular disease and diabetes. Apolipoproteins are found in varying amounts on the HDLs and activate enzyme or receptor sites that promote removal of fat from plasma, which is protective. The apolipoprotein A and apolipropotein B ratio must be done to predict CAD. Elevated HDLs are associated with a lower risk of CAD. Elevated total serum cholesterol must be calculated with HDL for a ratio over time to determine an increased risk of CAD.

7. d. All of this patient's results are abnormal. The patient in option c is close to being at risk, as all of that patient's results are at or near the cutoff for being acceptable. If this patient is a woman, the HDL is too low. The other patients' results are at acceptable levels.

8. a. Increased exercise without an increase in caloric intake will result in weight loss, reducing the risk associated with obesity. Exercise increases lipid metabolism and increases HDL, thus reducing CAD risk. Exercise may also indirectly reduce the risk of CAD by controlling hypertension, promoting glucose metabolism in diabetes, and reducing stress. Although research is needed to determine whether a decline in homocysteine can reduce the risk of heart disease, it appears that dietary modifications are indicated for risk reduction.

9. a, c, e. Therapeutic Lifestyle Changes diet recommendations emphasize reduction in saturated fat and cholesterol intake. Red meats, whole milk products, and eggs as well as butter, stick margarine, lard, and solid shortening should be reduced or eliminated from diets. If triglyceride levels are high, alcohol and simple sugars should be reduced.

10. a. The Therapeutic Lifestyle Changes diet includes recommendations for all people, not just those with risk factors, to decrease the risk for CAD.

11. c. Diet therapy and smoking cessation are indicated for a patient without CAD who has prehypertension and an LDL level ≥130 mg/dL. When the patient's LDL level is ≥160 mg/dL, drug therapy would be added to diet therapy. Because tobacco use is related to increased BP and LDL level, the benefit of smoking cessation is almost immediate. Exercise is indicated to reduce risk factors throughout treatment.

12. c, d, e. Unstable angina, ST-segment-elevation myocardial infarction (STEMI), and non–ST-segment-elevation myocardial infarction (NSTEMI) are conditions that are manifestations of acute coronary syndrome (ACS). The other options are not manifestations of ACS.

13. b, d, e, f. Increased oxygen demand is caused by increasing the workload of the heart, including left ventricular hypertrophy with hypertension, sympathetic nervous stimulation, and anything precipitating angina. Hypovolemia, anemia, and narrowed coronary arteries contribute to decreased oxygen supply.

14. c. When the coronary arteries are occluded, contractility ceases after several minutes, depriving the myocardial cells of glucose and oxygen for aerobic metabolism. Anaerobic metabolism begins and lactic acid accumulates, irritating myocardial nerve fibers that then transmit a pain message to the cardiac nerves and upper thoracic posterior roots. The other factors may occur during vessel occlusion but are not the source of pain.

15. c, d. Prinzmetal's angina and microvascular angina may occur in the absence of CAD but with arterial spasm in Prinzmetal's angina or abnormalities of the coronary microcirculation. Silent ischemia is prevalent in persons with diabetes mellitus and contributes to asymptomatic myocardial ischemia. Nocturnal angina occurs only at night. Chronic stable angina refers to chest pain that occurs with the same pattern of onset, duration, and intensity intermittently over a long period of time.

16. b, c. Unstable angina is unpredictable and unrelieved by rest and has progressively increasing severity. Chronic stable angina is usually precipitated by exertion. Angina decubitus

occurs when the person is recumbent. Prinzmetal's angina is frequently caused by a coronary artery spasm.

17. d. An increased heart rate (HR) decreases the time the heart spends in diastole, which is the time of greatest coronary blood flow. Unlike other arteries, coronary arteries are perfused when the myocardium relaxes and blood backflows from the aorta into the sinuses of Valsalva, which have openings to the right and left coronary arteries. Thus the heart has a decreased oxygen supply at a time when there is an increased oxygen demand. Tachycardia may also lead to ventricular dysrhythmia. The other options are incorrect.

18. b, c, d. Nitrates decrease preload and afterload to decrease the coronary workload and dilate coronary arteries to increase coronary blood supply. The other options are not attributed to nitrates.

19. b. Captopril (Capoten) would be added. It is an angiotensin-converting enzyme (ACE) inhibitor that vasodilates and decreases endothelial dysfunction and may prevent ventricular remodeling. Clopidogrel (Plavix) is an antiplatelet agent used as an alternative for a patient unable to use aspirin. Diltiazem (Cardizem), a calcium channel blocker, may be used to decrease vasospasm but is not known to prevent ventricular remodeling. Metoprolol (Lopressor) is a β-adrenergic blocker that inhibits sympathetic nervous stimulation of the heart.

20. a. A common complication of nitrates is dizziness caused by orthostatic hypotension, so the patient should sit or lie down and place the tablet under the tongue. The tablet should be allowed to dissolve under the tongue. To prevent the tablet from being swallowed, water should not be taken with it. The recommended dose for the patient for whom nitroglycerin (NTG) has been prescribed is one tablet taken sublingually (SL) or one metered spray for symptoms of angina. If symptoms are unchanged or worse after 5 minutes, the patient should contact the emergency medical services (EMS) system before taking additional NTG. If symptoms are significantly improved by one dose of NTG, instruct the patient or caregiver to repeat NTG every 5 minutes for a maximum of three doses and contact EMS if symptoms have not resolved completely. Headache is also a common complication of nitrates but usually resolves with continued use of nitrates and may be controlled with mild analgesics.

21. a. Orthostatic hypotension may cause dizziness and falls in older adults taking antianginal agents that decrease preload. Patients should be cautioned to change positions slowly. Daily exercise programs are indicated for older adults and may increase performance, endurance, and ability to tolerate stress. A change in lifestyle behaviors may increase the quality of life and reduce the risks of CAD, even in the older adult. Aspirin is commonly used in these patients and is not contraindicated.

22. c. Unstable angina is associated with the rupture of a once-stable atherosclerotic plaque, exposing the intima to blood and stimulating platelet aggregation and local vasoconstriction with thrombus formation. Patients with unstable angina require immediate hospitalization and monitoring because the lesion is at increased risk of complete thrombosis of the lumen with progression to MI. Any type of angina may be associated with severe pain, ECG changes, and dysrhythmias. Prinzmetal's angina is characterized by coronary artery spasm.

23. a. One of the primary differences between the pain of angina and the pain of an MI is that angina pain is usually relieved by rest or nitroglycerin, which reduces the oxygen demand of the heart, whereas MI pain is not. Both angina and MI pain can cause a pressure or squeezing sensation; may or may not radiate to the neck, back, arms, fingers, and jaw; and may be precipitated by exertion.

24. b. An exercise stress test will reveal ECG changes that indicate impaired coronary circulation when the oxygen demand of the heart is increased. A single ECG is not conclusive for CAD and negative findings do not rule out CAD. Coronary angiography can detect narrowing of coronary arteries but is an invasive procedure. Echocardiograms of various types may identify abnormalities of myocardial wall motion under stress but are indirect measures of CAD.

25. d. The subjective report of the pain from an MI is usually severe. It usually is unrelieved by nitroglycerin, rest, or position change and usually lasts more than the 15 or 20 minutes typical of angina pain. All of the other symptoms may occur with angina as well as with an MI.

26. c. At 10 to 14 days after MI, the myocardium is considered especially vulnerable to increased stress because of the unstable state of healing at this point, as well as the increasing physical activity of the patient. At 2 to 3 days, removal of necrotic tissue is taking place by phagocytic cells. By 4 to 10 days, the necrotic tissue has been cleared and a collagen matrix for scar tissue has been deposited. Healing with scar-tissue replacement of the necrotic area is usually complete by 6 weeks.

27. c. The most common complication of MI is cardiac dysrhythmias. Continuous cardiac monitoring allows identification and treatment of dysrhythmias that may cause further deterioration of the cardiovascular status or death. Measurement of hourly urine output and vital signs is indicated to detect symptoms of the complication of cardiogenic shock. Crackles, dyspnea, and tachycardia may indicate the onset of heart failure.

28. b. Heart failure, which can escalate to cardiogenic shock, initially occurs with mild dyspnea, restlessness, agitation, pulmonary congestion with crackles, S_3 or S_4 heart sounds, and jugular vein distention. Pericarditis is a common complication identified with chest pain that is aggravated by inspiration, coughing, and moving the upper body. Ventricular aneurysm is manifested with heart failure, dysrhythmias, and angina. Papillary muscle dysfunction is suspected with a new systolic apical murmur.

29. d. Creatine kinase–muscle and brain subunits band (CK-MB) is a tissue enzyme that is specific to cardiac muscle and is released into the blood when myocardial cells die. CK-MB levels begin to rise about 6 hours after an acute MI, peak in about 18 hours, and return to normal within 24 to 36 hours. This increase can identify the presence of and quantify myocardiac damage. Cardiac troponin T and troponin I are released with myocardial damage, rise as quickly as CK-MB does, and remain elevated for 2 weeks. ECG changes are often not apparent immediately after infarct and may be normal when the patient seeks medical attention. An enlarged heart, determined by x-ray, indicates cardiac stress but is not diagnostic of acute MI.

30. c. A differentiation is made between MIs that have ST segment elevations on ECG and those that do not because chest pain accompanied by ST segment elevations

is associated with prolonged and complete coronary thrombosis and is treated with reperfusion therapy. The other options are incorrect.

31. c. Transmyocardial laser revascularization (TMR) is a treatment used for patients with inoperable CAD. It uses a high-energy laser to create channels in the heart to allow blood to flow to the ischemic area and can be done percutaneously or during surgery with a left anterior thoracotomy incision. A stent is the structure used to hold vessels open and requires anticoagulation following the procedure. Surgical construction of new vessels is done with a coronary artery bypass graft (CABG).

32. c. Emergent percutaneous coronary intervention (PCI) is the first treatment for patients with a confirmed MI within 90 minutes of arriving at the facility with an interventional cardiac catheterization lab. Stent placement, CABG, and TMR are usually done to facilitate circulation in non-emergency situations.

33. b. Unlicensed assistive personnel (UAP) can check vital signs and report results to the RN. The other actions include assessment, teaching, and monitoring of IV fluids, which are all responsibilities of the RN.

34. c. The most common method of coronary artery bypass involves leaving the internal mammary artery attached to its origin from the subclavian artery but dissecting it from the chest wall and anastomosing it distal to an obstruction in a coronary artery. Synthetic grafts are not commonly used as coronary bypass grafts, although research continues to investigate this option. Saphenous veins are used for bypass grafts when additional conduits are needed.

35. c. Because an NSTEMI is an acute coronary syndrome that indicates a transient thrombosis or incomplete coronary artery occlusion, treatment involves intensive drug therapy with antiplatelets, glycoprotein IIb/IIIa inhibitors, antithrombotics, and heparin to prevent clot extension. In addition, IV nitroglycerin is used. Reperfusion therapy using thrombolytics, CABG, or PCI is used for treatment of STEMI.

36. c. Decreasing level of consciousness (LOC) may reflect hypoxemia resulting from internal bleeding, which is always a risk with thrombolytic therapy. Oozing of blood is expected, as are reperfusion dysrhythmias. BP is low but not considered abnormal because the pulse is within normal range.

37. a. If chest pain is unchanged, it is an indication that reperfusion was not successful. Indications that the occluded coronary artery is patent and blood flow to the myocardium is reestablished following thrombolytic therapy include return of ST segment to baseline on the ECG; relief of chest pain; marked, rapid rise of the CK enzyme within 3 hours of therapy; and the presence of reperfusion dysrhythmias.

38. a. Morphine sulfate decreases anxiety and cardiac workload as a vasodilator and reduces preload and myocardial O_2 consumption, which relieves chest pain. Calcium channel blockers, amiodarone, and ACE inhibitors will not relieve chest pain related to an MI.

39. c. Docusate sodium (Colace) is a stool softener, which prevents straining and provoking dysrhythmias. It does not do any of the other options. Antidysrhythmics are used to control ventricular dysrhythmias; morphine sulfate is used to decrease cardiac workload and anxiety; and glycoprotein IIb/IIIa inhibitors and antiplatelets prevent the binding of fibrinogen to platelets.

40. b. It is recommended that patients with hypertension and after an MI be on β-adrenergic blockers indefinitely to decrease oxygen demand. They inhibit sympathetic nervous stimulation of the heart; reduce heart rate, contractility, and blood pressure; and decrease afterload. Although calcium channel blockers decrease heart rate, contractility, and blood pressure, they are not used unless the patient cannot tolerate β-adrenergic blockers. ACE inhibitors and angiotensin II receptor blockers (ARBs) are used for vasodilation.

41. a. This patient is indicating positive coping with a realization that recovery takes time and that lifestyle changes can be made as needed. The patient who is "just going to get on with life" is probably in denial about the seriousness of the condition and the changes that need to be made. Nervous questioning about the expected duration and effect of the condition indicates the presence of anxiety, as does the statement regarding the health care professional's role in treatment.

42. a. 6; b. 4; c. 3; d. 1; e. 5; f. 2. A patient having chest pain needs to have the pain assessed and relieved as quickly as possible. The administration of oxygen may help to relieve the pain. Following an assessment of the pain, medication may be administered. It is important to know if the pain is accompanied by a change in vital signs and if any other manifestations or ECG changes exist before the report is given to the physician.

43. d. Anger about the MI may be directed at family, staff, or the medical regimen. Stating that the chest pain is no big deal is denial. Relaying an inability to care for self relates to dependency. Questioning what will happen if there is another attack is expressing anxiety and fear. Depression may be expressed related to changes in lifestyle. Realistic acceptance is seen with actively engaging in changing modifiable risk factors.

44. a. Golfing is a moderate-energy activity that expends about 5 metabolic equivalent units (METs) and is within the 3 to 5 METs activity level desired for a patient by the time of discharge from the hospital following an MI. Walking at 5 mph and mowing the lawn by hand are high-energy activities and cycling at 13 mph is an extremely high–energy activity.

45. a. Any activity or exercise that causes dyspnea and chest pain should be stopped in the patient with CAD. The training target for a healthy 58-year-old is 80% of maximum HR, or 130 bpm. In a patient with cardiac disease undergoing cardiac conditioning, however, the HR should not exceed 20 bpm over the resting pulse rate. HR, rather than respiratory rate, determines the parameters for exercise.

46. b. Resumption of sexual activity is often difficult for patients to approach and it is reported that most cardiac patients do not resume sexual activity after MI. The nurse can give the patient permission to discuss concerns about sexual activity by introducing it as a physical activity when other physical activities are discussed. Health care providers may have preferences regarding the timing of resumption of sexual activity and the nurse should discuss this with the health care provider and the patient but addressing the patient's concerns is a nursing responsibility. Patients should be informed that impotence after MI is common but that it usually disappears after several attempts.

47. c. It is not uncommon for a patient who experiences chest pain on exertion to have some angina during sexual stimulation or intercourse and the patient should be instructed to use nitroglycerin prophylactically. Positions

during intercourse are a matter of individual choice and foreplay is desirable because it allows a gradual increase in HR. Sildenafil (Viagra) should be used cautiously in men with CAD and should not be used with nitrates.

48. a. Most patients who experience sudden cardiac death (SCD) as a result of CAD do not have an acute MI but have dysrhythmias that cause death, probably as a result of electrical instability of the myocardium. To identify and treat those specific dysrhythmias, continuous monitoring is important. The other assessments can be done but are not the most important after an episode of SCD.

Case Study

1. Diabetes mellitus, smoking history, obesity, physical inactivity, and stress response.
2. Anxiousness with fist clutching; radiation of the burning from epigastric area into the sternum; and prior episodes of chest pain with activity, relieved by rest.
3. Provide emotional support and explain all interventions and procedures. As well, position her in an upright position, administer oxygen per nasal cannula, obtain vital signs, initiate continuous ECG monitoring, auscultate heart and breath sounds, assess pain using PQRST, medicate as ordered, and obtain baseline laboratory values and a chest x-ray.
4. Depressed ST segment and T wave inversion would indicate myocardial ischemia.
5. The nurse should inform H.C. that she will have continuous cardiac monitoring while she walks on a treadmill with increasing speed and elevation to evaluate the effects of exercise on the blood supply to her heart. Her pulse, respiration, BP, and heart rhythm will be measured while she walks and after the test until they return to normal and the cardiac monitor will be used after the test until any changes return to normal.
6. This patient does not seem motivated to assume responsibility for her health and, in the absence of symptoms, has not had a desire to make lifestyle changes. First, the nurse should assist her to clarify her personal values. Then, by explaining the symptoms related to her risk factors and having her identify her personal vulnerability to various risks, the nurse may help her to recognize her susceptibility to CAD. Help the patient to set realistic goals and allow her to choose which risk factor to change first.

7. A: Antiplatelet, antianginal, and ACE inhibitor or ARB therapy
B: β-adrenergic blocker and blood pressure control
C: Cigarette smoking cessation, cholesterol management, calcium channel blockers, and cardiac rehabilitation
D: Diet for weight management, diabetes management, and depression screening
E: Education and exercise
F: Flu vaccination
Many of these measures can be used now to help the patient better manage her current health if she is motivated to do so.

8. **Nursing diagnoses:**
   - Acute pain *related to* imbalance between myocardial oxygen supply and demand
   - Anxiety *related to* possible diagnosis and uncertain future
   - Ineffective denial *related to* reluctance to receive medical care or change lifestyle
   - Ineffective coping *related to* lack of effective coping skills
   - Imbalanced nutrition: more than body requirements *related to* intake of calories in excess of calorie expenditure
   - Ineffective health maintenance *related to* lack of health insurance and motivation

   Collaborative problems:
   Potential complications: myocardial infarction, cardiac dysrhythmias

CHAPTER 35
Answer Key

1. a, b. Diastolic failure is characterized by abnormal resistance to ventricular filling. Coronary artery disease (CAD), advanced age, and hypertension are all risk factors for heart failure (HF). Ejection fraction is decreased in systolic HF. Dysrhythmia precipitates HF with decreased cardiac output (CO) and increased workload and oxygen requirements of the myocardium.

2.

Compensatory Mechanism	↑ Cardiac Output	Detrimental Effect
Cardiac dilation	Increased force of contraction by stretching of cardiac muscle	Overstrains the muscle fibers; mitral valve incompetence
Cardiac hypertrophy	Increased contractile force of muscle	Increased myocardial oxygen need
Sympathetic nervous system stimulation	Increased heart rate (HR) and force of contraction; increased preload	Increased myocardial oxygen need; overwhelming preload; increased afterload
Neurohormonal response • Renin-angiotensin-aldosterone system	Increased fluid retention and vasoconstriction to maintain blood pressure (BP)	Increased preload and afterload
• Antidiuretic hormone (ADH)	Increased water retention	Increased blood volume when already overloaded

3. c. Both the natriuretic peptides and nitric oxide contribute to vasodilation, decreased blood pressure, and decreased afterload. The natriuretic peptides also increase excretion of sodium by increasing glomerular filtration rate and diuresis (renal effects) as well as interfere with ADH release and inhibit aldosterone and renin secretion (hormonal effects).

4. d. FACES is used to teach patients signs and symptoms of worsening heart failure. F = Fatigue; A = Activity limitations; C = Congestion/cough; E = Edema; S = Shortness of breath. The other options are not correct.

5. b. In left-sided heart failure, blood backs up into the pulmonary veins and capillaries. This increased hydrostatic pressure in the vessels causes fluid to move out of the vessels and into the pulmonary interstitial space. When increased lymphatic flow cannot remove enough fluid from the interstitial space, fluid moves into the alveoli, resulting in pulmonary edema and impaired alveolar oxygen and carbon dioxide exchange. Initially the right side of the heart is not involved.

6. a. Clinical manifestations of acute left-sided heart failure are those of interstitial edema, with bubbling crackles and tachycardia, as well as tachypnea. Later frothy, blood-tinged sputum; severe dyspnea; and orthopnea develop with alveolar edema. Severe tachycardia and cool, clammy skin are present as a result of stimulation of the sympathetic nervous system from hypoxemia. Systemic edema reflected by jugular vein distention, peripheral edema, and hepatosplenomegaly are characteristic of right-sided heart failure.

7. d. Paroxysmal nocturnal dyspnea (PND) is awakening from sleep with a feeling of suffocation and a need to sit up to be able to breathe and patients learn that sleeping with the upper body elevated on several pillows helps to prevent PND. Orthopnea is an inability to breathe effectively when lying down and nocturia occurs with heart failure as fluid moves back into the vascular system during recumbency, increasing renal blood flow.

8. a. SpO$_2$ of 84% on 2 L/min via nasal cannula indicates impaired oxygen saturation. The patient is having trouble with gas exchange. Airway and breathing are the priority (follow ABCs).

   b. The nurse should place the patient in high Fowler's position, assess the patient immediately, recheck SpO$_2$, auscultate breath sounds, assess level of consciousness (LOC), check the oxygen connection and rate setting (2 L/min), and talk with the patient about her or his breathing.

9. b. Thrombus formation occurs in the heart when the chambers do not contract normally and empty completely. Both atrial fibrillation and very low left ventricular output (LVEF <20%) lead to thrombus formation, which is treated with anticoagulants to prevent the release of emboli into the circulation as well as antidysrhythmics or cardioversion to control atrial fibrillation.

10. c. B-type natriuretic peptide (BNP) is released from the ventricles in response to increased blood volume in the heart and is a good marker for heart failure. If BNP is elevated, shortness of breath is due to heart failure; if BNP is normal, dyspnea is due to pulmonary disease. BNP opposes the actions of the renin-angiotensin-aldosterone system, resulting in vasodilation and reduction in blood volume. Exercise stress testing and cardiac catheterization are more important tests to diagnose coronary artery disease and although the blood urea nitrogen (BUN) may be elevated in heart failure, it is a reflection of decreased renal perfusion. (See Table 32-6.)

11. d. Isosorbide dinitrate and hydralazine (BiDil) is currently used only with African American patients for hypertension and angina. Captopril (Capoten) is used only for hypertension by all patients. Nitroglycerin (Nitro-Bid) is used with hydralazine (Apresoline) for patients who cannot tolerate renin-angiotensin-aldosterone system inhibitors for heart failure management. Spironolactone (Aldactone) is used for hypertension.

12. c. Nesiritide (Natrecor) is a recombinant form of a natriuretic peptide that decreases preload and afterload by reducing pulmonary artery wedge pressure (PAWP) and systolic BP which decreases the workload of the heart for short-term emergency treatment of acute decompensated heart failure (ADHF). Digoxin (Lanoxin) requires a loading dose and time to work, so it is not recommended for emergency treatment of ADHF. Morphine sulfate relieves dyspnea but has more adverse events and mortality. Bumetanide (Bumex) will decrease fluid volume but also will decrease potassium levels and activate the sympathetic nervous system and renin-angiotensin-aldosterone system, which can exacerbate HF symptoms.

13. c. Dopamine (Intropin) is a β-adrenergic agonist that is a positive inotrope given IV, not orally, and used for acute HF. Losartan (Cozaar) is an angiotensin II receptor blocker used for patients who do not tolerate angiotensin-converting enzyme inhibitors. Carvedilol (Coreg) is the β-adrenergic blocker that blocks the sympathetic nervous system's negative effects on the failing heart. Hydrochlorothiazide (HCTZ) is the diuretic.

14. b, d. Furosemide is a diuretic that eliminates potassium and spironalactone is a potassium-sparing diuretic that retains potassium. The other treatments and medications are used for patients with HF but they do not directly affect serum potassium levels.

15. b. Hypokalemia is one of the most common causes of digitalis toxicity because low serum potassium levels enhance ectopic pacemaker activity. When a patient is receiving potassium-losing diuretics, such as hydrochlorothiazide or furosemide, it is essential to monitor the patient's serum potassium levels to prevent digitalis toxicity. Monitoring the heart rate (HR) assesses for complications related to digoxin but does not prevent toxicity.

16. a. Spironolactone is a potassium-sparing diuretic and when it is the only diuretic used in the treatment of heart failure, moderate to low levels of potassium intake should be maintained to prevent development of hyperkalemia. Sodium intake is usually reduced to at least 2400 mg/day in patients with heart failure but salt substitutes cannot be freely used because most contain high concentrations of potassium. Calcium intake is not increased.

17. d. Although all of these drugs may cause hypotension, nitroprusside is a potent dilator of both arteries and veins and may cause such marked hypotension that an inotropic agent (e.g., dobutamine) administration may be necessary to maintain the BP during its administration. Furosemide may cause hypotension because of diuretic-induced depletion of

intravascular fluid volume. Nitroglycerin is a vasodilator and can decrease BP but not as severely as nitroprusside. It primarily dilates veins and increases myocardial oxygen supply. Milrinone has a positive inotropic effect in addition to direct arterial dilation.

18. c. All foods that are high in sodium should be eliminated in a 2400-mg sodium diet, in addition to the elimination of salt during cooking. Examples include obviously salted snack foods as well as pickles, processed prepared foods, and many sauces and condiments.

19.

Cardiovascular Condition Leading to HF	Preventive Measures
Hypertension	Use medications, diet, and exercise to control
Valvular defects	Surgical replacement before heart failure occurs; prophylactic antibiotics
Ischemic heart disease	Percutaneous coronary intervention (PCI); coronary artery bypass surgery; fibrinolytic therapy for occlusions
Dysrhythmias	Antidysrhythmic agents, pacemakers, or defibrillators to control; also adequate treatment of pulmonary hypertension, hyperthyroidism, or myocarditis

20. c. Successful treatment of heart failure is indicated by an absence of symptoms of pulmonary edema and hypoxemia, such as clear lung sounds and a normal HR. Weight loss and diuresis, warm skin, less fatigue, and improved LOC may occur without resolution of pulmonary symptoms. Chest pain is not a common finding in heart failure unless coronary artery perfusion is impaired.

21. d. Further teaching is needed if the patient believes a weight gain of 2 to 3 pounds in 2 days is an indication for dieting. In a patient with heart failure, this type of weight gain reflects fluid retention and is a sign of heart failure that should be reported to the health care provider. The other options show patient understanding of the heart failure management teaching. (See Table 35-10.)

22. d. The 52-year-old woman does not have any contraindications for cardiac transplantation, even though she lacks the indication of adequate financial resources. The postoperative transplant regimen is complex and rigorous and patients who have not been compliant with other treatments or who might not have the means to understand the care would not be good candidates. A history of drug or alcohol abuse is usually a contraindication to heart transplant.

23. a. Because of the need for long-term immunosuppressant therapy to prevent rejection, the patient with a transplant is at high risk for infection, a leading cause of death in transplant patients. Acute rejection episodes may also cause death in patients with transplants but many can be treated successfully with augmented immunosuppressive therapy. Malignancies occur in patients with organ transplants after taking immunosuppressants for a number of years.

Case Study

1. Right-sided HF: jugular vein distention, peripheral edema, and hepatomegaly.
   Left-sided HF: dyspnea, $\downarrow$ SpO$_2$, point of maximal impulse (PMI) displacement, pulmonary crackles, frothy pink sputum, $\downarrow$ BP, and S$_3$, S$_4$ heart sounds
   Present with both types of HF: fatigue, $\uparrow$ HR, and dysrhythmias.
2. Nursing interventions:
   • Calm, reassuring approach because of his anxiety and critical condition

   • Explanations of rationales for all diagnostic tests and medications
   • Administration of oxygen, sitting upright with legs out straight or dependent
   • Emotional and physical rest
   • Constant monitoring of cardiovascular and respiratory function
   • Administration of ordered medications per parameters
   • Evaluation and documentation of the effects of medical interventions (i.e., to determine if HF is resolving)
   • Initiation of strict intake and ouput (I&O) measurements and daily weights
3. Appropriate diagnostic procedures include the following:
   • Chest x-ray: cardiomegaly, pulmonary venous hypertension, pleural effusion
   • 12-Lead electrocardiogram (ECG): tachycardia and dysrhythmias of conduction disturbances
   • Echocardiogram: to determine the presence of a low left ventricular ejection fraction (LVEF)
   • Cardiac catheterization and coronary angiography: normal coronary arteries, ventricular pressures
   • Nuclear imaging studies: cardiac contractility, myocardial perfusion, low ejection fraction
   • Blood analysis: arterial blood gases (ABGs), serum chemistries, cardiac enzymes to assess cardiac damage, BNP level to confirm dyspnea of cardiac source, oxygenation status, liver function tests, renal function tests
4. Continuous ECG monitoring; hemodynamic monitoring (intraarterial BP, SaO$_2$, PAWP, cardiac output); and BP, HR, RR, pulse oximetry, and urine output every hour.
5. The Joint Commission core measures include (1) discharge instructions, (2) evaluation of left ventricular systolic function, and (3) angiotensin-converting enzyme (ACE) inhibitors or angiotensin receptor blocker (ARB) for left ventricular systolic dysfunction. Nursing can be responsible for providing (1) written discharge instructions or teaching material that includes activity level, diet, discharge medications, follow-up appointment, weight monitoring, and symptom management as prescribed. Although smoking cessation counseling is no longer a core measure for heart failure patients, the 40-year history of smoking could make smoking cessation an important topic to include for this patient during hospitalization or at discharge.

6. CRT is a pacemaker that will stimulate both the right and left ventricles (chambers) of the heart so that they will contract in coordination (together) to improve the way the heart pumps blood with each heartbeat.

7. Slowing the progression of heart failure is important. Use FACES to remind the patient of the signs and symptoms to watch for and to notify the health care provider about. Weigh self daily. Teach the patient the expected actions of the prescribed medications and the signs of drug toxicity, as well as the dose and time(s) to take them. Teach the patient to take the pulse every day for 1 full minute if he is taking a digitalis preparation or β-adrenergic blocker and instruct him on the HR or rhythm at which he should hold the medication and notify the health care provider. If the patient is taking diuretics, he will be taught the symptoms of hypokalemia or hyperkalemia. Using the DASH diet, home BP monitoring, oxygen therapy, daily activity simplification and the need for rest after activity, cardiac rehabilitation, the use of telehealth monitoring technology, and home health care may all be needed. An annual flu vaccination should be obtained in the fall and the pneumococcal vaccine should be administered before dismissal.

8. **Nursing diagnoses:**
   - Death anxiety *related to* question: "Am I going to die?"
   - Impaired gas exchange *related to* alveolar-capillary membrane changes
   - Ineffective peripheral tissue perfusion *related to* pump failure
   - Decreased cardiac output *related to* altered contractility
   - Activity intolerance *related to* imbalance between oxygen supply and demand
   - Risk for impaired skin integrity *related to* edema
   - Deficient knowledge *related to* lack of information about complications, medications, and disease management
   - Deficient nutritional status *related to* lack of intake

   Collaborative problems:
   Potential complications: cardiogenic shock, ventricular dysrhythmias, emboli, liver or renal failure, cardiac arrest

CHAPTER 36

Answer Key

1. c. The V1 leads are placed toward each limb and centrally at the fourth intercostal space to the right of the sternal border. Depolarization of the ventricular cells produces the QRS interval on the ECG. The T wave is produced by repolarization of the ventricular cells. Abnormal cardiac impulses from the atria, ventricles, or atrioventricular (AV) junction create ectopic beats. Artifacts are seen with leads or electrodes that are not secure, with muscle activity or electrical interference. The rate produced by the AV node pacing in a junctional escape rhythm is 40 to 60 bpm. If the His-Purkinje system is blocked, the heart rate is 20 to 40 bpm.

2. d, f. The expected PR interval is 0.12 to 0.20 seconds and is measured from the beginning of the P wave to the beginning of the QRS complex. The T wave is 0.16 seconds, the QRS interval is <0.12 seconds, the P wave is 0.06 to 0.12 seconds, and the QT interval is the time of depolarization and repolarization of the ventricles.

3. 4 (beats per 3 seconds) + 4 = 8 × 10 = 80 bpm

4. 1500 ÷ 20 = 75 bpm

5. d. Automaticity describes the ability to discharge an electrical impulse spontaneously. Excitability is a property of myocardial tissue that enables it to be depolarized by an impulse. Contractility is the ability of the chambers to respond mechanically to an impulse. Conductivity is the ability to transmit an impulse along a membrane.

6. b. Refractoriness is the period in which heart tissue cannot be stimulated. Ectopic foci are abnormal electrical impulses. Reentrant excitation causing premature beats may occur when areas of the heart do not repolarize simultaneously with depressed conduction. Depolarization of cardiac cells occurs when sodium migrates rapidly into the cell.

7. d. The normal PR interval is 0.12 to 0.20 seconds and reflects the time taken for the impulse to spread through the atria, AV node and bundle of His, the bundle branches, and Purkinje fibers. A PR interval of six small boxes is 0.24 second and indicates that the conduction of the impulse from the atria to the Purkinje fibers is delayed.

8. d. Electrophysiologic testing involves electrical stimulation to various areas of the atrium and ventricle to determine the inducibility of dysrhythmias and frequently induces ventricular tachycardia or ventricular fibrillation. The patient may have "near-death" experiences and requires emotional support if this occurs. Dye and anticoagulants are used for coronary angiograms.

9. d. In type II second-degree AV block, a P wave is nonconducted without progressive P-R interval lengthening. It is usually from a block in a bundle branch, occurs in a ratio of 2 P waves–to–1 QRS complex, 3:1, and so on. Atrial fibrillation has a chaotic P wave. Asystole is absence of ventricular activity. First-degree AV block is a prolonged AV conduction time, so the P-R interval is prolonged.

10. d. Pulseless electrical activity (PEA) occurs when there is electrical activity on the ECG but no mechanical activity on assessment and therefore no heart rate. PEA is the most common dysrhythmia seen after defibrillation and may be caused by hypovolemia, hypoxia, metabolic acidosis, altered potassium level, hypoglycemia, hypothermia, toxins, cardiac tamponade, thrombosis, tension pneumothorax, and trauma. Dissociated atria and ventricles is third-degree AV block.

11. c. The premature atrial contraction (PAC) has a distorted P wave that may feel like a skipped beat to the patient. Atrial flutter is an atrial tachydysrhythmia with recurring, regular, saw-toothed flutter waves from the same focus in the right or possibly left atrium. Sinus bradycardia has a regular heart rate less than 100 bpm. Paroxysmal supraventricular tachycardia (PSVT) starts in an ectopic focus above the bundle of His and may be triggered by PAC. If seen, the P wave may have an abnormal shape and has a spontaneous start and termination with a rate of 150 to 220 bpm.

12. b. Third-degree or complete heart block is recognized with the atrial and ventricular dissociation and treated with a pacemaker. Sinus bradycardia does not have atrial and ventricular dissociation. Atrial fibrillation does not have normal P waves, as they are stimulated by ectopic foci. In type 1 second-degree AV heart block the P-R interval gradually lengthens and a QRS complex is dropped. Then the cycle begins again.

13. b. When premature ventricular contraction (PVC) falls on the T wave of the preceding beat, R-on-T phenomenon occurs. Because the ventricle is repolarizing and there is increased excitability of cardiac cells, there is an increased risk of ventricular tachycardia or ventricular fibrillation. The other options do not increase this risk.

14. d. Although many factors can cause a sinus tachycardia, in the patient who has had an acute MI, tachycardia increases myocardial oxygen need in a heart that already has impaired circulation and may lead to increasing angina and further ischemia and necrosis.

15. a. A distorted P wave with normal conduction of the impulse through the ventricles is characteristic of a premature atrial contraction. In a normal heart, this dysrhythmia is frequently associated with emotional stress or the use of caffeine, tobacco, or alcohol. Sedatives rarely slow the heart rate (HR). Aerobic conditioning and holding of breath during exertion (Valsalva maneuver) often cause bradycardia.

16. a. A rhythm pattern that is normal except for a prolonged P-R interval is characteristic of a first-degree heart block. First-degree heart blocks are not treated but are observed for progression to higher degrees of heart block. Atropine is administered for bradycardia. Synchronized cardioversion is used for atrial fibrillation with a rapid ventricular response or supraventricular tachycardia (SVT). Pacemakers are used for higher-degree heart blocks.

17. b. Symptoms of decreased cardiac output (CO) related to cardiac dysrhythmias include a sudden drop in BP and symptoms of hypoxemia, such as decreased mentation, chest pain, and dyspnea. Peripheral pulses are weak and the HR may be increased or decreased, depending on the type of dysrhythmia present.

18. c. Multifocal PVCs in a patient with an MI indicate significant ventricular irritability that may lead to ventricular tachycardia or ventricular fibrillation. Antidysrhythmics, such as β-adrenergic blockers, procainamide, amiodarone, or lidocaine, may be used to control the dysrhythmias. Valsalva maneuver may be used to treat paroxysmal supraventricular tachycardia. The nurse must always be ready to perform cardiopulmonary resuscitation (CPR).

19. a. PVC is an ectopic beat that causes a wide, distorted QRS complex ≥0.12 second because the impulse is not conducted normally through the ventricles. Because it is premature, it precedes the P wave and the P wave may be hidden in the QRS complex, or the ventricular impulse may be conducted retrograde and the P wave may be seen following the PVC but the rhythm is not regular. Continuous wide QRS complexes with a ventricular rate between 150 and 250 bpm are seen in ventricular tachycardia, whereas saw-toothed P waves are characteristic of atrial flutter.

20. c. The intent of defibrillation is to apply an electrical current to the heart that will depolarize the cells of the myocardium so that subsequent repolarization of the cells will allow the SA node to resume the role of pacemaker. An artificial pacemaker provides an electrical impulse that stimulates normal myocardial contractions. Synchronized cardioversion involves delivery of a shock that is programmed to occur during the QRS complex of the ECG but this cannot be done during ventricular fibrillation because there is no normal ventricular contraction or QRS complex.

21. a. In preparation for defibrillation the nurse should apply conductive materials (e.g., saline pads, electrode gel, defibrillator gel pads) to the patient's chest to decrease electrical impedance and prevent burns. For defibrillation, the initial shock is 200 joules with biphasic defibrillators and the synchronizer switch used for cardioversion must be turned off. Sedatives may be used before cardioversion if the patient is conscious but the patient in ventricular fibrillation is unconscious.

22. b. If the cardioverter-defibrillator delivers a shock, the patient has experienced a lethal dysrhythmia and needs to notify the cardiologist. The patient will want to lie down to allow recovery from the dysrhythmia. In the event that the patient loses consciousness or there is repetitive firing, a call should be placed to the emergency medical services (EMS) system by anyone who finds the patient.

23. b. The patient should avoid standing near antitheft devices in doorways of department stores and libraries but walking through them at normal pace is fine. High-output electrical generators or large magnets, such as those used in magnetic resonance imaging (MRI), can reprogram pacemakers and should be avoided. Microwave ovens pose no problems to pacemaker function but the arm should not be raised above the shoulder for 1 week after placement of the pacemaker. The pacing current of an implanted pacemaker is not felt by the patient but an external pacemaker may cause uncomfortable chest muscle contractions.

24. a. Until the defibrillator is available, the patient needs CPR. Defibrillation is needed as soon as possible, so someone should bring the crash cart to the room. Defibrillation would be with 360 joules for monophasic defibrillators and 120 to 200 joules for biphasic defibrillators. Amiodarone is an antidysrhythmic that is part of the advanced cardiac life support (ACLS) protocol for ventricular fibrillation.

25. c. Catheter ablation therapy uses radiofrequency energy to ablate or "burn" accessory pathways or ectopic sites in the atria, AV node, or ventricles that cause tachydysrhythmias.

26. c. ST segment elevation indicates injury or infarction of an area of the heart. An inverted T wave is most often associated with ischemia and resolves when blood flow is restored. Occasional PVCs may be normal or may be the result of electrolyte imbalance or hypoxia. They require continued observation. A PR interval of 0.18 second is within normal range.

27. d. One of the most common causes of syncope is neurocardiogenic syncope, or "vasovagal" syncope. In this type of syncope there is accentuated adrenergic activity in the upright position, with intense activation of cardiopulmonary receptors resulting in marked bradycardia and hypotension. Normally testing with the upright tilt table causes activation of the renin-angiotensin-aldosterone system and compensation to increase CO and maintain BP when blood pools in the extremities. However, patients with neurocardiogenic syncope experience a marked decrease in BP and HR.

28. d. ST segment elevation is seen in myocardial injury. An absent or buried P wave can occur with PVCs, ventricular tachycardia, or ventricular fibrillation. A wide pathologic Q wave may be seen with infarction. T wave inversion may be seen with cardiac ischemia or within hours following an MI.

29. a. Third-degree block, characterized by atrial and ventricular dissociation with regular atrial rate
    b. Atrial flutter, saw-toothed flutter waves from same ectopic foci
    c. PVC, unifocal bigeminal, early occurrence of wide, distorted QRS complex every other beat
    d. Sinus bradycardia, only abnormal in rate less than 60 bpm
    e. Second-degree block, type I, progressively lengthening P-R interval until a QRS complex is blocked
    f. PAC, irregular rate and rhythm and different P wave shape
    g. Second-degree block, type II, regular atrial rate and P-R interval, ventricular rate irregular with blocked QRS complexes
    h. Sinus tachycardia, only irregular in rate of 101 to 200 bpm
    i. First-degree block, prolonged P-R interval
    j. Ventricular fibrillation, irregular waveforms of varying shapes and amplitude
    k. PVC, trigeminal, unifocal, early occurrence of wide, distorted QRS complex every third beat
    l. Atrial fibrillation, accelerated atrial rate with chaotic fibrillatory waves and irregular ventricular rate
    m. PAC, irregular rate and rhythm and different shaped P waves
    n. Normal sinus rhythm, starts at sinoatrial (SA) node with rate of 60 to 100 bpm and follows normal conduction pathway
    o. Monomorphic ventricular tachycardia, rate of 150 to 250 bpm with wide distorted QRS complex

Case Study

1. Age, hypertension, caffeine intake, and stress of her husband's recent death.
2. Ensure ABCs, administer oxygen (O_2), obtain baseline vital signs and O_2 saturation, obtain 12-lead ECG, initiate continuous ECG monitoring, identify rate and rhythm and any dysrhythmia, establish IV access, and be prepared for CPR as with all patients.
3. During atrial fibrillation there is total disorganization of atrial electrical activity and no effective atrial contraction. Fibrillatory waves or undulations occur at a rate of 300 to 600 per minute in the atria and although not all electrical activity is conducted to the ventricles, the ventricular rate is usually 100 to 160 bpm and irregular when there is an uncontrolled ventricular response. "Atrial kick" is lost and the result is a 15% to 20% decrease in CO. CO is also decreased due to tachycardia.
4. Atrial rhythm is chaotic and although no definite P wave can be observed, fibrillatory waves can be seen as a jagged, irregular baseline between QRS complexes. The P-R interval cannot be measured. The ventricular rhythm is usually irregular but QRS complexes are usually of normal contour.
5. The immediate goal of drug therapy is to decrease the rapid ventricular response to the atrial fibrillation to less than 100 bpm because it leads to decreased CO.
6. Diltiazem is indicated for treatment of atrial fibrillation because it decreases the automaticity of the SA node, as it inhibits the influx of calcium ions during depolarization of cardiac cells and slows the AV nodal conduction time, decreasing the ventricular response. Since this patient is unstable, a bolus dose would be ordered followed by a continuous drip and then oral drugs would be started.

Digoxin is used to treat atrial fibrillation because it decreases the ventricular response by increasing the refractory period of the AV node and it also decreases atrial automaticity.

Lovenox and Coumadin are used to prevent thrombus formation or extension in the atria where blood pools because of ineffective atrial contraction. If thrombi form in the left atria, arterial embolization may occur causing a stroke or MI or deep vein thrombosis.

7. Cardioversion may be used to convert the fibrillation to a normal sinus rhythm. Cardioversion is administered with an initial dose of 70 to 75 joules with biphasic defibrillator and 100 joules with monophasic defibrillator synchronized with the QRS complex of the ECG and the patient may be sedated before the procedure. If medications and cardioversion do not convert the rhythm, radiofrequency catheter ablation or the Maze procedure may be used.
8. **Nursing diagnoses:**
   - Decreased cardiac output *related to* dysrhythmia
   - Activity intolerance *related to* inadequate cardiac output
   - Impaired gas exchange *related to* alveolar-capillary membrane changes
   - Anxiety *related to* vulnerability and cardiac disease

   Collaborative problems:
   Potential complications: embolism, heart failure, cardiogenic shock

CHAPTER 37

Answer Key

1. a, b, c, d, e. Recent dental, urologic, surgical, or gynecologic procedures and history of IV drug abuse, heart disease, cardiac catheterization or surgery, renal dialysis, and infections all increase the risk of infective endocarditis.
2. a. Blood cultures are the primary diagnostic tool for infective endocarditis. Although a complete blood count (CBC) will reveal a mild leukocytosis, this is a nonspecific finding. Transesophageal echocardiograms can identify vegetations on valves but are used when blood cultures are negative. Cardiac catheterizations are used when surgical intervention is being considered.
3. a. Petechiae are seen as small hemorrhages in the conjunctiva, lips, and buccal mucosa and over the ankles, feet, and antecubital and popliteal areas. Roth's spots are hemorrhagic retinal lesions seen with funduscopic examination. Osler's nodes are lesions on the fingertips or toes. The cause of Roth's spots and Osler's nodes is not clear. Splinter hemorrhages are black longitudinal streaks that occur on nail beds. They may be caused by vessel damage from vasculitis or microemboli.
4. d. Janeway's lesions are flat, painless, small red spots found on the palms of the hands and the soles of the feet. Black streaks on the nails are splinter hemorrhages. Hemorrhagic retinal lesions are Roth's spots. Painful lesions on the fingers and toes are Osler's nodes.
5. b. Early valve replacement followed by prolonged antibiotic and anticoagulant therapy is recommended for these patients. Drug therapy for patients who develop endocarditis of prosthetic valves is often unsuccessful in eliminating the infection and preventing embolization.

6. c. The dyspnea, crackles, and restlessness that the patient is manifesting are symptoms of heart failure and decreased cardiac output (CO) that occurs in up to 80% of patients with aortic valve endocarditis as a result of aortic valve incompetence. Vegetative embolization from the aortic valve occurs throughout the arterial system and may affect any body organ. Pulmonary emboli occur in right-sided endocarditis.

7. d. The patient with outpatient antibiotic therapy requires vigilant home nursing care and it is most important to determine the adequacy of the home environment for successful management of the patient. The patient is at risk for life-threatening complications, such as embolization and pulmonary edema, and must be able to access a hospital if needed. Bed rest will not be necessary for the patient without heart damage. Avoiding infections and planning diversional activities are indicated for the patient but are not the most important factors while he is on outpatient antibiotic therapy.

8. d. Prophylactic antibiotic therapy should be initiated before invasive dental, medical, or surgical procedures to prevent recurrence of endocarditis. Continuous antibiotic therapy is indicated only in patients with implanted devices or ongoing invasive procedures. Symptoms of infection should be treated promptly but antibiotics are not used for exposure to infection.

9. c. The stethoscope diaphragm at the left sternal border with the patient leaning forward is the best method to use to hear the high-pitched, grating sound of a pericardial friction rub. The sound does not radiate widely and occurs with the heartbeat. To differentiate a pericardial friction rub from a pleural friction rub, have the patient hold his or her breath. The rub will still be heard if it is cardiac in nature.

10. b. The patient is experiencing a cardiac tamponade that consists of excess fluid in the pericardial sac, which compresses the heart and the adjoining structures, preventing normal filling and cardiac output. Fibrin accumulation, a scarred and thickened pericardium, and adherent pericardial membranes occur in chronic constrictive pericarditis.

11. b, e. Pulsus paradoxus is measured with a manually operated sphygmomanometer. The cuff is deflated slowly until the first Korotkoff sound during expiration is heard and the number is noted. The slow deflation of the cuff is continued until sounds are heard throughout the respiratory cycle and that number is subtracted from the first number. When the difference is >10 mm Hg, cardiac tamponade may be present. The difference is normally <10 mm Hg.

12. b. Pneumothorax may occur as a needle is inserted into the pericardial space to remove fluid for analysis and relieve cardiac pressure with pericardiocentesis. Other complications could include dysrhythmias, further cardiac tamponade, myocardial laceration, and coronary artery laceration.

13. d. Relief from pericardial pain is often obtained by sitting up and leaning forward. Pain is increased by lying flat. The pain has a sharp, pleuritic quality that changes with respiration and patients take shallow breaths. Antiinflammatory medications may also be used to help control pain but opioids are not usually indicated.

14. b. Viruses are the most common cause of myocarditis in the United States and early manifestations of myocarditis are often those of systemic viral infections. Myocarditis may also be associated with systemic inflammatory and metabolic disorders as well as with other microorganisms, drugs, or toxins. The patient with myocarditis is predisposed to drug-related dysrhythmias and toxicity with digoxin, so it is used very cautiously, if at all, in treatment of the condition.

15. d. Initial attacks of rheumatic fever and the development of rheumatic heart disease can be prevented by adequate treatment of group A streptococcal pharyngitis. Because streptococcal infection accounts for only about 20% of acute pharyngitis, cultures should be done to identify the organism and direct antibiotic therapy. Viral infections should not be treated with antibiotics. Prophylactic therapy is indicated in those who have valvular heart disease or have had rheumatic heart disease.

16. a. Major criteria for the diagnosis of rheumatic fever include evidence of carditis, polyarthritis, chorea (often very late), erythema marginatum, and subcutaneous nodules. Minor criteria include all laboratory findings as well as fever, arthralgia, and a history of previous rheumatic fever. There also must be evidence of a previous group A streptococci infection (e.g., positive antistreptolysin O titer).

17.

Drug	Rationale for Use
Antibiotics	To eliminate any residual group A β-hemolytic streptococci; prevent spread of infection; prevent recurrent infection
Aspirin	Antiinflammatory effect to control fever and arthritic and joint manifestations
Corticosteroids	Antiinflammatory effect to control fever and inflammation of severe carditis
Nonsteroidal antiinflammatory drugs (NSAIDs)	Antiinflammatory effect to control fever and joint manifestations

18. b. When carditis is present in the patient with rheumatic fever, ambulation is postponed until any symptoms of heart failure are controlled with treatment and full activity cannot be resumed until antiinflammatory therapy has been discontinued. In the patient without cardiac involvement, ambulation may be permitted as soon as acute symptoms have subsided and normal activity can be resumed when antiinflammatory therapy is discontinued.

19. d. Valvular regurgitation causes a backward flow of blood and volume overload in the preceding chamber. Without treatment, eventually hypertrophy of that chamber occurs. Stenosis causes a pressure gradient difference and decreased blood flow and hypertrophy of the preceding chamber. A pericardial friction rub is not related to valvular regurgitation but would be heard at the lower left sternal border of the chest.

20. c. Monitoring vital signs before and after ambulation is the collection of data. Instructions should be provided to the licensed practical nurse (LPN) regarding what changes in these vital signs should be reported to the RN. The other actions listed are RN responsibilities.

21. c. Mitral valve prolapse is the ballooning of the valve leaflets into the left atrium during ventricular systole. The rapid onset that prevents left chamber dilation and the rapid development of pulmonary edema and cardiogenic shock occur with acute mitral regurgitation. Pulmonary hypertension may contribute to tricuspid valve disease.

22. d. Acute aortic regurgitation causes a sudden cardiovascular collapse. With mitral valve stenosis dyspnea is a prominent symptom and embolization may result from chronic atrial fibrillation. With tricuspid and pulmonic valve diseases, stenosis occurs more often than regurgitation. Tricuspid valve stenosis results in right atrial enlargement and elevated systemic venous pressures. Pulmonic valve stenosis results in right ventricular hypertension and hypertrophy.

23. b. Aortic valve stenosis is identified with the triad of angina, syncope, and dyspnea on exertion, as well as the systolic murmur and prominent S_4 heart sound. Mitral valve stenosis manifests as exertional dyspnea, hemoptysis, fatigue, atrial fibrillation, and a diastolic murmur. Acute mitral valve regurgitation has a new systolic murmur with pulmonary edema and cardiogenic shock rapidly developing. Chronic mitral valve regurgitation is identified with weakness, fatigue, exertional dyspnea, palpitations, an S_3 gallop, and holosystolic murmur.

24. b. Patients with mechanical valves have an increased risk for thrombus formation. Therefore prophylactic anticoagulation therapy is used to prevent thrombus formation and systemic or pulmonary embolization. Nitrates are contraindicated for the patient with aortic stenosis because an adequate preload is necessary to open the stiffened aortic valve. Antidysrhythmics are used only if dysrhythmias occur and β-adrenergic blocking drugs may be used to control the heart rate if needed.

25. b. Dysrhythmias frequently cause palpitations, lightheadedness, and dizziness and the patient should be carefully attended to to prevent falls. Hypervolemia and paroxysmal nocturnal dyspnea (PND) would be apparent in the patient with heart failure. Exercises will not prevent dysrhythmias.

26. c. This procedure has been used for repair of mitral, tricuspid, and pulmonic stenosis and less often for aortic stenosis. It is usually used for older patients and for those patients who are poor surgical risks because it is relatively easy and has good results and few complications.

27. c. Repair of mitral or tricuspid valves has a lower operative mortality rate than does replacement and is becoming the surgical procedure of choice for these valvular diseases. Open repair is more precise than closed repair and requires cardiopulmonary bypass during surgery. All types of valve surgery are palliative, not curative, and patients require lifelong health care. Anticoagulation therapy is used for all valve surgery for at least some time postoperatively.

28. c. Mechanical prosthetic valves require long-term anticoagulation and this is a factor in making a decision about the type of valve to use for replacement. Patients who cannot take anticoagulant therapy, such as women of childbearing age, patients at risk for hemorrhage, patients who may not be compliant with anticoagulation therapy, and patients over age 65 may be candidates for the less durable biologic valves.

29. d. The greatest risk to a patient who has an artificial valve is the development of endocarditis with invasive medical or dental procedures. Before any of these procedures, antibiotic prophylaxis is necessary to prevent infection. Planning of an exercise program and monitoring anticoagulant therapy will be done.

30. b. A secondary cause of restrictive cardiomyopathy (CMP) is radiation treatment to the thorax with stiffness of the ventricular wall occurring. Dilated CMP may have a genetic link, follow infectious myocarditis, or be related to an autoimmune process or excess alcohol ingestion. Takotsubo CMP is an acute stress-related syndrome that mimics acute coronary syndrome. It is most common in postmenopausal women. Hypertrophic CMP has a genetic link in about one half of all cases and is frequently seen in young athletic individuals.

31. d, e, f. Dilated CMP, the most common type of CMP, reveals cardiomegaly with thin ventricular walls on echocardiogram, as there is no ventricular hypertrophy, and may follow an infective myocarditis. As well, stasis of blood in the ventricles may contribute to systemic embolization. Restrictive CMP is the least common type and is characterized by ventricular stiffness. Hypertrophic CMP has hyperdynamic systolic function creating a diastolic failure, is characterized by massive thickening of intraventricular septum and ventricular wall, and may result in syncope during increased activity resulting from an obstructed aortic valve outflow.

32. c. Nursing interventions for the patient with hypertrophic CMP are to improve ventricular filling by reducing ventricular contractility and relieving left ventricular outflow obstruction to relieve symptoms and prevent complications. Strenuous activity and dehydration will increase systemic vascular resistance and should be avoided. Atrioventricular pacing will allow the septum to move away from the left ventricular wall and reduce the degree of outflow obstruction. Vasodilators may decrease venous return and further increase obstruction of blood flow from the heart. The surgery that could be done involves cutting into the thickened septal wall and removing some of the ventricular muscle.

33. a, c, d, e, f. These topics can apply to any patient with CMP.

Case Study

1. His age (incidence is higher in older adults) and the invasive endoscopic cholecystectomy.

2. Mitral valve prolapse and degenerative valve lesions (calcification degeneration of a bicuspid aortic valve or senile calcification degeneration of a normal aortic valve).

3. Stroke symptoms: Embolization of vegetations to cerebral circulation with cerebral infarction
Petechiae: Occur as a result of fragmentation and microembolization of vegetative lesions
New systolic, crescendo-decrescendo murmur: Aortic valve involvement
Fever: Infection; occurs in 90% of patients with infective endocarditis

4. The endoscopic surgery provided a route for introduction of bacteria into the bloodstream to trigger the infectious process.

5. Two blood cultures drawn 30 minutes apart from two different sites are positive in 90% of patients; usually

shows *Staphylococcus aureus or Steptococcus viridians;* mild leukocytosis, increased erythrocyte sedimentation rate (ESR), and elevated C-reactive protein (CRP); and echocardiogram may show vegetation on the heart valves.

6. Identification of the organism with blood cultures and appropriate IV antibiotic therapy; antipyretics to control fever; rest, with increase in activity after fever abates and if there are no symptoms of heart failure; and valve replacement if there is no response to antibiotic therapy.

7. Preoperative prophylactic antibiotic therapy.

8. **Nursing diagnoses:**
   - Hyperthermia *related to* infection, elevated temperature
   - Decreased cardiac output *related to* valvular insufficiency
   - Risk for impaired skin integrity *related to* immobility

   Collaborative problems:
   Potential complications: emboli, heart failure

CHAPTER 38

Answer Key

1. d. Regardless of the location, atherosclerosis is responsible for peripheral arterial disease (PAD) and is related to other cardiovascular disease and its risk factors, such as coronary artery disease (CAD) and carotid artery disease. Venous thrombosis, venous stasis ulcers, and pulmonary embolism are diseases of the veins and are not related to atherosclerosis.

2. $102 \div 132 = 0.77$; mild (see Table 38-3)

3. c. Oral anticoagulants (warfarin) are not recommended for treatment of PAD but all of the other statements are correct in relation to treatment of PAD.

4. a, c, e. Warm legs and feet increase circulation. The lower extremities should be assessed at regular intervals for changes. Walking exercise increases oxygen extraction in the legs and improves skeletal muscle metabolism. The patient with PAD should walk at least 30 minutes a day, preferably twice a day. Exercise should be stopped when pain occurs and resumed when the pain subsides. Nicotine in all forms causes vasoconstriction and must be eliminated.

5. b. PAD occurs as a result of atherosclerosis and the risk factors are the same as for other diseases associated with atherosclerosis, such as CAD, cerebrovascular disease, and aneurysms. Major risk factors are tobacco use, hyperlipidemia, elevated C-reactive protein, diabetes mellitus, and uncontrolled hypertension. The risk for amputation is high in patients with severe occlusive disease but this is not the best approach to encourage patients to make lifestyle modifications.

6. c. Loss of palpable pulses, numbness and tingling of the extremity, extremity pallor, cyanosis or cold, and decreasing ankle-brachial indices are indications of occlusion of the bypass graft and need immediate medical attention. Pain, redness, and serous drainage at the incision site are expected postoperatively.

7. a. Pain; b. pallor; c. pulselessness; d. paresthesia; e. paralysis; f. poikilothermia. The physician requires immediate notification to begin immediate intervention to prevent tissue necrosis and gangrene.

8. b, d, f. Arterial leg ulcers and/or gangrene of the leg due to PAD and chronic ischemic rest pain lasting more than 2 weeks characterize critical limb ischemia. Optimal therapy is revascularization via bypass surgery.

9. a, b, c, d, f. Raynaud's phenomenon is predominant in young females and may be associated with autoimmune disorders (e.g., rheumatoid arthritis, scleroderma, systemic lupus erythematosus). Incidents occur with cold, emotional upsets, and caffeine or tobacco use due to vasoconstrictive effects. Small cutaneous arteries are involved and cause color changes of the fingertips or toes. When conservative management is ineffective, it may be treated with nifedipine (Procardia).

10. d. The fusiform aneurysm is circumferential and relatively uniform in shape. The false aneurysm or pseudoaneurysm is not an aneurysm but a disruption of all of the arterial wall layers with bleeding that is contained by surrounding anatomic structures. Saccular aneurysms are the pouchlike bulge of an artery.

11. c. Although most abdominal aortic aneurysms (AAAs) are asymptomatic, on physical examination a pulsatile mass in the periumbilical area slightly to the left of the midline may be detected and bruits may be audible with a stethoscope placed over the aneurysm. Hoarseness and dysphagia may occur with aneurysms of the ascending aorta and the aortic arch. Severe back pain with flank ecchymosis is usually present on rupture of an AAA and neurovascular loss in the lower extremities may occur from pressure of a thoracic aneurysm.

12. d. A computed tomography (CT) scan is the most accurate test to determine the diameter of the aneurysm and whether a thrombus is present. The other tests may also be used but the CT scan yields the most descriptive results.

13. b. Increased systolic blood pressure (SBP) continually puts pressure on the diseased area of the artery, promoting its expansion. Small aneurysms can be treated by decreasing blood pressure (BP), modifying atherosclerosis risk factors, and monitoring the size of the aneurysm. Anticoagulants are used during surgical treatment of aneurysms but physical activity is not known to increase their size. Calcium intake is not related to calcification in arteries.

14. b. Because atherosclerosis is a systemic disease, the patient with an AAA is likely to have cardiac, pulmonary, cerebral, or lower extremity vascular problems that should be noted and monitored throughout the perioperative period. Postoperatively, the BP is balanced: high enough to keep adequate flow through the artery to prevent thrombosis but low enough to prevent bleeding at the surgical site.

15. a. With the aortic cross-clamping proximal and distal to the aneurysm, the open aneurysm repair (OAR) above the renal artery may cause kidney injury from lack of blood flow during the surgery. The saccular aneurysm may involve excising only the weakened area of the artery and suturing the artery closed but this will not decrease renal blood flow. Renal blood flow will not be directly obstructed using the bifurcated graft or the minimally invasive endovascular aneurysm repair.

16. a. Usually aortic surgery patients will have a bowel preparation, skin cleansing with an antimicrobial agent on the day before surgery, nothing by mouth after midnight on the day of the surgery, and IV antibiotics immediately before the incision is made. Patients with a history of cardiovascular disease will receive a β-adrenergic blocker preoperatively to reduce morbidity and mortality. Each surgeon's protocol may be different.

17. b. The BP and peripheral pulses are evaluated every hour in the acute postoperative period to ensure that BP is adequate and that extremities are being perfused. BP is kept within normal range. If BP is too low, thrombosis of the graft may occur; if it is too high, it may cause leaking or rupture at the suture line. Hypothermia is induced during surgery but the patient is rewarmed as soon as surgery is completed. Fluid replacement to maintain urine output at 100 mL/hr would increase the BP too much and only 30 mL/hr of urine is needed to show adequate renal perfusion.

18. c. During repair of an AAA, the blood supply to the carotid arteries may be interrupted, leading to neurologic complications manifested by a decreased level of consciousness (LOC) and altered pupil responses to light as well as changes in facial symmetry, speech, and movement of the upper extremities. The thorax is opened for ascending aortic surgery and shallow breathing, poor cough, and decreasing chest drainage are expected. Often, lower limb pulses are normally decreased or absent for a short time following surgery.

19. d. Decreased or absent pulses in conjunction with cool, painful extremities below the level of repair indicate graft thrombosis. Cardiac dysrhythmias or chest pain indicates myocardial ischemia. Absent bowel sounds, abdominal distention, diarrhea, or bloody stools indicate bowel infarction. Increased temperature and white blood cells, surgical site inflammation, or drainage indicates graft infection.

20. b. The decreasing urine output is evidence that either the patient needs volume or there is reduced renal blood flow. The physician will want to be notified as soon as possible of this change in condition and may order laboratory tests. The other options are incorrect.

21. d. Patients are taught to palpate peripheral pulses to identify changes in their quality or strength but the rate is not a significant factor in peripheral perfusion. The color and temperature of the extremities are also important for patients to observe. The remaining statements are all true.

22. c. The onset of an aortic dissection involving the distal descending aorta is usually characterized by a sudden, severe, tearing pain in the back; as it progresses down the aorta, the kidneys, abdominal organs, and lower extremities may begin to show evidence of ischemia. Aortic dissections of the ascending aorta and aortic arch may affect the heart and circulation to the head, with the development of cerebral ischemia, murmurs, ventricular failure, and pulmonary edema.

23. a. Although most initial treatment for aortic dissection involves a period of lowering the BP and myocardial contractility to diminish the pulsatile forces in the aorta, immediate surgery is indicated when complications (such as occlusion of the carotid arteries) occur. Anticoagulants would prolong and intensify the bleeding and blood is administered only if the dissection ruptures.

24. a. Relief of pain is an indication that the dissection has stabilized and it may be treated conservatively for an extended time with drugs that lower the BP and decrease myocardial contractility. Surgery is usually indicated for dissection of the ascending aorta or if complications occur.

25. b, d, e, f. Arterial disease is manifested in thick, brittle nails; decreased peripheral pulses; pallor when the legs are elevated; and ulcers over bony prominences on the toes and feet, as well as paresthesia. The other options are

characteristic of venous disease and paresthesia could occur with venous thromboembolism (VTE).

26. b. If left untreated, a superficial vein thrombosis (SVT) may extend to deeper veins and VTE may occur. VTE may embolize to the lungs and have tenderness to pressure and edema. SVTs usually occur in superficial leg veins and have tenderness, itchiness, redness, warmth, pain, inflammation, and induration along the course of the superficial vein.

27. a, b, d, e, f. This patient is a smoker and on hormone therapy, both of which increase blood hypercoagulability. She will have an IV, which can cause VTE by damaging the venous endothelium. She is an older patient who has had an orthopedic surgery and may have experienced prolonged immobility postinjury and through her "lengthy hip replacement surgery," which contributes to venous stasis. These are representative of Virchow's triad in this patient. The other options are also related to Virchow's triad but not present in this patient via the transfer report.

28. a. With manifestations of a VTE, the D-dimer is drawn to determine if a VTE exists and the duplex ultrasound is most widely used to diagnose VTE by identifying where a thrombus is located and its extent.

29. c. The RN could delegate to the unlicensed assistive personnel (UAP) the task to remind the patient to flex and extend the legs and feet every 2 hours while in bed. Measuring for elastic compression stockings may be delegated to the licensed practical nurse (LPN). The RN must assess and teach the patient.

30. d. Prevention of emboli formation can be achieved by bed rest and limiting movement of the involved extremity until the clot is stable, inflammation has receded, and anticoagulation is achieved. Dangling the legs promotes venous stasis and further clot formation and elevating the affected limb will promote venous return but it does not prevent embolization.

31. d. Low-molecular-weight heparin (nadroparin [Fraxiparine]) is only given subcutaneously and does not require routine coagulation testing. Unfractionated heparin is the only other indirect thrombin inhibitor option but it can be given subcutaneously or IV and therapeutic effects must be monitored with coagulation testing.

32. a, e. Warfarin (Coumadin) is a vitamin K antagonist, so vitamin K is the antidote. It is monitored with the international normalized ratio (INR). It is only administered orally. Protamine sulfate is the antidote for unfractionated heparin (Heparin), which can be administered subcutaneously or IV and is monitored with activated partial thromboplastin time (aPTT). Hirudin derivatives are given IV or subcutaneously, do not have an antidote, and are also monitored with aPTT. Argatroban (Acova), a synthetic direct thrombin inhibitor, is given only IV and is monitored with aPTT. Factor Xa inhibitor fondaparinux (Arixtra) is given subcutaneously and does not require routine coagulation testing. Rivaroxaban (Xarelto), another factor Xa inhibitor, is given orally.

33. b. Anticoagulant therapy with heparin or warfarin (Coumadin) does not dissolve clots but prevents propagation of the clot, development of new thrombi, and embolization. Clot lysis occurs naturally through the body's intrinsic fibrinolytic system or by the administration of fibrinolytic agents.

34. d. Exercise programs for patients recovering from VTE should emphasize swimming, which is particularly beneficial because of the gentle, even pressure of the water. Coumadin will not blacken stools. If this occurs, it could be a sign of gastrointestinal bleeding. Dark green and leafy vegetables have high amounts of vitamin K and should not be increased during Coumadin therapy but they do not need to be restricted. The legs must not be massaged because of the risk for dislodging any clots that may be present.

35. a. During walking, the muscles of the legs continuously knead the veins, promoting movement of venous blood toward the heart. Walking is the best measure to prevent venous stasis. The other methods will help venous return but they do not provide the benefit that ambulation does.

36. a. 2; b. 7; c. 9; d. 1; e. 6; f. 4; g. 5; h. 3; i. 8

37. b. Although leg elevation, moist dressings, and topical antibiotics are useful in treatment of venous stasis ulcers, the most important factor appears to be elastic compression stockings, which provide extrinsic compression to minimize venous stasis, venous hypertension, and edema.

Case Study

1. Male gender, age, smoking history, and history of atherosclerosis with CAD.

2. The primary causes of an AAA are degenerative, congenital, mechanical, inflammatory, or infections. This patient's atherosclerosis causes degenerative changes in the media lining of the aorta. The changes lead to loss of elasticity, weakening, and eventual dilation of the aorta.

3. The severe back pain and the shock symptoms: HR 114 bpm; BP 88/68; and cool, clammy extremities.

4. The first priority is to control the bleeding, which will require immediate surgical repair of the aneurysm. Fatal hemorrhage is likely if the bleeding is not controlled. If shock continues to develop, resuscitation will also be needed.

5. The patient most likely will be taken to surgery from the emergency department and emergency departments are not the most private or supportive environments. It is important for the nurse to provide privacy as much as possible and allow the patient and family to be together and ask questions as necessary. The nurse should also provide explanations of the procedures and interventions that are being implemented, explain the many tubes that will be connected to the patient postoperatively in the intensive care unit (ICU), and be supportive during this critical time.

6. Conservative therapy of small, asymptomatic AAAs consists of risk modification: tobacco cessation, decreasing BP, optimizing lipid profile, and annual monitoring of aneurysm size with ultrasound, CT, or magnetic resonance imaging (MRI). Growth rates may be lowered with β-adrenergic blocking drugs, statins, and antibiotics. The only effective treatment for AAA is surgery and the only way to prevent rupture is to repair the aneurysm surgically before it ruptures. Surgical repair is generally required when the aneurysm is greater than or equal to 5.5 cm for men and greater than or equal to 5 cm for women.

7. After AAA repair, discharge teaching will include a gradual increase of activities. Fatigue, poor appetite, irregular bowel habits, and sexual dysfunction in male patients are common.

The patient should avoid heavy lifting for 6 weeks after surgery and report to the health care provider any redness, swelling, increased pain, drainage from incisions, or fever greater than 100 °F (37.8 °C). The patient should also report changes in color or warmth of extremities and decreased strength of peripheral pulses. He should eat a well-balanced diet with protein, vitamins C and A, and zinc; high-fiber foods; fresh fruits and vegetables; fewer high-fat foods; and reduced salt intake. Follow-up visits and routine CT or MRI scans will be done to monitor for complications.

8. **Nursing diagnoses:**
   - Acute pain *related to* compression of internal structures with blood
   - Decreased cardiac output *related to* hypovolemia
   - Deficient knowledge *related to* lack of information about surgical aneurysm repair and postoperative care

   Collaborative problems:
   Potential complications: organ ischemia, hypovolemic shock, myocardial infarction

CHAPTER 39

Answer Key

1. a. Parotid gland; b. submandibular saliva gland; c. pharynx; d. trachea; e. esophagus; f. diaphragm; g. liver; h. hepatic flexure; i. transverse colon; j. ascending colon; k. small intestine; l. cecum; m. vermiform appendix; n. anal canal; o. rectum; p. sigmoid colon; q. descending colon; r. stomach; s. splenic flexure; t. spleen; u. larynx; v. sublingual gland; w. tongue

2. a. Gallbladder; b. cystic duct; c. ampulla of Vater; d. pancreas (head); e. main pancreatic duct; f. duodenum; g. pancreas (tail); h. pancreas (body); i. common bile duct; j. common hepatic duct; k. left hepatic duct; l. right hepatic duct

3. c. The parasympathetic nervous system stimulates activity of the gastrointestinal (GI) tract, increasing motility and secretions and relaxing sphincters to promote movement of contents. A drug that blocks this activity decreases secretions and peristalsis, slows gastric emptying, and contracts sphincters. The enteric nervous system of the GI tract is modulated by sympathetic and parasympathetic influence.

4. d. Cholecystokinin is secreted by the duodenal mucosa when fats and amino acids enter the duodenum and stimulate the gallbladder to release bile to emulsify the fats for digestion. The bile is produced by the liver but stored in the gallbladder. Secretin is responsible for stimulating pancreatic bicarbonate secretion and gastrin increases gastric motility and acid secretion.

5. c. The stomach secretes intrinsic factor, necessary for cobalamin (vitamin B_{12}) absorption in the intestine. When part or all of the stomach is removed, cobalamin must be supplemented for life. The other options will not be a problem.

6. d. When food enters the stomach and duodenum, the gastrocolic and duodenocolic reflexes are initiated and are more active after the first daily meal. Additional laxatives or laxative abuse contribute to constipation in older adults. Decreasing food intake is not recommended, as many older adults have a decreased appetite. Fiber and fluids should be increased.

7. b, c. Pepsinogen is changed to pepsin by acidity of the stomach, where it begins to break down proteins. Gastrin stimulates gastric acid secretion and motility and maintains lower esophageal sphincter tone. The stomach also secretes lipase for fat digestion. Bile is secreted by the liver and stored in the gallbladder for emulsifying fats. Maltase is secreted in the small intestine and converts maltose to glucose. Secretin is secreted by the duodenal mucosa and inhibits gastric motility and acid secretion. Amylase is secreted in the small intestine and by the pancreas for carbohydrate digestion.

8. a. Bacteria in the colon (1) synthesize vitamin K, which is needed for the production of prothrombin by the liver and (2) deaminate undigested or nonabsorbed proteins, producing ammonia, which is converted to urea by the liver. A reduction in normal flora bacteria by antibiotic therapy can lead to decreased vitamin K, resulting in decreased prothrombin and coagulation problems. Bowel bacteria do not influence protein absorption or the secretion of mucus.

9. c. The ampulla of Vater is the site where the pancreatic duct and common bile duct enter the duodenum and the opening and closing of the ampulla is controlled by the sphincter of Oddi. Because bile from the common bile duct is needed for emulsification of fat to promote digestion and pancreatic enzymes from the pancreas are needed for digestion of all nutrients, a blockage at this point would affect the digestion of all nutrients. Gastric contents pass into the duodenum through the pylorus or pyloric valve.

10. The bilirubin from hemoglobin (Hgb) is insoluble (unconjugated) and attached to albumin in the blood, removed by the liver, combined with glucuronic acid to become soluble (conjugated), and excreted in bile into the intestine. Bowel bacteria convert some of the bilirubin to urobilinogen. Urobilinogen is absorbed into the blood and a small amount of urobilinogen is excreted by the kidneys in urine, with the rest being removed by the liver and reexcreted in the bile.

11. d. There is decreased tone of the lower esophageal sphincter with aging and regurgitation of gastric contents back into the esophagus occurs, causing heartburn and belching. There is a decrease in hydrochloric acid secretion with aging. Jaundice and intolerance to fatty foods are symptoms of liver or gallbladder disease and are not normal age-related findings.

12.

Functional Health Pattern	Risk Factor for or Response to GI Problem
Health perception–health management	Excessive alcohol intake, smoking, exposure to hepatotoxins, recent foreign travel, family history of colorectal cancer, inflammatory bowel disease or breast cancer.
Nutritional-metabolic	Anorexia and weight loss, excessive weight gain, inadequate diet
Elimination	Change in bowel patterns, laxative or enema use, decreased fluid or fiber intake, external drainage systems
Activity-exercise	Immobility, weakness, fatigue, inability to procure and prepare food, inability to feed self
Sleep-rest	Interruption of sleep with GI symptoms
Cognitive-perceptual	Changes in taste or smell, use of pain medications, sensory problems that interfere with food preparation or intake
Self-perception–self-concept	Self-esteem and body image problems related to weight, symptoms affecting appearance
Role-relationship	Loss of employment because of chronic illness, altered relationships with others
Sexuality-reproductive	Anorexia, obesity, alcohol intake, decreased acceptance by sexual partner
Coping–stress tolerance	GI problems or symptoms induced by stress, depression
Value-belief	Religious dietary restrictions, vegetarianism

13. c. A thin, white coating of the dorsum (top) of the tongue is normal. A red, slick appearance is characteristic of cobalamin deficiency and scattered red, smooth areas on the tongue are known as geographic tongue. The uvula should remain in the midline while the patient is saying "Ahh."

14. b. The pulsation of the aorta in the epigastric area is a normal finding. Bruits indicate that blood flow is abnormal, the liver is percussed in the right midclavicular line, and a normal spleen cannot be palpated.

15. b. The pancreas is located in the left upper quadrant, the liver is in the right upper quadrant, the appendix is in the right lower quadrant, and the gallbladder is in the right upper quadrant.

16. a. Borborygmi are loud gurgles (stomach growling) that indicate hyperperistalsis. Normal bowel sounds are relatively high-pitched and are heard best with the diaphragm of the stethoscope. High-pitched, tinkling bowel sounds occur when the intestines are under tension, as in bowel obstructions. Absent bowel sounds may be reported when no sounds are heard for 2 to 3 minutes in each quadrant.

17. a. The abdomen should be assessed in the following sequence: inspection, auscultation, percussion, palpation. The patient should empty his or her bladder before assessment begins.

18.

Procedure	(1) NPO	(2) Bowel	(3) Consent	(4) Allergy
Upper GI series	X			
Barium enema	X	X		
Percutaneous transhepatic cholangiogram	X		X	X
Gallbladder ultrasound	X			
Hepatobiliary scintigraphy	X			
Upper GI endoscopy	X		X	
Colonoscopy	X	X	X	
Endoscopic retrograde cholangiopancreatography (ERCP)	X		X	

19. c. The aspartate aminotransferase (AST) level is elevated in liver disease but it is important to note that it is also elevated in damage to the heart and lungs and is not a specific test for liver function. Measurement of most of the transaminases involves nonspecific tests unless isoenzyme fractions are determined. Hepatic encephalopathy is related to elevated ammonia levels.

20. c, d, f. Because the liver is a vascular organ, vital signs are monitored to assess for internal bleeding. Prevention of bleeding is the reason for positioning on the right side for at least 2 hours and for splinting the puncture site. Again, because of the vasculature of the liver, coagulation status is checked before the biopsy is done. White stools occur with upper gastrointestinal (UGI) or barium swallow tests. No smoking is to be done after midnight before the study with an UGI. The bowel must be cleared before a lower GI or barium enema, a virtual colonoscopy, or a colonoscopy. Rectal bleeding may occur with a sigmoidoscopy or colonoscopy. A perforation may occur with an esophagogastroduodenoscopy (EGD), ERCP, or peritoneoscopy.

21. a. The left upper quadrant (LUQ) pain and nausea and vomiting could occur from perforation. The return of gag reflex is essential to prevent aspiration after an ERCP. The gag reflex is also assessed with an EGD. These are not relevant assessments for the colonoscopy and barium swallow.

CHAPTER 40

Answer Key

1. a.

Nutrient	Percentage of Total Calories from Nutrient
Protein	120 g × 4% = 480 cal 16% of 3000 cal
Fat	160 g × 9% = 1440 cal 48% of 3000 cal
Carbohydrates	270 g × 4% = 1080 cal 36% of 3000 cal

b. An average adult requires an estimated 20 to 35 calories per kilogram of body weight per day. In this patient, recommended calories would be between 1600 (80 kg × 20) and 2800 (80 kg × 35) calories per day.

c. Without knowing the activity level of the patient, the intake should be 2400 calories for a sedentary man and 3000 calories for an active man. Increase breads, cereals, rice, and pasta as sources of complex carbohydrate. Decrease the meat and egg group to 7 oz per day in three servings each day to lower protein and fat. Use 3 cups of low-fat milk to lower fat intake. Increase fruits to 2 to 2½ cups and vegetables to 3½ cups per day. Use all fats, oils, and sweets sparingly.

2. c. Patients who have surgery on the GI tract may be at risk for vitamin deficiencies because of inability to absorb or metabolize them. The strict vegan diet most often lacks cobalamin (vitamin B_{12}) and iron. Although the high intake of fat is a major nutritional problem in the United States, vitamin deficiencies are rare in developed countries except in those with eating disorders or chronic alcohol abusers. Some vitamin deficiencies in adults have neurologic manifestations.

3. d. In the United States, where protein intake is high and of good quality, protein-calorie malnutrition most commonly results from problems of the GI system. In developing countries, adequate food sources might not exist, the inhabitants may not be well educated about nutritional needs, and economic conditions can prevent purchase of balanced diets.

4.

Time Frame	Metabolism of Nutrients
First 18 hours	Carbohydrates stored in the liver and muscles in the form of glycogen are used and may be depleted quickly.
18 hours to 5 to 9 days	Protein, primarily the amino acids alanine and glutamine, is converted to glucose for energy and a negative nitrogen balance occurs.
9 days to 6 weeks	Body fat is mobilized and used as the primary source of energy, conserving protein.
Over 6 weeks	Fat stores are usually depleted in 4 to 6 weeks and body or visceral proteins, including those in internal organs and plasma, are used because they are the only source of energy available.

5. c. The sodium-potassium pump uses 20% to 50% of all calories ingested. When energy sources are decreased, the pump fails to function, sodium and water are left in the cell, and potassium remains in extracellular fluids. Hyperkalemia, as well as hyponatremia, can occur.

6. a. With surgery a patient will recover more rapidly with a balanced nutritional status before the surgery and increased protein is needed for healing after the surgery. Following a vegan diet does not put the patient at risk of low protein intake. A lowered temperature will not cause increased protein need. Following religious and cultural beliefs would not be expected to affect an increased need for protein.

7. a, b, c, e, f. In malnutrition, metabolic processes are slowed, leading to increased sensitivity to cold, decreased heart rate (HR) and cardiac output (CO), and decreased neurologic function. Because of slowed GI motility and absorption, the abdomen becomes distended and protruding and bowel sounds are decreased. Skin is rough, dry, and scaly whereas bone structures protrude because of muscle loss. Because the immune system is weakened, susceptibility to respiratory infections is increased.

8. d. Malnutrition that results from a decreased intake of food is most common in individuals with severe anorexia where there is a decreased desire to eat. Infections create a hypermetabolic state that increases nutritional demand, malabsorption causes loss of nutrients that are ingested, and draining decubitus ulcers are examples of disorders that cause both loss of protein and hypermetabolic states.

9. c. Serum transferrin is a protein that is synthesized by the liver and used for iron transport and decreases when there is protein deficiency. An increase in the protein would indicate a more positive nitrogen balance with amino acids available for synthesis. Decreased lymphocytes and serum prealbumin are indicators of protein depletion and increased serum potassium shows continuing failure of the sodium-potassium pump.

10. d. Anthropometric measurements, including mid-upper arm circumference and triceps skinfold measurements, are good indicators of lean body mass and skeletal protein reserves and are valuable in evaluating persons who may have been or are being treated for acute protein malnutrition. The other measurements do not specifically address muscle mass.

11. a. The breakfast with the eggs provides 24 g of protein, compared with 14 g for the protein-fortified cream of wheat and milkshake breakfast. Whole milk instead of skim milk helps to meet the calorie requirements. The toast has 10 g of protein and the pancakes have about 6 g. Bacon is considered a fat rather than a meat serving.

12. b. Although calorie intake should be decreased in the older adult because of decreased activity and basal metabolic rate, the need for specific nutrients, such as proteins and vitamins, does not change.

13. a. Socioeconomic conditions frequently have the greatest effect on the nutritional status of the healthy older adult. Limited income and social isolation can result in the "tea and toast" meals of the older adult. The other options do not interfere with nutritional status.

14. a. Standard nasogastric (NG) tubes are used for tube feedings for short-term feeding problems because prolonged therapy can result in irritation and erosion of the mucosa of the upper GI tract. Gastric reflux and the potential for aspiration can occur with both tubes that deliver fluids into the stomach. Both NG and gastrostomy tubes can become displaced and deprive the patient of the sensations associated with eating.

15.

Desired Outcome	Nursing Intervention
Prevention of aspiration	X-ray confirmation of tube location before feeding. Recheck the tube's insertion length at regular intervals. Position the patient with the head of the bed elevated 30 to 45 degrees during feedings. Following intermittent feedings, keep the head of the bed elevated for 30 to 60 minutes. Measure residual every 8 hours or per policy after the first 24 hours to validate gastric emptying. Hold tube feeding if residual is greater than 500 mL. Monitor for sensation of fullness, nausea, and vomiting.
Prevention of diarrhea	Start tube feedings with small amounts and/or decrease rate of infusion. Refrigerate and date opened solutions to prevent bacterial growth but warm them to room temperature before administration; discard outdated formula; use closed systems; use sterile water to flush; check for medications that may cause diarrhea; and provide free water with tube feedings to compensate for high-concentration enteral feedings.
Maintenance of tube patency	Flush the tube with 30 mL water before and after feedings and medication administration. Only administer medications that can be crushed and be sure that they are dissolved in water before administration. In continuous feedings, flush the tube with water every 4 hours; flush after residual measurements.
Maintenance of tube placement	Confirm placement initially with chest x-ray; mark exit point of tube following x-ray confirmation and routinely assess for changes in the external length of the tube. If lengthened, check pH of aspirate (<5).
Administration of medication	Stop feeding. Check tube placement. Flush with 15 mL of water, dilute medications, and use clean oral syringe to administer medications; flush again taking into account the patient's fluid status; separately dilute and administer medications; use liquid forms of medications, if available; use immediate release form, if liquid not available. Check to see if medications are to be given with meals or on an empty stomach and hold feeding if necessary.

16. b. With intermittent feedings, less than 250 mL residual does not require further action. With continuous feedings and a residual of 250 mL or more after the second residual check, a promotility agent should be considered.

17. a. RN; b. UAP; c. RN; d. RN; e. UAP; f. UAP; g. RN; h. UAP

18. a. PPN; b. CPN; c. CPN; d. PPN; e. CPN; f. PPN; g. CPN

19. c. In malabsorption syndromes, foods that are ingested into the intestinal tract cannot be digested or absorbed and tube feedings infused into the intestinal tract would not be absorbed. All of the other conditions can be treated with enteral or parenteral nutrition, depending on the patient's needs.

20.

Complication	Preventive Measure
Infection	Refrigerate solutions until 30 minutes before use; aseptically change dressing to catheter site per institutional protocol and assess for signs of infection; label date and time started; change filter and tubing every 24 hours if lipids are being administered or every 72 hours if amino acids and dextrose are being administered and label tubing with date and time attached; do not infuse solution in one bottle more than 24 hours; do not add anything to the solution.
Hyperglycemia	Start infusions slowly, gradually increasing rate for 24 to 48 hours; check capillary blood glucose levels every 4 to 6 hours; provide sliding-scale insulin as prescribed; do not speed up infusion rates or remove infusion from infusion controllers and pumps; visually check the amount infused every 30 to 60 minutes.
Air embolism	Place patient supine before changing the dressing with sterile technique; clamp the infusion line before changing the injection cap with sterile technique; if the line cannot be clamped, instruct the patient to perform the Valsalva maneuver when the catheter is open to air; do not inject air when flushing the catheter lumen(s).

21. a. Bacterial growth occurs at room temperature in nutritional solutions. Therefore solutions must not be infused for longer than 24 hours. Remaining solution should be discarded. Speeding up the solution may cause hyperglycemia and should not be done. The health care provider does not need to be notified.

22. a. AB; b. A; c. B; d. AB; e. AB; f. A; g. A; h. B

23. d. The potential life-threatening cardiac complications related to the hypokalemia are the most important immediate considerations in the patient's care. The other nursing diagnoses are important for the patient's care but do not pose the immediate risk that the hypokalemia does.

Case Study

1. Vital signs, R.M.'s position on the weight for height and body frame chart, and food intake history. Assessment of each body system. Ability to obtain and make food or a support system to help her do so.

2. The surgery, chemotherapy, and radiation have greatly increased nutritional need but R.M.'s food intake is decreased because of side effects of cancer treatment. Weakness may lead to an inability to procure and prepare food; the patient lives alone and has no socialization with meals. As well, she has feelings of hopelessness about treatment for cancer.

3. Edema and possible ascites indicated by hypoalbuminemia and paleness of skin and mucous membranes indicated by R.M.'s hemoglobin and hematocrit levels.

4. Liver damage with fatty infiltration; susceptibility to infection is very high because of chemotherapy and radiation immunosuppression in addition to malnutrition; and further muscle wasting from inactivity due to fatigue.

5. Easy-to-prepare foods. Use MyPlate to help R.M. plan nutritious meals within her cultural and individual preferences, as previously assessed. Use high-calorie, high-protein supplements. Teach her how to add a protein supplement or powdered milk to foods, decrease fluids with meals so that more calories are consumed, and eat small multiple feedings that are of nutritional value. Provide all written instructions in Spanish. Refer R.M. to community resources for socialization and Meals on Wheels.

6. **Nursing diagnoses:**
   - Imbalanced nutrition: less than body requirements *related to* anorexia and decreased food intake
   - Activity intolerance *related to* fatigue and weakness
   - Hopelessness *related to* belief that cancer therapy is ineffective
   - Risk for infection *related to* decreased host defense mechanisms

   Collaborative problems:
   Potential complications: liver failure, electrolyte imbalance

CHAPTER 41

Answer Key

1. a. $202 \times 703 = 142,006 \div 4225$ (65×65) = 33.6 kg/m^2; obesity

   b. $32 \div 36 = 0.88$; an increased risk for health complications

2. b. Twin studies and studies with adopted children have shown that body shape and weight gain are influenced by genetics but more research is needed. Older obese people do have exacerbated aging problems related to declines in physical function. African Americans and Hispanics have a higher incidence of obesity than whites. Women have a higher incidence of obesity and more difficulty losing weight than men because women have a higher percentage of metabolically less-active fat.

3. b. The 56-year-old woman has a body mass index (BMI) of 38 kg/m^2 (obese, Class II) with a waist-to-hip ratio of 1.1 with android obesity and is more at risk (very high) than the other patients. The 30-year-old woman has the least risk with a BMI of 27.3 kg/m^2 (overweight) and gynoid shape. The 42-year-old man has a BMI of 24.2 kg/m^2 (normal weight) with one risk factor in the waist-to-hip ratio of 1.0 and the 68-year-old man has a BMI of 27.9 kg/m^2 (overweight) with a waist-to-hip ratio of 0.9.

4. b. A patient who is obese (BMI of 32.2) but has a waist-to-hip ratio of less than 0.8, indicating gynoid obesity, has an increased risk for osteoporosis. The other conditions are risks associated with android obesity. (See Table 41-2.)

5. a. Motivation is essential. Focus on the reasons for wanting to lose weight. The rest of the options will assist in planning the weight loss if the patient is motivated.

6. a, b, c, d, e, f. Normally ghrelin and neuropeptide Y stimulate appetite. Leptin suppresses appetite and hunger. Insulin decreases appetite. Peptide YY and cholecystokinin inhibit appetite by slowing gastric emptying and sending satiety signals to the hypothalamus.

7. a, c. To restrict dietary intake so that it is below energy requirements, the moderately obese woman should limit or avoid alcohol intake because it increases caloric intake and has low nutritional value. Portion sizes have increased over the years and are larger than they should be. Teach the patient to determine portion sizes by weight or learn equivalencies such as that a serving of fruit is the size of a baseball. A progressive exercise program will increase energy requirements and a diet with an initial 800- to 1200-calorie limit would decrease calorie intake. Overeaters Anonymous would not restrict dietary intake below energy requirements, although it may offer support for the patient.

8. c. With reducing diets that severely restrict carbohydrates, the body's glycogen stores become depleted within a few days. The glycogen normally binds to water in fat cells and it is this water loss that causes weight loss in the first few days. Fat is not burned until the glycogen-water pool is depleted. Although psychosocial components (i.e., using food for comfort or reward and inability to buy high–nutritional quality food) may have an influence on weight gain, these factors along with lack of physical exercise, underestimation of portion size, and genetics contribute to weight gain. Weekly weighing is recommended as a more reliable indicator of weight loss because daily weighing shows frequent fluctuation from retained water (including urine) and elimination of feces. Men are able to lose weight more quickly than women because women have a higher percentage of metabolically less-active fat.

9. a. Plateau periods during which no weight is lost are normal occurrences during weight reduction and may last for several days to several weeks but weight loss will resume if the prescribed weight reduction plan is continued. Weight loss may stop if former eating habits are resumed but this is not the most common cause of plateaus.

10. d. A chicken breast the size of a deck of cards is about 3 oz, a recommended portion size of meat. Other normal portions include a 3-inch bagel, ½ cup of chopped vegetables, and a piece of cheese the size of six dice.

11. b. Medications are used only as adjuncts to diet and exercise programs in the treatment of obesity. Drugs do not cure

obesity; without changes in food intake and physical activity, weight gain will occur when the medications are discontinued. The medications used work in a variety of ways to control appetite but over-the-counter (OTC) drugs are probably the least effective and most abused of these drugs.

12. a. Qsymia is a combination of phentermine and topiramate. It must not be used in patients with glaucoma or hyperthyroidism.

13. d. People who have undergone behavior therapy are more successful in maintaining weight losses over time because most programs deemphasize the diet, focus on how and when the person eats and education, and provide support from others. Weighing daily is not recommended and plateaus may not allow for consistent weight loss. A goal for weight loss must be set and 1 to 2 pounds a week is realistic. A more rapid loss often causes skin and underlying tissue to lose elasticity and become flabby folds of tissue. Exercising more often depresses appetite and exercise need not be limited.

14. b. The Roux-en-Y gastric bypass is a common combination of restrictive (limiting the size of the stomach) and malabsorptive (less food is absorbed) surgery. Lipectomy is used to remove unsightly flabby folds of adipose tissue. Adjustable gastric banding is the most common restrictive procedure. Vertical sleeve gastrectomy is a restrictive procedure that preserves stomach function.

15. b, e. The adjustable gastric banding procedure is reversible and allows a change in gastric stoma size by inflation or deflation of the band around the fundus of the stomach. The vertical sleeve gastrectomy removes 85% of the stomach and eliminates the hormones produced in the stomach that stimulate hunger. The biliopancreatic diversion is a maladaptive surgery that prevents absorption of nutrients, including fat-soluble vitamins. The Roux-en-Y gastric bypass reduces the stomach size with a gastric pouch anastomosed to the small intestine, so it is both restrictive and malabsorptive.

16. c. Special considerations are needed for the care of the severely obese patient because most hospital units are not prepared with beds, chairs, BP cuffs, and other equipment that will need to be used with the very obese patient. Consideration of all aspects of care should be made before implementing care for the patient, including extra time and perhaps assistance for positioning, physical assessment, and transferring the patient.

17. c, e, f. Obese patients are at higher risk for cancer, sleep apnea and sleep deprivation, type 2 diabetes mellitus, gastroesophageal reflux disease (GERD), nonalcoholic steatohepatitis, osteoarthritis, and cardiovascular problems. The other options are not related to obesity.

18. b. Patients with histories of untreated depression or psychosis are not good candidates for surgery. All other historical information includes medical complications of severe obesity that would help to qualify the patient for the surgery.

19. d. Turning, coughing, and deep breathing are essential to prevent postoperative complications. Protecting the incision from strain is important since wound dehiscence is a problem for obese patients. If a nasogastric (NG) tube that is present following gastric surgery for severe obesity becomes blocked or needs repositioning, the health

care provider should be notified. Ambulation is usually started on the evening of surgery and additional help will be needed to support the patient. Respiratory function is promoted by keeping the head of the bed elevated at an angle of 35 to 40 degrees.

20. a. Fluids and foods high in carbohydrates tend to promote diarrhea and symptoms of dumping syndrome in patients with gastric bypass surgery. The diet generally should be high in protein and low in carbohydrates, fat, and roughage and consist of six small feedings a day because of the small stomach size. Liquid diets are likely to be used longer for the patient with a gastroplasty.

21. b. Three of the following five measures are needed for a woman to be diagnosed with metabolic syndrome: waist circumference >35 in, triglycerides >150 mg/dL, high-density lipoproteins < 50 mg/dL, BP >130 mm Hg systolic or >85 mm Hg diastolic, fasting blood glucose > 110 mg/dL. Although the other options have some abnormal measures, none has all three measures in the diagnostic ranges. The criteria for metabolic syndrome for both women and men are listed in Table 41-10.

22. a, c, d, e. Patients with metabolic syndrome need to lower their risk factors by reducing and maintaining weight, increasing physical activity, establishing healthy diet habits, and smoking cessation. Some patients with metabolic syndrome are diabetic and would need to monitor glucose levels frequently. When monitoring weight reduction, it is recommended to check weight weekly, not daily.

23. c. Insulin resistance is the main underlying risk factor for metabolic syndrome. Aging is associated with metabolic syndrome. High cholesterol, hypertension, and increased clotting risk are characteristics of metabolic syndrome.

Case Study

1. L.C.'s BMI is about 45 kg/m^2: 296 × 703 ÷ 4624 [68 × 68].
2. L.C. has a risk for almost all health problems associated with obesity: type 2 diabetes, obesity hypoventilation syndrome, osteoarthritis, gout, lumbar disc disease, chronic low back pain, sudden cardiac death, heart failure, coronary artery disease (CAD), deep vein thrombosis (DVT), gallstones, nonalcoholic steatohepatitis, renal disease, and cancer. He already has hypertension, hyperlipidemia, sleep apnea, metabolic syndrome, impaired mobility, and depression.
3. L.C. would qualify for bariatric surgery. He has a BMI >40 kg/m^2, has one or more obesity-related medical complications, is age 18 years or older, understands the risks and benefits of the surgery, has tried and failed other methods of weight loss, has no serious endocrine problems that are causing the obesity, is psychiatrically and socially stable, and is able to follow up on a long-term basis. Surgery would lessen the risks for obesity complications.

4.

Surgical Procedure	Advantages	Disadvantages
Roux-en-Y gastric bypass	Excellent patient tolerance, sustained long-term weight loss, low complication rates, most commonly used bariatric procedure, improved glucose control or type 2 diabetes reversal, normalization of BP, decreased total cholesterol and triglycerides, decreased GERD, decreased sleep apnea	Absorption deficiencies of iron, cobalamin, folic acid, and calcium; mortality rate of 2% in first month; dumping syndrome with vomiting, nausea, weakness, sweating, and faintness; irreversible
Adjustable gastric banding	Stomach remains intact, an earlier sense of fullness with smaller stomach accommodation, small stoma size delays stomach emptying that provides further satiety, digestion is not altered, successful weight loss, can be modified or reversed	Possible intractable vomiting, distention of pouch wall, rupture of staple line, erosion of the band into the stomach

5. This patient needs to be instructed in proper coughing technique, deep breathing, and turning methods. He should be taught to use an incentive spirometer. He will also need to take several showers per day for a few days before surgery. If he uses a continuous positive airway pressure (CPAP) machine at home, he should also use one at the hospital. He should be told what to expect postoperatively: an IV, NG tube, and urinary catheter. He also should be prepared for frequent assessment, early ambulation, active and passive range of motion, the use of antiembolism stockings or pneumatic compression devices, low-dose heparin administered subcutaneously, the need for pain medication, and initiation of oral liquids (30 mL every 2 hours while awake).

6. On discharge this patient needs to be taught about the signs of infection, wound dehiscence, and delayed healing; the need for a measured amount of a high-protein liquid diet, to eat slowly and stop eating when feeling full, and to avoid consuming liquids with solids. The patient also needs to be instructed on the need for a multivitamin with iron and calcium supplements to prevent deficiencies. The dietitian's contact information will also be helpful for him. A progressive exercise program will need to be included as well.

7. **Nursing diagnoses:**
   - Activity intolerance *related to* fatigue
   - Sense of powerlessness *related to* lack of control of eating
   - Ineffective breathing pattern *related to* obesity
   - Ineffective individual coping *related to* changes in social participation
   - Health-seeking behavior: expressed desire for weight loss and health maintenance mechanisms

   Collaborative problems:

   Potential complications: CAD, respiratory complications, type 2 diabetes, renal failure, liver failure, musculoskeletal problems, skin breakdown, postoperative wound infection, pain

CHAPTER 42

Answer Key

1. d. The parasympathetic nervous system causes increased salivation and gastric mobility as well as relaxation of the lower esophageal sphincter. The acid-base imbalance that occurs with vomiting is metabolic alkalosis from the loss of hydrochloric acid. The vomiting center in the chemoreceptor trigger zone (CTZ) can be caused by chemical stimuli of drugs, toxins, and labyrinthine stimulation. Vomiting requires the coordination of closing the glottis, deep inspiration with contraction of the diaphragm in the inspiratory position, closure of the pylorus, relaxation of the stomach and lower esophageal sphincter, and contraction of abdominal muscles.

2. c. The loss of gastric hydrochloric acid causes metabolic alkalosis and an increase in pH; loss of potassium, sodium, and chloride; and loss of fluid, which increases the hematocrit.

3. b. The patient with severe or persistent vomiting requires IV replacement of fluids and electrolytes until able to tolerate oral intake to prevent serious dehydration and electrolyte imbalances. Oral fluids are not given until vomiting has been relieved and parenteral antiemetics are often not used until a cause of the vomiting can be established. Nasogastric (NG) intubation may be indicated in some cases but fluid and electrolyte replacement is the first priority.

4. a. Water is the fluid of choice for rehydration by mouth. Very hot or cold liquids are not usually well tolerated and although broth and Gatorade have been used for the patient with severe vomiting, these substances are high in sodium and should be administered with caution.

5. d. Ondansetron (Zofran) is one of several serotonin antagonists that act both centrally and peripherally to reduce vomiting: centrally on the vomiting center in the brainstem and peripherally by promoting gastric emptying. Dronabinol (Marinol) is an orally active cannabinoid that causes sedation and has a potential for abuse and it is used when other therapies are ineffective. Antihistamines used as antiemetics also cause sedation.

6. c. Implementing safety precautions (placement close to the nurses' station, call bell in reach, hourly visual checks, use of sitters) is the priority. The patient would not be kept in a flat position because of the potential for aspiration of vomitus. Because the older patient is more likely to have cardiac or renal insufficiency, the patient's fluid and electrolyte status are monitored more closely (laboratory, intake and output). Monitor vital signs along with breath sounds. Assess mucous membranes, skin turgor, and color to assess for dehydration. Assess level of consciousness closely. Check dosing of antiemetics. Assess for weakness and fatigue.

7. a. When gingivitis is untreated, abscesses form and teeth are loosened with periodontitis. Herpes simplex is the viral infection related to the upper respiratory system and has shallow, painful vesicular ulcerations of lips and mouth. Aphthous stomatitis has infectious ulcers of the mouth and lips with a defined erythematous base occurring as a result of systemic disease.

8. b. Stomatitis is inflammation of the mouth related to systemic diseases and cancer chemotherapy medications. There is excessive salivation, halitosis, and a sore mouth. Parotitis is a *Staphylococcus* infection that may occur with prolonged NPO status and results in decreased saliva and ear pain. Oral candidiasis is seen with prolonged antibiotic or corticosteroid therapy; it has white membranous lesions on the mucosa of the mouth and larynx. Vincent's infection is a bacterial infection predisposed by fatigue, stress, and poor oral hygiene. There are painful, bleeding gums and increased metallic-tasting saliva.

9. c. A positive history of use of tobacco and alcohol is the most significant etiologic factor in oral cancer. Excessive exposure to ultraviolet radiation from the sun is a factor in the development of cancer of the lip. Herpes simplex infections have not been associated with oral cancer. Difficulty swallowing and ear pain are symptoms of advanced oral cancer, not risk factors.

10. b. Because surgical treatment of oral cancers involves extensive excision, a tracheostomy is usually performed with the radical dissections. The first goal of care is that the patient will have a patent airway. The other goals are appropriate but of lesser priority.

11. b. Measures to assess and treat withdrawal from alcohol should be implemented with patients who have heavy use of this substance because alcohol is a strong risk factor and withdrawal can be life threatening. Tobacco withdrawal also may be uncomfortable for the patient. Nutritional needs may need to be addressed with tube feedings postoperatively and pain medications may need to be increased because of cross-tolerance. Counseling about lifestyle changes is not a priority in the early postoperative course.

12. a, c, e, f. Alcohol, chocolate, fatty foods, and cola sodas (caffeine) as well as peppermint and spearmint will decrease lower esophageal sphincter (LES) pressure. Root beer and herbal tea do not have caffeine. Citrus fruits will not affect LES pressure.

13. c. The use of blocks to elevate the head of the bed facilitates gastric emptying by gravity and is strongly recommended to prevent nighttime reflux. Liquids should be taken between meals to prevent gastric distention with meals. Small meals should be eaten frequently but patients should not eat at bedtime or lie down for 2 to 3 hours after eating. Activities that involve increasing intraabdominal pressure, such as bending over, lifting, or wearing tight clothing, should be avoided.

14. c. Eating a high-calorie, high-protein diet, perhaps in liquid form, is the highest priority preoperatively. Because of dysphagia, the patient frequently has poor nutritional status because of the inability to ingest adequate amounts of food before surgery. An esophageal stent may be placed to improve the nutritional status. Turning and deep breathing will be done and the patient will need to know about postoperative care but these are not the priorities. Meticulous oral care is done but it may be done with swabs or gauze pads to prevent the injury and pain brushing may incur.

15. b. Following esophageal surgery, the patient should be positioned in semi-Fowler's or Fowler's position to prevent reflux and aspiration of gastric sections. NG drainage is

expected to be bloody for 8 to 12 hours postoperatively. Abdominal distention is not a major concern following esophageal surgery and even though the thorax may be opened during the surgery, clear breath sounds should be expected in all areas of the lungs.

16. b. Barrett's esophagus is an esophageal metaplasia primarily related to gastroesophageal reflux disease (GERD). Achalasia is a rare chronic disorder with the absence of peristalsis of the lower two thirds of the esophagus. Esophageal strictures are narrowing of the esophagus from scarring by many causes. Esophageal diverticula are saclike outpouchings of one or more layers of the esophagus commonly seen above the esophageal sphincter.

17. d. Eosinophilic esophagitis is swelling of the esophagus caused by infiltration of eosinophils in response to food triggers or environmental allergens. Esophageal cancer is usually caused by adenocarcinoma, with the remainder being squamous cell tumors. Esophageal varices are dilated vessels in the esophagus caused by portal hypertension. Esophagitis is inflammation of the esophagus commonly seen with GERD.

18. a. Acute gastritis is most likely to occur with an isolated drinking binge. Chronic gastritis is usually caused by *Heliobacter pylori* or viral and fungal infections. Autoimmune gastritis is an inherited condition.

19. b. A nonirritating diet with six small meals a day is recommended to help control the symptoms of gastritis. Nonsteroidal antiinflammatory drugs (NSAIDs) are often as irritating to the stomach as aspirin and should not be used in the patient with gastritis. Antacids are often used for control of symptoms but have the best neutralizing effect if taken after meals. Alcohol and caffeine should be eliminated entirely because they may precipitate gastritis.

20. a, c, f. Duodenal ulcers have increased gastric secretion, which causes the burning and cramping in the midepigastric area, and the pain is relieved with food. The other options occur with both duodenal and gastric ulcers.

21. a. The 55-year-old female smoker experiencing nausea and vomiting is more likely to have a gastric ulcer. The other patients are not in the highest-risk age range or do not have enough risk factors. Although lower socioeconomic status, smoking, and drug use do increase the risk of gastric ulcers, these patients are more likely to experience duodenal ulcers but further assessment is needed.

22. c. Corticosteroids decrease the rate of mucous cell renewal. *H. pylori* produces the enzyme urease. Alcohol ingestion increases the secretion of hydrochloric acid. Aspirin and NSAIDs inhibit the synthesis of mucus and prostaglandins.

23. a. The ultimate damage to the tissues of the stomach and duodenum, precipitating ulceration, is acid back diffusion into the mucosa. The gastric mucosal barrier is protective of the mucosa but without the acid environment and damage, ulceration does not occur. Ammonia formation by *H. pylori* and release of histamine impair the barrier but are not directly responsible for tissue injury.

24. b. Back pain is a common manifestation of ulcers located on the posterior aspect of the duodenum and is important for nurses to keep in mind during assessment of the patient, because the more typical epigastric burning and pain may not be present. Duodenal ulcers are more often relieved by food than are gastric ulcers and when epigastric discomfort occurs, it is lower than that of gastric ulcers. Eating stimulates gastric acid production, increasing discomfort for patients with gastric ulcers, whereas the pain of duodenal ulcers usually occurs several hours after eating.

25. c. There is no specific diet used for the treatment of peptic ulcers and patients are encouraged to eat as normally as possible, eliminating foods that cause discomfort or pain. Eating six meals a day prevents the stomach from being totally empty and is also recommended. Caffeine and alcohol should be eliminated from the diet because they are known to cause gastric irritation. Milk and milk products do not need to be avoided but they can add fat content to the diet.

26. d. NG intubation is used with acute exacerbation of peptic ulcer disease to remove the stimulation for hydrochloric acid (HCl) and pepsin secretion by keeping the stomach empty. Stopping the spillage of GI contents into the peritoneal cavity is used for peritonitis. Removing excess fluids and undigested food from the stomach is the rationale for using NG intubation for gastric outlet obstruction.

27. b, c, f. Antacids need a high dose and frequency, which may lead to noncompliance; prevent the conversion of pepsinogen to pepsin; and may stimulate the release of gastrin. Amoxicillin/clarithromycin/omeprazole are used in patients with verified *H. pylori*. Sucralfate (Carafate) covers the ulcer to protect it from acid erosion.

28. a, c, d, e. Famotidine (Pepcid) reduces HCl secretion by blocking histamine and omeprazole (Prilosec) decreases gastric acid secretion by blocking adenosine triphosphatase (ATPase) enzyme. Sucralfate (Carafate) coats the ulcer to protect it from acid erosion. Misoprostol (Cytotec) mixture has antisecretory effects. Amoxicillin/clarithromycin/omeprazole are used in patients with verified *H. pylori*.

29. c. Increased vagal stimulation from emotional stress causes hypersecretion of hydrochloric acid and stress reduction is an important part of the patient's management of peptic ulcers, especially duodenal ulcers. If side effects to medications develop, the patient should notify the health care provider before altering the drug regimen. Although effective treatment will promote pain relief in several days, the treatment regimen should be continued until there is evidence that the ulcer has healed completely. Interchanging brands and preparations of antacids and histamine (H_2)-receptor blockers without checking with health care providers may cause harmful side effects and patients should take only prescribed medications.

30. c. Perforation of an ulcer causes sudden, severe abdominal pain that is often referred to the back, accompanied by a rigid, boardlike abdomen and other signs of peritonitis. Vomiting of blood indicates hemorrhage of an ulcer and gastric outlet obstruction is characterized by projectile vomiting of undigested food, hyperactive stomach sounds, and upper abdominal swelling.

31. a. If symptoms of gastric outlet obstruction, such as nausea, vomiting, and stomach distention, occur while the patient is on NPO status or has an NG tube, the patency of the NG tube should be assessed. A recumbent position should not be used in a patient with a gastric outlet obstruction because it increases abdominal pressure on the stomach and vital signs and circulatory status assessment are important if hemorrhage or perforation is suspected. Deep breathing and relaxation may help some patients with nausea but not when stomach contents are obstructed from flowing into the small intestine.

32. d. Abdominal pain that causes the knees to be drawn up and shallow, grunting respirations in a patient with peptic ulcer disease are characteristic of perforation and the nurse should assess the patient's vital signs and abdomen before notifying the health care provider. Irrigation of the NG tube should not be performed because the additional fluid may be spilled into the peritoneal cavity and the patient should be placed in a position of comfort, usually on the side with the head slightly elevated.

33. a. 3; b. 4; c. 2; d. 1

34. d. Because there is no sphincter control of food taken into the stomach following a Billroth II procedure, concentrated food and fluid move rapidly into the small intestine, creating a hypertonic environment that pulls fluid from the bowel wall into the lumen of the intestine, reducing plasma volume and distending the bowel. Postprandial hypoglycemia occurs when the concentrated carbohydrate bolus in the small intestine results in hyperglycemia and the release of excessive amounts of insulin into the circulation, resulting in symptoms of hypoglycemia. Irritation of the stomach by bile salts causes epigastric distress after meals, not dumping syndrome.

35. a. Dietary control of dumping syndrome includes small, frequent meals with low carbohydrate content and elimination of fluids with meals. The patient should also lie down for 30 to 60 minutes after meals. These measures help to delay stomach emptying, preventing the rapid movement of a high-carbohydrate food bolus into the small intestine.

36. d. If the patient's NG tube becomes obstructed following a gastrectomy with an intestinal anastomosis, gastric secretions may put a strain on the sutured anastomosis and cause serious complications. Be sure that the suction is working and the health care provider may order periodic gentle irrigation with normal saline solution. Because of the danger of perforating the gastric mucosa or disrupting the suture line, the nurse should notify the health care provider if the tube needs to be repositioned or replaced.

37. b. A total gastrectomy removes the parietal cells responsible for secreting intrinsic factor necessary for absorption of cobalamin. Lifelong administration of cobalamin is necessary to prevent the development of pernicious anemia. Wound healing is usually impaired in the patient with a total gastrectomy performed for gastric cancer because of impaired nutritional status before surgery. Following a total gastrectomy, the patient also requires diet modifications as a result of dumping syndrome and postprandial hypoglycemia. Peptic ulcers are not a common finding after total gastrectomy.

38. a. Melena is black, tarry stools from slow bleeding from an upper GI source when blood passes through the GI tract and is digested. Occult blood is the presence of guaiac-positive stools or gastric aspirate. Coffee-ground emesis is blood that has been in the stomach for some time and has reacted with gastric secretions. Profuse bright-red hematemesis is arterial blood that has not been in contact with gastric secretions, as in esophageal or oral bleeding.

39. b. Although all of the interventions may be indicated when a patient has upper GI bleeding, the first nursing priority with bright-red (arterial) blood is to perform a focused assessment of the patient's condition, with emphasis on blood pressure (BP), pulse, and peripheral perfusion to determine the presence of hypovolemic shock.

40. d. Octreotide is a somatostatin analog that has been shown to reduce upper GI bleeding and inhibit the release of GI hormones such as gastrin, thereby decreasing hydrochloric acid secretion. Nizatidine is a histamine (H2)-receptor blocker that decreases acid secretion and omeprazole inhibits the proton pump necessary for the secretion of hydrochloric acid. Vasopressin has a vasoconstriction action useful in controlling upper GI bleeding.

41. b. All over-the-counter (OTC) drugs should be avoided because their contents may include drugs that are contraindicated because of the irritating effects on the gastric mucosa. Patients are taught to test suspicious vomitus or stools for occult blood but all stools do not need to be tested. Antacids cannot be taken with all medications because they prevent the absorption of many drugs. Misoprostol is used to protect the gastric mucosa in patients who must take NSAIDs for other conditions because it inhibits acid secretion stimulated by NSAIDs.

42. d. The patient's blood urea nitrogen (BUN) is usually elevated with a significant hemorrhage because blood proteins are subjected to bacterial breakdown in the GI tract. With control of bleeding, the BUN will return to normal. During the early stage of bleeding, the hematocrit (Hct) is not always a reliable indicator of the amount of blood lost or the amount of blood replaced and may be falsely high or low. A urinary output of ≤20 mL/hr indicates impaired renal perfusion and hypovolemia and a urine specific gravity of 1.030 indicates concentrated urine typical of hypovolemia.

43. b. Food poisoning caused by *Escherichia coli* is characterized by profuse diarrhea, abdominal cramping, and bloody stools and is most often associated with contaminated beef, especially ground beef. Salmonella contamination most often occurs with poultry, staphylococcal infections occur with milk and salad dressings, and botulism occurs with fish and low-acid canned products.

Case Study

1. Infiltration of the gastric wall by a tumor causes epigastric discomfort. Growth of the tumor into the gastric lumen can cause anorexia and weight loss. Release of substances by cancer cells also contributes to anorexia, nausea, and vomiting. Nausea and vomiting may also be caused if the tumor obstructs the gastric outlet. Fatigue and other symptoms of anemia occur because of chronic blood loss as the lesion erodes through the mucosa.

2. Malnutrition is indicated in this patient by weight loss, decreased hemoglobin and hematocrit, decreased serum albumin, skin changes and discoloration, and her emaciated appearance.
3. Other factors that may contribute to S.E.'s malnutrition include the increased metabolic demands of tumor cells; responses to radiation therapy, such as vomiting, stomatitis, esophagitis, diarrhea, and decreased bone marrow function; and perhaps pernicious anemia resulting from the lack of intrinsic factor common with gastric cancer.
4. Malnourished patients do not respond well to radiation therapy and normal cells do not recover from radiation damage when malnutrition is present. Depletion of protein stores also places S.E. at risk for impaired immune function.
5. A plan for this patient and her family should include the following:
   - Increasing nutrition with bland, warm, high-calorie, high-protein foods; small, frequent feedings; and nutritional supplements as tolerated
   - Oral care to prevent stomatitis and make eating more pleasurable
   - Skin care for radiation therapy
   - Anticipatory planning for pain relief and continuing care as she becomes more impaired
   - Discussion of feelings and concerns of the patient and her family, with explanations of realistic expectations of outcome of her condition
6. In responding to S.E., the nurse should provide accurate information in a way that will decrease her stress and promote her decision making and coping skills. It is important to tell her that although it is unlikely she will recover from her cancer, the radiation treatment can help to shrink the tumor mass, improve her nutritional status, and promote a feeling of well-being. She should be told that her family and health care providers will help her to function effectively for as long as possible.
7. **Nursing diagnoses:**
   - Imbalanced nutrition: less than body requirements *related to* inability to ingest, digest, and absorb nutrients
   - Fatigue *related to* anemia and effects of radiation therapy
   - Activity intolerance *related to* generalized weakness
   - Impaired skin integrity *related to* malnutrition and radiation therapy
   - Ineffective self-health management *related to* lack of knowledge regarding disease progression
   - Nausea *related to* radiation therapy
   - Grieving *related to* perceived unfavorable diagnosis and impending death

   Collaborative problems:
   Potential complications: sepsis related to immuno-suppression, negative nitrogen balance, organ failure

CHAPTER 43

Answer Key

1. c. Antiperistaltic agents, such as loperamide (Imodium) and paregoric, should not be used in infectious diarrhea because of the potential of prolonging exposure to the infectious agent. Demulcent agents may be used to coat and protect mucous membranes in these cases. The other options are all appropriate measures to use in cases of infectious diarrhea.
2. c. Wearing gloves will avoid hand contamination and washing hands with soap and water will remove more *Clostridium difficile* spores than alcohol-based hand cleaners and ammonia-based disinfectants. The entire room will need to be disinfected with a 10% solution of household bleach. Probiotics may help to prevent diarrhea in the patient on antibiotics by replacing normal intestinal bacteria.
3. d. The first intervention to establish bowel regularity includes promoting bowel evacuation at a regular time each day, preferably by placing the patient on the bedpan, using a bedside commode, or walking the patient to the bathroom. To take advantage of the gastrocolic reflex, an appropriate time is 30 minutes after the first meal of the day or at the patient's usual individual time. Perianal pouches are used to protect the skin only when regularity cannot be established and evacuation suppositories are also used only if other techniques are not successful.
4. d. Ignoring the urge to defecate causes the muscles and mucosa in the rectal area to become insensitive to the presence of feces and drying of the stool occurs. The urge to defecate is decreased and stool becomes more difficult to expel. Taking a bulk-forming agent with fluids or high-fiber diet with fluids prevent constipation. Hemorrhoids are the most common complication of chronic constipation, caused by straining to pass hardened stool. The straining may cause problems in patients with hypertension but these do not cause constipation. Other things that may cause constipation are a history of diverticulosis, which is seen in individuals with low fiber intake, small stool mass, and hard stools. Chronic laxative use and chronic dilation and loss of colonic tone may also cause chronic constipation.
5. c. Of the foods listed, dried beans contain the highest amount of dietary fiber and are an excellent source of soluble fiber. Bran and berries also have large amounts of fiber.
6. a. Enemas are fast acting and beneficial in the immediate treatment of acute constipation but should be limited in their use. Bulk-forming medication stimulates peristalsis but takes 24 hours to act. Stool softeners have a prolonged action, taking up to 72 hours for an effect, and fluids can help to decrease the incidence of constipation.
7. a. The patient with an acute abdomen may have significant fluid or blood loss into the abdomen and evaluation of blood pressure (BP) and heart rate (HR) should be the first intervention, followed by assessment of the abdomen and the nature of the pain. Analgesics should be used cautiously until a diagnosis can be determined so that symptoms are not masked.
8. b, c, e, f. An immediate surgical consult is needed for acute ischemic bowel, foreign-body perforation, ruptured ectopic pregnancy, or ruptured abdominal aneurysm. A diagnostic laparoscopy may be done or a laparotomy may be done to repair a ruptured abdominal aneurysm or remove the appendix. Surgery is not needed for pancreatitis or pelvic inflammatory disease, as these can be diagnosed and treated without surgery.

9. c. An adequately functioning nasogastric (NG) tube should prevent nausea and vomiting because stomach contents are continuously being removed. The first intervention in this case is to check the amount and character of the recent drainage and check the tube for patency. Decreased or absent bowel sounds are expected after a laparotomy and the Jackson-Pratt drains only fluid from the tissue of the surgical site. Antiemetics may be given if the NG tube is patent because anesthetic agents may cause nausea.

10. a. The abdominal pain and distention that occur from the decreased motility of the bowel should be treated with increased ambulation and frequent position changes to increase peristalsis. If the pain is severe, cholinergic drugs, rectal tubes, or application of heat to the abdomen may be prescribed. Assessment of bowel sounds is not an intervention to relieve the pain and a high Fowler's position is not indicated. Opioids may still be necessary for pain control and motility can be increased by other means.

11. d. The patient is having symptoms of an acute abdomen and should be evaluated by a health care provider immediately. The patient's age, location of pain, and other symptoms are characteristic of appendicitis. Heat application and laxatives should not be used in patients with undiagnosed abdominal pain because they may cause perforation of the appendix or other inflammations. Fluids should not be taken until vomiting is controlled, nor should they be taken in the event that surgery may be performed.

12. b. Because there is no definitive treatment for irritable bowel syndrome (IBS) and patients become frustrated and discouraged with uncontrolled symptoms, it is important to develop a trusting relationship that will support the patient as different treatments are implemented and evaluated. Diagnosis of IBS can be established by Rome criteria and by elimination of other problems. Although IBS can be precipitated and aggravated by stress and emotions, it is not a psychogenic illness. High-fiber diets may help but they might also increase the bloating and gas pains of IBS. Medications are available but usually used as a last resort because of side effects.

13. a. It is likely that the patient could be developing a peritonitis, which could be life-threatening, and assessment of vital signs for hypovolemic shock should be done to report to the health care provider. If an IV line is not in place, it should be inserted and pain may be eased by flexing the knees.

14. b. The patient's manifestations are characteristic of appendicitis. After laboratory test and CT scan confirmation, the patient will have surgery. Laxatives are not used. The 6 hours of fluids and antibiotics preoperatively would be used only if the appendix was ruptured. The NG tube is more likely to be used with abdominal trauma.

15. c. IV fluid replacement along with antibiotics, NG suction, analgesics, and surgery would be expected. Peritoneal lavage may be used to determine abdominal trauma. Peritoneal dialysis would not be performed. Oral fluids would be avoided with peritonitis.

16. a, c, e, f. Crohn's disease may have severe weight loss, segmented distribution through the entire wall of the bowel, and crampy abdominal pain. Rectal bleeding and toxic megacolon are more often seen with ulcerative colitis.

17. c. In the patient with ulcerative colitis, decreased Na^+, K^+, Mg^+, Cl^-, and HCO_3^- are a result of diarrhea and vomiting. Hypoalbuminemia may be present. Elevated WBCs occur with toxic megacolon. Decreased hemoglobin (Hgb) and hematocrit (Hct) occur with bloody diarrhea.

18. d. Ulcerative colitis and Crohn's disease have many of the same extraintestinal symptoms, including erythema nodosum and osteoporosis, as well as gallstones, uveitis, and conjunctivitis. Colonic dilation and celiac disease are not extraintestinal.

19. a, b, e, f. With an acute exacerbation of inflammatory bowel disease (IBD), to rest the bowel the patient will be NPO, receive IV fluids and parenteral nutrition, and have nasogastric suction. Sedatives would be used to alleviate stress. Enteral nutrition will be used as soon as possible.

20. c. Cobalamin and iron injections will help to correct malnutrition. Correcting malnutrition will also indirectly help to improve quality of life and fight infections.

21. c. Antidiarrheal agents only relieve symptoms. Corticosteroids, 6-mercaptopurine, and sulfasalazine (Azulfidine) are used to treat and control inflammation with various diseases.

22. b. The initial procedure for a total proctocolectomy with ileal pouch and anal anastomosis includes a colectomy, rectal mucosectomy, ileal reservoir construction, ileoanal anastomosis, and a temporary ileostomy. A loop ileostomy is the most common temporary ileostomy and it may be held in place with a plastic rod for the first week. A rectal tube to suction is not indicated in any of the surgical procedures for ulcerative colitis. A colostomy is not used and an NG tube would not be used to irrigate the pouch. A permanent ileostomy stoma would be expected following a total proctocolectomy with a permanent ileostomy.

23. a. Initial output from a newly formed ileostomy may be as high as 1500 to 2000 mL daily and intake and output must be accurately monitored for fluid and electrolyte imbalance. Ileostomy bags may need to be emptied every 3 to 4 hours but the appliance should not be changed for several days unless there is leakage onto the skin. A terminal ileum stoma is permanent and the entire colon has been removed. A return to a normal, presurgical diet is the goal for the patient with an ileostomy, with restrictions based only on the patient's individual tolerances.

24. a. Signs of malnutrition include pallor from anemia, hair loss, bleeding, cracked gingivae, and muscle weakness, which support a nursing diagnosis that identifies impaired nutrition. Diarrhea may contribute to malnutrition but is not a defining characteristic. Anorectal excoriation and pain relate to problems with skin integrity. Hypotension relates to problems with fluid deficit.

25. b. Volvulus is the bowel twisting on itself. The bowel folding on itself is intussusception. Emboli of arterial blood supply to the bowel is vascular obstruction. Protrusion of bowel in a weak or abnormal opening is a hernia.

26. c. Intermittent crampy abdominal pain, nausea, projectile vomiting, and dehydration are characteristics of mechanical upper small intestinal obstruction. With continued vomiting, metabolic alkalosis may occur. Large bowel obstruction is

characterized by constipation, low-grade abdominal pain, and abdominal distention. Fecal vomiting is seen with lower small intestinal obstruction.

27. b. Mouth care should be done frequently for the patient with a small intestinal obstruction who has an NG tube because of vomiting, fecal taste and odor, and mouth breathing. No ice chips are allowed when a patient is NPO because of a bowel obstruction. The NG tube should be checked for patency and irrigated as ordered. The position of the patient should be one of comfort.

28. c. Although all polyps are abnormal growths, the most common type of polyp (hyperplastic) is non-neoplastic, as are inflammatory, lipomas, and juvenile polyps. However, adenomatous polyps are characterized by neoplastic changes in the epithelium and most colorectal cancers appear to arise from these polyps. Only patients with a family history of familial adenomatous polyposis (FAP) have close to a 100% lifetime risk of developing colorectal cancer.

29. a. A diet high in red meat and low fruit and vegetable intake is associated with development of colorectal cancer (CRC), as are alcohol intake and smoking. Family and personal history of CRC also increases the risk. Other environmental agents are not known to be related to colorectal cancer. Long-term use of nonsteroidal antiinflammatory drugs (NSAIDs) is associated with reduced CRC risk.

30. d. With an abdominal perineal-resection (APR), an abdominal incision is made and the proximal sigmoid colon is brought through the abdominal wall and formed into a permanent colostomy. The patient is repositioned, a perineal incision is made, and the distal sigmoid colon, rectum, and anus are removed through the perineal incision, which may be left open, packed, and have drains.

31. d. The ileostomy drainage is extremely irritating to the skin, so the skin must be cleaned and a new solid skin barrier and pouch applied as soon as a leak occurs to prevent skin damage. The pouch is usually worn for 4 to 7 days unless there is a leak. Because the initial drainage from the ileostomy is high, the fluid intake must not be decreased. The pouch must always be worn, as the liquid drainage, not formed bowel movements, is frequent.

32. b. A normal new colostomy stoma should appear bright red, have mild to moderate edema, and have a small amount of bleeding or oozing of blood when touched. A purplish stoma indicates inadequate blood supply and should be reported. The colostomy will not have any fecal drainage for 2 to 4 days but there may be some earlier mucus or serosanguineous drainage. Bowel sounds after extensive bowel surgery will be diminished or absent.

33. d, e. The licensed practical nurse (LPN) can monitor and record observations related to the drainage and can measure and record the amount. The LPN could also monitor the skin around the stoma for breakdown. LPNs can irrigate a colostomy in a stable patient but this patient is only 2 days postoperative. The other actions are responsibilities of the RN (teaching, assessing stoma, and developing a care plan).

34. d. Sexual dysfunction may result from an anterior-posterior repair but the nurse should discuss with the patient that different nerve pathways affect erection, ejaculation, and orgasm and that a dysfunction of one does not mean total sexual dysfunction and also that an alteration in sexual activity does not have to alter sexuality. Simple reassurance of desirability and ignoring concerns about sexual function do not help the patient to regain positive feelings of sexuality.

35. d. The patient with a transverse colostomy has semiliquid to semiformed stools needing a pouch and needs to have fluid balance monitored. The ascending colostomy has semiliquid stools needing a pouch and increased fluid. The ileostomy has liquid to semiliquid stools needing a pouch and increased fluid. The sigmoid colostomy has formed stools and may or may not need a pouch but will need irrigation.

36. a. Encouraging the patient to share concerns and ask questions will help the patient to begin to adapt to living with the colostomy. The other options do not support the patient and do not portray the nurse's focus on helping the patient or treating the patient as an individual.

37. b. Following infusion of the fluid into the stoma, the solution and feces will take about 30 to 45 minutes to return and the patient can plan to read or perform other quiet activities during the wait time. Between 500 and 1000 mL of warm tap water should be used. A cone tip on the end of the tubing prevents bowel damage that could occur if a stiff plastic catheter is used. Fluid should be elevated about 18 to 24 inches above the stoma, or to about shoulder level, to prevent too rapid infusion of the solution and cramping.

38. c. Formation of diverticula is common when decreased bulk of stool, combined with a more narrowed lumen in the sigmoid colon, causes high intraluminal pressures that result in saccular dilation or outpouching of the mucosa through the muscle of the intestinal wall. To prevent the high intraluminal pressure, fecal volume should be increased with use of high-fiber diets and bulk laxatives, such as psyllium (Metamucil). Anticholinergic drugs are used only during an acute episode of diverticulitis and the lesions are not premalignant.

39. a. The inflammation and infection of diverticula cause small perforations with spread of the inflammation to the surrounding area in the intestines. Abscesses may form or complete perforation with peritonitis may occur. Systemic antibiotic therapy is often used but medicated enemas would increase intestinal motility and increase the possibility of perforation, as would the application of heat. Surgery is only necessary to drain abscesses or to resect an obstructing inflammatory mass.

40. a, d. The ventral or incisional hernia is due to a weakness of the abdominal wall at the site of a previous incision. It is reducible when it returns to the abdominal cavity. Inguinal hernias are at the weak area of the abdominal wall where the spermatic cord in men or the round ligament in women emerges. A femoral hernia is a protrusion through the femoral ring into the femoral canal. Incarcerated hernias do not reduce.

41. c. A strangulated femoral hernia obstructs intestinal flow and blood supply, thus requiring emergency surgery. The other options are incorrect.

42. b. Scrotal edema is a common and painful complication after an inguinal hernia repair and can be relieved in part by

application of ice and elevation of the scrotum with a scrotal support. Heat would increase the edema and the discomfort and a truss is used to keep unrepaired hernias from protruding. Coughing is discouraged postoperatively because it increases intraabdominal pressure and stress on the repair site.

43. b. The most common type of malabsorption syndrome is lactose intolerance and it is managed by restricting the intake of milk and milk products. Antibiotics are used in cases of bacterial infections that cause malabsorption, pancreatic enzyme supplementation is used for pancreatic insufficiency, and restriction of gluten is necessary for control of adult celiac disease (celiac sprue, gluten-induced enteropathy).

44. c. The autoimmune process associated with celiac disease continues as long as the body is exposed to gluten, regardless of the symptoms it produces, and a lifelong gluten-free diet is necessary. The other statements regarding celiac disease are all true.

45. b. Short bowel syndrome results from extensive resection of portions of the small bowel and would occur if a patient had an extensive resection of the ileum. The other conditions primarily affect the large colon and result in fewer and less severe symptoms.

46. b. An anorectal abscess is a collection of perianal pus. An ulcer in the anal wall is an anal fissure. Sacrococcygeal hairy tract describes a pilonidal sinus. A tunnel leading from the anus or rectum is an anorectal fistula.

47. c. Human papillomavirus (HPV) is associated with about 80% of anal cancer cases. Other risk factors include multiple sexual partners, smoking, receptive anal sex, and HIV infection, as well as being female, age 60, and African American. The other options are not considered risk factors for anal cancer.

48. d. Warm sitz baths provide comfort, healing, and cleansing of the area following all anorectal surgery and may be done three or four times a day for 1 to 2 weeks. Stool softeners may be prescribed for several days postoperatively to help keep stools soft for passage but laxatives may cause irritation and trauma to the anorectal area and are not used postoperatively. Early passage of a bowel movement, although painful, is encouraged to prevent drying and hardening of stool, which would result in an even more painful bowel movement.

Case Study

1. Changes in bowel patterns with alternating constipation and diarrhea, changes in stool caliber with ribbon or pencil stools, rectal bleeding, sensation of incomplete evacuation, unexplained weight loss, and vague abdominal pain.

2. Assess drains placed in the wound and the type and amount of drainage. Assess the skin around the drain for inflammation and keep the area clean and dry. Assess the incision for suture integrity and signs and symptoms of wound infection. Assess drainage from the wound for amount, color, and characteristics. Monitor for edema, erythema, and drainage around the suture line as well as fever and elevated WBC count. Take warm sitz baths at 100.4 °F to 106 °F (38 °C to 41.1 °C) for 10 to 20 minutes three to four times a day and use pressure-reducing chair cushions for comfort. Make sterile dressing changes.

3. To be able to manage care independently; have normal skin integrity; adapt to new dietary needs to manage bloating, gas, diarrhea, and bowel evacuation; and adjust to altered body image.

4. It appears that C.D. is depersonalizing the stoma and, to preserve his body image, is seeing it as something separate from him, with a name and personality of its own.

5. Anxiety, ineffective coping, and fear may influence C.D.'s tolerance of pain.

6. With stage III rectal cancer, adjuvant therapy is recommended. Current chemotherapy protocols include 5-fluorouracil (5-FU) and folinic acid (leucovorin) alone or in combination with oxaliplatin (Eloxatin). Oral fluoropyrimidines (capecitabine [Xeloda]) may also be used alone or with oxaliplatin. Metastatic colorectal cancer may be treated with bevacizumab (Avastin), an angiogenesis inhibitor, to prevent blood supply to the tumors. Cetuximab (Erbitux) and panitumumab (Vectibix) block the epidermal growth factor.

7. Care of the perineal wound; importance of fluids and diet and dietitian contact information; care for colostomy, including skin care, odor control, supplies needed, and where to obtain supplies; signs and symptoms of complications to report and when to seek medical care; name and contact information for the wound, ostomy, and continence (WOC) nurse; name and contact information for the ostomy association and community resources; follow-up appointments with the surgeon and WOC nurse; and potential effects of ostomy on sexual activity, social life, work, and recreation and strategies to manage these situations.

8. **Nursing diagnoses:**
   - Disturbed body image *related to* presence of stoma
   - Acute pain *related to* surgical incisions and inadequate pain-control measures
   - Risk for impaired skin integrity *related to* stoma drainage and open perineal wound
   - Fear and anxiety *related to* diagnosis and further treatment of rectal cancer and possible terminal illness

   Collaborative problems:
   Potential complications: perineal infection; stomal necrosis, retraction, prolapse, or obstruction

CHAPTER 44

Answer Key

1. c. Gallstones cause obstructive or posticteric jaundice and may elevate both conjugated and unconjugated bilirubin.

2. d. Hemolytic jaundice from a blood transfusion reaction is from increased breakdown of RBCs producing increased unconjugated bilirubin in the blood. Hepatocellular jaundice results from hepatocellular disease. Hemolytic jaundice occurs with malaria. Obstructive jaundice is from obstructed bile flow through the liver or biliary duct system.

3. d. Hepatitis E virus (HEV) is associated with poor sanitation and contaminated water in developing countries.

4. b. Hepatitis B virus (HBV) is a DNA virus that is transmitted via infectious blood and body products and is required for hepatitis D virus (HDV) replication, and

chronic HBV along with chronic hepatitis C virus (HCV) accounts for 80% of hepatocellular cancer cases. Hepatitis A virus (HAV), HCV, HDV, and HEV are all RNA viruses.

5. c. Immunization to HBV after vaccination is identified with the hepatitis B surface antibody Anti-HBs. Anti-HBcIgG indicates previous or ongoing HBV infection. Surface antigen HBsAg is present in acute and chronic infection. Core antigen Anti-HBcIgM indicates acute infection and does not appear after vaccination.

6. d. HBV DNA quantitation is the best indicator of viral replication and effectiveness of therapy for chronic HBV. HBsAg is present in acute or chronic infection. HBeAg indicates high infectivity and can also be used to determine clinical management of patients with chronic HBV. Anti-HBcIgM indicates acute infection and anti-HBcIgG indicates ongoing infection. Anti-HDV is present in past or current infection with HDV and therefore HBV. Anti-HBs indicate previous infection with HBV or immunization.

7. d. Anti-HAV immunoglobulin M (IgM) indicates acute HAV infection. Anti-HBc immunoglobulin G (IgG) indicates previous or ongoing infection with HBV. Anti-HBc IgM indicates acute HBV infection. Anti-HAV IgG indicates previous infection with HAV.

8. b. HCV genotyping is done to predict HCV response to drug therapy. Anti-HCV and HCV RNA quantitation are tests completed to diagnose HCV. Recombinant immunoblot assays are used to confirm anti-HCV reactivity.

9. d. The systemic manifestations of rash, angioedema, arthritis, fever, and malaise in viral hepatitis are caused by the activation of the complement system by circulating immune complexes. Liver manifestations include jaundice from hepatic cell damage and cholestasis as well as anorexia. Impaired portal circulation usually does not occur in uncomplicated viral hepatitis but would be a liver manifestation.

10. c. Incubation symptoms occur before the onset of jaundice and include a variety of gastrointestinal (GI) symptoms as well as discomfort and heaviness in the upper right quadrant of the abdomen. Pruritus, dark urine, and light-colored stools occur with the onset of jaundice in the acute phase. Easy fatigability and malaise are seen in the convalescent phase as jaundice disappears.

11. d. The most common cause of acute liver failure is drugs, usually acetaminophen in combination with alcohol abuse. HBV is the second most common cause.

12. d. HBV vaccine and hepatitis B immune globulin (HBIG) are used together prophylactically after a needle stick. Interferon is used to treat chronic HBV.

13. c. Individuals who have been exposed to hepatitis A through household contact or foodborne outbreaks should be given immune globulin within 1 to 2 weeks of exposure to prevent or modify the illness. Hepatitis A vaccine is used to provide preexposure immunity to the virus and is indicated for individuals at high risk for hepatitis A exposure. Although hepatitis A may be spread by sexual contact, the risk is higher for transmission with the oral-fecal route.

14. c. Nucleoside and nucleotide analogs (e.g., lamivudine), ribavirin, and pegylated interferon are used to treat chronic hepatitis B or C. Protease inhibitors are also used to treat chronic hepatitis C. No specific drugs are effective in treating acute viral hepatitis, although supportive drugs, such as antiemetics, sedatives, or antipruritics, may be used for symptom control.

15. b. The patient with hepatitis B is infectious for 4 to 6 months and precautions to prevent transmission through percutaneous and sexual contact should be maintained until tests for HbsAg or Anti-HBcIgM are negative. Close contact does not have to be avoided but close contacts of the patient should be vaccinated. Alcohol should not be used for at least a year and rest with increasing activity during convalescence is recommended.

16. a. Adequate nutrition is especially important in promoting regeneration of liver cells but the anorexia of viral hepatitis is often severe, requiring creative and innovative nursing interventions. Strict bed rest is not usually required, and the patient usually has only minor discomfort with hepatitis. Diversional activities may be required to promote psychologic rest but not during periods of fatigue.

17. c. Immunosuppressive agents are indicated in hepatitis associated with immune disorders to decrease liver damage caused by autoantibodies. Autoimmune hepatitis is similar to viral hepatitis in presenting signs and symptoms and may become chronic and lead to cirrhosis.

18. c. Corneal Fleischer rings, brownish red rings in the cornea near the limbus, are the hallmark of Wilson's disease. Pruritus (not seen with Wilson's disease) is commonly seen with jaundice or primary biliary cirrhosis. Renal failure associated with hepatorenal syndrome is not seen with Wilson's disease. Elevated serum iron levels are seen with hemochromatosis.

19. d. The majority of patients with primary sclerosing cholangitis (PSC) also have ulcerative colitis. The manifestations are otherwise similar to cirrhosis and PSC may lead to cirrhosis, liver failure, and liver cancer.

20. a, c, d. The anemia of cirrhosis is related to overactivity of the enlarged spleen that removes blood cells from circulation. Vitamin B deficiencies from altered intake and metabolism of nutrients and decreased prothrombin production can increase bleeding tendencies. The other options do not contribute to anemia in the patient with cirrhosis.

21. a, b, d. There is no treatment for nonalcoholic fatty liver disease (NAFLD) except to control the other diseases that are frequently diagnosed in these individuals. These measures include weight loss for obesity, control of blood glucose for diabetes, control of hyperlipidemia, and treating hypertension if it is present. Ulcerative colitis is unrelated to NAFLD.

22. c. Esophageal varices occur when collateral channels of circulation develop inelastic fragile veins as a result of portal hypertension. Portal hypertension is from scarring and nodular changes in the liver leading to compression of the veins and sinusoids, causing resistance of blood flow through the liver from the portal vein. It contributes to peripheral edema and ascites. Jaundice is from the inability of the liver to conjugate bilirubin. Biliary cirrhosis causes the loss of small bile ducts and ultimate cholestasis in patients with other autoimmune disorders.

23. d. Blood flow through the portal system is obstructed and causes portal hypertension that increases the blood pressure in the portal venous system. Decreased albumin production leads to decreased serum colloidal oncotic pressure that contributes to ascites. Hyperaldosteronism increases sodium and water retention and contributes to increased fluid retention, hypokalemia, and decreased urinary output. The retained fluid has low oncotic colloidal pressure and it escapes into the interstitial spaces, causing peripheral edema. Portal hypertension also contributes to esophageal varices. Reduced renal blood flow and increased serum levels of antidiuretic hormone (ADH) also contribute to impaired water excretion and ascites.

24. b. Serum bilirubin, both direct and indirect, would be expected to be increased in cirrhosis. Serum albumin and cholesterol are decreased and liver enzymes, such as aspartate aminotransferase (AST) and alanine aminotransferase (ALT), are initially elevated but may be normal in end-stage liver disease.

25. a. Oral hygiene may improve the patient's taste sensation. Food preferences are important but some foods may be restricted if the patient is on a low-sodium diet. The patient will feel more independent with self-feeding and will be more likely to increase intake by having someone sit with the patient while the patient eats. Snacks and supplements should be available whenever the patient desires them but should not be forced on the patient.

26. b, c. With diuretic therapy, fluid and electrolyte balance must be monitored; serum levels of sodium, potassium, chloride, and bicarbonate must be monitored, especially hypokalemia. Renal function must be monitored with blood urea nitrogen and serum creatinine. Water excess is manifested by muscle cramping, weakness, lethargy, and confusion. GI bleeding, body image disturbances, and bleeding tendencies seen with cirrhosis are not related to diuretic therapy.

27. d. Early signs (grade 1) of this neurologic condition include changes in mentation (e.g., depression, apathy, irritability, confusion, agitation, drowsiness, lethargy). Loss of consciousness (grade 4) is usually preceded by asterixis (grades 2 and 3), disorientation, hyperventilation, hypothermia, and alterations in reflexes. Increasing oliguria is a sign of hepatorenal syndrome.

28. c. Ammonia must be reduced to treat hepatic encephalopathy. The laxative, lactulose, decreases ammonia by trapping the ammonia and eliminating it in the feces. A β-adrenergic blocker will be used to decrease portal venous pressure and decrease variceal bleeding. The proton pump inhibitor will decrease gastric acidity but will not eliminate blood already in the GI tract. The rifaximin will decrease bacterial flora and therefore decrease ammonia formation from protein metabolism.

29. c. The patient may not be oriented or able to walk to the bathroom alone because of hyperreflexia, asterixis, or decreased motor coordination. Turning should be done every 2 hours to prevent skin breakdown. Activity is limited to decrease ammonia as a by-product of protein metabolism. Although constipation will be prevented, it will not keep the patient safe.

30. b. The patient with advanced, complicated cirrhosis requires a high-calorie, high-carbohydrate diet with moderate to low fat. Patients with cirrhosis are at risk for edema and ascites and their sodium intake may be limited. The tomato sandwich with salt-free butter best meets these requirements. Rough foods, such as popcorn, may irritate the esophagus and stomach and lead to bleeding. Peanut butter is high in sodium and fat and canned chicken noodle soup is very high in sodium.

31. d. Monitoring for viral, fungal, and bacterial infection after the liver transplant is essential, as only fever may be present with an infection. Alcohol will not be any better for the patient after the transplant than it was before the transplant. HBIG is given for postexposure protection from HBV. The head of the bed is elevated to improve ventilation with severe ascites.

32. c. Bleeding esophageal varices are a medical emergency. During an episode of bleeding, management of the airway and prevention of aspiration of blood are critical factors. Occult blood as well as fresh blood from the GI tract would be expected. Vasopressin causes vasoconstriction, decreased heart rate, and decreased coronary blood flow. IV nitroglycerin may be given with the vasopressin to counter these side effects. Portal shunting surgery is performed for esophageal varices but not during an acute hemorrhage.

33. d. By shunting fluid sequestered in the peritoneum into the venous system, pressure on esophageal veins is decreased and more volume is returned to the circulation, improving cardiac output and renal perfusion. However, because ammonia is diverted past the liver, hepatic encephalopathy continues. These procedures do not prolong life or promote liver function.

34. c. Abstinence from alcohol is very important in alcoholic cirrhosis and may result in improvement if started when liver damage is limited. Although further liver damage may be reduced by rest and nutrition, most changes in the liver cannot be reversed. Exercise does not promote portal circulation and very moderate exercise is recommended. Acetaminophen should not be used by the patient with alcoholic cirrhosis because this liver is more sensitive to the hepatotoxicity of acetaminophen.

35. c. Because the prognosis for cancer of the liver is poor and treatment is largely palliative, supportive nursing care is appropriate. The patient exhibits clinical manifestations of liver failure, as seen in any patient with advanced liver failure. Whether the cancer is primary or metastatic, there is usually a poor response to chemotherapy and surgery is indicated in the few patients that have localization of the tumor when there is no evidence of invasion of hepatic blood vessels.

36. d. Liver transplantation is indicated for patients with cirrhosis as well as for many adults and children with other irreversible liver diseases. Although health care providers make the decisions regarding the patient's qualifications for transplantation, nurses should be knowledgeable about the indications for transplantation and be able to discuss the patient's questions and concerns related to transplantation. Rejection is less of a problem in liver transplants than with other organs such as the kidney.

37. d. A pancreatic abscess is a collection of pus that must be drained to prevent infection of adjacent organs and sepsis. Tetany from hypocalcemia is treated with IV calcium gluconate (10%). Although pseudocysts usually resolve spontaneously, they may be treated with surgical, percutaneous catheter, or endoscopic drainage to prevent perforation. Pleural effusion is treated by treating the cause (pancreatitis) and monitoring for respiratory distress and oxygen saturation.

38. d. The predominant symptom of acute pancreatitis is severe, deep abdominal pain that is usually located in the left upper quadrant (LUQ) but may be in the midepigastrium. Bowel sounds are decreased or absent, temperature is elevated only slightly, and the patient has hypovolemia and may manifest symptoms of shock.

39. b. Although serum lipase levels and urinary amylase levels are increased, an increased serum amylase level is the criterion most commonly used to diagnose acute pancreatitis in the first 24 to 72 hours. Serum calcium levels are decreased.

40. c. Pancreatic rest and suppression of secretions are promoted by preventing any gastric contents from entering the duodenum, which would stimulate pancreatic activity. Surgery is not indicated for acute pancreatitis but may be used to drain abscesses or cysts. An endoscopic retrograde cholangiopancreatography (ERCP) pancreatic sphincterotomy may be performed when pancreatitis is related to gallstones. Pancreatic enzyme supplements are necessary in chronic pancreatitis if a deficiency in secretion occurs.

41. c. Positions that flex the trunk and draw the knees up to the abdomen help to relieve the pain of acute pancreatitis and positioning the patient on the side with the head elevated decreases abdominal tension. Diversional techniques are not as helpful as positioning in controlling the pain. The patient is usually NPO because food intake increases the pain and inflammation. Bed rest is indicated during the acute attack because of hypovolemia and pain.

42. c. Sodium restriction is not indicated for patients recovering from acute pancreatitis but the stools should be observed for steatorrhea, indicating that fat digestion is impaired, and glucose levels may be monitored for indication of impaired β-cell function. Alcohol is a primary cause of pancreatitis and should not be used.

43. c. Chronic damage to the pancreas causes a deficiency of digestive enzymes and insulin resulting in malabsorption and diabetes mellitus. Abstinence from alcohol is necessary in both types of pancreatitis, as is a high-carbohydrate, high-protein, and low-fat diet. Although abdominal pain is a major manifestation of chronic pancreatitis, more commonly a constant heavy, gnawing feeling occurs.

44. a, b, c. Measures to prevent attacks of pancreatitis are those that decrease the stimulation of the pancreas. Lower fat intake and foods that are less stimulating and irritating (bland) should be encouraged. Higher carbohydrates are less stimulating. Avoid alcohol and nicotine, since both stimulate the pancreas. Monitor for steatorrhea to determine effectiveness of the enzymes and because it may indicate worsening pancreatic function. Pancreatic enzymes should be taken with, not after, meals.

45. b. Major risk factors for pancreatic cancer are cigarette smoking, high-fat diet, diabetes, and exposure to benzidine. Pancreatic cancer is not directly associated with alcohol intake, as pancreatitis is. Chronic pancreatitis is a risk factor for pancreatic cancer.

46. d. In a Whipple procedure the head of the pancreas, gallbladder, part of the duodenum adjacent to the pancreas, and sometimes the pylorus of the stomach are removed. The duodenum is responsible for the breakdown of food in the small intestine and regulates the rate of stomach emptying, which affects the patient's nutritional status.

47. a, b, c, e, f. Incidence of cholelithiasis is higher in women, multiparous women, persons over 40 years of age, and those with family history and obesity. Postmenopausal women taking estrogen therapy have a higher incidence than women taking oral contraceptives. Alcohol intake and diet do not increase the incidence of cholelithiasis.

48. a, c, d. Acalculous cholecystitis is associated with prolonged immobility, fasting, prolonged parenteral nutrition, and diabetes mellitus. Hypothyroidism, *Streptococcus pneumoniae*, and absence of bile in the intestine are unrelated to this condition.

49. b. Absence of bile salts in the intestine and duodenum lead to clay-colored stools and steatorrhea. Soluble bilirubin in the blood excreted into the urine leads to dark urine. Contraction of the inflamed gallbladder leads to pain with fatty food intake. Obstruction of the common bile duct prevents bile drainage into the duodenum, with congestion of bile in the liver. Bilirubin absorption in the blood leads to jaundice.

50. a. Ultrasonography is 90% to 95% accurate in detecting gallstones and is a noninvasive procedure. An IV cholangiogram uses radiopaque dye to outline the gallbladder and the ducts. Liver function tests will be elevated if liver damage has occurred but do not indicate gallbladder disease.

51. a. NPO and nasogastric (NG) suction prevent gallbladder stimulation by food or fluids moving into the duodenum. Incisional choleycystectomy removes the gallbladder, not its stimulation. Administration of antiemetics decreases nausea and vomiting but does not decrease gallbladder stimulation. Anticholinergics counteract the smooth muscle spasms of the bile ducts to decrease pain.

52. d. The laparoscopic cholecystectomy requires one to four small abdominal incisions to visualize and remove the gallbladder and the patient has small dressings placed over these incisions. The patient with an incisional cholecystectomy is usually hospitalized for 2 to 3 days, whereas the laparoscopic procedure allows same-day or next-day discharge with return to work within 1 week. A T-tube is placed in the common bile duct after exploration of the duct during an incisional cholecystectomy.

53. c. After removal of the gallbladder, bile drains directly from the liver into the duodenum and a low-fat diet is recommended until adjustment to this change occurs. Most patients tolerate a regular diet with moderate fats but should avoid excessive fats, as large volumes of bile previously stored in the gallbladder are not available. Steatorrhea could occur with a large fat intake.

54. a. The T-tube drains bile from the common bile duct until swelling from trauma has subsided and bile can freely enter the duodenum. The tube is placed to gravity drainage and should be kept open and free from kinks to prevent bile from backing up into the liver. The tube is not normally irrigated.

55. c. Bile-colored drainage or pus from any incision may indicate an infection and should be reported to the health care provider immediately. The bandages on the puncture sites should be removed the day after surgery, followed by bathing or showering. Referred shoulder pain is a common and expected problem following laparoscopic procedures, when carbon dioxide used to inflate the abdominal cavity is not readily absorbed by the body. Nausea and vomiting are not expected postoperatively and may indicate damage to other abdominal organs and should be reported to the health care provider.

Case Study

1. Some etiologic factor causes injury to pancreatic cells or activation of the pancreatic enzymes in the pancreas rather than in the intestine and the activated enzymes digest the pancreas itself, a process known as autodigestion. Activated trypsin can digest the protein of the pancreas and activate other enzymes that cause damage to the pancreas. The pancreas may be edematous or it may become necrotic.

2. The two most common causes are gallbladder disease and alcohol abuse. After these, causes include cigarette smoking, biliary sludge, hypertriglyceridemia, trauma, certain drugs, metabolic disorders, and vascular diseases.

3. The serum and urinary amylase levels and serum lipase levels are elevated, indicating release of these enzymes into the blood circulating through the pancreas. The WBC count is high, indicating marked inflammation. The blood glucose level is elevated, indicating impairment of insulin production and release by the β-cells. The decreased calcium indicates hypocalcemia, a sign of severe pancreatitis.

4. Hypocalcemia occurs in part because calcium combines with fatty acids released during fat necrosis of the pancreas. The nurse should observe for symptoms of tetany, such as jerking, irritability, muscular twitching, and positive Chvostek's and Trousseau's signs. Numbness or tingling around the lips and in the fingers is an early indicator of hypocalcemia.

5. The pain is usually located in the LUQ but may be in the midepigastric area and frequently radiates to the back. It has a sudden onset and is described as severe, deep, piercing, and continuous. It is aggravated by eating and often begins when the patient is recumbent. It is not relieved by vomiting and may be accompanied by flushing, cyanosis, and dyspnea.

6. Hypovolemia, shock, and the local complications of pseudocysts and abscesses; paralytic ileus with abdominal distention; and crackles in the lungs. Seepage of blood-stained exudates may cause Grey Turner's or Cullen's signs.

7. NPO status and suction with an NG tube prevent gastric contents from entering the duodenum and stimulating pancreatic secretion.

8. Morphine is for pain relief. Pantoprazole (proton pump inhibitor) is to decrease hydrochloric acid production by the stomach because hydrochloric acid stimulates pancreatic activity. Omeprazole (Prilosec) may be taken orally when the patient is no longer NPO.

9. **Nursing diagnoses:**
   - Acute pain *related to* distention of the pancreas and peritoneal irritation
   - Deficient fluid volume *related to* nausea, vomiting, NG suction, and restricted oral intake
   - Impaired oral mucous membrane *related to* NG tube and NPO status
   - Imbalanced nutrition: less than body requirements *related to* dietary restrictions, nausea and vomiting, and impaired digestion

   Collaborative problems:
   Potential complications: hypovolemia and shock, hypocalcemia, hyperglycemia, fluid and electrolyte imbalance

CHAPTER 45

Answer Key

1. a. Adrenal gland; b. hilus; c. vena cava; d. bladder; e. urethra; f. ureter; g. aorta; h. kidney; i. fibrous capsule; j. calyx; k. renal pelvis; l. papilla; m. medulla; n. cortex; o. ureter; p. renal vein; q. renal artery; r. pyramid

2. a, 1; b, 4; c, 3; d, 6; e, 5; f, 2. Blood is filtered in the glomerulus and the ultrafiltrate flows from the Bowman's capsule to the tubules for reabsorption of essential materials and secretion of nonessential ones. In the proximal convoluted tubule, most electrolytes, glucose, amino acids, and small proteins are reabsorbed. Water is conserved in the loop of Henle with chloride and sodium reabsorbed in the ascending loop. The distal convoluted tubules complete final water balance and acid-base balance.

3. a, c, e, f. The distal tubules regulate water and acid-base balance by reabsorption of water under antidiuretic hormone (ADH) influence, secreting H^+ and reabsorbing bicarbonate, reabsorption of Na^+ in exchange for K^+, and reabsorption of Ca^{+2} with the influence of parathormone. The reabsorption of water without ADH occurs in the proximal convoluted tubule and the descending loop of Henle. The reabsorption of glucose and amino acids occurs in the proximal convoluted tubule. Active reabsorption of Cl^- and passive reabsorption of Na^+ occurs in the ascending loop of Henle.

4. a, c. Atrial natriuretic peptide (ANP) responds to increased atrial distention by increasing sodium excretion and inhibiting renin, ADH, and angiotensin action. Aldosterone secretion is also suppressed. ANP also causes afferent arteriole relaxation that increases the glomerular filtration rate (GFR).

5. c. GFR is primarily dependent on adequate blood flow and hydrostatic pressure. The glomerulus filters the blood. The GFR is the amount of blood filtered each minute by the glomeruli, which determines the concentration of urea in the blood. Increased permeability in the glomerulus causes loss of proteins in the urine. The prostaglandins increase the GFR with increased renal blood flow.

6. a. Renin is released in response to decreased arterial blood pressure (BP), renal ischemia, decreased extracellular fluid (ECF), decreased serum Na^+ concentration, and increased urinary Na^+ concentration. It is the catalyst of the renin-angiotensin-aldosterone system, which raises BP when

stimulated. ADH is secreted by the posterior pituitary in response to serum hyperosmolality and low blood volume. Aldosterone is secreted only after stimulation by angiotensin II. Kidney prostaglandins lower BP by causing vasodilation.

7. a. Erythropoietin is released when the oxygen tension of the renal blood supply is low and stimulates production of red blood cells in the bone marrow. Hypotension causes activation of the renin-angiotensin-aldosterone system, as well as release of ADH. Hyperkalemia stimulates the release of aldosterone from the adrenal cortex and fluid overload does not directly stimulate factors affecting the erythropoietin release by the kidney.

8. a, b, e. Testing would include urinalysis to see crystals and look for red blood cells. Abdominal ultrasound and CT scan may also be done.

9. b. When the amount of urine in the bladder has reached 1200 mL, the person would need relief and probably catheterization. The bladder capacity ranges from 600 to 1000 mL. When there is 250 mL of urine in the bladder, the person will usually feel the urge to urinate and 400 to 600 mL will be uncomfortable.

10. c. Relaxation of female urethra, bladder, vagina, and pelvic floor muscles may contribute to stress and urge incontinence and urinary tract infections. The short urethra of women allows easier ascension and colonization of bacteria in the bladder than occurs in men and the urethra does not lengthen with age. The bladder capacity of men and women is the same but decreases with aging.

11. d. Decreased renal blood flow and altered hormone levels result in a decreased ability to concentrate urine that results in an increased volume of dilute urine, which does not maintain the usual diurnal elimination pattern. A decrease in bladder capacity also contributes to nocturia but decreased bladder muscle tone results in urinary retention. Decreased renal mass decreases renal reserve but function is generally adequate under normal circumstances.

12.

Functional Health Pattern	Risk Factor for or Response to Urinary Problem
Health perception–health management	Smoking history, occupational history and history of exposure to carcinogenic and nephrotoxic chemicals, family history of kidney disease, geographic residence
Nutritional-metabolic	Low fluid intake or loss of fluids, high calcium and purine intake; caffeine, alcohol, carbonated beverage, artificial sweetener, or spicy food intake; weight gain resulting from fluid retention; anorexia, nausea, or vomiting; supplements and herbal therapy
Elimination	Change in appearance and amount of urine, change in urinary patterns, necessary assistance in emptying bladder, bowel function
Activity-exercise	Change in energy level, sedentary lifestyle, urine leakage during activity
Sleep-rest	Sleep deprivation from nocturia
Cognitive-perceptual	Pain in flank, groin, or suprapubic area; dysuria; absence of pain with other urinary symptoms; cognitive impairment affecting continence; mobility, visual acuity, and dexterity
Self-perception–self-concept	Decreased self-esteem and body image because of urinary problems
Role-relationship	Problems maintaining job and social relationships
Sexuality-reproductive	Change in sexual pleasure or performance
Coping–stress tolerance	Withdrawal or ineffective coping with incontinence or urinary problem
Value-belief	Any treatment decisions that are affected by value syste

13. c. To assess for kidney tenderness, the nurse strikes the fist of one hand over the dorsum of the other hand at the posterior costovertebral angle. The upper abdominal quadrants and costovertebral angles are auscultated for vascular bruits in the renal vessels and aorta and an empty bladder is not palpable. The kidneys are palpated through the abdomen, with the patient supine.

14. d. Stress incontinence is involuntary urination with increased pressure when sneezing or coughing and is seen with weakness of sphincter control. Nocturia is frequent urination at night. Micturition is the evacuation of urine. Urge incontinence is involuntary urination is preceded by urinary urgency.

15. a. Retention is the inability to void. Anuria is no urine formation. Polyuria is a large amount of urine output over time. Frequency is increased incidence of urination.

16. b. Hesitancy is difficulty starting the urine stream and is common with benign prostatic hyperplasia (BPH). Oliguria is scanty urine formation and output. Hematuria is blood in the urine. Pneumaturia is urine containing gas, as is caused by a fistula between the bowel and bladder.

17. c. Enuresis is involuntary urination at night. Ascites is excess fluid in the intraperitoneal cavity. Dysuria is painful urination. Urgency is the feeling of needing to void immediately.

18. b. Bacteria in warm urine specimens multiply rapidly and false or unreliable bacterial counts may occur with urine that has been sitting for periods of time. Glucose, specific gravity, and WBCs do not change in urine specimens but pH becomes more alkaline, RBCs are hemolyzed, and casts may disintegrate.

19. b. Cloudiness in a fresh urine specimen, WBC count above 5 per high-power field (hpf), and the presence of casts are all indicative of urinary tract infection (UTI). The pH is usually elevated because bacteria in urine split the urea alkaline ammonia. Cloudy, brown urine usually indicates hematuria or the presence of bile. Colorless urine is usually very dilute. Option a is characteristic of normal urine.

20. a. A urine specific gravity of 1.002 is low, indicating dilute urine and the excretion of excess fluid. Fluid overload, diuretics, or lack of ADH can cause dilute urine. Normal urine specific gravity is 1.003 to 1.030. A high urine specific gravity indicates concentrated urine that would be seen in dehydration.

21. d. During a renal arteriogram, a catheter is inserted, most commonly at the femoral artery. Following the procedure the patient is positioned with the affected leg extended with a pressure dressing applied. Peripheral pulse monitoring is essential to detect the development of thrombi around the insertion site, which may occlude blood supply to the leg. Gross bleeding in the urine is a complication of a renal biopsy. Allergy to the contrast medium should be established before the procedure.

22. c. The rate at which creatinine is cleared from the blood and eliminated in the urine approximates the GFR and is the most specific test of renal function. The renal scan is useful in showing the location, size, and shape of the kidney and general blood perfusion.

23. a. The blood urea nitrogen (BUN) is increased in patients with renal problems. It may also be increased when there is rapid or extensive tissue damage from other causes. Low protein intake may cause a low BUN.

24.

Laboratory Finding	Impaired Kidney Function
Serum Ca²⁺: 7.2 mg/dL (1.8 mmol/L)	Impaired conversion of inactive vitamin D to active vitamin D results in poor calcium absorption from the bowel, resulting in hypocalcemia.
Hb: 9.6 g/dL (96 g/L)	Loss of cells that produce erythropoietin results in lack of stimulation of bone marrow to produce RBCs.
Serum creatinine: 3.2 mg/dL (283 mmol/L)	This serum creatinine level is high, indicating the loss of tubular secretion (passage of substances from the blood into the tubule) by the kidney.

25. b. Bleeding from the kidney following a biopsy is the most serious complication of the procedure and urine must be examined for both gross and microscopic blood, in addition to vital signs and hematocrit levels being monitored. Following a cystoscopy the patient may have burning with urination and warm sitz baths may be used. Urinary infections are a complication of any procedure requiring instrumentation of the bladder.

26. a, d, e. A clean-catch urine specimen is obtained in a sterile container after cleaning the meatus. The patient will void a small amount in the toilet, stop, and then void in the container to catch the urine midstream. The first morning specimen is best for a urinalysis. A full bladder is necessary for a urine flow study. A urinary catheter is inserted immediately after voiding to assess residual urine.

27. c. A cathartic the evening before the procedure and sensitivity to iodine are important for both intravenous pyelogram (IVP) and renal arteriogram but the salty taste is only a possibility with IVP. The cystometrogram involves filling the bladder with water or saline to measure tone and stability. The kidneys, ureters, and bladder (KUB) is an x-ray that may have bowel preparation.

CHAPTER 46

Answer Key

1. a. An upper urinary tract infection (UTI) affects the renal parenchyma, renal pelvis, and ureters. A lower UTI is an infection of the bladder and/or urethra. A complicated UTI exists in the presence of obstruction, stones, or preexisting diseases. An uncomplicated UTI occurs in an otherwise normal urinary tract.

2. c. The usual classic manifestations of UTI are often absent in older adults, who tend to experience nonlocalized abdominal discomfort and cognitive impairment characterized by confusion or decreased level of consciousness rather than dysuria and suprapubic pain.

3. c. Unless a patient has a history of recurrent UTIs or a complicated UTI, trimethoprim-sulfamethoxazole (TMP-SMX) or nitrofurantoin (Macrodantin) is usually used to empirically treat an initial UTI without a culture and sensitivity or other testing. Asymptomatic bacteriuria does not justify treatment but symptomatic UTIs should always be treated.

4. b. The bladder should be emptied at least every 3 to 4 hours. Fluid intake should be increased to about 2000 mL/day without caffeine, alcohol, citrus juices, and chocolate drinks, because they are potential bladder irritants. Cleaning the urinary meatus with an antiinfective agent after voiding will irritate the meatus but the perineal area should be wiped from front to back after urination and defecation to prevent fecal contamination of the meatus.

5. c. Ascending infections from the bladder to the kidney are prevented by the normal anatomy and physiology of the urinary tract unless a preexisting condition, such as vesicoureteral reflux or lower urinary tract dysfunction (bladder tumors, prostatic hyperplasia, strictures, or stones), is present. Resistance to antibiotics and failure to take a full prescription of antibiotics for a UTI usually result in relapse or reinfection of the lower urinary tract.

6. a. Systemic manifestations of fever and chills with leukocytosis and nausea and vomiting are more common in pyelonephritis than in a lower UTI. Dysuria, frequency, and urgency can be present with both.

7. d. A urine specimen specifically obtained for culture and sensitivity is required to diagnose pyelonephritis because it will show pyuria, the specific bacteriuria, and what drug the bacteria is sensitive to for treatment. The renal biopsy is used to diagnose chronic pyelonephritis or cancer. Blood cultures would be done if bacteremia is suspected. Intravenous pyelogram (IVP) would increase renal irritation, but CT urograms may be used to assess for signs of infection in the kidney and complications of pyelonephritis.

8. d. The symptoms of interstitial cystitis (IC) imitate those of an infection of the bladder but the urine is free of infectious agents. Unlike a bladder infection, the pain with IC increases as urine collects in the bladder and is temporarily relieved by urination. Acidic urine is very irritating to the bladder in IC and the bladder is small but urinary retention is not common.

9. d. Calcium glycerophosphate (Prelief) alkalinizes the urine and can help to relieve the irritation from acidic foods. A diet low in acidic foods is recommended and if a multivitamin is used, high-potency vitamins should be avoided because these products may irritate the bladder. A voiding diary is useful in diagnosis but does not need to be kept indefinitely.

10. c. Glomerulonephritis is not an infection but rather an antibody-induced injury to the glomerulus, where either autoantibodies against the glomerular basement membrane (GBM) directly damage the tissue or antibodies reacting with nonglomerular antigens are randomly deposited as immune complexes along the GBM. Prior infection by bacteria or viruses may stimulate the antibody production but is not present or active at the time of glomerular damage.

11. d. An elevated blood urea nitrogen (BUN) indicates that the kidneys are not clearing nitrogenous wastes from the blood and protein may be restricted until the kidney recovers. Proteinuria indicates loss of protein from the blood and possibly a need for increased protein intake. Hypertension is treated with sodium and fluid restriction, diuretics, and antihypertensive drugs. The hematuria is not specifically treated.

12. a. Most patients recover completely from acute poststreptococcal glomerulonephritis (APSGN) with supportive treatment. Chronic glomerulonephritis that progresses insidiously over years and rapidly progressive glomerulonephritis that results in renal failure within weeks or months occur in only a few patients with APSGN. In Goodpasture syndrome, antibodies are present against both the GBM and the alveolar basement membrane of the lungs and dysfunction of both renal and pulmonary are present.

13. c. The massive proteinuria that results from increased glomerular membrane permeability in nephrotic syndrome leaves the blood without adequate proteins (hypoalbuminemia) to create an oncotic colloidal pressure to hold fluid in the vessels. Without oncotic pressure, fluid moves into the interstitium, causing severe edema. Hypercoagulability occurs in nephrotic syndrome but is not a factor in edema formation and glomerular filtration rate (GFR) is not necessarily affected in nephrotic syndrome.

14. a. 6; b. 3; c. 1; d. 4; e. 8; f. 5; g. 2; h. 7

15. b. The manifestations of renal tuberculosis are described. Urosepsis is when the UTI has spread systemically. Urethral diverticula are localized outpouching of the urethra and occur more often in women. Goodpasture syndrome manifests with flu-like symptoms with pulmonary symptoms that include cough, shortness of breath, and pulmonary insufficiency and renal manifestations that include hematuria, weakness, pallor, anemia, and renal failure.

16. c. Because crystallization of stone constituents can precipitate and unite to form a stone when in supersaturated concentrations, one of the best ways to prevent stones of any type is by drinking adequate fluids to keep the urine dilute and flowing (e.g., an output of about 2 L of urine a day). Sedentary lifestyle is a risk factor for renal stones but exercise also causes fluid loss and a need for additional fluids. Protein foods high in purine should be restricted only for the small percentage of patients with uric acid stones and although UTIs contribute to stone formation, prophylactic antibiotics are not indicated.

17. c. Calcium oxalate calculi are most common and small enough to get trapped in the ureter.

18. b. Struvite calculi are most common in women and always occur with UTIs. They are also usually large staghorn type.

19. b, e. This patient is most likely to have uric acid calculi, which have a high incidence in Jewish men, and gout is a predisposing factor. The treatment will include allopurinol and reducing animal protein intake to reduce purine, as uric acid is a waste product from purine metabolism. Reducing oxalate and using thiazide diuretics help to treat calcium oxalate calculi. Administration of α-penicillamine and tiopronin prevent cystine crystallization for cystine calculi. Reducing intake of milk products to reduce calcium intake may be used with calcium calculi.

20. a. Calcium phosphate calculi are typically mixed with struvite or oxalate stones and related to alkaline urine. Cystine calculi are associated with a genetic autosomal recessive defect and defective GI and kidney absorption of cystine. Struvite calculi are three to four times more common in women than in men.

21. c. A classic sign of the passage of a calculus down the ureter is intense, colicky back pain that may radiate into the testicles, labia, or groin and may be accompanied by mild shock with cool, moist skin. Many patients with renal stones do not have a history of chronic UTIs. Stones obstructing a calyx or at the ureteropelvic junction may produce dull costovertebral flank pain and large bladder stones may cause bladder fullness and lower obstructive symptoms.

22. d. Oxalate-rich foods should be limited to reduce oxalate excretion. Foods high in oxalate include spinach, rhubarb, asparagus, cabbage, and tomatoes, in addition to chocolate, coffee, and cocoa. Currently, it is believed that high dietary calcium intake may actually lower the risk for renal stones by reducing the intestinal oxalate absorption and therefore the urinary excretion of oxalate. Milk, milk products, dried beans, and dried fruits are high sources of calcium. Organ meats are high in purine, which contributes to uric acid lithiasis.

23. b. A high fluid intake maintains dilute urine, which decreases bacterial concentration in addition to washing stone fragments and expected blood through the urinary system following lithotripsy. High urine output also prevents supersaturation of minerals. Moist heat to the flank may be helpful to relieve muscle spasms during renal colic and all urine should be strained in patients with renal stones to collect and identify stone composition but these are not related to infection.

24. b. The patient with urethral stricture will benefit from being taught to dilate the urethra by self-catheterization every few days. Renal trauma is treated related to the severity of the injury with bed rest, fluids, and analgesia. Renal artery stenosis includes control of hypertension

with possible surgical revascularization. Accelerated nephrosclerosis is associated with malignant hypertension that must be aggressively treated as well as monitoring kidney function.

25. b. Adult-onset polycystic kidney disease is an inherited autosomal dominant disorder that often manifests after the patient has children but the children should receive genetic counseling regarding their life choices. The disease progresses slowly, eventually causing progressive renal failure. Hereditary medullary cystic disease causes poor concentration ability of the kidneys and classic Alport syndrome is a hereditary nephritis that is associated with deafness and deformities of the optic lens.

26. d. Systemic lupus erythematosus causes connective tissue damage that affects the glomerulus. Gout deposits uric acid crystals in the kidney. Amyloidosis deposits hyaline bodies in the kidney. Diabetes mellitus causes microvascular damage affecting the kidney.

27. a. Both cancer of the kidney and cancer of the bladder are associated with smoking. A family history of renal cancer is a risk factor for kidney cancer and cancer of the bladder has been associated with the use of phenacetin-containing analgesics and recurrent upper UTIs.

28. c. There are no early characteristic symptoms of cancer of the kidney and gross hematuria, flank pain, and a palpable mass do not occur until the disease is advanced. The treatment of choice is a partial or radical nephrectomy, which can be successful in early disease. Many kidney cancers are diagnosed as incidental imaging findings. Targeted therapy is the preferred treatment for metastatic kidney cancer. Radiation is palliative. The most common sites of metastases are the lungs, liver, and long bones.

29. d, e, f. Urge incontinence is involuntary urination preceded by urgency caused by overactivity of the detrusor muscle when the bladder contracts by reflex, which overrides central inhibition. Treatment includes treating the underlying cause and retraining the bladder with urge suppression, anticholinergic drugs, or containment devices. The other options are characteristic of stress incontinence. Patients may have a combination of urge and stress incontinence.

30. a. Reflex incontinence occurs with no warning, equally during the day and night, and with spinal cord lesions above S2. Overflow incontinence is when the pressure of urine in the overfull bladder overcomes sphincter control and is caused by bladder or urethral outlet obstruction. Functional incontinence is loss of urine resulting from cognitive, functional, or environmental factors. Incontinence after trauma or surgery occurs when fistulas have occurred or after a prostatectomy.

31. c, d, e. α-Adrenergic blockers block the stimulation of the smooth muscle of the bladder, 5α-reductase inhibitors decrease outlet resistance, and bethanechol enhances bladder contractions. Baclofen or diazepam is used to relax the external sphincter for reflex incontinence. Anticholinergics are used to relax bladder tone and increase sphincter tone with urge incontinence.

32. c. Pelvic floor exercises (Kegel exercises) increase the tone of the urethral sphincters and should be done in sets of 10 or more contractions four to five times a day (total of 40 to 50 per day). Frequent bladder emptying is recommended for patients with urge incontinence and an increase in pressure on the bladder is recommended for patients with overflow incontinence. Absorptive perineal pads should be only a temporary measure because long-term use discourages continence and can lead to skin problems.

33. c. All urinary catheters in hospitalized patients pose a very high risk for infection, especially antibiotic-resistant, health care–associated infections, and scrupulous aseptic technique is essential in the insertion and maintenance of all catheters. Routine irrigations are not performed. Turning the patient to promote drainage is recommended only for suprapubic catheters. Cleaning the insertion site with soap and water should be performed for urethral and suprapubic catheters but lotion or powder should be avoided and site care for other catheters may require special interventions.

34. b. Output from ureteral catheters must be monitored every 1 to 2 hours because an obstruction will cause overdistention of the renal pelvis and renal damage. The renal pelvis has a capacity of only 3 to 5 mL and if irrigation is ordered, no more than 5 mL of sterile saline is used. The patient with a ureteral catheter is usually kept on bed rest until specific orders for ambulation are given. Suprapubic tubes may be milked to prevent obstruction of the catheter by sediment and clots.

35. b. A nephrectomy incision is usually in the flank, just below the diaphragm or in the abdominal area. Although the patient is reluctant to breathe deeply because of incisional pain, the lungs should be clear. Decreased sounds and shallow respirations are abnormal and would require intervention.

36. a. The Kock pouch is a continent diversion created by formation of an ileal pouch with an external stoma requiring catheterization. Ileal conduit is the most common incontinent diversion using a stoma of resected ileum with implanted ureters. Orthotopic neobladder is a new bladder from a reshaped segment of intestine in the anatomic position of the bladder with urine discharged through the urethra. A cutaneous ureterostomy diverts the ureter from the bladder to the abdominal skin but there is frequent scarring and strictures of the ureters, so ileal conduits are used more often.

37. d. Urine drains continuously from an ileal conduit and the drainage bag must be emptied every 2 to 3 hours and measured to ensure adequate urinary output. Fitting for a permanent appliance is not done until the stoma shrinks to its normal size in a few weeks. With an ileal conduit, mucus is present in the urine because it is secreted by the ileal segment as a result of the irritating effect of the urine but the surgery causes paralytic ileus and the patient will be NPO for several days postoperatively. Self-catheterization is performed when patients have formation of a continent Kock pouch.

38. b. Because the stoma continuously drains urine, a wick formed of a rolled-up 4 × 4 gauze or a tampon is held against the stoma to absorb the urine while the skin is cleaned and a new appliance is attached. The skin is cleaned with warm water only because soap and other agents cause drying and irritation and clean, not sterile, technique is used. The appliance should be left in place for as long as possible before it loosens and allows leakage onto the skin, perhaps up to 14 days.

39. e, f. The unlicensed assistive personnel (UAP) may assist the incontinent patient to void at regular intervals and provide perineal care. An RN should perform the assessments and teaching. In long-term care and rehabilitation facilities, UAP may use bladder scanners after they are trained.

Case Study

1. The staging of bladder cancer is determined by the depth of invasion of the bladder wall and surrounding tissue. Stage II indicates that the tumor has grown into the muscle layer of the bladder but not passed completely through it. The TNM grading system indicates the characteristics of the tumor (T), the nodal involvement (N), and the presence of distant metastasis (M). (See Chapter 16 for TNM classification.)

2. Opioids and stool softeners may be used for a short time after the procedure. P.G. will be taught to drink a large volume of fluid and monitor the color and consistency of the urine. The urine will be pink at first but should not be red or contain clots. Seven to 10 days after the tumor resection P.G. may observe dark red or rust-colored flecks in the urine from the healing tumor resection sites.

3. The drug will be instilled into the empty bladder via a urethral catheter at weekly intervals for 6 to 12 weeks. The drug needs to be retained for about 2 hours with P.G.'s position changed about every 15 minutes to ensure that the drug comes into maximum contact with all areas of the bladder. He may have irritative symptoms, such as frequency, urgency, and bladder spasms, in addition to hematuria during the weeks of treatment. Bacille Calmette-Guérin (BCG) therapy may cause flu-like symptoms or systemic infection because BCG stimulates the immune system rather than directly destroying cancer cells. The usual side effects of cancer chemotherapy are not experienced with BCG therapy or with intravesical chemotherapy.

4. P.G. should stop smoking; it is the only significant risk factor in his history. Maintenance therapy after the initial induction regimen may be beneficial, as there is a high rate of disease recurrence.

5. Follow-up cystoscopies on a regular basis are essential to evaluate the effectiveness of the treatment and detect any new tumors while they are in a superficial stage. Two thirds of patients have tumor recurrence within 5 years and nearly 95% have recurrence by 15 years.

6. A cystectomy with urinary diversion would be indicated. This could be an incontinent urinary diversion or a continent urinary diversion.

7. The patient's ability and readiness to learn must be considered. His anxiety and fear may affect the teaching. Psychosocial aspects of living with a stoma may affect the choice. Acceptance of the surgery and of alterations in body image is needed to ensure the patient's best adjustment. If a continent diversion is used, the patient must be able to catheterize the pouch every 4 to 6 hours and irrigate it daily. Orthotopic bladder reconstruction may be considered if the cancer did not involve the bladder neck or urethra and the patient has normal renal and liver function, a longer than 1- to 2-year life expectancy, adequate motor skills, and no history of inflammatory bowel disease or colon cancer. Obese patients are not good candidates for orthotopic bladder reconstruction.

8. **Nursing diagnoses:**
   - Anxiety *related to* unknown outcome
   - Impaired urinary elimination *related to* effects of treatment
   - Acute pain *related to* effects of treatment
   - Risk for infection *related to* effects of treatment
   - Risk for sexual dysfunction *related to* reactions to treatment

   Collaborative problems:
   Potential complication: bladder injury, impaired skin integrity

CHAPTER 47

Answer Key

1. d, e, f. Intrarenal causes of acute kidney injury (AKI) include conditions that cause direct damage to the kidney tissue, including nephrotoxic drugs, acute glomerulonephritis, and tubular obstruction by myoglobin, or prolonged ischemia. Anaphylaxis and other prerenal problems are frequently the initial cause of AKI. Renal stones and bladder cancer are among the postrenal causes of AKI.

2. c, e. Because the patient has had nothing to eat or drink for 2 days, she is probably dehydrated and hypovolemic. Decreased cardiac output (CO) is most likely because she is older and takes heart medicine, which is probably for heart failure or hypertension. Both hypovolemia and decreased CO cause prerenal AKI. Anaphylaxis is also a cause of prerenal AKI but is not likely in this situation. Nephrotoxic drugs would contribute to intrarenal causes of AKI and renal calculi would be a postrenal cause of AKI.

3. d. Acute tubular necrosis (ATN) is primarily the result of ischemia, nephrotoxins, or sepsis. Major surgery is most likely to cause severe kidney ischemia in the patient requiring a blood transfusion. A blood transfusion hemolytic reaction produces nephrotoxic injury if it occurs. Diabetes mellitus, hypertension, and acetaminophen overdose will not contribute to ATN.

4. b. Injury is the stage of RIFLE classification when urine output is less than 0.5 mL/kg/hr for 12 hours, the serum creatinine is increased times two or the glomerular filtration rate (GFR) is decreased by 50%. This stage may be reversible by treating the cause or, in this patient, the dehydration by administering IV fluid and a low dose of a loop diuretic, furosemide (Lasix). Assessing the daily weight will be done to monitor fluid changes but it is not the first treatment the nurse should anticipate. IV administration of insulin and sodium bicarbonate would be used for hyperkalemia. Checking the urinalysis will help to determine if the AKI has a prerenal, intrarenal, or postrenal cause by what is seen in the urine but with this patient's dehydration, it is thought to be prerenal to begin treatment.

5. d. In prerenal oliguria, the oliguria is caused by a decrease in circulating blood volume and there is no damage yet to the renal tissue. It can be reversed by correcting the precipitating factor, such as fluid replacement for hypovolemia. Prerenal oliguria is characterized by urine with a high specific gravity and a low sodium concentration, whereas oliguria of intrarenal failure is characterized by urine with a low specific gravity and a high sodium

concentration. Malignant hypertension causes damage to renal tissue and intrarenal oliguria.

6. b. A urine specific gravity that is consistently 1.010 and a urine osmolality of about 300 mOsm/kg is the same specific gravity and osmolality as plasma. This indicates that tubules are damaged and unable to concentrate urine. Hematuria is more common with postrenal damage. Tubular damage is associated with a high sodium concentration (greater than 40 mEq/L).

7. a. Metabolic acidosis occurs in AKI because the kidneys cannot synthesize ammonia or excrete acid products of metabolism, resulting in an increased acid load. Sodium is lost in urine because the kidneys cannot conserve sodium. Impaired excretion of potassium results in hyperkalemia. Bicarbonate is normally generated and reabsorbed by the functioning kidney to maintain acid-base balance.

8. d. The blood urea nitrogen (BUN) and creatinine levels remain high during the oliguric and diuretic phases of AKI. The recovery phase begins when the glomerular filtration returns to a rate at which BUN and creatinine stabilize and then decrease. Urinary output of 3 to 5 L/day, decreasing sodium and potassium levels, and fluid weight loss are characteristic of the diuretic phase of AKI.

9. d. Hyperkalemia is a potentially life-threatening complication of AKI in the oliguric phase. Muscle weakness and abdominal cramping are signs of the neuromuscular impairment that occurs with hyperkalemia. In addition, hyperkalemia can cause the cardiac conduction abnormalities of peaked T wave, prolonged PR interval, prolonged QRS interval, and depressed ST segment. Urine output of 300 mL/day is expected during the oliguric phase, as is the development of peripheral edema.

10. d. Measuring daily weights with the same scale at the same time each day allows for the evaluation and detection of excessive body fluid gains or losses. Infection is the leading cause of death in AKI, so meticulous aseptic technique is critical. The fluid limitation in the oliguric phase is 600 mL plus the prior day's measured fluid loss. Dietary sodium and potassium intake are managed according to the plasma levels.

11. b. This patient has at least three of the six common indications for renal replacement therapy (RRT), including (1) high potassium level, (2) metabolic acidosis, and (3) changed mental status. The other indications are (4) volume overload, resulting in compromised cardiac status (this patient has a history of hypertension), (5) BUN greater than 120 mg/dL, and (6) pericarditis, pericardial effusion, or cardiac tamponade. Although the other treatments may be used, they will not be as effective as RRT for this older patient. Loop diuretics and increased fluid are used if the patient is dehydrated. Insulin and sodium bicarbonate can be used to temporarily drive the potassium into the cells. Sodium polystyrene sulfonate (Kayexalate) is used to actually decrease the amount of potassium in the body.

12. a, b, c, d, e. High-risk patients include those exposed to nephrotoxic agents and advanced age (a), massive trauma (b), prolonged hypovolemia or hypotension (possibly b and c), obstetric complications (c), cardiac failure (d), preexisting chronic kidney disease, extensive burns, or sepsis. Patients with prostate cancer may have obstruction of the outflow tract, which increases risk of postrenal AKI (e).

13. a. Dysrhythmias may occur with an elevated potassium level and are potentially lethal. Monitor the rhythm while contacting the physician or calling the rapid response team. Vital signs should be checked. Depending on the patient's history and cause of increased potassium, instruct the patient about dietary sources of potassium; however, this would not help at this point. The nurse may want to recheck the value but until then the heart rhythm needs to be monitored.

14. b. During acidosis, potassium moves out of the cell in exchange for H^+ ions, increasing the serum potassium level. Correction of the acidosis with sodium bicarbonate will help to shift the potassium back into the cells. A decrease in pH and the bicarbonate and $PaCO_2$ levels would indicate worsening acidosis.

15. b. Stages of chronic kidney disease are based on the GFR. No specific markers of urinary output, mental status, or azotemia classify the degree of chronic kidney disease (CKD).

16. a, b, d. Pruritus is common in patients receiving dialysis. It causes scratching from dry skin, sensory neuropathy, and calcium-phosphate deposition in the skin. Vascular calcifications contribute to cardiovascular disease, not to itching skin. Uremic frost rarely occurs without BUN levels greater than 200 mg/dL, which should not occur in a patient on dialysis; urea crystallizes on the skin and also causes pruritis.

17. c. Uremic fetor, or the urine odor of the breath, is caused by high urea content in the blood. Increased ammonia from bacterial breakdown of urea leads to stomatitis and mucosal ulcerations. Irritation of the gastrointestinal (GI) tract from urea in CKD contributes to anorexia, nausea, and vomiting. Ingestion of iron salts and calcium-containing phosphate binders, limited fluid intake, and limited activity cause constipation.

18. c. Kussmaul respirations occur with severe metabolic acidosis when the respiratory system is attempting to compensate by removing carbon dioxide with exhalations. Uremic pleuritis would cause a pleural friction rub. Decreased pulmonary macrophage activity increases the risk of pulmonary infection. Dyspnea would occur with pulmonary edema.

19. d. As GFR decreases, BUN and serum creatinine levels increase. Although elevated BUN and creatinine indicate that waste products are accumulating, the calculated GFR is considered a more accurate indicator of kidney function than BUN or serum creatinine.

20. b. Hyperkalemia can lead to life-threatening dysrhythmias. Hypocalcemia leads to an accelerated rate of bone remodeling and potentially to tetany. Hyponatremia may lead to confusion. Elevated sodium levels lead to edema, hypertension, and heart failure. Hypermagnesemia may decrease reflexes, mental status, and blood pressure.

21. c. The calcium-phosphorus imbalances that occur in CKD result in hypocalcemia, from a deficiency of active vitamin D and increased phosphorus levels. This leads to an increased rate of bone remodeling with a weakened bone matrix. Aluminum accumulation is also believed to

contribute to the osteomalacia. Osteitis fibrosa involves replacement of calcium in the bone with fibrous tissue and is primarily a result of elevated levels of parathyroid hormone resulting from hypocalcemia.

22. d. A patient with CKD may have unlimited intake of sugars and starches (unless the patient is diabetic) and hard candy is an appropriate snack and may help to relieve the metallic and urine taste that is common in the mouth. Raisins are a high-potassium food. Ice cream contains protein and phosphate and counts as fluid. Pickled foods have high sodium content.

23. a. Erythropoietin is used to treat anemia, as it stimulates the bone marrow to produce red blood cells.

24. b. Nifedipine (Procardia) is a calcium channel blocker and furosemide (Lasix) is a loop diuretic. Both are used to treat hypertension.

25. a, b, d. Cinacalcet (Sensipar), a calcimimetic agent to control secondary hyperparathyroidism; sevelamer (Renagel), a noncalcium phosphate binder; and calcium acetate (PhosLo), a calcium-based phosphate binder are used to treat mineral and bone disorder in CKD. IV glucose and insulin and IV 10% calcium gluconate along with sodium polystyrene sulfonate (Kayexalate) are used to treat the hyperkalemia of CKD.

26. d. In the patient with CKD, when serum calcium levels are increased, calcium-based phosphate binders are not used. The nutrient supplemented for patients on dialysis is folic acid. The various body system manifestations occur with uremia, which includes azotemia. Meperidine is contraindicated in patients with CKD related to possible seizures.

27. c. The most common causes of CKD in the United States are diabetes mellitus and hypertension. The nurse should obtain information on long-term health problems that are related to kidney disease. The other disorders are not closely associated with renal disease.

28. c, e. Peritoneal dialysis is less stressful for the cardiovascular system and requires fewer dietary restrictions. Peritoneal dialysis actually contributes to more protein loss and increased hyperlipidemia. The fluid and creatinine removal are slower with peritoneal dialysis than hemodialysis.

29. c. Dextrose or icodextrin or amino acid is added to dialysate fluid to create an osmotic gradient across the membrane to remove excess fluid from the blood. The dialysate fluid has no potassium so that potassium will diffuse into the dialysate from the blood. Dialysate also usually contains higher calcium to promote its movement into the blood. Dialysate sodium is usually less than or equal to that of blood to prevent sodium and fluid retention.

30. a. 3; b. 2; c. 1

31. b. Automated peritoneal dialysis (APD) is the type of dialysis in which the patient dialyzes during sleep and leaves the fluid in the abdomen during the day. Long nocturnal hemodialysis occurs while the patient is sleeping and is done up to six times per week. Continuous venovenous hemofiltration (CVVH) is a type of continuous renal replacement therapy used to treat AKI. Continuous ambulatory peritoneal dialysis (CAPD) is dialysis that is done with exchanges of 1.5 to 3 L of dialysate at least four times daily.

32. b. Peritonitis is a common complication of peritoneal dialysis (PD) and may require catheter removal and termination of dialysis. Infection occurs from contamination of the dialysate or tubing or from progression of exit-site or tunnel infections and strict sterile technique must be used by health professionals as well as the patient to prevent contamination. Too-rapid infusion may cause shoulder pain and pain may be caused if the catheter tip touches the bowel. Difficulty breathing, atelectasis, and pneumonia may occur from pressure of the fluid on the diaphragm, which may be prevented by elevating the head of the bed and promoting repositioning and deep breathing.

33. c. A more permanent, soft, flexible Silastic double-lumen catheter is used for long-term access when other forms of vascular access have failed. These catheters are tunneled subcutaneously and have Dacron cuffs that prevent infection from tracking along the catheter.

34. a. While patients are undergoing hemodialysis, they can perform quiet activities that do not require the limb that has the vascular access. Blood pressure is monitored frequently and the dialyzer monitors dialysis function but cardiac monitoring is not usually indicated. The hemodialysis machine continuously circulates both the blood and the dialysate past the semipermeable membrane in the machine. Graft and fistula access involve the insertion of two needles into the site: one to remove blood from and the other to return blood to the dialyzer.

35. b. A patent arteriovenous fistula (AVF) creates turbulent blood flow that can be assessed by listening for a bruit or palpated for a thrill as the blood passes through the graft. Assessment of neurovascular status in the extremity distal to the graft site is important to determine that the graft does not impair circulation to the extremity but the neurovascular status does not indicate whether the graft is open.

36. c. Continuous renal replacement therapy (CRRT) is indicated for the patient with AKI as an alternative or adjunct to hemodialysis to slowly remove solutes and fluid in the hemodynamically unstable patient. It is especially useful for treatment of fluid overload, but hemodialysis is indicated for treatment of hyperkalemia, pericarditis, or other serious effects of uremia.

37. d. Extensive vascular disease is a contraindication for renal transplantation, primarily because adequate blood supply is essential for the health of the new kidney. Other contraindications include disseminated malignancies, refractory or untreated cardiac disease, chronic respiratory failure, chronic infection, or unresolved psychosocial disorders. Coronary artery disease (CAD) may be treated with bypass surgery before transplantation and transplantation can relieve hypertension. Hepatitis B or C infection is not a contraindication.

38. a. Fluid and electrolyte balance is critical in the transplant recipient patient, especially because diuresis often begins soon after surgery. Fluid replacement is adjusted hourly based on kidney function and urine output. Urine-tinged drainage on the abdominal dressing may indicate leakage from the ureter implanted into the bladder and the health care provider should be notified. The donor patient may have a flank or laparoscopic incision(s) where the kidney

was removed. The recipient has an abdominal incision where the kidney was placed in the iliac fossa. The urinary catheter is usually used for 2 to 3 days to monitor urine output and kidney function.

39. a. Infection is a significant cause of morbidity and mortality after transplantation because the surgery, the immunosuppressive drugs, and the effects of CKD all suppress the body's normal defense mechanisms, thus increasing the risk of infection. The nurse must assess the patient as well as use aseptic technique to prevent infections. Rejection may occur but for other reasons. Malignancy occurrence increases later due to immunosuppressive therapy. Cardiovascular disease is the leading cause of death after renal transplantation but this would not be expected to cause death within the first month after transplantation.

Case Study

1. The kidney is recognized as foreign and, as a foreign substance, stimulates activation of the immune system. T helper cells are activated to produce interleukin-2 (IL-2) and T cytotoxic lymphocytes are sensitized. After T cytotoxic lymphocytes proliferate, they attack the transplanted kidney, setting in process the activation of the inflammatory and complement systems. This usually occurs 4 days to 6 months after the transplant but it may occur later. It is not uncommon to have at least one rejection episode.

2. All laboratory test results are abnormal, except potassium at high normal, and are typical of renal insufficiency that occurs during acute rejection:
   • Serum creatinine—decreased excretory function of kidneys
   • BUN—decreased ability of the kidney to excrete urea
   • Glucose—D.B. has diabetes and the combination of this disease and the insulin resistance that occurs in CKD may be increasing the glucose levels. In addition, the corticosteroid therapy and stress response from the disease increase glucose levels.
   • Potassium—decreased ability of the kidney to excrete potassium
   • Bicarbonate—impaired generation and reabsorption by the kidney, as it is being used to buffer acid load
   Nursing care includes monitoring for central nervous system (CNS) depression and skin and oral mucous breakdown from high urea; monitoring capillary blood glucose and administering insulin to keep glucose within normal range; and monitoring for increasing weakness and cardiac changes related to hyperkalemia and for symptoms of metabolic acidosis, such as Kussmaul respirations.

3. *Immunosuppressive therapy* is designed to reduce proliferation and action of T cytotoxic lymphocytes that are responsible for acute rejection.
   • Muromonab-CD3 (Orthoclone OKT3) is a monoclonal antibody that binds to CD3 receptors on T cells, causing cell lysis. It inhibits the function of T cytotoxic cells and is given via IV push to treat acute rejection.
   • Mycophenolate mofetil (CellCept) is a cytotoxic antiproliferative drug that inhibits purine synthesis and suppresses proliferation of T and B cells.
   • Methylprednisolone (Solu-Medrol) is a corticosteroid that suppresses inflammatory response. It inhibits cytokine production and T-cell activation and proliferation.
   • Tacrolimus (Prograf) is a calcineurin inhibitor that prevents production and release of IL-2 and γ-interferon in addition to inhibiting production of T cytotoxic lymphocytes and B cells.
   Supportive therapy is designed to treat underlying disease and control the symptoms produced by renal insufficiency.
   • Furosemide (Lasix) is a loop diuretic that is not influenced by GFR and is used to promote sodium, potassium, and fluid loss through the kidney. It helps to relieve hypervolemia and hypertension.
   • Nifedipine (Procardia) is a calcium channel blocker that reduces cardiac output to control blood presssure.
   • Sodium bicarbonate helps to control the metabolic acidosis of renal insufficiency and replaces that which is not produced or reabsorbed by the kidney.
   • Metformin and IV insulin control the hyperglycemia resulting from diabetes and insulin resistance of CKD.

4. Many side effects may occur from immunosuppressive therapy but the most common is decreased resistance to infection and increased incidence of cancer because of depression of T cytotoxic lymphocytes.
   • Muromonab-CD3 causes fever, chills, dyspnea, chest pain, nausea, and vomiting. Anaphylactic reactions include pulmonary edema and cardiac or respiratory arrest.
   • Mycophenolate mofetil causes gastrointestinal toxicity with diarrhea, nausea, and vomiting; severe neutropenia; thrombocytopenia; increased risks of infection; and malignancy.
   • As a corticosteroid, methylprednisolone may cause Cushing syndrome with sodium and water retention, redistribution of fat, muscle weakness with protein wasting, hyperglycemia, hypertension, osteoporosis, delayed healing, easy bruising, and increased risk of infection.
   • Tacrolimus is nephrotoxic, hepatotoxic, and neurotoxic with headaches, seizures, and tremors; hypertension; hirsutism; leukopenia; gingival hyperplasia; and lymphoma.

5. Long-term problems include increased risk for infections and malignancies; chronic liver disease; increased risk for atherosclerosis, with CAD a major cause of death; joint necrosis from chronic steroid therapy; psychologic adjustment (constant fear of rejection and wondering how long the transplant will last); and depression if there is failure and a return to dialysis.

6. **Nursing diagnoses:**
   • Excess fluid volume *related to* inability of kidney to excrete fluid
   • Grieving *related to* threat of loss of kidney
   • Risk for acute confusion *related to* CNS changes induced by uremic toxins and immunosuppressive drugs
   • Risk for infection *related to* suppressed immune system
   Collaborative problems:
   Potential complications: hypertension, hyperkalemia with cardiac dysrhythmias, hyperglycemia, metabolic acidosis, infection

CHAPTER 48

Answer Key

1. a. Pineal; b. hypothalamus; c. pituitary; d. parathyroids; e. thyroid; f. thymus; g. adrenals; h. pancreatic islets of Langerhans; i. ovaries (female); j. testes (male)

2. a, e, f, h, i, j. The anterior pituitary gland secretes prolactin, growth hormone (GH), gonadotropic hormones, melanocyte-stimulating hormone, thyroid-stimulating hormone (TSH), and adrenocorticotropic hormone (ACTH). The pineal gland secretes melatonin. The delta cells of the islets of Langerhans secrete somatostatin. The parathyroid secretes parathormone. The posterior pituitary secretes antidiuretic hormone (ADH).

3. c. The α-cells in the islets of Langerhans in the pancreas produce and secrete the hormone glucagon. The F cells secrete pancreatic polypeptide. The β-cells produce and secrete insulin and amylin. The delta cells produce and secrete somatostatin.

4. c. Cortisol is secreted by the adrenal cortex in a diurnal pattern. Ovaries secrete estrogen and progesterone to maintain a woman's secondary sex characteristic function. The thyroid secretes thyroxine (T_4) and triiodothyronine (T_3) in response to TSH, and calcitonin in response to high serum calcium levels. The adrenal medulla secretes epinephrine and norepinephrine in response to stress.

5. d. Epinephrine and norepinephrine are hormones from the adrenal medulla. Androgens and cortisol are from the adrenal cortex. The thyroid and adrenal cortex are controlled by negative feedback but the adrenal medulla's hormone production is controlled by the central nervous system.

6. a. 3, 2; b. 1, 4; c. 13, 14; d. 6, 5; e. 9, 10; f. 11, 12; g. 8, 7; h. 10, 9; i. 7, 8

7. b. ADH release is controlled by the osmolality of the blood. As the osmolality rises, ADH is released from the posterior pituitary gland and acts on the kidney to cause reabsorption of water from the kidney tubule, resulting in more dilute blood and more concentrated urine. Aldosterone, the major mineralocorticoid, causes sodium reabsorption from the kidney and potassium excretion. Calcium levels are not a factor in serum osmolality.

8. d. Atrial natriuretic peptide (ANP) is secreted in response to high blood volume and high serum sodium levels and has an inhibiting effect on ADH and the renin-angiotensin-aldosterone system, the effects of which would make the blood volume even higher. The relationship between cortisol and insulin is indirect; cortisol raises blood glucose levels and insulin secretion is stimulated by high glucose levels. Glucagon secretion inhibits insulin secretion but insulin does not inhibit glucagon. Testosterone and estrogen have no reciprocal action and both are secreted by the body in response to tropic hormones.

9. d. Usually insulin and glucagon function in a reciprocal manner, except after a high-protein, carbohydrate-free meal, in which both hormones are secreted. Glucagon increases gluconeogenesis and insulin facilitates transport of amino acids across muscle membranes for protein synthesis.

10. a. Hypokalemia inhibits aldosterone release as well as insulin release.

11.

Functional Health Pattern	Risk Factor for or Response to Endocrine Problem
Health perception–health management	Decreased energy level in relation to the past; family history of similar problems
Nutritional-metabolic	Changes in appetite and weight, difficulty swallowing; changes in hair distribution, color, and texture; skin changes; hot and cold intolerances
Elimination	Increased thirst with frequent urination; kidney stones; frequent defecation or constipation; change in stool consistency or pattern
Activity-exercise	Decrease in previous activity levels; fatigue, hyperactivity
Sleep-rest	Sleep disturbances, nightmares, sweating, nocturia, insomnia, excessive sleep, or snoring
Cognitive-perceptual	Memory deficits, depression, inability to concentrate; visual disturbances or exophthalmos; apathy; headaches
Self-perception–self-concept	Changes in body appearance and self-perception
Role-relationship	Changes in ability to maintain usual roles
Sexuality-reproductive	Menstrual irregularity and infertility; history of delivering large babies; male sexual dysfunction; changes in secondary sex characteristics
Coping–stress tolerance	Perception of stress in life and usefulness of previous coping mechanisms, changes in response to stress; lack of support system
Value-belief	Commitment to lifestyle changes, value of health management

12. a. Although cortisol is a glucocorticoid, it has action on mineralocorticoid receptors, which causes sodium retention and potassium excretion from the kidney, resulting in hypokalemia. Because water is reabsorbed with the sodium, serum sodium remains normal. In its effect on glucose and fat metabolism, cortisol causes an elevation in blood glucose as well as increases in free fatty acids and triglycerides.

13. b. Many symptoms of hypothyroidism, such as fatigue, mental impairment, dry skin, and constipation, that would be apparent in younger persons are attributed to general aging in the older adult; as a result, hypothyroidism goes unrecognized as a treatable condition.

14. c. Assessment of the endocrine system is often difficult because hormones affect every body tissue and system,

causing great diversity in the signs and symptoms of endocrine dysfunction. Weight loss, fatigue, and depression are signs that may occur with many different endocrine problems or other diseases. Goiter, exophthalmos, and the three "polys" are specific findings of endocrine dysfunction.

15. c. In the patient with thyroid disease, palpation can cause the release of thyroid hormone into circulation, increasing the patient's symptoms and potentially causing a thyroid storm. Examination should be deferred to a more experienced clinician if possible. Pressure should not be so great as to damage the cricoid cartilage or laryngeal nerve and if the thyroid is palpated correctly, the carotid arteries are not compressed.

16. b, c, e. Heat intolerance, exophthalmos, and a goiter are all related to thyroid dysfunction. Tetanic muscle spasms are related to hypofunction of the parathyroid. Hyperpigmentation is related to hypofunction of the adrenal gland. Increased hand and foot size is related to excess growth hormone secretion.

17. a. Endocrine disorders related to hormone secretion from glands that are stimulated by tropic hormones can be caused by a malsecretion of the tropic hormone or of the target gland. If the problem is in the target gland, it is known as a primary endocrine disorder; a problem with tropic hormone secretion is known as a secondary endocrine disorder. Serum levels of tropic hormones can illustrate the status of the negative feedback system in relation to target organ hormone levels. Normally, if a target organ produces low amounts of hormone, tropic hormones will be increased; if a target organ is overproducing hormones, tropic hormones will be low or undetectable.

18. c. To ensure that the level is a fasting level, a minimum of 8 hours should be allowed. Water may be taken, however, and does not affect the glucose level. Many medications also may influence results, which will need to be evaluated.

19. b, d, e. Luteinizing hormone (LH) and follicle-stimulating hormone (FSH) are used to distinguish gonad problems from pituitary insufficiency. LH and FSH are low in pituitary insufficiency and high in gonadal failure. The MRI would be used to identify tumors involving the pituitary gland or hypothalamus. Thyroglobulin is a tumor marker for thyroid cancer. Parathyroid hormone (PTH), along with calcium and phosphorus levels, are checked for parathyroid function. The ACTH suppression test assesses adrenal function, especially with hyperactivity.

20. d. The elevated cortisol of Cushing syndrome manifests in elevated blood pressure and blood glucose. Also seen are moon face, hirsutism, decreased muscle mass from protein wasting, increased weight, and fragile skin with striae across the abdomen.

21. d. Glycosylated hemoglobin (A1C) is used to assess blood glucose control during the previous 3 months. Water deprivation (ADH stimulation) is used to differentiate causes of diabetes insipidus. Fasting blood glucose will measure only the current blood glucose result. The oral glucose tolerance test is used to diagnose diabetes when abnormal fasting blood glucose levels do not clearly indicate diabetes.

CHAPTER 49

Answer Key

1. d. Insulin is an anabolic hormone that is responsible for growth, repair, and storage. It facilitates movement of amino acids into cells, synthesis of protein, storage of glucose as glycogen, and deposition of triglycerides and lipids as fat into adipose tissue. Glucagon is responsible for hepatic glycogenolysis and gluconeogenesis. Fat is used for energy when glucose levels are depleted.

2. c, e. Adipose tissue and skeletal muscle require insulin to allow the transport of glucose into the cells. Brain, liver, and blood cells require adequate glucose supply for normal function but do not depend directly on insulin for glucose transport.

3. b. The counter regulatory hormones have the opposite effect of insulin by stimulating glucose production and output by the liver and by decreasing glucose transport into the cells. The counter regulatory hormones and insulin together regulate the blood glucose level.

4. a, b, c, d, e, f. Type 2 diabetes is characterized by insulin resistance, β-cell exhaustion, altered production of adipokines, genetic predisposition, inherited defect in insulin receptors, and inappropriate glucose production by the liver.

5. d. Prediabetes is defined as impaired glucose tolerance and impaired fasting glucose or both. Fasting blood glucose results between 100 mg/dL (5.56 mmol/L) and 125 mg/dL (6.9 mmol/L) indicate prediabetes. A diagnosis of impaired glucose tolerance is made if the 2-hour oral glucose tolerance test (OGTT) results are between 140 mg/dL (7.8 mmol/L) and 199 mg/dL (11.0 mmol/L).

6. a, e. To reduce the risk of developing diabetes, the patient with prediabetes should learn to monitor for symptoms of diabetes, have blood glucose and glycosylated hemoglobin (A1C) tested regularly, maintain a healthy weight, exercise regularly, and eat a healthy diet.

7. b. Polydipsia is caused by fluid loss from polyuria when high glucose levels cause osmotic diuresis. Cellular starvation from lack of glucose and the use of body fat and protein for energy contribute to fatigue, weight loss, and polyphagia in type 1 diabetes.

8. c. Type 2 diabetes has a strong genetic influence and offspring of parents who both have type 2 diabetes have an increased chance of developing it. In contrast, type 1 diabetes is associated with a genetic susceptibility that is related to human leukocyte antigens (HLAs). Offspring of parents who both have type 1 diabetes have a 1% to 4% chance of developing the disease. Other risk factors for type 2 diabetes include obesity; being a Native American, Hispanic, or African American; and being 55 years or older. Although 50% of people with a parent with maturity-onset diabetes of the young (MODY) will develop MODY, it is autosomal dominant and treatment depends on which genetic mutation caused it. It is not associated with obesity or hypertension and is not currently considered preventable.

9. a. Metabolic syndrome is a cluster of abnormalities that include elevated glucose levels, abdominal obesity, elevated blood pressure, high levels of triglycerides, and low levels of high-density lipoproteins (HDLs). Overweight individuals with metabolic syndrome can prevent or delay the onset of diabetes through a program of weight loss. Exercise is also important but normal weight is most important.

10. a, c. The patient has one prior test result that meets criteria for a diagnosis of diabetes but this test must be confirmed on a subsequent day. The A1C is greater than 6.5% so it also indicates diabetes according to criteria for diabetes diagnosis. These criteria include a fasting plasma glucose (FPG) level ≥126 mg/dL (7.0 mmol/L), A1C ≥6.5%, or a 2-hour OGTT level ≥200 mg/dL (11.1 mmol/L), or in a patient with classic symptoms of hyperglycemia (polyuria, polydipsia, unexplained weight loss) or hyperglycemic crisis, a random plasma glucose ≥200 mg/dL (11.0 mmol/L).

11. d. Impaired glucose tolerance exists when a 2-hour OGTT level is higher than normal but lower than the level diagnostic for diabetes (i.e., >200). Impaired fasting glucose exists when fasting glucose levels are greater than the normal of 100 mg/dL but less than the 126 mg/dL diagnostic of diabetes. Both abnormal values are diagnostic for a condition known as prediabetes.

12. b. U100 insulin must be used with a U100 syringe but for those using low doses of insulin, syringes that have increments of 1 unit instead of 2 units are available. Errors can be made in dosing if patients switch back and forth between different sizes of syringes. Aspiration before injection of the insulin is not recommended, nor is the use of alcohol to clean the skin. Because the rate of peak serum concentration varies with the site selected for injection, injections should be rotated within a particular area, such as the abdomen, before changing to another area.

13. c. A split-mixed dose of insulin requires that the patient adhere to a set meal pattern to provide glucose for the peak action of the insulin and a bedtime snack is usually required when patients take an intermediate-acting insulin late in the day to prevent nocturnal hypoglycemia. Hypoglycemia is most likely to occur with this dose late in the afternoon and during the night. When premixed formulas are used, flexible dosing based on glucose levels is not recommended.

14. d. Lispro is a rapid-acting insulin that has an onset of action of approximately 15 minutes and should be injected at the time of the meal to within 15 minutes of eating. Regular insulin is short acting with an onset of action in 30 to 60 minutes following administration and should be given 30 to 45 minutes before meals.

15. a. When mixing regular and intermediate-acting insulin, regular insulin should always be drawn into the syringe first to prevent contamination of the regular insulin vial with intermediate-acting insulin additives. Air is added to the neutral protamine Hagedorn (NPH) vial. Then air is added to the regular vial and the regular insulin is withdrawn, bubbles are removed, and the dose of NPH is withdrawn.

16. b. Checking the temperature of the bath water is part of assisting with activities of daily living (ADLs) and within the scope of care for unlicensed assistive personnel (UAP). This is important for the patient with neuropathy. Discussion of complications, teaching, and assessing learning are appropriate for RNs.

17. d. Insulin glargine (Lantus), a long-acting insulin that is continuously released with no peak of action, cannot be diluted or mixed with any other insulin or solution. Mixed insulins should be stored needle-up in the refrigerator and warmed before administration. Currently used bottles of insulin can be kept at room temperature out of sunlight.

18. a. Insulin pumps provide tight glycemic control by continuous subcutaneous insulin infusion based on the patient's basal profile, with bolus doses at mealtime at the patient's discretion and related to blood glucose monitoring. Errors in insulin dosing and complications of insulin therapy are still potential risks with insulin pumps.

19. c. The patient's elevated glucose on arising may be the result of either dawn phenomenon or Somogyi effect. The best way to determine whether the patient needs more or less insulin is by monitoring the glucose at bedtime, between 2:00 AM and 4:00 AM, and on arising. If predawn levels are below 60 mg/dL, the insulin dose should be reduced. If the 2:00 AM to 4:00 AM blood glucose is high, the insulin should be increased.

20. b. Biguanides (e.g., metformin [Glucophage]) are most commonly used with type 2 diabetes. They reduce glucose production by the liver and increase insulin sensitivity at the tissue level that improves glucose transport into the cells. Insulin is not taken orally, as it is ineffective. Meglitinides and sulfonylureas increase insulin production from the pancreas.

21. a, d, e. Acarbose (Precose) is an α-glucosidase inhibitor that is taken with the first bite of each meal. The effectiveness is measured with 2-hour postprandial blood glucose testing, as it delays glucose absorption from the GI tract. The other options describe thiazolidinediones.

22. c. Rapid deep respirations are symptoms of diabetic ketoacidosis (DKA), so this is the priority of care. Stage II pressure ulcers and bilateral numbness are chronic complications of diabetes. The lumps and dents on the abdomen indicate a need to teach the patient about site rotation.

23. a. The body requires food at regularly spaced intervals throughout the day and omission or delay of meals can result in hypoglycemia, especially for the patient using conventional insulin therapy or oral hypoglycemic agents. Weight loss may be recommended in type 2 diabetes if the individual is overweight but many patients with type 1 diabetes are thin and do not require a decrease in caloric intake. Fewer than 7% of total calories should be from saturated fats and simple sugar should be limited but moderate amounts can be used if counted as a part of total carbohydrate intake.

24. b. Maintenance of near-normal blood glucose levels and achievement of optimal serum lipid levels with dietary modification are believed to be the most important factors in preventing both short- and long-term complications of diabetes. There is no longer a specific "diabetic diet" and use of dietetic foods is not necessary for diabetes control. Most diabetics eat three meals a day and some require a bedtime snack for control of nighttime hypoglycemia. Loss of weight, which may or may not be to ideal body weight, may improve insulin resistance. The other goals of nutrition therapy include prevention of chronic complications of diabetes, attention to individual nutritional needs, and maintenance of the pleasure of eating.

25. b. During exercise, a diabetic person needs both adequate glucose to prevent exercise-induced hypoglycemia and adequate insulin, because counter regulatory hormones are produced during the stress of exercise and may cause hyperglycemia. Exercise after meals is best but a 15-g carbohydrate snack may be taken if exercise is performed before meals or is prolonged. Blood glucose levels should be monitored before, during, and after exercise to determine the effect of exercise on the levels.

26. c. Cleaning the puncture site with alcohol is not necessary and may interfere with test results and lead to drying and splitting of the fingertips. Washing the hands with warm water is adequate cleaning and promotes blood flow to the fingers. Blood flow is also increased by holding the hand down. Punctures on the side of the finger pad are less painful. Self-monitored blood glucose (SMBG) should be performed before and after exercise.

27. b. The American Diabetes Association recommends that testing for type 2 diabetes with a FPG, A1C, or 2-hour OGTT should be considered for all individuals at the age of 45 and above and, if normal, repeated every 3 years. Testing for immune markers of type 1 diabetes is not recommended. Testing at a younger age or more frequently should be done for members of a high-risk ethnic population, including African Americans, Hispanics, Native Americans, Asian Americans, and Pacific Islanders. Overweight adults with additional risk factors should be tested.

28. a. During minor illnesses, the patient with diabetes should continue drug therapy and food intake. Insulin is important because counter regulatory hormones may increase blood glucose during the stress of illness. Food or a carbohydrate liquid substitution is important because during illness the body requires extra energy to deal with the stress of the illness. Blood glucose monitoring should be done every 4 hours and the health care provider should be notified if the level is greater than 240 mg/dL (13.9 mmol/L) or if fever, ketonuria, or nausea and vomiting occur.

29. c. When insulin is insufficient and glucose cannot be used for cellular energy, the body releases and breaks down stored fats and protein to meet energy needs. Free fatty acids from stored triglycerides are released and metabolized in the liver in such large quantities that ketones are formed. Ketones are acidic and alter the pH of the blood, causing acidosis. Osmotic diuresis occurs as a result of elimination of both glucose and ketones in the urine.

30. a, b, c, d, e, f. In DKA, ketosis leads to ketonuria in trying to decrease the blood glucose and ketonemia. The metabolic acidosis leads to the Kussmaul respirations trying to decrease the acid in the system. The sweet, fruity breath odor is from DKA. Thirst and dehydration are found with both DKA and hyperosmolar hyperglycemic syndrome (HHS).

31. c. The management of DKA is similar to that of HHS except that HHS requires greater fluid replacement because of the severe hyperosmolar state. Bicarbonate is not usually given in DKA to correct acidosis unless the pH is <7.0 because administration of insulin will reverse the abnormal fat metabolism. Total body potassium deficit is possible in both conditions, requiring potassium administration, and in both conditions glucose is added to IV fluids when blood glucose levels fall to 250 mg/dL (13.9 mmol/L).

32. c. Hypoglycemia causes epinephrine release that contributes to shakiness and irritability from nervousness and anxiety. Without glucose in the brain, the patient may have difficulty speaking, visual disturbances, stupor, confusion, or coma. It is better to treat for hypoglycemia when unsure of the actual blood glucose level.

33. a, c, e, f. Manifestations of hyperglycemia include abdominal cramps, polyuria, weakness, fatigue, and headache. The headache can also be seen with hypoglycemia that is manifested by the remaining options.

34. d. If a diabetic patient is unconscious, immediate treatment for hypoglycemia must be given to prevent brain damage and IM or subcutaneous administration of 1 mg of glucagon should be done. If the unconsciousness has another cause, such as ketosis, the rise in glucose caused by the glucagon is not as dangerous as the low glucose level. Following administration of the glucagon, the patient should be transported to a medical facility for further treatment and evaluation. Insulin is contraindicated without knowledge of the patient's glucose level and oral carbohydrates cannot be given when patients are unconscious.

35. a. 3; b. 2; c. 1; d. 5; e. 4; f. 6. As with all patients, first establish an airway. With a patient with diabetes and abnormal behavior, the blood glucose must then be checked to determine if the patient's symptoms are related to the diabetes. In this case, it is hyperglycemia, so an IV must be started for fluid resuscitation and insulin administration. The last food intake and times at which medications were recently taken may establish a cause for the hyperglycemia and aid in determining further treatment.

36. a. Blood glucose levels of 80 to 90 mg/dL (4.4 to 5 mmol/L) are within the normal range and are desired in the patient with diabetes, even following a recent hypoglycemic episode. Hypoglycemia is often caused by a single event, such as skipping a meal, taking too much insulin, or vigorous exercise. Once corrected, normal glucose control should be maintained.

37. b. The development of atherosclerotic vessel disease seems to be promoted by the altered lipid metabolism common in diabetes. Although tight glucose control may help to delay the process, it does not prevent it completely. Atherosclerosis in patients with diabetes does respond somewhat to a reduction in general risk factors, as it does in nondiabetics, and reduction in fat intake, control of hypertension, abstention from smoking, maintenance of normal weight, and regular exercise should be carried out by all patients.

38. b, d. Macrovascular disease causes coronary artery disease and ulceration and results in amputation of the lower extremities. However, neuropathy may also contribute to not feeling ulcerations. The remaining options are related to microvascular complications of diabetes.

39. b, e, f. Autonomic neuropathy affects most body systems. Manifestations of autonomic neuropathy include erectile dysfunction in men and decreased libido, gastroparesis (nausea, vomiting, gastroesophageal reflux and feeling full), painless myocardial infarction, postural hypotension, and resting tachycardia. The remaining options would occur with sensory neuropathy.

40. d. Complete or partial loss of sensitivity of the feet is common with peripheral neuropathy of diabetes and patients with diabetes may suffer foot injury and ulceration without ever having pain. Feet must be inspected during daily care for any cuts, blisters, swelling, or reddened areas.

41. a. Older adults have more conditions that may be treated with medications that impair insulin action. Hypoglycemic unawareness is more common, so these patients are more likely to suffer adverse consequences from blood glucose–lowering therapy. Because the clinical manifestations of long-term complications of diabetes take 10 to 20 years to develop, the goals for glycemic control are not as rigid as in the younger population. Treatment is indicated and insulin may be used if the patient does not respond to oral agents. The patient's needs rather than age determine the responsibility of others in care.

Case Study

1. The hypoglycemia might have been prevented by F.W. taking time to eat breakfast and perhaps increasing food intake in anticipation of strenuous exercise. She also should have checked her glucose level before exercising. She should be carrying a quick-acting carbohydrate with her and taking advantage of the snacks or drinks offered along the marathon route.

2. Sympathetic response to hypoglycemia:
   - Weakness, nervousness, tremor
   - Vasoconstriction with pallor, numbness, coldness, headache, tachycardia

   Low glucose levels in the brain:
   - Confusion, slurred speech, unsteady gait

3. The hypoglycemia should be treated with 15 g of a fast-acting carbohydrate: 120 to 180 mL of orange juice or regular soda, five or six hard candies, 1 tbs syrup or honey, or 4 tsp jelly. Repeat the carbohydrate in 15 minutes if symptoms are still present or if blood glucose remains less than 70 mg/dL (3.9 mmol/L). When glucose is above 70 mg/dL, a regularly scheduled meal or snack of complex carbohydrate and protein should be eaten. The blood glucose should be checked again about 45 minutes after treatment to ensure that hypoglycemia does not recur.

4. F.W. should be taught how to recognize situations that lead to hypoglycemia; the effects of exercise on glucose levels and the need for both adequate glucose and insulin; and how to balance exercise, food, and insulin. Have the patient discuss insulin dosage for running and racing with her health care provider.

5. F.W. should monitor her blood glucose before, during, and after exercise; increase dietary intake before exercise; manage insulin doses with her health care provider; exercise 60 to 90 minutes after meals; and carry simple carbohydrates to take at first symptoms of hypoglycemia.

6. **Nursing diagnoses:**
   Ineffective self-health management *related to* non-compliance with recommended regimen
   Collaborative problems:
   Potential complications: brain damage, coma, seizures, death

CHAPTER 50

Answer Key

1. d. A normal response to growth hormone (GH) secretion is stimulation of the liver to produce somatomedin C, or insulin-like growth factor-1 (IGF-1), which stimulates growth of bones and soft tissues. The increased levels of somatomedin C normally inhibit GH but in acromegaly the pituitary gland secretes GH despite elevated IGF-1 levels. When both GH and IGF-1 levels are increased, overproduction of GH is confirmed. GH also causes elevation of blood glucose and normally GH levels fall during an oral glucose challenge but not in acromegaly.

2. c. The increased production of GH in acromegaly causes an increase in thickness and width of bones and enlargement of soft tissues, resulting in marked changes in facial features, oily and coarse skin, and speech difficulties. Infertility is not a common finding because GH is usually the only pituitary hormone involved in acromegaly. Height is not increased in adults with GH excess because the epiphyses of the bones are closed.

3. a. A transsphenoidal hypophysectomy involves entry into the sella turcica through an incision in the upper lip and gingiva into the floor of the nose and the sphenoid sinuses. Postoperative clear nasal drainage with glucose content indicates cerebrospinal fluid (CSF) leakage from an open connection to the brain, putting the patient at risk for meningitis. After surgery, the patient is positioned with the head elevated to avoid pressure on the sella turcica. Coughing and straining are avoided to prevent increased intracranial pressure and CSF leakage. Although mouth care is required every 4 hours, toothbrushing should not be performed because injury to the suture line may occur.

4. d. Compression of the optic chiasm can cause visual problems as well as signs of increased intracranial pressure, including headache, nausea, and vomiting. About 30% of prolactinomas will have excess prolactin secretion with manifestations of impotence in men, galactorrhea or amenorrhea in women without relationship to pregnancy, and decreased libido in both men and women. There is decreased follicle-stimulating hormone (FSH) and luteinizing hormone (LH).

5. a, b, d, e. With panhypopituitarism, lifetime hormone replacement is needed for cortisol, vasopressin, thyroid, and GH. Sex hormones will not be replaced because of the patient's history of breast cancer. Dopamine agonists will not be used because they reduce secretion of GH, which has already been achieved with the radiation.

6. b. With increased antidiuretic hormone (ADH), the permeability of the renal distal tubules is increased, so water is reabsorbed into circulation. Decreased output of concentrated urine with increased urine osmolality and specific gravity occur. In addition, fluid retention with weight gain, serum hypoosmolality, dilutional hyponatremia, and hypochloremia occur.

7. a. The patient with syndrome of inappropriate antidiuretic hormone (SIADH) has marked dilutional hyponatremia and should be monitored for decreased neurologic function and seizures every 2 hours. Sodium intake is supplemented because of the hyponatremia and sodium loss caused by diuretics. ADH release is reduced by keeping the head of the bed flat to increase left atrial filling pressure. A reduction in blood pressure (BP) indicates a reduction in total fluid volume and is an expected outcome of treatment.

8. b. The patient with SIADH has water retention with hyponatremia, decreased urine output, and concentrated urine with high specific gravity. Improvement in the patient's condition is reflected by increased urine output, normalization of serum sodium, and more water in the urine, thus decreasing the specific gravity.

9. c. Patients with diabetes insipidus (DI) excrete large amounts of urine with a specific gravity of less than 1.005. Blood glucose would be tested to diagnose diabetes mellitus. The serum sodium level is expected to be low with DI but is not diagnostic. To diagnose central DI a water deprivation test is required. Then a CT of the head may be done to determine the cause. Nephrogenic DI is differentiated from central DI with determination of the level of ADH after an analog of ADH is given.

10. d. A patient with central diabetes insipidus has a deficiency of ADH with excessive loss of water from the kidney, hypovolemia, hypernatremia, and dilute urine with a low specific gravity. When vasopressin is administered, the symptoms are reversed, with water retention, decreased

urinary output that increases urine osmolality, and an increase in BP.

11. c. Normal urine specific gravity is 1.005 to 1.025 and urine with a specific gravity of 1.002 is very dilute, indicating that there continues to be excessive loss of water and that treatment of diabetes insipidus is inadequate. Headache, weight gain, and oral intake greater than urinary output are signs of volume excess that occur with overmedication. Nasal irritation and nausea may also indicate overdosage.

12. b. In nephrogenic diabetes insipidus, the kidney is unable to respond to ADH, so vasopressin or hormone analogs are not effective. Thiazide diuretics slow the glomerular filtration rate (GFR) in the kidney and produce a decrease in urine output. Low-sodium diets (<3 g/day) are also thought to decrease urine output. Fluids are not restricted because the patient could easily become dehydrated.

13. d. In Hashimoto's thyroiditis, thyroid tissue is destroyed by autoimmune antibodies. An enlarged thyroid gland is a goiter. Viral-induced hyperthyroidism is subacute granulomatous thyroiditis. Acute thyroiditis is caused by bacterial or fungal infection.

14. a. Exophthalmos or protrusion of the eyeballs may occur in Graves' disease from increased fat deposits and fluid in the orbital tissues and ocular muscles, forcing the eyeballs outward. Graves' disease is the most common form of hyperthyroidism. Increased metabolic rate and sensitivity of the sympathetic nervous system lead to the clinical manifestations. Thyroid-stimulating hormone (TSH) level is decreased in Graves' disease.

15. d. In Graves' disease, antibodies to the TSH receptor are formed, attach to the receptors, and stimulate the thyroid gland to release triiodothyronine (T_3), thyroxine (T_4), or both, creating hyperthyroidism. The disease is not directly genetic but individuals appear to have a genetic susceptibility to develop autoimmune antibodies. Goiter formation from insufficient iodine intake is usually associated with hypothyroidism.

16. c. A hyperthyroid crisis results in marked manifestations of hyperthyroidism, with severe tachycardia, heart failure, shock, hyperthermia, restlessness, irritability, abdominal pain, vomiting, diarrhea, delirium, and coma. Although exophthalmos may be present in the patient with Graves' disease, it is not a significant factor in hyperthyroid crisis. Hoarseness and laryngeal stridor are characteristic of the tetany of hypoparathyroidism and lethargy progressing to coma is characteristic of myxedema coma, a complication of hypothyroidism.

17. b. The β-adrenergic blocker atenolol is used to block the sympathetic nervous system stimulation by thyroid hormones. Potassium iodide is used to prepare the patient for thyroidectomy or for treatment of thyrotoxic crisis to inhibit the synthesis of thyroid hormones. Antithyroid medications inhibit the synthesis of thyroid hormones. Radioactive iodine (RAI) therapy destroys thyroid tissue, which limits thyroid hormone secretion.

18. a, d, e. RAI causes hypothyroidism over time by damaging thyroid tissue and is the treatment of choice for nonpregnant adults. Potassium iodide decreases the release of thyroid hormones and decreases the size of the thyroid gland preoperatively. Propylthiouracil (PTU) blocks peripheral conversion of T_4 to T_3 and may be used with iodine to produce a euthyroid state before surgery.

19. a. To prevent strain on the suture line postoperatively, the patient's head must be manually supported while turning and moving in bed but range-of-motion exercises for the head and neck are also taught preoperatively to be gradually implemented after surgery. There is no contraindication for coughing and deep breathing and these should be carried out postoperatively. Tingling around the lips or fingers is a sign of hypocalcemia, which may occur if the parathyroid glands are inadvertently removed during surgery. This sign should be reported immediately.

20. a. A tracheostomy tray is in the room to use if vocal cord paralysis occurs from recurrent laryngeal nerve damage or for laryngeal stridor from tetany. The oxygen equipment may be useful but will not improve oxygenation with vocal cord paralysis without a tracheostomy. IV calcium salts will be used if hypocalcemia occurs from parathyroid damage. The paper and pencil for communication may be helpful, especially if a tracheostomy is performed, but will not aid in emergency oxygenation of the patient.

21. d. With the decrease in thyroid hormone postoperatively, calories need to be reduced substantially to prevent weight gain. When a patient has had a subtotal thyroidectomy, thyroid replacement therapy is not given because exogenous hormone inhibits pituitary production of TSH and delays or prevents the restoration of thyroid tissue regeneration. Regular exercise stimulates the thyroid gland and is encouraged. Saltwater gargles are used for dryness and irritation of the mouth and throat following radioactive iodine therapy.

22. d. Both Graves' disease and Hashimoto's thyroiditis are autoimmune disorders that eventually destroy the thyroid gland, leading to primary hypothyroidism. Thyroid tumors most often result in hyperthyroidism. Secondary hypothyroidism occurs as a result of pituitary failure and iatrogenic hypothyroidism results from thyroidectomy or radiation of the thyroid gland.

23. b. Cardiorespiratory response to activity is important to monitor in this patient to determine the effect of activities and plan activity increases. Monitoring changes in orientation, cognition, and behavior are interventions for impaired memory. Monitoring bowels is needed to plan care for the patient with constipation. Assisting with meal planning will help the patient with imbalanced nutrition: more than body requirements to lose weight if needed.

24. d. All these manifestations may occur with treatment of hypothyroidism. However, as a result of the effects of hypothyroidism on the cardiovascular system, when thyroid replacement therapy is started myocardial oxygen consumption is increased and the resultant oxygen demand may cause angina, cardiac dysrhythmias, and heart failure, so monitoring for dysrhythmias is most important.

25. b. Because of the mental sluggishness, inattentiveness, and memory loss that occur with hypothyroidism, it is important to provide written instructions and repeat information when teaching the patient. Replacement therapy must be taken for life and alternate-day dosing is not therapeutic. Although most patients return to a normal state with treatment, cardiovascular conditions and psychoses may persist.

26. d. The patient with hyperparathyroidism may have calcium nephrolithiasis, skeletal pain, decreased bone density, psychomotor retardation, or cardiac dysrhythmias. The other endocrine problems would not be related to calcium kidney stones or decreased bone density.

27. b. A high fluid intake is indicated in hyperparathyroidism to dilute the hypercalcemia and flush the kidneys so that calcium stone formation is reduced. Seizures are not associated with hyperparathyroidism. Impending tetany of hypoparathyroidism after parathyroidectomy can be noted with Trousseau's and Chvostek's signs. The patient with hyperparathyroidism is at risk for pathologic fractures resulting from decreased bone density but mobility is encouraged to promote bone calcification.

28. b, c, d, e, f. In hypoparathyroidism the patient has inadequate circulating parathyroid hormone (PTH) that leads to hypocalcemia from the inability to maintain serum calcium levels. With hypocalcemia there is muscle stiffness and spasms, which can lead to cardiac dysrhythmias and abdominal cramps. There can also be personality and visual changes and dry, scaly skin.

29. b. Rebreathing in a paper bag promotes carbon dioxide retention in the blood, which lowers pH and creates an acidosis. An acidemia enhances the solubility and ionization of calcium, increasing the proportion of total body calcium available in physiologically active form and relieving the symptoms of hypocalcemia. Saline promotes calcium excretion, as does furosemide. Phosphate levels in the blood are reciprocal to calcium and an increase in phosphate promotes calcium excretion.

30. c. The hypocalcemia that results from PTH deficiency is controlled with calcium and vitamin D supplementation and possibly oral phosphate binders. Replacement with PTH is not used because of antibody formation to PTH, the need for parenteral administration, and cost. Milk products, although good sources of calcium, also have high levels of phosphate, which reduce calcium absorption. Whole grains and foods containing oxalic acid also impair calcium absorption.

31. a. The effects of adrenocortical hormone excess, especially glucocorticoid excess, include weight gain from accumulation and redistribution of adipose tissue, sodium and water retention, glucose intolerance, protein wasting, loss of bone structure, loss of collagen, and capillary fragility leading to petechiae. Clinical manifestations of adrenocortical hormone deficiency include hypotension, dehydration, weight loss, and hyperpigmentation of the skin.

32. c. Although the patient with Cushing syndrome has excess corticosteroids, removal of the glands and the stress of surgery require that high doses of corticosteroids (cortisone) be administered postoperatively for several days before weaning the dose. The nurse should monitor the patient's vital signs postoperatively to detect whether large amounts of hormones were released during surgical manipulation, obtain morning urine specimens for cortisol measurement to evaluate the effectiveness of the surgery, and provide dressing changes with aseptic technique to avoid infection as usual inflammatory responses are suppressed.

33. b. Vomiting and diarrhea are early indicators of Addisonian crisis and fever indicates an infection, which is causing additional stress for the patient. Treatment of a crisis requires immediate glucocorticoid replacement and IV hydrocortisone, fluids, sodium, and glucose are necessary for 24 hours. Addison's disease is a primary insufficiency of the adrenal gland and adrenocorticotropic hormone (ACTH) is not effective, nor would vasopressors be effective with the fluid deficiency of Addison's disease. Potassium levels are increased in Addison's disease and KCl would be contraindicated.

34. b. A weight reduction in the patient with Addison's disease may indicate a fluid loss and a dose of replacement therapy that is too low rather than too high. Because vomiting and diarrhea are early signs of crisis and because fluid and electrolytes must be replaced, patients should notify their health care provider if these symptoms occur. Patients with Addison's disease are taught to take two to three times their usual dose of steroids if they become ill, have teeth extracted, or engage in rigorous physical activity and should always have injectable hydrocortisone available if oral doses cannot be taken.

35. c. Alendronate (Fosamax) is used to prevent corticosteroid-induced osteoporosis. Potassium is used to prevent the mineralocorticoid effect of hypokalemia. Furosemide (Lasix) is used to decrease sodium and fluid retention from the mineralocorticoid effect. Pantoprazole (Protonix) is used to prevent gastrointestinal (GI) irritation from an increase in secretion of pepsin and hydrochloric acid.

36. c. Taking corticosteroids on an alternate-day schedule for pharmacologic purposes is less likely to suppress ACTH production from the pituitary and prevent adrenal atrophy. Normal adrenal hormone balance is not maintained during glucocorticoid therapy because excessive exogenous hormone is used.

37. a. Hyperaldosteronism is an excess of aldosterone, which is manifested by sodium and water retention and potassium excretion. Furosemide is a potassium-wasting diuretic that would increase the potassium deficiency. Aminoglutethimide blocks aldosterone synthesis. Spironolactone and amiloride are potassium-sparing diuretics.

38. b. Pheochromocytoma is a catecholamine-producing tumor of the adrenal medulla, which may cause severe, episodic hypertension; severe, pounding headache; and profuse sweating. Monitoring for a dangerously high BP before surgery is critical, as is monitoring for BP fluctuations during medical and surgical treatment.

Case Study

1. All of the blood tests are altered because of the effect of elevated glucocorticoids:
   - Elevated glucose—increased gluconeogenesis by liver and induced insulin resistance
   - Elevated white blood cell (WBC) count—leukocytosis
   - Decreased lymphocytes—lymphocytopenia
   - Increased red blood cell (RBC) count—polycythemia
   - Decreased K+—increased mineralocorticoid effect causing sodium retention and potassium excretion

2. Cushing syndrome has several causes:
   - ACTH-secreting pituitary adenoma is the most common cause of endogenous Cushing syndrome.
   - Ectopic ACTH production by tumors outside the hypothalamic-pituitary-adrenal axis (usually of the lung or pancreas) is most common in men.
   - The pathophysiology of Cushing syndrome reflects an excess of normal glucocorticoid and mineralocorticoid activity, an exaggeration of normal functions.
   - Adrenal tumors are most common in women 20 to 40 years of age.
   - Iatrogenic administration of exogenous corticosteroids is the most common cause but unrelated to this patient.

3. A 24-hour urine collection for free cortisol is done, with elevated levels indicating Cushing syndrome. Plasma ACTH levels would be measured; high or normal levels

of ACTH indicate Cushing disease from ACTH-secreting pituitary adenoma and low or undetectable levels of ACTH indicate an adrenal or ectopic cause.

4. Treatment depends on the cause of the syndrome. With a pituitary cause, transsphenoidal hypophysectomy is performed; with an adrenal cause, adrenalectomy is performed or drug therapy is used; with an ectopic cause, the tumor is located and removed if possible. If exogenous corticosteroid therapy is the cause, discontinue or alter the dose of the exogenous corticosteroids.

5. A medical adrenalectomy involves treatment with ketoconazole, aminoglutethimide, or mitotane to suppress cortisol production, alter peripheral metabolism of steroids, and decrease plasma and urine steroid levels by actually killing adrenocortical cells.

6. Priority nursing responsibilities include the following:
   - Emotional support
   - Assessment of signs and symptoms of hormone toxicity:
     - Vital signs q4hr
     - Daily weights
     - Glucose monitoring
     - Changes in mental status
     - Administer medications (e.g., IV corticosteroids, analgesics)
   - Assessment for complications:
     - Manifestations of gynecomastia or testicular atrophy
     - Manifestations of increased gastrointestinal secretions
     - Manifestations of infection, such as pain or purulent drainage, because fever and inflammation may be minimal or absent
     - Manifestations of thromboembolic phenomena, such as chest pain, dyspnea, and tachypnea
     - Manifestations of bone pain or limitations in motion, indicating pathologic fractures
     - Manifestations of nephrolithiasis from increased calcium excretion
   - Preoperative preparation
   - Instruction about exercises, coughing, and deep breathing
   - Possible presence of nasogastric tube, urinary catheter, IV therapy, and leg sequential compression devices
   - Explanations about early monitoring for circulatory instability
   - Explanations about hormone replacement

7. **Nursing diagnoses:**
   - Risk for infection *related to* lowered resistance to stress and suppression of immune system
   - Imbalanced nutrition: more than body requirements *related to* increased appetite, high caloric intake, and inactivity
   - Situational low self-esteem *related to* altered body image and diminished physical capabilities

   Collaborative problems:
   Potential complications: thromboembolism, cardiac dysrhythmias, pathologic fractures, nephrolithiasis, diabetes mellitus, hypertensive crisis, impaired skin integrity

CHAPTER 51

Answer Key

1. a. Seminal vesicle; b. ejaculatory duct; c. prostate gland; d. rectum; e. Cowper's gland; f. anus; g. epididymis; h. testis; i. scrotum; j. glans; k. penis; l. urethra; m. ductus deferens; n. bladder; o. ureter; p. fallopian tube; q. ovary; r. body of

uterus; s. fundus of uterus; t. bladder; u. vagina; v. vaginal introitus; w. anus; x. rectum; y. urethra; z. cervix; aa. ureter

2. a. Prepuce; b. labia minora; c. vaginal introitus; d. vestibule; e. perineum; f. anus; g. labia majora; h. urethral meatus; i. clitoris; j. mons pubis; k. pectoralis major muscle; l. alveoli; m. areola; n. nipple

3. a. 3; b. 8; c. 2; d. 6; e. 1; f. 7; g. 4; h. 5

4. a. Ducts carry milk from the alveoli to the lactiferous sinuses. The areola is the pigmented center of the breast, the nipple is the erectile tissue that contains pores, and adipose tissue makes up the majority of the nonlactating breast tissue.

5. c. Montgomery's tubercles are similar to sebaceous glands and lubricate the nipple. The alveoli secrete milk during lactation and it is stored in the lactiferous sinuses. The nipple has erectile tissue and contains pores for milk delivery.

6. c. Menopause is identified after 1 year of amenorrhea. A Papanicolaou (Pap) test includes cells from both the endocervix and the ectocervix. The ovum is fertilized by the sperm in the fallopian tube. The reabsorption of oocytes by the body is called atresia. Follicle-stimulating hormone (FSH) stimulates the initial stage of follicular maturation, while luteinizing hormone (LH) must be present for complete maturation and ovulation to occur.

7. b, c, f. LH completes follicle maturation, stimulates testosterone production, and is called interstitial cell-stimulating hormone (ICSH) in men. Progesterone maintains an implanted egg. Prolactin stimulates the growth of the mammary glands. Estrogen develops and maintains secondary sex characteristics of women as well as the proliferative phase of the menstrual cycle after menstruation and the uterine changes essential to pregnancy.

8. b, c, f. FSH is elevated at menopause. In men it is responsible for spermatogenesis. FSH stimulates growth and maturity of ovarian follicles. Testosterone is produced by the testes and produces male sex characteristics. Gonadotropin-releasing hormone (GnRH) is stimulated by elevated estrogen levels and decreased testosterone levels.

9. b. Age-related changes in sexual function in men include a need for increased stimulation for an erection, a decreased need to ejaculate, and a possible decreased response to sexual stimuli. There is a decreased ability to attain an erection but it is not related to prostatic changes. A negative social attitude toward sexuality in older adults may also affect the sexual activity of people in this age-group.

10.

Factor	Problem Identified During Assessment
Rubella	Potential congenital anomalies if rubella occurs during the first trimester of pregnancy
Mumps	Increased sterility in young men with mumps because of testicular atrophy resulting from orchitis
Diabetes mellitus	Impotence and retrograde ejaculation in male diabetics in addition to erectile problems from neuropathies. In women, sexual performance and health of mother and fetus may be affected if diabetes mellitus is uncontrolled
Antihypertensive agents	Many may cause impotence in men

11. d. The prostate is palpated through the wall of the rectum with a digital rectal examination. Inguinal hernias are detected by palpating the inguinal ring while the patient bears down and scrotal palpation is done to detect testicular masses or tumors. No specific conditions are indicated by enlargement at the base of the penis.
12. a. A decrease in the size of the penis is a normal finding in the older man. Loss of pubic hair is not normal, nor is any enlargement of the breasts. The normally darker color of the scrotum does not change with aging.
13. c. Vaginal dryness occurs with decreased estrogen and increased androgens circulating in the aging female. This also leads to breast and genital atrophy, reduction in bone mass, and increased atherosclerosis. A rectocele may occur and cause sexual or fecal elimination problems for the patient that will need treatment.

14.

Functional Health Pattern	Risk Factor for or Patient Response to Reproductive Problem
Health perception–health management	Lack of Pap testing, breast self-examination, prostate examinations, or testicular self-examination; smoking, alcohol, and caffeine use; family history of breast, ovarian, uterine, or prostate cancer
Nutritional-metabolic	History of anorexia nervosa, obesity, anemia, decreased calcium intake
Elimination	Urge and stress incontinence; difficulty urinating in male patients; vaginal and bladder infections
Activity-exercise	Fatigue and activity intolerance related to menorrhagia
Sleep-rest	Sleep interruption related to hot flashes and sweating; nocturia
Cognitive-perceptual	Pelvic pain; dyspareunia
Self-perception–self-concept	Changes in self-concept related to sexuality and aging
Role-relationship	Occupational hazards related to sexual functioning and reproductive capacity; dysfunctional or changing roles and relationships with others
Sexuality-reproductive	Recent changes in sexual practices; dissatisfaction with sexual expression; reproductive problems that affect sexual satisfaction; changes in menstrual patterns; multiple sexual partners; no protection against sexually transmitted infections (STIs)
Coping–stress tolerance	Effect of STI on sex partners; stress of sexual problems or changes; infertility
Value-belief	Conflict between value system and treatment; abortion issues; infertility issues

15. b. Candidiasis is a white, thick or curdy discharge and causes itching and inflammation. Cancer would be more likely to produce a bloody discharge. Trichomonas vaginalis produces a malodorous frothy green or yellow discharge. Bacterial vaginosis infection produces copious amounts of thin gray or white drainage with a fishy odor.
16. d. The vulva should be the color of the skin or slightly pink. Redness indicates inflammation. A small amount of clear vaginal discharge is normal in females, as are episiotomy scars in women who have had children. Skene's glands should not be palpable.
17. b, d. Gram stain smears and the nucleic acid amplification test (NAAT) can screen for *Chlamydia* from vaginal, endocervical, urinary, and urethral samples. The NAAT can also be used to detect gonorrhea. A Pap test detects potentially cancerous cells. The rapid plasma reagin (RPR), the Venereal Disease Research Laboratory (VDRL), and fluorescent treponemal antibody absorption (FTA-Abs) tests all screen for syphilis.
18. c. Serum estradiol measures ovarian function to assess estrogen-secreting tumors and precocious female puberty or to confirm perimenopausal status in women. It may also be indicative of testicular tumors in men. Pregnancy is detected with urinary or serum human chorionic gonadotropin (hCG). Prostate cancer is detected with prostate-specific antigen (PSA). Gonadal failure secondary to pituitary dysfunction is identified with urine or serum FSH studies.
19. b. The risk for bleeding is increased following a dilation and curettage (D&C) because the endometrial lining is scraped and injury to the uterus can occur. The nurse should closely assess the amount of bleeding with frequent pad checks for the first 24 hours. Infection following D&C is uncommon and the urinary system is not affected.
20. a, b, c, e. A culdoscopy involves insertion of an endoscope through an incision made through the posterior fornix of the cul-de-sac and requires surgical anesthesia, as does the removal of cervical tissue during a conization. A D&C and laparoscopy are also operative procedures requiring surgical anesthesia. Colposcopy and endometrial biopsies do not require surgical anesthesia.
21. a. Huhner (or Sims-Huhner) test involves examination of a mucus sample of the cervix within 2 to 8 hours after intercourse to determine the number and mobility of sperm in the cervical mucus. A semen analysis is a simple examination of semen for the number, mobility, and structure of sperm. An endometrial biopsy provides a sample of endometrium to evaluate its changes under the influence of progesterone. A hysterosalpingogram is a contrast x-ray of the uterine cavity and fallopian tubes.

CHAPTER 52

Answer Key

1. b. The value of breast self-examination (BSE) in reducing mortality rates from breast cancer in women is currently controversial and under review. However, it is still a useful tool in helping women to become self-aware of how their breasts normally look and feel. None of the other options has been validated at this time.

2. a. Annual screening mammogram every year starting at the age of 40.
   b. Clinical breast examination (CBE) every 3 years in their 20s and 30s and every year for women beginning at age 40.
   c. Optional monthly BSE starting at age 20 and reporting changes.
   d. In women with increased risk, decisions for additional and more frequent testing to be determined with the health care provider.

3. a. One of the major reasons why women do not examine their breasts regularly is because of a lack of confidence in BSE skill. A teaching program should include allowing time for women to use models to identify problems and perform a return demonstration of the examination on themselves. Fear and denial often interfere with BSE even when women know that the perceived risk for cancer is high, know the statistics, and know that they should seek medical care if an abnormality is detected. Examinations in premenopausal women should be done right after the menstrual period and specific dates are set for postmenopausal women or those who have had hysterectomies.

4. d. A definitive diagnosis of breast cancer can be made only by a histologic examination of biopsied tissue. A core (core needle) biopsy is as reliable as a surgical biopsy and has the advantages of decreased length of time for the procedure and recovery and reduced cost. A limitation of fine-needle aspiration is that if negative results are found, more definitive biopsy procedures are required.

5. d. MammaPrint is used in early-stage breast cancer with estrogen receptor–positive or estrogen receptor–negative breast cancer without nodal involvement to assess risk of recurrence within 10 years without additional treatment and the likely benefit of chemotherapy. CA 27-29 is a cancer marker produced by the *MUC1* gene. TNM is not a genomic assay but rather a system for staging cancer using tumor size, nodal involvement, and the presence of metastasis. Oncotype DX genomic assay is used in newly diagnosed early-stage estrogen receptor–positive breast cancer treated with hormonal therapy to assess risk of occurrence and the need for treatment with chemotherapy to prevent recurrence.

6. d. Most breast lesions are benign and many mobile cystic lesions change in response to the menstrual cycle, whereas most malignant tumors do not. Caffeine has been associated with fibrocystic changes in some women but research has not established caffeine as a cause of breast pain or cysts. Questions regarding a patient's last mammogram or family history are not closely related to the nurse's findings.

7. c. Fibrocystic changes make breasts difficult to examine because of fibrotic changes and multiple lumps. A woman with this condition should be familiar with the characteristic changes in her breasts and monitor them closely for new lumps that do not respond in a cyclic manner over 1 to 2 weeks. Estrogen antagonizes the condition and fibrocystic changes are not precancerous.

8. d, e, f. Intraductal papilloma is associated with increased cancer risk, is more common in women 40 to 60 years old, and is a wartlike growth in mammary ducts beneath the areola. Fat necrosis is associated with breast trauma. Fibroadenoma occurs in 10% of young women. Multicolored, sticky nipple discharge is seen in ductal ectasia.

9. a. Mastitis occurs during lactation and is caused by *Staphylococcus aureus*. Ductal ectasia involves subareolar area ducts and has multicolored sticky nipple discharge and inflammatory signs. It is not associated with malignancy. Fibroadenoma occurs in 10% of women ages 15 to 40 and has well-delineated, very mobile tumors. A biopsy must be done to exclude malignancy. Senescent gynecomastia occurs in older men, probably from increased conversion of androgens to estrogens in peripheral circulation. It generally regresses in 6 to 12 months.

10. d. After the age of 60, the incidence of breast cancer increases dramatically and advanced age is the highest risk factor for females. Ninety-nine percent of breast cancer cases occur in women. A first-degree relative with breast cancer is a contributing factor for breast cancer. Obesity and lack of physical activity are other contributing factors. Genetic mutations in *BRCA1, BRCA2, p53, ATM,* and *CHEK2* genes may increase the risk of breast cancer. Fibrocystic breast changes are neither a precursor of breast cancer nor a known risk factor for cancer.

11. b. On palpation, malignant lesions are characteristically hard, irregularly shaped, poorly delineated, nontender, and nonmobile and the most common site is the upper outer quadrant of the breast. A fibroadenoma is firm, defined, and mobile. Fibrocystic lesions are usually large, tender, moveable masses found throughout the breast tissue. A painful, immobile mass under a reddened area of skin is most typical of a local abscess.

12. a. Axillary lymph node status is one of the most important prognostic factors in primary breast cancer; the more nodes involved, the higher the risk for relapse or metastasis. Aneuploid DNA tumor content indicates that cells have abnormally high or low DNA content compared with normal cells and is associated with tumor aggressiveness. Cells in S-phase have a higher risk for recurrence and can produce earlier cancer death. Hormone receptor–negative tumors are usually poorly differentiated histologically, frequently recur, and are usually unresponsive to hormonal therapy.

13. b. Either treatment choice is indicated for women with early-stage breast cancer because the 10-year survival rate with lumpectomy with radiation is about the same as that with modified radical mastectomy. Each procedure has advantages and disadvantages that the patient must consider in making an informed choice and the nurse should make that information available to the patient to assist in decision making.

14. d. Sentinel lymph node dissection (SLND) has become the standard of care, with axillary lymph node dissection reserved for patients with clinical indications of disease in the axilla. SLND provides prognostic information and helps to determine further treatment. A lumpectomy, or breast-conservation surgery, is followed by radiation therapy to

the entire breast and the use of chemotherapy or hormone therapy depends on the characteristics of the tumor and evidence of metastases.

15. c. Lymphatic mapping with SLND identifies one to four lymph nodes that drain first from the tumor site. Those nodes are examined for malignant cells. If any of the nodes have malignant cells, a complete axillary lymph node dissection is done. If the sentinel nodes are negative, no additional lymph nodes are removed.

16. a, c. High-dose brachytherapy may be completed in 5 days and is an alternative to traditional radiation for early-stage breast cancer. Primary radiation follows local excision of a tumor. Radiation as an adjuvant to surgery is used to treat possible residual cancer cells postmastectomy. Palliative radiation is used to reduce tumor size and relieve pain.

17. c. Tamoxifen is an antiestrogen agent that blocks the estrogen-receptor sites of malignant cells and is the usual first choice of treatment in postmenopausal women with hormone receptor–positive tumors, with or without nodal involvement. Tamoxifen reduces the risk for recurrent breast cancer and also that for new primary tumors. The side effects of the drug are minimal and are those commonly associated with decreased estrogen.

18. c. As early as in the recovery room following a modified radical mastectomy, the patient should start flexing and extending the fingers and wrist of the affected arm with daily increases in activity. Postoperative mastectomy exercises, such as hair care, wall climbing with the fingers, and shoulder rotation and extension, are instituted gradually to prevent disruption of the wound.

19. b. Removal of the axillary lymph nodes impairs lymph drainage from the affected arm and predisposes the patient to infection of the arm. The arm must be protected from even minor trauma and blood pressure, venipunctures, and injections should not be done on the arm. The arm should never be dependent, even during sleep, and should be elevated to promote lymph drainage.

20. c. The Reach to Recovery program consists of volunteers, all women, who have had breast cancer and can answer questions about what to expect at home, how to tell people about the surgery, and what prosthetic devices are available. It is a valuable resource for patients who have breast cancer and should be used if available in the community. If a volunteer is not available, the nurse is responsible for assisting the patient in the same manner. Although the nurse should stress the importance of wearing a prosthesis, a permanent prosthesis cannot be used until healing is complete and inflammation is resolved.

21. b. It is most important for the patient planning a mammoplasty that she have a realistic idea about what the surgery can accomplish and about possible complications. Currently surgery cannot restore nipple sensation or erectility and the breast will not fully resemble its premastectomy appearance but the outcome is usually more acceptable than the mastectomy scar. The woman's motives for breast reconstruction should not be questioned. There have been allegations of immune-related diseases associated with the use of silicone gel implants but after further evaluation the Food and Drug Administration (FDA) has approved these implants for use.

22. a. When an expander is used to stretch the skin and muscle at the mastectomy site, the expander is gradually increased in size by weekly injections of water or saline until the site is large enough to hold an implant. Placement of the expander can be at the time of mastectomy or at a later date. A musculocutaneous flap procedure is a type of reconstruction using the patient's own tissue. The nipple of the affected breast is removed at mastectomy and a new nipple can be reconstructed after breast reconstruction from various normal tissues.

23. b. Vinorelbine (Navelbine) is used to treat metastatic breast cancer and is better tolerated with fewer and milder side effects than other chemotherapy medications. Capecitabine (Xeloda) is used in women whose metastatic breast cancer has not responded to started chemotherapy. Doxorubicin (Adriamycin) is a first-line chemotherapy medication and has severe side effects, especially cardiotoxicity. Eribulin mesylate (Halaven) is used in metastatic breast cancer patients who have received at least two prior chemotherapy regimens.

Case Study

1. It is likely that micrometastases to distant sites have occurred at the time of the diagnosis of breast cancer, even in stage I disease and almost certainly in stage III disease, supporting indications for systemic treatment of the cancer following local surgical treatment. Breast cancer is one of the solid tumors that is most responsive to chemotherapy and destruction or control of tumor cells that have spread to distant sites is the goal of systemic chemotherapy.

2. a. Cyclophosphamide [C]: alkylating agent, cell cycle–phase nonspecfic
   Side effects: Myelosuppression, nausea and vomiting, alopecia, hemorrhagic cystitis
   b. Doxorubicin: Antitumor antibiotic, cell cycle–phase nonspecfic
   Side effects: Myelosuppression, mucositis, nausea and vomiting, alopecia, cardiotoxicity
   c. 5-Fluorouracil: antimetabolite, cell cycle–phase specific
   Side effects: Myelosuppression, mucositis, nausea and vomiting, alopecia, photosensitivity

3. Teach this patient to perform the following activities as necessary:
   - *Myelosuppression:*
     - Monitor her temperature every day.
     - Report any chilling; sore throat; cough; or rectal, urinary, or chest pain.
     - Keep the venous access catheter site clean and dry.
     - Avoid crowds and anyone with communicable diseases.
     - Wash the hands after toileting and before eating.
     - Report any bleeding, serious bruising, or persistent headaches.
     - Avoid using aspirin products.
     - Examine the mouth daily for blood-filled lesions.
     - Guard against bumping and other injury that might cause bleeding.
   - *Mucositis:*
     - Examine the mouth daily for bleeding, redness, or ulcers.
     - Use a mouthwash of baking soda or salt water every 2 hours as needed.
     - Use a soft-bristled toothbrush or sponge-tipped applicators for oral care.

- ○ Avoid hot, spicy, acidic foods and alcohol and tobacco.
  - ○ Drink water frequently during the day.
  - • *Nausea and vomiting*:
    - ○ Use antiemetic medications as prescribed.
    - ○ Use small, frequent meals that include bland, lukewarm, high-calorie, high-protein foods and use liquid nutritional supplements if necessary.
    - ○ Avoid strong odors and sights that increase nausea.
    - ○ Eat and drink slowly.
    - ○ Use gum, tea, or any food that stimulates salivation without causing nausea.
  - • *Alopecia*:
    - ○ Select a wig and begin to wear it before hair loss begins.
    - ○ Wear a scarf or turban to conceal hair loss.
    - ○ Use a mild, protein-based shampoo and hair conditioner every 4 to 7 days to avoid drying remaining hair.
    - ○ Avoid excessive shampooing, brushing, and combing of hair.
    - ○ Avoid the use of curling irons, curlers, blow dryers, and hair spray.

4. An estrogen receptor–positive tumor is estrogen-dependent and estrogen can promote growth of these breast cancer cells. Hormone receptor–positive cells usually are well differentiated, have low proliferative indices, and have a DNA content equal to that of normal cells. Medications such as tamoxifen (Nolvadex) or toremifene (Fareston) that block the estrogen receptor site of malignant cells can cause tumor regression and are widely used to treat recurrent or metastatic cancer that is estrogen-dependent. Fulvestrant (Faslodex) may be used with advanced breast cancer in women who no longer respond to tamoxifen. Aromatase inhibitors interfere with the enzyme aromatase, which is needed for the synthesis of estrogen. These medications include anastrozole (Arimidex), letrozole (Femara), and exemestane (Aromasin) and are used to treat breast cancer in postmenopausal women. Raloxifene (Evista) may also be prescribed. It is a selective estrogen receptor modulator that produces both estrogen-agonistic effects on bone and estrogen-antagonistic effects on breast tissue.

5. The nurse should do the following:
   - • Assist the patient to develop a positive but realistic attitude.
   - • Help her to identify sources of support and strength.
   - • Encourage her to verbalize her guilt and anger and fears about her diagnosis and the impact it is having on her life.
   - • Promote open communication between the patient and her husband.
   - • Provide accurate and complete answers to the patient's questions about her disease.
   - • Offer information about community resources and local support groups.

6. Fear, denial, embarrassment, and being too busy are common reasons that women do not perform BSE or have a mammogram and a lack of practice and skill at BSE undermines their confidence in performing the examination. Denial was probably a big factor for P.T. in view of the value of her breasts in her relationship with her husband.

7. The nurse should explain that some patients undergoing chemotherapy can have changes in maintaining focus, attention, and memory and difficulties in concentration. We currently do not know why this happens but research is being performed to determine the cause of chemobrain.

8. The nurse should teach her that she will need follow-up for the rest of her life at regular intervals. She should expect to have a professional examination every 3 to 6 months for 5 years and annually thereafter. She should be taught to perform BSE of both breasts every month and report any changes to her health care provider. Breast imaging should also be done at regular intervals, as recurrence of breast cancer is likely to happen.

9. **Nursing diagnoses:**
   - • Ineffective self-health management *related to* lack of compliance and information regarding breast cancer surveillance
   - • Ineffective coping *related to* reported feelings of guilt and perceived expectations of husband
   - • Impaired physical mobility *related to* decreased arm and shoulder mobility
   - • Disturbed body image *related to* physical and emotional effects of treatment modalities

   Collaborative problems:
   Potential complications: vascular access catheter displacement or infection, hyperuricemia, bleeding, septicemia, tumor recurrence, lymphedema

CHAPTER 53

Answer Key

1. c. Although many factors relate to the current sexually transmitted infections (STI) rates, one major factor is the widespread use of oral contraceptives instead of condoms (both male and female). Condoms are the only contraceptive device that protects against STIs.

2. c. *Chlamydia trachomatis* can cause nongonococcal urethritis in men and cervicitis in women. Herpes simplex virus causes genital herpes. *Treponema pallidum* causes syphilis. *Neisseria gonorrhoeae* causes gonorrhea.

3. c. Genital warts are caused by human papillomavirus (HPV). Syphilis is caused by *T. pallidum*. Gonorrhea is caused by *N. gonorrhoeae*. Genital herpes are caused by herpes simplex virus.

4. c. An established diagnosis of gonorrhea is treated with cefixime (Suprax) orally or with a single dose of IM ceftriaxone (Rocephin). If chlamydia is also present, azithromycin (Zithromax) or doxycycline (Vibramycin) may also be used. Gram stain smears are not useful in diagnosing gonorrhea in women because the female genitourinary tract normally harbors a large number of organisms that resemble *N. gonorrhoeae* and cultures must be performed to confirm the diagnosis in women. Penicillin was used to treat gonorrhea but gonorrhea is now resistant to penicillin. Penicillin G is used to treat syphilis. Although gonorrhea may lead to pelvic inflammatory disease (PID), its diagnosis would not necessarily indicate that the patient has PID.

5. a. Upward extension of gonorrhea or chlamydia commonly causes PID, which can cause adhesions and fibrous scarring, leading to tubal pregnancies and infertility. Disseminated gonococcal infection is rare and endocarditis and aneurysms are associated with syphilis. Polyarthritis and adenopathy are not seen in gonorrhea or chlamydia.

6. d. All sexual contacts of patients with gonorrhea must be notified, evaluated, and treated for STIs. The other information may be helpful in diagnosis and treatment but the nurse must try to identify the patient's sexual partners.

7. a, b, c, d, f. In the tertiary (or late) stage of syphilis there can be gummas (chronic destructive lesions), cardiovascular problems (heart failure, aneurysms, valve insufficiency), and neurosyphilis manifestations (mental deterioration, tabes dorsalis, and speech disturbances). Generalized cutaneous rash occurs in the secondary stage of syphilis, a few weeks after the chancre appears.

8. a. Lack of clinical manifestations but a positive treponemal antibody test with normal cerebrospinal fluid (CSF) occurs in the latent stage. The primary stage is characterized by a chancre, regional lymphadenopathy, and genital ulcers. The secondary stage has flu-like symptoms and cutaneous lesions. The late or tertiary stage is characterized by gummas, cardiovascular changes, and neurosyphilis.

9. c. Many other diseases or conditions may cause false-positive test results on nontreponemal Venereal Disease Research Laboratory (VDRL) or rapid plasma reagent (RPR) tests and additional testing is needed before a diagnosis is confirmed or treatment is administered. The diagnosis is confirmed by specific treponemal tests, such as the fluorescent antibody absorption (FTA-Abs) test or the TP-PA test. Analysis of CSF is used to diagnose asymptomatic neurosyphilis.

10. c. The risk factors of drug abuse and sexual promiscuity are found in patients with both syphilis and human immunodeficiency virus (HIV) infection and persons at highest risk for acquiring syphilis are also at high risk for acquiring HIV. Syphilitic lesions on the genitals enhance HIV transmission. Also, HIV-infected patients with syphilis appear to be at greatest risk for central nervous system (CNS) involvement and may require more intensive treatment with penicillin to prevent this complication of HIV.

11. b. Notification and treatment of sexual partners are necessary to prevent recurrence and the "ping-pong effect" of passing STIs between partners. Vibramycin is prescribed twice a day for 7 days and although alcohol may cause more urinary irritation in the patient with chlamydia, it will not interfere with treatment.

12. b. The nucleic acid amplification test (NAAT) is more sensitive than other diagnostic tests, can be done with a urine sample, and has results within 24 hours. A cell culture can be used to detect chlamydia organisms but it requires specific handling and is not as easy or as fast to perform as the NAAT. Gonorrhea and chlamydia have very similar symptoms in men and frequently occur together. Gram stain smears and cultures for *N. gonorrhoeae* do not definitively diagnose *Chlamydia*. Manifestations of epididymitis or proctitis may be present, as with other STIs, but are not diagnostic.

13. c, e. Sexual activity and stress may precipitate the recurrence of genital herpes symptoms of painful vesicular lesions that rupture and ulcerate. Acyclovir only decreases recurrences of genital herpes. Herpes simplex virus type 2 (HSV-2) may cause oral or genital lesions. Prevention of the spread of genital herpes is best done with avoidance of sexual activity when lesions are present.

14. d. HPV is responsible for causing genital warts, which manifest as discrete single or multiple white to gray warts that may coalesce to form large cauliflower-like masses on the vulva, vagina, cervix, and perianal area. Purulent vaginal discharge is associated with gonorrhea or chlamydia. Painful perineal vesicles and ulcerations are characteristic of genital herpes and a chancre of syphilis is a painless indurated lesion on the vulva, vagina, lips, or mouth.

15. a. There is a strong association of genital warts with the development of dysplasia and neoplasia of the genital tract, especially when lesions involve the cervix, introitus, and perianal and intraanal mucosa of women or the penis and perianal and anal mucosa of men. Regular Papanicolaou (Pap) tests in women are critical in detecting early malignancies of the cervix. Oral acyclovir is used to treat HSV-2 but topical use has no value in treating viral STIs. Sexual partners of patients with HPV should be examined and treated but because treatment does not destroy the virus, condoms should always be used during sexual activity. Genital warts often grow more rapidly during pregnancy but pregnancy is not contraindicated.

16. d. Women with an active herpes simplex virus (HSV) genital lesion at the time of delivery have the highest risk of transmitting genital herpes to the neonate, so delivery will be done with a cesarean section (C-section). Syphilis is spread to the fetus in utero and has a high risk of stillbirth but C-sections are not required. Treatment with parenteral penicillin will cure both the mother and the fetus. *Chlamydia* spread to the fetus can be prevented by treating the pregnant woman, so a C-section is not required. Prevention of the spread of gonorrhea to the neonate's eyes is done with erythromycin ophthalmic ointment or silver nitrate aqueous solution.

17. c. A vaccine is available for HPV types 6, 11, 16, and 18 that protects against genital warts and cervical cancer. Although sexual abstinence is the most certain method of avoiding all STIs, it is not usually a feasible alternative. Undamaged condoms also serve to protect against infection. Conscientious hand washing and voiding after intercourse are positive hygienic measures that will help to prevent secondary infections but will not prevent STIs.

18. a. STIs, such as syphilis, that can be treated with a single dose or short course of antibiotic therapy often lead to a casual attitude about the outcome of the disease, which leads to nonadherence with instructions and delays in treatment. This is particularly true of diseases that initially show few distressing or uncomfortable symptoms, such as syphilis.

Case Study

1. The nurse should tell C.J. that he must tell his fiancée the truth about the sexual encounter and that it is most important for her to be evaluated for the disease. She may have the disease without symptoms and yet be at risk for developing PID and infertility as a result of the gonorrhea. The nurse may offer a counseling referral, if necessary, for them to work through problems in their relationship.

2. Females often do not have any symptoms but Ms. A could have vaginal discharge, dysuria, urinary frequency, or changes in her menstrual patterns.

3. For the patient, the diagnosis can be confirmed by a positive Gram stain smear of urethral drainage. For the fiancée, a positive culture of cervical secretions or the urethra, anus, or oropharynx is necessary for confirmation of the diagnosis.

4. Support and counseling may be needed from the nurse and the couple should be assisted to verbalize their feelings and concerns. Active listening with a nonjudgmental attitude is important. Referral for professional counseling may be indicated.

5. Cefixime (Suprax) orally in a single dose or ceftriaxone (Rocephin) administered intramuscularly in a single dose and doxycycline (Vibramycin) or azithromycin (Zithromax) twice daily for 7 days is the recommended treatment for gonorrhea with a possible concurrent chlamydia infection. Because chlamydia infections are closely associated with gonococcal infections, both infections are usually treated concurrently, even without diagnostic evidence. Sexual activity is avoided during treatment and for 7 days after treatment.

6. *Men:* Prostatitis, urethral strictures, and sterility from orchitis or epididymitis
   Women: PID, Bartholin's abscess, ectopic pregnancy, infertility from tubal stricture
   Both men and women: Possible development of disseminated gonococcal infection

7. **Nursing diagnoses:**
   - Anxiety *related to* impact of condition on relationships and disease outcomes
   - Disturbed body image *related to* symptoms associated with gonorrhea
   - Risk for infection *related to* failure to practice precautionary measures
   Collaborative problem:
   Potential complication: infertility

CHAPTER 54

Answer Key

1. a. The initial visit of a couple seeking assistance with infertility includes a history and physical for both partners, testing for medical problems and sexually transmitted infections (STIs), a cervical Papanicolaou (Pap) test, possible semen analysis, and instruction for at-home ovulation testing. A discussion of possible future testing options and cost is also done. If the couple decides to continue with treatment, further visits will include more intensive evaluation, including postcoital testing, a hysterosalpingogram, pelvic ultrasound, and midluteal progesterone and prolactin levels.

2. c. Drug therapy will be used before more invasive treatments. Drugs may include selective estrogen receptor modulators, menotropin (human menopausal gonadotropin), follicle-stimulating hormone agonists, gonadotropin-releasing hormone (GnRH) antagonists, GnRH agonists, or human chorionic gonadotropin (hCG). If the husband's reproductive system is functioning, intrauterine insemination with his sperm will be done. The assisted reproductive technologies may be used if this is not successful. The surgery for endometriosis could be done if this was diagnosed but that is not included in this question.

3. b. In the presence of a confirmed pregnancy, uterine cramping with vaginal bleeding is the most important sign of spontaneous abortion. Other conditions causing vaginal bleeding, such as an incompetent cervix, do not usually cause cramping. There is no evidence that any medical treatment improves the outcome for spontaneous abortion. Blood loss can be significant and the loss of the pregnancy may cause long-term grieving. Dilation and curettage (D&C) (if needed) is performed after the abortion to minimize blood loss and reduce the chance of infection.

4. d. There is physical and emotional pain and grieving after an abortion that puts the patient in need of support. D&C is needed only if the products of conception do not pass completely or bleeding becomes excessive. The time it takes for the products of conception to pass depends on the type of abortion being done and is immediate with surgical abortion and slower with medical abortion.

5. d. Premenstrual syndrome (PMS) is diagnosed when other possible causes for symptoms have been eliminated. A diagnosis is based on a symptom diary that indicates the same symptoms during the luteal phase, approximately 1 week before menses, for two or three consecutive menstrual cycles. Oral contraceptives may be used to control the symptoms of PMS by suppressing ovulation and although progesterone may also relieve the symptoms of PMS, its effectiveness is not associated with the diagnosis of PMS. There are no laboratory findings that account for the premenstrual symptoms.

6. b. Limitation of refined sugar and caffeine in the diet has been shown to decrease the PMS symptoms of abdominal bloating, increased appetite, and irritability. Exercise is encouraged because it increases the release of endorphins, which elevates the mood, and also has a tranquilizing effect on muscle tension. Estrogen is not used during the luteal phase but progesterone may be tried. Vitamin B_6 and foods high in tryptophan may promote serotonin production, which improves symptoms.

7. c. The release of excess prostaglandin $F_2\alpha$ ($PGF_2\alpha$) from the endometrium at the time of menstruation or increased sensitivity to the prostaglandin is responsible for symptoms of primary dysmenorrhea and drugs that inhibit prostaglandin production and release, such as nonsteroidal antiinflammatory drugs (NSAIDs), are effective in many patients with primary dysmenorrhea. Oral contraceptives may be used for primary dysmenorrhea by reducing endometrial hyperplasia.

8. c. Young female athletes may experience amenorrhea related to excessive exercise, low body weight, or severe dieting as well as stress. If she had increased sexual activity, she would be assessed for pregnancy but decreased sexual activity will not affect her menses. Excess prostaglandin production leads to dysmenorrhea. Metrorrhagia is associated with endometrial cancer or uterine fibroids.

9. c. When ovulation does not occur, estrogen continues to be unopposed by progesterone and excessive buildup of the endometrium occurs. To prevent the risk of endometrial cancer by the buildup of the endometrium or to prevent menorrhagia from an unstable endometrium, progesterone or birth control pills are prescribed to ensure that the patient's endometrial lining will be shed at least four to six times a year. Balloon therapy to treat menorrhagia is contraindicated in women who desire future fertility.

10. d. Menorrhagia is increased duration or amount of bleeding with menses. Pain with menses is called dysmenorrhea. Metrorrhagia is excessive bleeding at irregular intervals or spotting between menstrual periods.

11. b. Ectopic pregnancy is a life-threatening condition. If the fallopian tube ruptures, profuse bleeding can lead to hypovolemic shock. All of the interventions are indicated but the priority is monitoring the vital signs and pain for evidence of bleeding.

12. a, c. The lack of estrogen in menopause contributes to many of the signs of aging, including cessation of menses, vasomotor instability (hot flashes), atrophic changes of vaginal and external genitalia and breast tissue, increased risks for coronary artery disease and osteoporosis, redistribution of fat, muscle and joint pain, loss of skin elasticity, and atrophic lower urinary tract changes.

13. b. Taking combination hormone therapy (HT) increases bone marrow density and decreases fractures. Both progestin and estrogen are recommended for a menopausal woman with a uterus. The risk for breast cancer, cardiovascular disease, and stroke are increased and the risk for endometrial cancer is decreased with combination HT.

14. c. Bacterial vaginosis is characterized by watery vaginal discharge with a fishy odor. Cervicitis displays mucopurulent discharge and postcoital spotting. Trichomoniasis has frothy greenish or gray discharge. Vulvovaginal candidiasis has thick, white, curdy discharge.

15. a, d. "Yeast infection" or vulvovaginal candidiasis has intense itching and dysuria from urine coming in contact with fissures or irritated areas in the vulva. The discharge is thick, white, and curdlike. Hemorrhagic cervix and vagina occur with trichomoniasis and produce a pruritic, frothy greenish or gray discharge. Mucopurulent discharge and postcoital spotting from cervical inflammation is seen with cervicitis.

16. a. *Gardnerella vaginalis* infection is a bacterial vaginosis that may be sexually transmitted and both partners may be infected. Treatment of the condition includes vaginal treatment with metronidazole (Flagyl) or clindamycin (Cleocin) or treatment via the oral route. Sexual activity is avoided until both partners are infection free. Minipads may be used to contain vaginal secretions but they do not prevent reinfection. Vaginal suppositories and creams are used at bedtime so that the medication remains in the vagina for a long period of time.

17. b. Sexual activity with multiple partners increases the risk for pelvic inflammatory disease (PID) and there is often a history of an acute infection of the lower genital tract caused by gonococcal or chlamydial microorganisms. The only significant contraceptive issue related to PID is that condom use will help to prevent STIs that may lead to PID.

18. b. Bed rest in semi-Fowler's position promotes drainage of the pelvic cavity by gravity and may prevent the development of abscesses high in the abdomen. Coitus, douching, and tampon use should be avoided to prevent spreading infection upward from the vagina, although frequent perineal care should be performed to remove infectious drainage.

19. c. The risk for infertility following PID is high and the nurse should allow time for the patient to express her feelings, clarify her concerns, and begin problem solving with regard to the outcomes of the disease. Responses that do not allow for discussion of feelings and concerns or that tell the patient how she should feel or what she should worry about are not therapeutic.

20. c. The treatment of endometriosis and leiomyomas is surgical when the patient does not tolerate the symptoms, with the type of surgery for endometriosis dependent on the desire for pregnancy. Endometriosis and leiomyomas subside with the onset of menopause. Therefore the medications to treat them create a pseudomenopause. The ectopic uterine tissue is endometriosis, while leiomyomas are fibrous smooth muscle tumors.

21. d. Left untreated, polycystic ovary syndrome (PCOS) may lead to cardiovascular disease and abnormal insulin resistance with type 2 diabetes mellitus. Hirsutism may be treated with spironolactone. Leuprolide is used to treat hyperandrogenism but PCOS cannot be cured. Severity of symptoms is associated with obesity but the hormone abnormalities will be treated along with the obesity to prevent complications. If this treatment is not successful, a hysterectomy with bilateral salpingectomy and oophorectomy may be performed.

22. b. A stage 0 cervical cancer indicates cancer in situ that is confined to the epithelial layer of the cervix and requires treatment. Stage 0 is the least invasive. Stage I is confined to the cervix. Stage II has spread beyond the cervix to the upper two thirds of the vagina but not the tissues around the uterus. Stage III involves the pelvic wall, lower third of the vagina, and/or kidney problems. Stage IV indicates spread to distant organs.

23. c. Conization (an excision of a cone-shaped section of the cervix) and laser treatment both are effective to locally remove or destroy malignant cells of the cervix and preserve fertility. Radiation treatments frequently impair ovarian and uterine function and lead to sterility. A subtotal hysterectomy would be contraindicated in the treatment of cervical cancer because the cervix would be left intact in this procedure.

24. a. Postmenopausal vaginal bleeding is the first sign of endometrial cancer. When it occurs, a sample of endometrial tissue must be taken to exclude cancer. An endometrial biopsy can be done as an office procedure and is indicated in this case. Abdominal x-rays and Pap tests are not reliable tests for endometrial cancer. Laser treatment of the cervix is indicated only for cervical dysplasia.

25. b. Treatment of ovarian cancer is determined by staging from the results of laparoscopy with multiple biopsies of the ovaries and other tissue throughout the pelvis and lower abdomen. The patient's desire for fertility is not a consideration because of the high mortality rate associated with ovarian cancer. Although diagnosis of ovarian tumors may be made by transvaginal ultrasound or computed tomography (CT) scan, the treatment of ovarian cancer depends on the staging of the tumor.

26. a. Vaginal cancer is usually related to metastases of other cancers or intrauterine exposure to diethylstilbestrol (DES).

27. a, b, f. Endometrial cancer is at higher risk in obese patients because adipose cells store estrogen, which is the major risk factor, especially unopposed estrogen. Smoking is a risk factor for endometrial and cervical cancer. Early sexual activity is a risk factor for cervical cancer. Family history and early menarche and late menopause causing increased menstrual cycles are risk factors for ovarian cancer.

28. a. Early signs of cancer of the vulva include pruritus, soreness of the vulva, unusual odor, and discharge or bleeding of the vulva, with edema of the vulva and lymphadenopathy occurring as the disease progresses. Labial lesions and excoriation more commonly occur with infections and nodules are more often cysts or lipomas.

29. c. A total hysterectomy involves the removal of the uterus and possibly the cervix but the fallopian tubes and ovaries are left intact. Although menstruation is terminated, normal ovarian production of estrogen continues. When the tubes and ovaries are removed, it is called a bilateral salpingo-oophorectomy. A panhysterectomy is the procedure in which the uterus and cervix as well as the tubes and ovaries are removed.

30. c. A pelvic exenteration is the most radical gynecologic surgery and results in removal of the uterus, ovaries, fallopian tubes, vagina, bladder, urethra, and pelvic lymph nodes and, in some situations, also the descending colon, rectum, and anal canal. There are urinary and fecal diversions on the abdominal wall, the absence of a vagina, and the onset of menopausal symptoms, all of which result in severe altered body structure and changes in body image. The patient and family will need much understanding and support during the long recovery period, including verbalization of feelings.

31. d. To prevent displacement of the intrauterine implant, the patient is maintained on absolute bed rest with turning from side to side. Bowel elimination is discouraged during the treatment by cleaning the colon before implantation and urinary elimination is maintained by an indwelling catheter. Because the patient is radioactive, no individual nurse should spend more than 30 minutes daily with the patient and visitors are restricted to less than 3 hours each day at a minimum of 6 feet from the patient.

32. a. The muscles that should be exercised are those affected by trying to stop a flow of urine. Kegel exercises help to strengthen muscular support of the perineum, pelvic floor, and bladder and are also beneficial for problems with pelvic support and stress incontinence.

33. c. A uterine prolapse occurs when the uterus is displaced through the vagina, causing the feeling of something coming down her vagina, a backache, dyspareunia, or a heavy feeling in the pelvis.

34. d. The primary goal of care is to prevent wound infection and pressure on the vaginal incision, which requires perineal cleansing at least twice daily and after each urination and defecation. An ice pack and stool softener will be used but they are not the priority. The enema would have been done preoperatively.

35. a. An anterior colporrhaphy involves repair of a cystocele and an indwelling urinary catheter is left in place for several days postoperatively while healing occurs. Bowel function should not be altered and is maintained with a low-residue diet and a stool softener if necessary to avoid straining and pressure on the incision.

36. b. Sexual assault is an act of violence and the first priority of care for the patient should be assessment and treatment of serious injuries involving extragenital areas, such as fractures, subdural hematomas, cerebral concussions, and intraabdominal injuries. All of the other options are appropriate treatments but treatment for shock and urgent medical injuries is the first priority.

37. a. Specific informed consent must be obtained from the rape victim before any examination can be made or rape data collected. Following consent, the patient is advised not to wash, eat, drink, or urinate before the examination so that evidence can be collected for medicolegal use. Prophylaxis for STIs, hepatitis B, and tetanus is administered following examination and follow-up testing for pregnancy and human immunodeficiency virus (HIV) is done in several weeks.

Case Study

1. The gonococcus spreads directly along the endometrium to the tubes and into the peritoneum, resulting in salpingitis, pelvic peritonitis, or tubo-ovarian abscesses.

2. Clinical manifestations include crampy or continuous bilateral lower abdominal pain that is increased with movement or ambulation. Other manifestations are irregular menstrual bleeding and vaginal discharge that is purulent with a foul odor, dyspareunia, fever and chills, and possible nausea and vomiting.

3. Outpatient management would include oral antibiotics, increased fluid intake, good nutrition, restriction of activities, rest with the head elevated, and examination and treatment of her partner(s). She should be instructed to avoid intercourse, douching, and tampons and to return for follow-up in 48 to 72 hours. She should be instructed to return to the hospital if the pain is not relieved, if symptoms of Fitz-Hugh-Curtis syndrome (e.g., right upper quadrant pain, pelvic or generalized peritonitis) occur, or if symptoms of septic shock (e.g., shortness of breath, decreased urination, confusion) occur.

4. Chronic pelvic pain occurs in up to one third of women who have PID. There may be severe steady pain, intermittent pain, dull and achy pain, pelvic pressure or heaviness, and sharp pains or cramping as well as pain during intercourse or while having a bowel movement.

5. Elevating the head of the bed promotes drainage of the pelvic cavity by gravity and may prevent the development of abscesses high in the abdomen. Monitoring vital signs for septic shock is also a priority.

6. Clarify the possible course and outcomes of the disease with the patient. Although early treatment may help to prevent complications, it is realistic that sterility often results from PID because of adhesions and strictures of the fallopian tubes. She is at increased risk for ectopic pregnancies. Discuss and listen to her concerns about her future childbearing ability.

7. **Nursing diagnoses:**
   • Ineffective health maintenance *related to* lack of protective measures against STIs
   • Pain *related to* movement and sexual intercourse
   • Anxiety *related to* outcome of disease on reproductive status
   • Risk for impaired skin integrity *related to* vaginal drainage
   Collaborative problems:
   Potential complications: peritonitis, septic shock, thromboembolism, Fitz-Hugh-Curtis syndrome

CHAPTER 55

Answer Key

1. d. Hyperplasia is an increase in the number of cells and in benign prostatic hyperplasia (BPH), it is thought that the enlargement caused by the increase in new cells results from hormonal changes associated with aging. Hypertrophy refers to an increase in the size of existing cells. The hyperplasia is not considered a tumor, nor has BPH been proven to predispose to cancer of the prostate.

2. c. Classic symptoms of uncomplicated BPH are those associated with irritative symptoms, including nocturia, frequency, urgency, dysuria, bladder pain, and incontinence associated with inflammation or infection. Urinary obstruction symptoms include diminished caliber and force of the urinary stream, hesitancy, difficulty initiating voiding, intermittent urination, dribbling at the end of urination, and a feeling of incomplete bladder emptying because of urinary retention.

3. c. Urinary flow meters are used to measure the urinary flow rate, which is slowed with increased obstruction. Cystourethroscopy may also evaluate the degree of obstruction but a cystometrogram measures bladder tone. A transrectal ultrasound may determine the size and configuration of the prostate gland. Postvoiding catheterization measures residual urine.

4. a. Finasteride results in suppression of androgen formation by inhibiting the formation of the testosterone metabolite dihydroxytestosterone, the principal prostatic androgen, and results in a decrease in the size of the prostate gland. α-Adrenergic blockers are used to cause smooth muscle relaxation in the prostate that improves urine flow. Drugs affecting bladder tone are not indicated.

5. c. Because of edema, urinary retention, and delayed sloughing of tissue that occurs with a laser prostatectomy, the patient will have postprocedure catheterization for up to 7 days. The procedure is done under local anesthetic, and incontinence or urinary retention is not usually a problem with laser prostatectomy.

6. d. The prostate gland can be easily palpated by rectal examination and enlargement of the gland is detected early if yearly examinations are performed. If symptoms of prostatic hyperplasia are present, further diagnostic testing, including a urinalysis, prostate-specific antigen (PSA), and cystoscopy, may be indicated.

7. b. The transurethral needle ablation (TUNA) uses low-wave radiofrequency to heat the prostate, causing necrosis. Laser prostatectomy uses a laser beam. Transurethral microwave thermotherapy (TUMT) uses microwave radiating heat to produce coagulative necrosis of the prostate and is not used for men with rectal problems. Transurethral electrovaporization of prostate (TUVP) uses electrosurgical vaporization and desiccation to destroy prostate tissue.

8. e, f. The transurethral resection of the prostate (TURP) is the most common surgical procedure to treat BPH and uses a resectoscopic excision and cauterization of prostate tissue. A simple open prostatectomy is used for a large prostate and has an external incision. Transurethral incision into the prostate to expand the urethra for a small to moderate-sized prostate is done with a transurethral incision of the prostate (TUIP).

9. b, c, d. TUNA, TUIP, and TUMT are currently done on an outpatient basis or in a health care provider's office.

10. b. Because of injury to the internal urinary sphincter, there is usually some degree of retrograde ejaculation following most transurethral surgeries, especially following TURP. The semen is ejaculated into the bladder and is eliminated with the next voiding. Urinary incontinence, erectile dysfunction, and continued catheterization are uncommon following TURP.

11. c. Bleeding and blood clots from the bladder are expected after prostatectomy and continuous irrigation is used to keep clots from obstructing the urinary tract. The rate of the irrigation may be titrated to keep the clots from forming, if ordered, but the nurse should also check the vital signs because hemorrhage is the most common complication of prostatectomy. The traction on the catheter applies pressure to the operative site to control bleeding and should be relieved only if specific orders are given. The catheter does not need to be manually irrigated unless there are signs that the catheter is obstructed and clamping the drainage tube is contraindicated because it would cause distention of the bladder.

12. b. The nurse should first check for the presence of clots obstructing the catheter or tubing and then may administer a belladonna and opium (B&O) suppository if one is ordered. The patient should not try to void around the catheter because this will increase the spasms. The flow rate of the irrigation fluid may be decreased if orders permit because fast-flowing, cold fluid may also contribute to spasms.

13. b. Activities that increase intraabdominal pressure should be avoided until the surgeon approves these activities at a follow-up visit. Stool softeners and high-fiber diets may be used to promote bowel elimination but enemas should not be used because they increase intraabdominal pressure and may initiate bleeding. Because TURP does not remove the entire prostate gland, the patient needs annual prostatic examinations to screen for cancer of the prostate. Fluid intake should be high but caffeine and alcohol should not be used because they have a diuretic effect and increase bladder distention.

14. c. Most prostate cancers (about 75%) are considered sporadic. About the only modifiable risk factor for prostate cancer is its association with a diet high in red and processed meat and high-fat dairy products along with a low intake of vegetables and fruits. Age, ethnicity, and family history are risk factors for prostate cancer but are not modifiable. Simple enlargement or hyperplasia of the prostate is not a risk factor for prostate cancer.

15. c. A prostatectomy performed with a perineal approach has a high risk for infection because of the proximity of the wound to the anus, so wound care is the priority. Chemotherapy is usually not the first choice of drug therapy following surgery, nor is sildenafil. The catheter size would not be changed but the catheter would be removed. Urinary incontinence is a bigger problem than retention.

16. a, b, f. Pelvic or perineal pain, fatigue, malaise, and a hard asymmetric prostate may be present with prostate cancer. Annual prostate examination is recommended starting at a younger age for African American men because of increased diagnosis and mortality from prostate cancer in this ethnic group. An orchiectomy may be done with prostatectomy or for metastatic stages of prostate cancer.

Hormonal treatment includes androgen deprivation therapy, luteinizing hormone–releasing hormone agonists, and androgen receptor blockers. Early detection of prostate cancer is best detected with annual rectal exams and serum PSA. Elevated prostatic acid phosphatase (PAP) will be seen with metastasis, not a new diagnosis.

17. d. The prostate with chronic bacterial prostatitis feels enlarged and firm, often described as boggy, and is tender. The other options are true of both chronic and acute prostatitis.

18. c. Hypospadias is the urethral meatus located on the ventral surface of the penis. Scrotal lymphedema is called a hydrocele. An undescended testicle is cryptorchidism. Inflammation of the prepuce or foreskin is called phimosis.

19. d. Paraphimosis is tightness of the foreskin and the inability to pull it forward from a retracted position to return it over the glans. It is usually associated with poor hygiene techniques. Painful, prolonged erection is priapism. Epididymitis is inflammation of the epididymis. A painful downward curvature of an erect penis is chordee.

20. d. The cremasteric reflex is elicited by light stroking of the inner aspect of the thigh in a downward direction with a tongue blade. In testicular torsion, or a twisted spermatic cord that supplies blood to the testes and epididymis, this reflex is absent on the swollen side. Varicocele is dilation of the veins that drain the testes. Hydrocele is scrotal lymphedema from interference with lymphatic drainage of the scrotum. Spermatocele is a sperm-containing cyst of the epididymis.

21. b. α-Fetoprotein (AFP) and human chorionic gonadotropin (hCG) are glycoproteins that may be elevated in testicular cancer. If they are elevated before surgical treatment, the levels are noted, and if response to therapy is positive, the levels will decrease. Lactate dehydrogenase (LDH) may also be elevated. Tumor necrosis factor (TNF) is a normal cytokine responsible for tumor surveillance and destruction. C-reactive protein (CRP) is found in inflammatory conditions and widespread malignancies. PSA and PAP are used for screening of prostatic cancer. Carcinoembryonic antigen (CEA) is a tumor marker for cancers of the GI system. Antinuclear antibody (ANA) is found most frequently in autoimmune disorders.

22. d. Testicular tumors most often present on the testis as a lump or nodule that is very firm, is nontender, and cannot be transilluminated. There may also be scrotal swelling and a feeling of heaviness. All of the other options are normal findings.

23. c. Until sperm distal to the anastomotic site is ejaculated or absorbed by the body, the semen will contain sperm and alternative contraceptive methods must be used. When a postoperative semen examination reveals no sperm, the patient is considered sterile. Following vasectomy, there is rarely noticeable difference in the amount of ejaculate because ejaculate is primarily seminal fluid. Vasectomy does not cause erectile dysfunction, nor does it affect testicular production of sperm or hormones.

24. a. Before treatment for erectile dysfunction is initiated, the cause must be determined so that appropriate treatment can be planned. Only a small percentage of erectile dysfunction is caused by psychologic factors. In the case of the 80% to 90% of erectile dysfunction that is of physiologic causes,

interventions are directed at correcting or eliminating the cause or restoring function by medical means. New invasive or experimental treatments are not widely used and should be limited to research centers and patients with systemic diseases can be treated medically if the cause cannot be eliminated.

25. d. Intraurethral devices include the use of vasoactive drugs administered as a topical gel, an injection into the penis (intracavernosal self-injection), or a medication pellet (alprostadil) inserted into the urethra (intraurethral) using a medicated urethral system for erection (MUSE) device. A medication pellet inserted into the urethra using a MUSE device, a topical gel, or the intracavernosal self-injection of vasoactive drugs may be used for erectile dysfunction. The vasoactive drugs enhance blood flow into the penile arteries for erection. Erectogenic drugs (e.g., tadalafil [Cialis]) cause smooth muscle relaxation and increase blood flow to promote an erection. Blood drawn into corporeal bodies and held with a ring is achieved with a vacuum constriction device (VCD). Devices implanted into corporeal bodies to firm the penis are penile implants. Androgen or testosterone replacement therapy may also be used for erectile dysfunction.

26. a. The gel may spread the testosterone to others if it is not washed off of his hands after application. If his wife applies the gel, she should wear gloves to prevent absorption of the testosterone and its effects on her body. Clothing over the area until it has dried is recommended. The gel is only topical; a buccal testosterone tablet is called Striant.

27. d. Varicocele is the most common testicular cause of infertility. Surgical ligation of the spermatic vein is done to correct the problem. Antibiotics are used if there is an infection but this is not as common as a varicocele. Semen analysis is the first study done when investigating male infertility but it is not a treatment. Avoidance of scrotal heat is a lifestyle change that may be used with idiopathic infertility.

Case Study

1. Testicular tumors develop either from the cellular components of the testis (very rare and usually benign) or from the embryonal precursors (germinal tumors that are almost always malignant). Risk factors include age between 15 and 35, a history of cryptorchidism, family history of testicular cancer, orchitis, human immunodeficiency virus (HIV) infection, maternal exposure to diethylstilbestrol (DES), and testicular cancer in the contralateral testis.

2. The primary difference on testicular examination between a spermatocele and a testicular cancer is that spermatocele will transilluminate whereas cancer cannot be transilluminated.

3. About 95% of patients with testicular cancer that is found in early stages obtain a complete remission. This patient has no back pain or gynecomastia, which are manifestations that would indicate metastatic disease. His prognosis is positive but he will need careful monitoring to detect any relapse early.

4. AFP and hCG are frequently elevated in testicular cancer and should be noted before treatment. If these markers are elevated before treatment and then decrease after treatment,

a positive response to treatment is indicated. The levels of AFP and hCG are monitored during long-term follow-up to detect any relapse of the tumor.

5. The nurse should initiate conversation with him about his concerns and allow him to talk about them. It is important to discuss the option of sperm banking before his surgery in case he later wants to have children.

6. The orchiectomy and lymph node resection will most likely be followed by radiation of the remaining lymph nodes and/or a single or multiple chemotherapy regimens. The surgery will cause sterility but the surgery and additional treatment should not alter his sexual function.

7. Seminoma germ cell tumors are very sensitive to radiation and germ cell tumors are more sensitive to systemic chemotherapy than other adult solid tumors, so its use is recommended.

8. Spermatogenesis may return but because of the high risk for infertility, sperm may be cryopreserved in a sperm bank before treatment begins. However, ejaculatory dysfunction may be impaired.

9. **Nursing diagnoses:**
   • Anxiety *related to* effects of surgery
   • Fear *related to* outcome of disease process and prognosis
   • Deficient knowledge *related to* unfamiliarity with information

CHAPTER 56

Answer Key

1. a. Mitochondrion; b. nucleolus; c. nucleus; d. axon; e. Schwann cell; f. myelin sheath; g. collateral axon; h. node of Ranvier; i. telodendria; j. synaptic knobs; k. neuron cell body; l. dendrites

2. a. Dura mater; b. arachnoid; c. pia mater; d. ventral root; e. dorsal root; f. white matter; g. central canal; h. spinal cord; i. gray matter; j. anterior horn; k. spinal ganglia; l. spinal nerves; m. transverse process of vertebra; n. sympathetic ganglion; o. body of vertebra

3. d. The protective fluid of the central nervous system (CNS) is cerebrospinal fluid (CSF). The synaptic cleft is the space where neurotransmitters cross from neuron to neuron. The limbic system is the area of the brain concerned with emotion, aggression, feeding behavior, and sexual response. Myelin is the white insulator for the conduction of impulses in the CNS and peripheral nervous system (PNS).

4. c. Schwann cells are the macroglial cells that myelinate peripheral nerve fibers. Astrocytes provide structural support to neurons and form the blood-brain barrier with the endothelium of blood vessels. Ependymal cells line the brain ventricles and aid in secretion of CSF. Neurons are not glial cells.

5. c. The presynaptic terminal submits neurotransmitter impulses through the synaptic cleft to the receptor site on the postsynaptic cell, either another neuron or a gland or muscles. If there are enough presynaptic cells releasing excitatory neurotransmitters on a single neuron, the sum of their input is enough to generate an action potential. The synapse is not a physical connection between neurons, as there is a space between them where the neurotransmitter goes from one to the other.

6. b. The dendrite carries impulses to the nerve cell body. The gap in the peripheral nerve axons is the node of Ranvier that allows an action potential to travel faster by jumping from node to node without traversing the insulated membrane segment. The axon carries impulses from the nerve cell body. Regeneration may occur with damage to peripheral axons.

7. b. The fasciculus gracilis and fasciculus cuneatus tracts carry information and transmit impulses concerned with touch, deep pressure, vibration, position sense, and kinesthesia. Spinothalamic tracts carry pain and temperature sensations. The spinocerebellar tracts carry subconscious information about muscle tension and body position. Descending corticobulbar tracts carry impulses responsible for voluntary impulses from the cortex to the cranial and peripheral nerves.

8. a. The cell bodies of lower motor neurons that send impulses to skeletal muscles in the arms, legs, and trunk are located in the anterior horn of the spinal cord and lesions generally cause weakness or paralysis, decreased muscle tone, hyporeflexia, and flaccidity. Upper motor neurons include the brainstem and cerebral cortex motor neurons that influence skeletal muscle movement. Lesions at this point cause weakness and paralysis with hyperreflexia and spasticity.

9. a. The medulla contains the vital centers concerned with respiratory, vasomotor, and cardiac function. The cerebellum maintains trunk stability and equilibrium but is not related to respiratory or cardiac function. The parietal lobe interprets spatial information and controls the sensory cortex. Wernicke's area is responsible for language comprehension.

10. b. The occipital lobes are responsible for visual perception. This patient may experience inability to identify colors, hallucinations, vision loss, or total blindness. Heat is sensed with the sensory part of the cerebrum. The olfactory nerve is responsible for identifying smells. Broca's area regulates verbal expression.

11. c. Endocrine and autonomic nervous system (ANS) function is regulated by the hypothalamus. The basal ganglia function includes initiation, execution, and completion of voluntary movements, learning, emotional response, and automatic movements associated with skeletal muscle activity. The temporal lobe integrates somatic, visual, and auditory data and contains Wernicke's area. The reticular activating system regulates arousal and sleep-wake transitions with communication among the brainstem, reticular formation in the brainstem, and the cerebral cortex.

12. c. The thalamus relays sensory and motor input to and from the cerebrum. Auditory input is registered by the superior temporal gyrus. Past experiences are integrated by the anterior temporal lobe. The basal ganglia controls and facilitates learned and automatic movements.

13. d. Some cranial nerves (CNs) are only efferent motor nerves (e.g., III, IV, VI, VII, XI, XII), some are only afferent sensory nerves (e.g., I, II, VIII), and some have both motor and sensory functions (e.g., V, IX, X) but spinal nerves always have both sensory and motor fibers. Both cranial and spinal nerves occur in pairs and whereas most cell bodies of CNs are located in the brain, the primary cell bodies of CN I, II, and XI are located outside of the brain.

14. b, c, d, e. Descriptions or characteristics of the sympathetic nervous system (SNS) include being necessary for male ejaculation, increases heart rate (HR) and dilates coronary arteries. Most postganglionic fibers release norepinephrine and preganglionic cell bodies are located in spinal segments T1–L2.

15. b. The circle of Willis is a vascular circle formed by the arteries that join the basilar artery and the internal carotid arteries. It may act as an anastomotic pathway when occlusion of a major artery on one side of the brain occurs. The middle cerebral artery supplies the outer portions of the frontal, parietal, and superior temporal lobes but the circle of Willis may accommodate for plaque in this artery.

16. b. The falx cerebri is a fold of the dura that separates the cerebral hemispheres and slows expansion of brain tissue. The ventricles produce CSF. The arachnoid layer is a membrane that forms a space with the pia mater for blood vessels and nerves to pass through. The tentorium cerebella is a fold of dura that separates the cerebral hemispheres from the posterior fossa that contains the brainstem and cerebellum.

17. b. The blood-brain barrier physiologically protects the brain from harmful agents in the blood. The skull protects the brain from external trauma. The vertebral column allows flexibility while protecting the spinal cord. The dura mater is the outer protective membrane.

18. c. A decrease in sensory receptors caused by degenerative changes leads to a diminished sense of touch, temperature, and pain in the older adult. Reflexes are decreased but not normally absent and intelligence does not decrease, although there may be some loss of memory. Hypothalamic modifications lead to increased frequency of spontaneous awakening with interrupted sleep and insomnia.

19. a, c, e. When taking the history of a patient with a neurologic problem, avoid suggesting symptoms or asking leading questions. The mode of onset and course of the illness are especially important. Validate the history if the patient's mental status causes question as to the reliability of the history. The other options are part of the physical assessment and will depend on the patient's history and manifestations.

20.

Functional Health Pattern	Risk Factor for or Patient Response to Neurologic Problem
Health perception–health management	Uncontrolled hypertension, lack of appropriate helmet or seat belt use, family history of neurologic problems, substance abuse, smoking, malnutrition, mental or physical changes noticed by others
Nutritional-metabolic	Difficulty chewing and swallowing, B-vitamin deficiency
Elimination	Bowel or bladder incontinence, constipation; frequency of episodes, sensations and measures to control
Activity-exercise	Problems in mobility, strength, and coordination; history of falling; activities of daily living (ADL) performance
Sleep-rest	Sleep disturbances from pain or immobility; insomnia, frequent awakening; hallucinations
Cognitive-perceptual	Pain; sensory changes, dizziness; cognitive changes; language difficulties
Self-perception–self-concept	Decreased self-worth and body image; unkempt physical appearance and hygiene
Role-relationship	Changes in roles at work or in family from neurologic problems
Sexuality-reproductive	Decreased sexual desire, stimulation, function, or response
Coping–stress tolerance	Sense of being overwhelmed, inadequate coping patterns
Value-belief	Life-changing effects; religious or cultural beliefs that interfere or assist with planned treatment

21. b, d, e. The trochlear (CN IV), abducens (CN VI), and oculomotor (CN III) nerves cause oblique eye movement. The optic nerve (CN II) is for vision. The trigeminal nerve (CN V) provides sensation from the face and the motor function of mastication.

22. c. The trigeminal (CN V) and facial (CN VII) nerves both respond to the corneal reflex test. The optic (CN II) nerve responds to confrontation. The vagus (CN X) nerve provides the gag reflex with the glossopharyngeal (CN IX) nerve. The spinal accessory (CN XI) nerve is tested with the resistive shoulder shrug.

23. c, e, f. The facial (CN VII) nerve is assessed with the corneal reflex test; smile, frown, and close eyes; and salt and sugar discrimination. Gag reflex is used to evaluate the glossopharyngeal (CN IX) and vagus (CN X) nerves.

Confrontation is used to assess the optic (CN II) nerve. Light touch to the face and the corneal reflex test are used to evaluate the trigeminal (CN V) nerve.

24. c. The hypoglossal (CN XII) nerve is tested with tongue protrusion. The vagus (CN X) and glossopharyngeal (CN IX) nerves are tested with the gag reflex. The olfactory (CN I) nerve is tested with odor identification.

25. d. The cochlear branch of the acoustic (CN VIII) nerve should enable the patient to hear. The patient may be distracted or hard of hearing but the damage to the nerve is most likely the cause of the inability to hear the ticking watch, as the nurse should ensure that there are no distractions or extraneous noise when performing this test. The vagus (CN X) nerve is unrelated to hearing.

26. c. The primary purposes of the nursing neurologic examination are to determine the effects of neurologic dysfunction on daily living and the patient's and the family's ability to cope with neurologic deficits. The examination should be viewed in terms of functional disabilities rather than dysfunction of component parts of the nervous system. Findings of the examination should be used to plan appropriate care for deficits in self-care and in ADLs.

27. b. The heel-to-shin test tests coordination and cerebellar function. Muscle tone is assessed by passively moving limbs through their range of motion. Plantar stimulation tests extensor plantar response. Loss of proprioception (or position sense) is assessed by placing the thumb and forefinger on either side of the patient's forefinger or great toe and gently moving it up and down, then asking the patient to indicate the direction in which the digit was moved.

28. d. Extinction is assessed by simultaneously stimulating both sides of the body; it is abnormal if the patient extinguishes one stimulus and perceives the stimulus only on one side. Pain sensation is assessed by touching the sharp and dull end of a pin to each of the patient's limbs with the patient responding "sharp" or "dull" each time. The cotton wisp assesses light touch. A tuning fork to bony prominences assesses vibration sense.

29. c. A positive Romberg test is demonstrated when the patient is unable to maintain balance with the feet together and then closing the eyes. Pronator drift is observed when the patient holds both arms fully extended at shoulder level in front of him with the palms upward but the patient is unable to maintain the position. Absent patellar reflex is when there is no response to striking the patellar tendon just below the patella. Absence of two-point discrimination is seen when the two points of a calibrated compass are on the tips of the fingers and are not recognized as two distinct points.

30. b. The normal response of the triceps reflex is extension of the arm or visible contraction of the triceps. The normal response of the biceps reflex is flexion of the arm at the elbow whereas the presence of the brachioradialis reflex is seen with flexion and supination at the elbow.

31. b. This is a normal patellar reflex response. Deep-tendon grading is as follows: 0/5 = absent; 1/5 = weak response; 2/5 = normal response; 3/5 = exaggerated response; 4/5 = hyperreflexia with clonus.

32. d. To facilitate insertion of the spinal needle between the third and fourth lumbar vertebrae, the patient should round the spine by flexing the knees, hips, and neck while in a lateral recumbent position. Sitting on the edge of the bed and bending only the spine does not separate the vertebrae as efficiently. Stimulants are withheld for 8 hours before an electroencephalogram (EEG) and sedation is used for more invasive tests, such as myelograms and angiography.

33. a. A spinal headache, which may be caused by loss of CSF at the puncture site, is common following a lumbar puncture or a myelogram and nuchal rigidity may also occur as a result of meningeal irritation. The patient is not in danger of paralysis with a lumbar puncture, nor does hemorrhage from the site occur. Contrast media are not used with a lumbar puncture.

34. b. Following a myelogram (and a lumbar puncture), the patient is positioned flat in bed for several hours to avoid a spinal headache and fluids are encouraged to help in the excretion of the contrast medium. Pain at the insertion site is rare and the most common complaint after a myelogram is a headache.

35. b. Cerebral angiography involves the injection of contrast media through a catheter inserted into the femoral or brachial artery and passed into the base of a carotid or vertebral artery and is performed when vascular lesions or tumors are suspected. Allergic reactions to the contrast medium may occur and vascular spasms or dislodgement of plaques is possible. Neurologic and vital signs must be monitored every 15 to 30 minutes for 2 hours, every hour for the next 6 hours, and then every 2 hours for 24 hours following the test. EEGs and transcranial Doppler sonography are not invasive studies.

36. d. Normal glucose levels in CSF are 40 to 70 mg/dL. All types of organisms consume glucose, and a decreased glucose level reflects bacterial activity. Increased levels are associated with diabetes. The other values are all normal.

CHAPTER 57

Answer Key

1. a, c, e. Blood adapts with increased venous outflow, decreased cerebral blood flow (CBF), and collapse of veins and dural sinuses. Brain tissue adapts with distention of the dura, slight compression of tissue, or herniation. Cerebrospinal fluid (CSF) adapts with increased absorption, decreased production, and displacement into the spinal canal. Skull bone and scalp tissue do not adapt to changes in intracranial pressure (ICP).

2. 56 mm Hg
   Mean arterial pressure (MAP) = diastolic blood pressure (DBP) + ⅓ (systolic blood pressure [SBP] – DBP) = 52 + 18 = 70
   Cerebral perfusion pressure (CPP) = MAP – ICP = 70 – 14 = 56

3. 45 mm Hg
   MAP = DBP + ⅓ (SBP – DBP) = 64 + 15 = 79
   CPP = MAP – ICP = 79 – 34 = 45

4. c, e. Cerebral blood flow is decreased when the MAP and the $PaCO_2$ are decreased. The other options increase cerebral blood flow.

5. b, e. Vasogenic cerebral edema, the most common type of edema, occurs mainly in the white matter and is characterized by leakage of macromolecules from the capillaries into the surrounding extracellular space. This results in an osmotic gradient that favors the flow of fluid from the intravascular to the extravascular space. A variety of insults, such as brain tumors, abscesses, and ingested toxins, may cause an increase in the permeability of the blood-brain barrier and produce an increase in the extracellular fluid volume. Hydrocephalus causes interstitial cerebral edema.

6. a, b, d. Increased ICP is caused by vasodilation and edema from the initial brain insult or necrotic tissue. Blood vessel compression and brainstem compression and herniation occur as a result of increased ICP.

7. c. One of the most sensitive signs of increased ICP is a decreasing level of consciousness (LOC). A decrease in LOC will occur before changes in vital signs, ocular signs, or projectile vomiting occur.

8. c. Cushing's triad consists of three vital sign measures that reflect ICP and its effect on the medulla, hypothalamus, pons, and thalamus. Because these structures are very deep, Cushing's triad is usually a late sign of ICP. The signs include an increasing SBP with a widening pulse pressure, a bradycardia with a full and bounding pulse, and irregular respirations.

9. c. The dural structures that separate the two hemispheres and the cerebral hemispheres from the cerebellum influence the patterns of cerebral herniation. A cingulate herniation occurs where there is lateral displacement of brain tissue beneath the falx cerebri. Uncal herniation occurs when there is lateral and downward herniation. Tentorial herniation occurs when the brain herniates down through the opening created by the brainstem. The temporal lobe can be involved in central herniation.

10. a. An intraventricular catheter is a fluid-coupled system that can provide direct access for microorganisms to enter the ventricles of the brain and aseptic technique is a very high nursing priority to decrease the risk for infection. Constant monitoring of ICP waveforms is not usually necessary and removal of CSF for sampling or to maintain normal ICP is done only when specifically ordered.

11. b. An inaccurate ICP reading can be caused by CSF leaks around the monitor device, obstruction of the intraventricular catheter, kinks or bubbles in the tubing, and incorrect height of the transducer or drainage system relative to the patient's reference point. The P2 wave being higher than the P1 wave indicates poor ventricular compliance. The transducer height should be at the tragus of the ear. The drain of the CSF drainage device should be closed for 6 minutes preceding the reading.

12. b. The normal pressure of oxygen in brain tissue ($PbtO_2$) is 20 to 40 mm Hg. The normal jugular venous oxygen saturation ($SjvO_2$) is 55% to 75% and indicates total venous brain tissue extraction of oxygen; this is used for short-term monitoring. The MAP of 70 to 150 mm Hg is needed for effective autoregulation of CBF. The normal range for PaO_2 is 80 to 100 mm Hg.

13. c. Mannitol (Osmitrol) (25%) is an osmotic diuretic that expands plasma and causes fluid to move from tissues into the blood vessels. Hypertonic saline reduces brain swelling by moving water out of brain tissue. Oxygen administration is done to maintain brain function. Pentobarbital (Nembutal) and other barbiturates are used to reduce cerebral metabolism. The corticosteroid dexamethasone (Decadron) is used to treat vasogenic edema to stabilize cell membranes and improve neuronal function by improving CBF and restoring autoregulation.

14. d. A patient with increased ICP is in a hypermetabolic and hypercatabolic state and needs adequate glucose to maintain fuel for the brain and other nutrients to meet metabolic needs. Malnutrition promotes cerebral edema and if a patient cannot take oral nutrition, other means of providing nutrition should be used, such as tube feedings or parenteral nutrition. Glucose alone is not adequate to meet nutritional requirements and 5% dextrose solutions may increase cerebral edema by lowering serum osmolarity. Patients should remain in a normovolemic fluid state with close monitoring of clinical factors such as urine output, fluid intake, serum and urine osmolality, serum electrolytes, and insensible losses.

15. a. The Glasgow Coma Scale (GCS) is used to quickly assess the LOC with a standardized system. The three areas assessed are the patient's ability to speak, obey commands, and open eyes to verbal or painful stimulus. Although best motor response is an indicator, it is not used to assess coordination.

16. b. No opening of eyes = 1; incomprehensible words = 2; flexion withdrawal = 4. Total = 7

17. d. Of the body functions that should be assessed in an unconscious patient, cardiopulmonary status is the most vital function and gives priorities to the ABCs (airway, breathing, and circulation).

18. c. One of the functions of cranial nerve (CN) III, the oculomotor nerve, is pupillary constriction and testing for pupillary constriction is important to identify patients at risk for brainstem herniation caused by increased ICP. The corneal reflex is used to assess the functions of CN V and VII and the oculocephalic reflex tests all cranial nerves involved with eye movement. Nystagmus is commonly associated with specific lesions or chemical toxicities and is not a definitive sign of ICP.

19. a. Nursing care activities that increase ICP include hip and neck flexion, suctioning, clustering care activities, and noxious stimuli. They should be avoided or performed as little as possible in the patient with increased ICP. Lowering the $PaCO_2$ below 20 mm Hg can cause ischemia and worsening of ICP.

20. c. A PaO_2 of 70 mm Hg reflects hypoxemia that may lead to further decreased cerebral perfusion. PaO_2 should be maintained at greater than or equal to 100 mm Hg. The pH and SaO_2 are within normal range and a $PaCO_2$ of 35 mm Hg reflects a normal value.

21. a, b, d, e. The first sign of increased ICP is a change in LOC. Other manifestations are dilated ipsilateral pupil, changes in motor response such as posturing, and fever, which may indicate pressure on the hypothalamus. Changes in vital signs would be an increased SBP with widened pulse pressure and bradycardia.

22. b. If reflex posturing occurs during range of motion (ROM) or positioning of the patient, these activities should be done less frequently until the patient's condition stabilizes because posturing can cause increases in ICP and may indicate herniation. Neither restraints nor central nervous system (CNS) depressants would be indicated.

23. d. A cerebral concussion may include a brief disruption in LOC, retrograde amnesia, and a headache, all of short duration. A basilar skull fracture may have a dural tear with CSF or brain otorrhea, rhinorrhea, hearing difficulty, vertigo, and Battle's sign. A temporal fracture would have a boggy temporal muscle because of extravasation of blood, Battle's sign, or CSF otorrhea.

24. c. The posterior fossa fracture causes occipital bruising resulting in cortical blindness or visual field defects. A cerebral contusion is bruising of brain tissue within a focal area. An orbital skull fracture would cause periorbital ecchymosis (raccoon eyes) and possible optic nerve injury. A frontal lobe skull fracture would expose the brain to contaminants through the frontal air sinus and the patient would have CSF rhinorrhea or pneumocranium.

25. c. The compound skull fracture is a depressed skull fracture and scalp lacerations with communicating pathway(s) to the intracranial cavity. A linear skull fracture is a straight break in the bone without alteration in the fragments. A depressed skull fracture is an inward indentation of the skull that may cause pressure on the brain. A comminuted skull fracture has multiple linear fractures with bone fragmented into many pieces.

26. b. Testing clear drainage for CSF in nasal or ear drainage may be done with a Dextrostik or Tes-Tape strip but if blood is present, the glucose in the blood will produce an unreliable result. To test bloody drainage, the nurse should test the fluid for a "halo" or "ring" that occurs when a yellowish ring encircles blood dripped onto a white pad or towel within a few minutes.

27. d. An arterial epidural hematoma is the most acute neurologic emergency and typical symptoms include unconsciousness at the scene with a brief lucid interval followed by a decrease in LOC. An acute subdural hematoma manifests signs within 48 hours of an injury. A chronic subdural hematoma develops over weeks or months.

28. d. When there is a depressed fracture or a fracture with loose fragments, a craniotomy is indicated to elevate the depressed bone and remove free fragments. A craniotomy is also indicated in cases of acute subdural and epidural hematomas to remove the blood and control the bleeding. Burr holes may be used in an extreme emergency for rapid decompression or to aid in removing a bone flap but with a depressed fracture, surgery would be the treatment of choice.

29. a. In addition to monitoring for a patent airway during emergency care of the patient with a head injury, the nurse must always assume that a patient with a head injury may have a cervical spine injury. Maintaining cervical spine precautions in all assessment and treatment activities with the patient is essential to prevent additional neurologic damage.

30. a. Residual mental and emotional changes of brain trauma with personality changes are often the most incapacitating problems following head injury and are common in patients who have been comatose for longer than 6 hours. Families must be prepared for changes in the patient's behavior to avoid family-patient friction and maintain family functioning and professional assistance may be required. There is no indication the patient will be dependent on others for care but he likely will not return to pretrauma status.

31. d. The positron emission tomography (PET) scan or magnetic resonance imaging (MRI) are used to reliably detect very small tumors. The computed tomography (CT) and brain scans are used to identify the location of a lesion. Angiography could be used to determine blood flow to the tumor and further localize it. Electroencephalography (EEG) would be used to rule out seizures.

32. b. Frontal lobe tumors often lead to loss of emotional control, confusion, memory loss, disorientation, seizures, and personality and judgment changes that are very disturbing and frightening to the family. Physical symptoms, such as blindness, speech disturbances, or disturbances in sensation and perception that occur with other tumors, are more likely to be understood and accepted by the family.

33. d. A craniectomy is excision of cranial bone without replacement, so the patient will need to protect the brain from trauma in this surgical area. Burr holes are opened into the cranium with a drill to remove blood and fluid. A craniotomy is opening the cranium with removal of a bone flap to open the dura. The replaced bone flap is wired or sutured after surgery. A cranioplasty replaces part of the cranium with an artificial plate.

34. b. A stereotactic radiosurgery technique uses precisely focused radiation to destroy tumor cells. The radiation is computer and imagery guided. Radioactive seeds are used to deliver radiation. Ventricular shunts are used to redirect CSF from one area to another. A craniotomy is done by first making burr holes and then opening the cranium by connecting the holes to remove a flap of bone to expose the dura mater.

35. a. To prevent undue concern and anxiety about hair loss and postoperative self-esteem disturbances, a patient undergoing cranial surgery should be informed preoperatively that the head is usually shaved in surgery while the patient is anesthetized and that a turban, scarf, or cap may be used after the dressings are removed postoperatively and a wig also may be used after the incision has healed to disguise the hair loss. In the immediate postoperative period the patient is very ill and the focus is on maintaining neurologic function but preoperatively the nurse should anticipate the patient's postoperative need for self-esteem and maintenance of appearance.

36. d. The primary goal after cranial surgery is prevention of increased ICP and interventions to prevent ICP and infection postoperatively are nursing priorities. The residual deficits, rehabilitation potential, and ultimate function of the patient depend on the reason for surgery, the postoperative course, and the patient's general state of health.

37. c. The symptoms of brain abscess closely resemble those of meningitis and encephalitis, including fever, headache, nausea, vomiting, and increased ICP, except that the patient also may have some focal symptoms that reflect the local area of the abscess.

38. b, c, e. Encephalitis is usually caused by a virus that inflames the brain and can be transmitted by ticks and mosquitoes. The other options are characteristics of meningitis.

39. d. Meningitis is often a result of an upper respiratory infection or a penetrating wound of the skull, where organisms gain entry to the CNS. Epidemic encephalitis is transmitted by ticks and mosquitoes and nonepidemic encephalitis may occur as a complication of measles, chickenpox, or mumps. Encephalitis caused by the herpes simplex virus carries a high fatality rate.

40. b. High fever, severe headache, nuchal rigidity, nausea, and vomiting are key signs of meningitis. Other symptoms, such as papilledema, generalized seizures, hemiparesis, and decreased LOC, and cranial nerve dysfunction may occur as complications of increased ICP in meningitis.

41. b. LOC must be monitored because it will decrease with the increased brain metabolism that the fever causes. Analgesics will not aid in lowering the body temperature, although acetaminophen will be used as an antipyretic. Rapid cooling may lead to shivering that increases metabolism. Monitoring cerebral edema will be done. Peripheral edema is unrelated and there will not be a rapid

fluid infusion for the fever. Fluid replacement will be calculated with 800 mL/day for respiratory losses and 100 mL for each degree of temperature above 100.4°F (38°C).

42. c. Any warm-blooded mammal, including livestock, can carry rabies. Worldwide, dogs are the most common carrier of rabies; however, in developed countries raccoons, skunks, bats, and foxes are the primary animal carriers. Because rabies is usually fatal, it is much better to prevent its spread.

Case Study

1. The temperature elevation and nuchal rigidity in the presence of increased ICP and decreasing LOC indicate that this patient has developed a meningeal infection.

2. The risks for meningitis after head injury and surgery include penetrations into the intracranial cavity with the compound fracture that involves a depressed skull fracture with scalp lacerations with a communicating pathway to the intracranial cavity and the incisions necessary for craniotomy for hematoma evacuation. Postoperative drains, invasive monitoring, environmental pathogens, and impaired immune response also contribute to the development of meningitis.

3. Acute inflammation and infection of the pia mater and the arachnoid membrane cause nuchal rigidity, a sign of meningeal irritation, and fever. The inflammatory response increases CSF production with an increase in pressure and as the purulent secretion produced by microbial infection spreads to other areas of the brain, cerebral edema and increased ICP occur. Increased ICP is thought to be a result of swelling around the dura, increased CSF volume, and endotoxins produced by the bacteria.

4. Priority interventions include reduction of fever, reduction of ICP, maintaining antibiotic schedule to keep therapeutic levels, maintaining fluid balance, protection from injury if seizures occur, and minimizing environmental stimuli.

5. Access to the meninges could have occurred from facial and cranial fractures, sinuses, and the surgical incisions.

6. **Nursing diagnoses:**
   - Risk for ineffective cerebral tissue perfusion *related to* cerebral tissue swelling
   - Hyperthermia *related to* infection and abnormal temperature regulation
   - Ineffective breathing pattern *related to* decreased LOC and immobility
   - Risk for injury *related to* potential for seizures
   - Imbalanced nutrition: less than body requirements *related to* hypermetabolism and inability to ingest food and fluids
   - Risk for impaired skin integrity *related to* immobility
   Collaborative problems:
   Potential complications: increased ICP, seizures, hydrocephalus, disseminated intravascular coagulation, brain herniation

CHAPTER 58

Answer Key

1. c. The highest risk factors for thrombotic stroke are hypertension and diabetes. African Americans have a higher risk for stroke than do white persons, probably because they have a greater incidence of hypertension, diabetes mellitus,

and obesity. Factors such as diet high in saturated fats and cholesterol, cigarette smoking, metabolic syndrome, sedentary lifestyle, and excessive alcohol use are also risk factors but carry less risk than hypertension.

2. c. The communication between the anterior and posterior cerebral circulation in the circle of Willis provides a collateral circulation, which may maintain circulation to an area of the brain if its original blood supply is obstructed. All areas of the brain require constant blood supply and atherosclerotic plaques are not readily reversed. Neurologic deficits can result from ischemia caused by many factors.

3. d. A transient ischemic attack (TIA) is a temporary focal loss of neurologic function caused by ischemia of an area of the brain, usually lasting an hour or less. TIAs may be due to microemboli that temporarily block blood flow and are a warning of progressive cerebrovascular disease. Evaluation is necessary to determine the cause of the neurologic deficit and provide prophylactic treatment if possible.

4. a, b, e. Strokes from intracerebral hemorrhage have a poor prognosis, are caused by the rupture of a blood vessel, are frequently atherosclerotic, and create a mass that compresses the brain. Thrombotic strokes are related to hypertension and occur during sleep or after sleep.

5. a. Embolic strokes are associated with endocardial disorders such as atrial fibrillation, have a rapid onset, and are unrelated to activity.

6. c. Clinical manifestations of altered neurologic function differ, depending primarily on the specific cerebral artery involved and the area of the brain that is perfused by the artery. The degree of impairment depends on rapidity of onset, the size of the lesion, and the presence of collateral circulation.

7. a. L; b. R; c. R; d. L; e. R; f. R; g. L

8. c. Receptive aphasia is the lack of comprehension of both verbal and written language. Dysarthria is disturbance in muscular control of speech. In fluent dysphasia speech is present but contains little meaningful communication. Expressive aphasia is the loss of the production of language.

9. c. MRI could be used to rapidly distinguish between ischemic and hemorrhagic stroke and determine the size and location of the lesion. A noncontrast CT scan could also be used. Lumbar punctures are not performed routinely because of the chance of increased intracranial pressure causing herniation. Cerebral arteriograms are invasive and may dislodge an embolism or cause further hemorrhage. They are performed only when no other test can provide the needed information.

10. c. A carotid endarterectomy is the removal of an atherosclerotic plaque in the carotid arteries that may impair circulation enough to cause a stroke. The other procedures described may also be used to prevent strokes. An extracranial-intracranial bypass involves cranial surgery to bypass a sclerotic intracranial artery. Stenting may improve circulation in the brain. A percutaneous transluminal angioplasty uses a balloon to compress stenotic areas in the carotid and vertebrobasilar arteries and often includes inserting a stent to hold the artery open.

11. c. The administration of antiplatelet agents, such as aspirin, ticlopidine (Ticlid), clopidogrel (Plavix), dipyridamole (Persantine), and combined dipyridamole and aspirin (Aggrenox), reduces the incidence of stroke in those at risk. Anticoagulants are also used for prevention of embolic strokes but increase the risk for hemorrhage. Diuretics are not indicated for stroke prevention other than for their role

in controlling blood pressure (BP) and antilipidemic agents have not been found to have a significant effect on stroke prevention. The calcium channel blocker nimodipine is used in patients with subarachnoid hemorrhage to decrease the effects of vasospasm and minimize tissue damage.

12. d. The first priority in acute management of the patient with a stroke is preservation of life. Because the patient with a stroke may be unconscious or have a reduced gag reflex, it is most important to maintain a patent airway for the patient and provide oxygen if respiratory effort is impaired. IV fluid replacement, treatment with osmotic diuretics, and avoiding hyperthermia may be used for further treatment.

13. b. Surgical management with clipping of an aneurysm to decrease rebleeding and vasospasm is an option for a stroke caused by rupture of a cerebral aneurysm. Placement of coils into the lumens of the aneurysm via interventional neuroradiology can also be done to prevent the blood from circulating through the aneurysm and to reduce the risk of rupture. Hyperventilation therapy would increase vasodilation and the potential for hemorrhage. Thrombolytic therapy would be absolutely contraindicated and if a vessel is patent, osmotic diuretics may leak into tissue, pulling fluid out of the vessel and increasing edema.

14. a. The body responds to the vasospasm and decreased circulation to the brain that occurs with a stroke by increasing the BP, frequently resulting in hypertension. The other options are important cardiovascular factors to assess but they do not result from impaired cerebral blood flow.

15. a, b, c, d, f. The secondary assessment and ongoing neurologic monitoring include the gaze, facial palsy, distal motor function (part of the NIH Stroke Scale), sensation, proprioception, cognition, motor abilities, cerebellar function, and deep tendon reflexes. Current medications and history of hypertension are part of the primary assessment.

16. d. Active range of motion (ROM) should be initiated on the unaffected side as soon as possible and passive ROM of the affected side should be started on the first day. Having the patient actively exercise the unaffected side provides the patient with active and passive ROM as needed. Use of footboards is controversial because they stimulate plantar flexion. The unaffected arm should be supported but immobilization may precipitate a painful shoulder-hand syndrome. The patient should be positioned with each joint higher than the joint proximal to it to prevent dependent edema.

17. a. The presence of homonymous hemianopia in a patient with right hemisphere brain damage causes a loss of vision in the left field bilaterally. Early in the care of the patient, objects should be placed on the right side of the patient in the field of vision and the nurse should approach the patient from the right side. Later in treatment, patients should be taught to turn the head and scan the environment and should be approached from the affected side to encourage head turning. Eye patches are used if patients have diplopia (double vision).

18. a. Usually the speech therapist will have completed a swallowing study before a diet is ordered. The first step in providing oral feedings for a patient with a stroke is ensuring that the patient has an intact gag reflex because oral feedings will not be provided if the gag reflex is impaired. After placing the patient in an upright position, the nurse should then evaluate the patient's ability to swallow ice chips or ice water.

19. c. Soft foods that provide enough texture, flavor, and bulk to stimulate swallowing should be used for the patient with dysphagia. Thin liquids are difficult to swallow and patients may not be able to control them in the mouth. Pureed foods are often too bland and too smooth and milk products should be avoided because they tend to increase the viscosity of mucus and increase salivation.

20. d. Recombinant tissue plasminogen activator (tPA) dissolves clots and increases the risk for bleeding. It is not used with hemorrhagic strokes. If the patient had a thrombotic or embolic stroke, the timeframe of 3 to 4.5 hours after onset of clinical signs of the stroke would be important as well as a history of surgery. The nurse should answer the question as accurately as possible and then encourage the wife to talk with the physician if she has further questions.

21. a, d, e, f. The patient's rehabilitation potential and the expectations of the patient and caregiver related to the rehabilitation program will have a big impact on planning and carrying out the rehabilitation plan. The other things the rehabilitation nurse will assess are the physical status of all of the patient's body systems, presence of complications caused by the stroke or other chronic conditions, the cognitive status of the patient, and the family (including the patient and caregiver) resources and support.

22. b. During rehabilitation, the patient with aphasia needs frequent, meaningful verbal stimulation that has relevance for him or her. Conversation by the nurse and family should address activities of daily living (ADLs) that are familiar to the patient. Gestures, pictures, and simple statements are more appropriate in the acute phase, when patients may be overwhelmed by verbal stimuli. Flashcards are often perceived by the patient as childish and meaningless. Not responding verbally does not promote communication.

23. c. Unilateral neglect, or neglect syndrome, occurs when the patient with a stroke is unaware of the affected side of the body, which puts the patient at risk for injury. During the acute phase, the affected side is cared for by the nurse with positioning and support but during rehabilitation the patient is taught to care consciously for and attend to the affected side of the body to protect it from injury. Patients may be positioned on the affected side for up to 30 minutes.

24. c. Patients with left-brain damage from stroke often experience emotional lability, inappropriate emotional responses, mood swings, and uncontrolled tears or laughter disproportionate to or out of context with the situation. The behavior is upsetting and embarrassing to both the patient and the family and the patient should be distracted to minimize its presence. Maintaining a calm environment and avoiding shaming or scolding the patient is important. Patients with right-brain damage often have impulsive, rapid behavior that requires supervision and direction.

25. d. The patient and family need accurate and complete information about the effects of the stroke to problem-solve and make plans for chronic care of the patient. It is uncommon for patients with major strokes to return completely to prestroke function, behaviors, and role and both the patient and family will mourn these losses. The patient's specific needs for care must be identified and rehabilitation efforts should be continued at home. Family therapy and support groups may be helpful for some patients and families.

26. c. Medication administration is within the scope of practice for a licensed practical nurse (LPN). Assessment and teaching are within the scope of practice for the RN.

Case Study

1. A noncontrast CT or MRI scan would be able to determine the size and location of a lesion and to differentiate between an infarction and a hemorrhage. A lumbar puncture would not be indicated because of the chance that hemorrhage had increased intracranial pressure (ICP). Other tests that might be used when hemorrhage is evident include cerebral angiography to identify the source of subarachnoid hemorrhage; intraarterial digital subtraction angiography, which is considered safer than cerebral angiography; transcranial Doppler ultrasonography that measures the velocity of blood flow in the major cerebral arteries; and carotid duplex scanning.
2. Unconsciousness, Glasgow Coma Scale score of 5, and wide pulse pressure with a decrease in pulse and respiration all indicate increased ICP.
3. The loss of consciousness is associated with a poor prognosis for recovery and the family should be told that her condition is very guarded.
4. The highest priorities for interventions are those that support the patient's life processes: airway and respiratory function with oxygen administration, fluid management without overloading the vascular system, and measures that decrease ICP.
5. Anything that impairs clotting is contraindicated in a hemorrhagic stroke: anticoagulants, antiplatelet agents, and thrombolytic therapy. Hyperosmolar diuretics are also contraindicated because they may escape from an injured vessel, causing increased edema in brain tissue.
6. Hypothermia and barbiturate therapy may be used but these treatments have not proved effective. Surgery is the only other option and clipping or coiling of an aneurysm may be performed or the aneurysm may be wrapped or reinforced with muscle.
7. **Nursing diagnoses:**
   * Decreased intracranial adaptive capacity *related to* increase in ICP secondary to hemorrhage
   * Risk for ineffective cerebral tissue perfusion *related to* hemorrhage
   * Ineffective airway clearance *related to* unconsciousness
   * Risk for aspiration *related to* decreased level of consciousness
   * Impaired physical mobility *related to* unconsciousness
   * Self-care deficit *related to* altered mental state
   * Risk for injury *related to* inability to monitor personal safety
   * Risk for infection *related to* immobility
   Collaborative problems:
   Potential complications: increased ICP, brain herniation, seizures

CHAPTER 59

Answer Key

1. b. Migraine headaches are frequently unilateral and usually throbbing. They may be preceded by a prodrome and frequently there is a family history. Cluster headaches are also unilateral with severe bone-crushing pain but there is no prodrome or family history. Frontal-type headache is not a functional type of headache. Tension-type headaches are bilateral with constant, squeezing tightness without prodrome or family history.
2. b, c, d, f. Cluster headaches have only alcohol as a dietary trigger and have an abrupt onset lasting 5 minutes to 3 hours with severe, sharp, penetrating pain. Cluster headaches may be accompanied by unilateral ptosis, lacrimation, rhinitis, facial flushing or pallor and commonly recur several times each day for several weeks, with months or years between clustered attacks. Family history and nausea, vomiting, or irritability may be seen with migraine headaches. Bilateral pressure occurring between migraine headaches and intermittent occurrence over long periods of time are characteristics of tension-type headaches.
3. d. The primary way to diagnose and differentiate between headaches is with a careful history of the headaches, requiring assessment of specific details related to the headache. Electromyelography (EMG) may reveal contraction of the neck, scalp, or facial muscles in tension-type headaches but this is not seen in all patients. CT scans and cerebral angiography are used to rule out organic causes of the headaches.
4. d. Triptans (sumatriptan [Imitrex]) affect selected serotonin receptors that decrease neurogenic inflammation of the cerebral blood vessels and produce vasoconstriction. Both migraine headaches and cluster headaches appear to be related to vasodilation of cranial vessels and drugs that cause vasoconstriction are useful in treatment of migraine and cluster headaches. Methysergide blocks serotonin receptors in the central and peripheral nervous systems and is used for prevention of migraine and cluster headaches. β-adrenergic blockers and tricyclic antidepressants are used prophylactically for migraine headaches but are not effective for cluster headaches.
5. a. When the anxiety is related to a lack of knowledge about the etiology and treatment of a headache, helping the patient to identify stressful lifestyle patterns and other precipitating factors and ways of avoiding them are appropriate nursing interventions for the anxiety. Interventions that teach alternative therapies to supplement drug therapy also give the patient some control over pain and are appropriate teaching regarding treatment of the headache. The other interventions may help to reduce anxiety generally but they do not address the etiologic factor of the anxiety.
6. c. The unlicensed assistive personnel (UAP) is able to obtain equipment from the supply cabinet or department. The RN may need to provide a list of necessary equipment and should set up the equipment and ensure proper functioning. The RN is responsible for the initial history and assessment as well as teaching the patient about the room's call system. Padded tongue blades are no longer used and no effort should be made to place anything in the patient's mouth during a seizure.
7. d. Generalized seizures have bilateral synchronous epileptic discharge affecting the entire brain at onset of the seizure. Loss of consciousness is also characteristic but many focal seizures also include an altered consciousness. Focal seizures begin in one side of the brain but may spread to involve the entire brain. Focal seizures that start with a local focus and spread to the entire brain, causing a secondary generalized seizure, are associated with a transient residual neurologic deficit postictally known as Todd's paralysis.

8. c. The typical absence seizure is also known as petit mal and the child has staring spells that last for a few seconds. Atonic seizures occur when the patient falls from loss of muscle tone accompanied by brief unconsciousness. Simple focal seizures have focal motor, sensory, or autonomic symptoms related to the area of the brain involved without loss of consciousness. Staring spells in atypical absence seizures last longer than those in typical absence seizures and are accompanied by peculiar behavior during the seizure or confusion after the seizure.

9. c, d, f. Complex focal seizures are psychomotor seizures with automatisms such as lip smacking. They cause altered consciousness or loss of consciousness producing a dreamlike state and may involve behavioral, emotional, or cognitive experiences without memory of what was done during the seizure. In generalized tonic-clonic seizures (previously known as grand mal seizures) there is loss of consciousness and stiffening of the body with subsequent jerking of extremities. Incontinence or tongue or cheek biting may also occur.

10. d. Tonic-clonic status epilepticus is most dangerous because the continuous seizing can cause respiratory insufficiency, hypoxemia, cardiac dysrhythmia, hyperthermia, and systemic acidosis, which can all be fatal. Subclinical seizures may occur in a patient who is sedated, so there is no physical movement. Myoclonic seizures may occur in clusters and have a sudden, excessive jerk of the body that may hurl the person to the ground. Psychogenic seizures are psychiatric in origin and diagnosed with video-electroencephalography (EEG) monitoring. They occur in patients with a history of emotional abuse or a specific traumatic episode.

11. c. A seizure is a paroxysmal, uncontrolled discharge of neurons in the brain, which interrupts normal function, but the factor that causes the abnormal firing is not clear. Seizures may be precipitated by many factors and although scar tissue may make the brain neurons more likely to fire, it is not the usual cause of seizures. Epilepsy is established only by a pattern of spontaneous, recurring seizures.

12. b. Most patients with seizure disorders maintain seizure control with medications but if surgery is considered, three requirements must be met: the diagnosis of epilepsy must be confirmed, there must have been an adequate trial with drug therapy without satisfactory results, and the electroclinical syndrome must be defined. The focal point must be localized but the presence of scar tissue is not required.

13. c. Serum levels of antiseizure drugs are monitored regularly to maintain therapeutic levels of the drug, above which patients are likely to experience toxic effects and below which seizures are likely to occur. Many newer drugs do not require drug level monitoring because of large therapeutic ranges. A daily seizure log and urine testing for drug levels will not measure compliance or monitor for toxicity. EEGs have limited value in diagnosis of seizures and even less value in monitoring seizure control.

14. c. If antiseizure drugs are discontinued abruptly, seizures can be precipitated. Missed doses should be made up if the omission is remembered within 24 hours and patients should not adjust medications without professional guidance because this also can increase seizure frequency and may cause status epilepticus. Antiseizure drugs have numerous interactions with other drugs and the use of other medications should be evaluated by health professionals. If side effects occur, the physician should be notified and drug regimens evaluated.

15. a, b, c. The focus is on maintaining a patent airway and preventing patient injury. The nurse should not place objects in the patient's mouth or restrain the patient.

16. b. In the postictal phase of generalized tonic-clonic seizures, patients are usually very tired and may sleep for several hours and the nurse should allow the patient to sleep as long as necessary. Suctioning is performed only if needed and decreased level of consciousness is not a problem postictally unless a head injury has occurred during the seizure.

17. b. One of the most common complications of a seizure disorder is the effect it has on the patient's lifestyle. This is because of the social stigma attached to seizures, which causes patients to hide their diagnosis and to prefer not to be identified as having epilepsy. Medication regimens usually require only once- or twice-daily dosing and the major restrictions of lifestyle usually involve driving and high-risk environments. Job discrimination against the handicapped is prevented by federal and state laws and patients only need to identify their disease in case of medical emergencies.

18. c. Restless legs syndrome that is not related to other pathologic processes, such as diabetes mellitus or rheumatic disorders, may be caused by a dysfunction in the basal ganglia circuits that use the neurotransmitter dopamine, which controls movements. Dopamine precursors and dopamine agonists, such as those used for parkinsonism, are effective in managing sensory and motor symptoms. Polysomnography studies during sleep are the only tests that have diagnostic value and although exercise should be encouraged, excessive leg exercise does not have an effect on the symptoms.

19. c. Huntington's disease (HD) involves deficiency of acetylcholine and γ-aminobutyric acid (GABA) in the basal ganglia and extrapyramidal system that causes the opposite symptoms of parkinsonism. Myasthenia gravis involves autoimmune antibody destruction of cholinergic receptors at the neuromuscular junction. Amyotrophic lateral sclerosis (ALS) involves degeneration of motor neurons in the brainstem and spinal cord.

20. a. Most patients with multiple sclerosis (MS) have remissions and exacerbations of neurologic dysfunction or a relapsing-remitting initial course followed by progression with or without occasional relapses, minor remissions, and plateaus that progressively cause loss of motor, sensory, and cerebellar functions. Intellectual function generally remains intact but patients may experience anger, depression, or euphoria. A few people have chronic progressive deterioration and some may experience only occasional and mild symptoms for several years after onset.

21. c. Specific neurologic dysfunction of MS is caused by destruction of myelin and replacement with glial scar tissue at specific areas in the nervous system. Motor, sensory, cerebellar, and emotional dysfunctions, including paresthesias as well as patchy blindness, blurred vision, pain radiating along the dermatome of the nerve, ataxia, and severe fatigue, are the most common manifestations of MS. Constipation and bladder dysfunctions, short-term memory loss, sexual dysfunction, anger, and depression or euphoria may also occur. Excessive involuntary movements and tremors are not seen in MS.

22. d. There is no specific diagnostic test for MS. A diagnosis is made primarily by history and clinical manifestations. Certain diagnostic tests may be used to help establish a diagnosis of MS. Positive findings on MRI include evidence of at least two inflammatory demyelinating lesions in at least two different locations within the central nervous system (CNS). Cerebrospinal fluid (CSF) may have increased immunoglobulin G and the presence of oligoclonal banding. Evoked potential responses are often delayed in persons with MS.

23. b. Mitoxantrone (Novantrone) cannot be used for more than 2 to 3 years because it is an antineoplastic drug that causes cardiac toxicity, leukemia, and infertility. It is a monoclonal antibody given IV monthly when patients have inadequate responses to other drugs. It increases the risk of progressive multifocal leukoencephalopathy.

24. c. The main goal in care of the patient with MS is to keep the patient active and maximally functional and promote self-care as much as possible to maintain independence. Assistive devices encourage independence while preserving the patient's energy. No care activity that the patient can do for himself or herself should be performed by others. Involvement of the family in the patient's care and maintenance of social interactions are also important but are not the priority in care.

25. b. Corticosteroids used in treating acute exacerbations of MS should not be abruptly stopped by the patient because adrenal insufficiency may result and prescribed tapering doses should be followed. Infections may exacerbate symptoms and should be avoided and high-protein diets with vitamin supplements are advocated. Long-term planning for increasing disability is also important.

26. d. The degeneration of dopamine-producing neurons in the substantia nigra of midbrain and basal ganglia lead to this triad of signs. Muscle soreness, pain, and slowness of movement are patient function consequences related to rigidity. Shuffling gait, lack of postural stability, absent arm swing while walking, absent blinking, masked facial expression, and difficulty initiating movement are all related to bradykinesia. Impaired handwriting and hand activities are related to the tremor of Parkinson's disease (PD).

27. b. Although clinical manifestations are characteristic in PD, no laboratory or diagnostic tests are specific for the condition. A diagnosis is made when at least two of the three signs of the classic triad are present and it is confirmed with a positive response to antiparkinsonian medication. Research regarding the role of genetic testing and MRI to diagnose PD is ongoing. Essential tremors increase during voluntary movement whereas the tremors of PD are more prominent at rest.

28. c. The bradykinesia of PD prevents automatic movements and activities such as beginning to walk, rising from a chair, or even swallowing saliva cannot be executed unless they are consciously willed. Handwriting is affected by the tremor and results in the writing trailing off at the end of words. Specific limb weakness and muscle spasms are not characteristic of PD.

29. c. Peripheral dopamine does not cross the blood-brain barrier but its precursor, levodopa, is able to enter the brain, where it is converted to dopamine, increasing the supply that is deficient in PD. Other drugs used to treat PD include bromocriptine, which stimulates dopamine receptors in the basal ganglia, and amantadine, which blocks the reuptake of dopamine into presynaptic neurons. Carbidopa is an agent that is usually administered with levodopa to prevent the levodopa from being metabolized in peripheral tissues before it can reach the brain.

30. c. The shuffling gait of PD causes the patient to be off balance and at risk for falling. Teaching the patient to use a wide stance with the feet apart, to lift the toes when walking, and to look ahead helps to promote a more balanced gait. Use of an elevated toilet seat and rocking from side to side will enable a patient to initiate movement. Canes and walkers are difficult for patients with PD to maneuver and may make the patient more prone to injury.

31. b. The reduction of the acetylcholine (ACh) effect in myasthenia gravis (MG) is treated with anticholinesterase drugs, which prolong the action of ACh at the neuromuscular synapse, but too much of these drugs will cause a cholinergic crisis with symptoms very similar to those of MG. To determine whether the patient's manifestations are due to a deficiency of ACh or to too much anticholinesterase drug, the anticholinesterase drug edrophonium chloride (Tensilon) is administered. If the patient is in cholinergic crisis, the patient's symptoms will worsen; if the patient is in a myasthenic crisis, the patient will improve.

32. c. The patient in myasthenic crisis has severe weakness and fatigability of all skeletal muscles, affecting the patient's ability to breathe, swallow, talk, and move. However, the priority of nursing care is monitoring and maintaining adequate ventilation.

33. b. In ALS there is gradual degeneration of motor neurons with extreme muscle wasting from lack of stimulation and use. However, cognitive function is not impaired and patients feel trapped in a dying body. Chorea manifested by writhing, involuntary movements is characteristic of HD. As an autosomal dominant genetic disease, HD also has a 50% chance of being passed to each offspring.

34. c. Many chronic neurologic diseases involve progressive deterioration in physical or mental capabilities and have no cure, with devastating results for patients and families. Health care providers can only attempt to alleviate physical symptoms, prevent complications, and assist patients in maximizing function and self-care abilities for as long as possible.

Case Study

1. The cause of MS is unknown, although research findings suggest that MS is related to genetic susceptibility with precipitating factors including infectious, immunologic, and environmental factors. T cells are activated by some unknown factor and these T cells migrate to the CNS and cause a disruption in the blood-brain barrier. Subsequent antigen-antibody reaction within the CNS results in activation of the inflammatory response and through multiple mechanisms, demyelination of axons occurs. There is loss of myelin, disappearance of oligodendrocytes, and eventual damage to the underlying axon. The nerve impulse transmission is disrupted, resulting in permanent loss of nerve function. As inflammation subsides, glial scar formation replaces the damaged tissue, resulting in characteristic hard sclerotic plaque formation scattered through the CNS.

2. The risk factors this patient has are being female between 20 and 50 years of age and being a European American from the northern United States.

3. The role of precipitating factors, such as exposure to pathogenic agents, in the etiology of MS is controversial. It is possible that their association with MS is random and that there is no cause-and-effect relationship. Possible precipitating factors for this patient include emotional stress, fatigue, pregnancy, and a poorer state of health. It is also possible that the viral neuritis was a precipitating factor.

4. Because there is no definitive diagnostic test for MS, diagnosis is based primarily on history and clinical manifestations. Although MRI can detect sclerotic plaques, her initial symptoms were so nonspecific and transient that a "wait-and-see" approach is often taken. The evidence of at least two plaques in the white matter seen with MRI and several attacks occurring support the current diagnosis of MS.

5. Patient teaching should focus on preventing exacerbations (e.g., upper respiratory tract infection, trauma, immunization, delivery after pregnancy) or worsening of the disease. Building general resistance to illness, including avoiding fatigue, stress, extremes of heat and cold, and exposure to infection, is an important measure in maintaining general health. Vigorous and early treatment of infection is critical if it does occur. It is important to teach the patient to achieve a good balance of exercise and rest, minimize caffeine intake, and eat nutritious, well-balanced meals with roughage to avoid constipation. Patients should know their treatment regimens, side effects of medications, and drug interactions with over-the-counter medications. The patient should consult a health care provider before taking nonprescription medications.

6. Because there is no cure for MS, treatment is aimed at slowing the disease process and providing individualized symptomatic relief. The disease process is treated with drugs and symptoms are controlled with a variety of medications and other forms of therapy.
   - *Immunomodulator drugs:* Interferon β-1b (Betaseron), interferon β-1a (Avonex or Rebif), and glatiramer acetate (Copaxone) are used to modify the disease progression and prevent relapses but the drugs are administered parenterally. Teriflunomide (Aubagio) is an immunomodulatory agent with antiinflammatory properties. The exact mechanism of action is unknown but may involve a reduction in the number of activated lymphocytes in the CNS.
   - *Immunosuppressant* for aggressive MS: The antineoplastic drug mitoxantrone (Novantrone) reduces both B and T lymphocytes and macrophages.
   - *Sphingosine1-phosphate receptor modulator:* Oral fingolimod (Gilenya) reduces the rate of relapses in relapsing-remitting MS but has serious side effects.
   - *Monoclonal antibody:* Natalizumab (Tysabri) is used when patients have an inadequate response to other drugs.
   - *Corticosteroids:* These are most helpful in treating acute exacerbations of MS by reducing edema and acute inflammation at the site of demyelination but the ultimate outcome is not affected.

   However, the potential benefits of these drugs in patients with MS need to be weighed against the potentially serious side effects. Physical therapy and speech therapy may also help to improve neurologic function.

7. **Nursing diagnoses:**
   - Interrupted family processes *related to* shift in health status, potential financial problems, and fluctuating physical condition
   - Ineffective self-health management *related to* knowledge deficit regarding management of MS
   - Anxiety *related to* diagnosis of a chronic disabling illness
   - Disturbed sensory perception: visual *related to* prolonged visual evoked potential in right eye
   - Risk for impaired parenting *related to* fatigue and numbness and tingling on left side

   Collaborative problems:
   Potential complication: blindness, impaired physical mobility, urinary incontinence

CHAPTER 60

Answer Key

1. a, d, e. Manifestations of delirium include cognitive impairment with reduced awareness, reversed sleep/wake cycle, and distorted thinking and perception. The other options are characteristic of dementia.

2. d. The diagnosis of vascular dementia can be aided by neuroimaging studies showing vascular brain lesions along with exclusion of other causes of dementia. Overproduction of β-amyloid protein contributes to Alzheimer's disease (AD). Vascular dementia can be prevented or slowed by treating underlying diseases (e.g., diabetes mellitus, cardiovascular disease). Dementia caused by hepatic or renal encephalopathy potentially can be reversed.

3. a. Depression is often associated with AD, especially early in the disease when the patient has awareness of the diagnosis and the progression of the disease. When dementia and depression occur together, intellectual deterioration may be more extreme. Depression is treatable and use of antidepressants often improves cognitive function.

4. c. The Mini-Mental State Examination is a tool to document the degree of cognitive impairment and it can be used to determine a baseline from which changes over time can be evaluated. It does not evaluate mood or thought processes but can detect dementia and delirium and differentiate these from psychiatric mental illness. It cannot help to determine etiology.

5. c. Hypothyroidism can cause dementia but it is a treatable condition if it has not been long standing. The other conditions are causes of irreversible dementia.

6. d. In mild cognitive impairment people frequently forget people's names and begin to forget important events. Delirium changes usually occur abruptly. In Alzheimer's disease the patient may not remember knowing a person and loses the sense of time and which day it is. Normal forgetfulness includes momentarily forgetting names and occasionally forgetting to run an errand.

7. b. The only definitive diagnosis of AD can be made on examination of brain tissue during an autopsy but a clinical diagnosis is made when all other possible causes of dementia have been eliminated. Patients with AD may have β-amyloid proteins in the blood, brain atrophy, or isoprostanes in the urine but these findings are not exclusive to those with AD.

8. c. In the moderate stage of AD, the patient may need help with getting dressed. In the severe stage, patients will be unable to dress or feed themselves and are usually incontinent.

9. b. Because there is no cure for AD, collaborative management is aimed at controlling the decline in cognition, controlling the undesirable manifestations that the patient may exhibit, and providing support for the family caregiver. Anticholinesterase agents help to increase acetylcholine (ACh) in the brain but a variety of other drugs are also used to control behavior. Memory-enhancing techniques have little or no effect in patients with AD, especially as the disease progresses. Patients with AD have limited ability to communicate health symptoms and problems, leading to a lack of professional attention for acute and other chronic illnesses.

10. c. Lorazepam (Ativan) is a benzodiazepine used to manage behavior with AD. Sertraline (Zoloft) is a selective serotonin reuptake inhibitor used to treat depression. Donepezil (Aricept) is a cholinesterase inhibitor used for decreased memory and cognition. Risperidone (Risperdal) is an antipsychotic used for behavior management.

11. d. Memantine (Namenda) is the *N*-methyl-D-aspartate (NMDA) receptor antagonist frequently used for AD patients with decreased memory and cognition. Trazodone (Desyrel) is an atypical antidepressant that may help with sleep problems. Olanzapine (Zyprexa) is an antipsychotic medication used for behavior management. Rivastigmine (Exelon) is a cholinesterase inhibitor used for decreased memory and cognition.

12. b. Patients with moderate to severe AD frequently become agitated but because their short-term memory loss is so pronounced, distraction is a very good way to calm them. "Why" questions are upsetting to them because they don't know the answer and they cannot respond to normal relaxation techniques.

13. a, b, f. Avoiding trauma to the brain, treating depression early, and exercising regularly can maintain cognitive function. Staying socially active, avoiding intake of harmful substances, and challenging the brain to keep its connections active and create new ones also help to keep the brain healthy.

14. a. The risk of early-onset AD for the children of parents with it is 50%. Women do get AD more often than men but that is more likely related to women living longer than men than to the type of AD. *ApoE* gene testing is used for research with late-onset AD but does not predict who will develop the disease. Late-onset AD is more genetically complex than early-onset AD and is more common in those over age 60 but because his parent has early-onset AD he is at a 50% risk of getting it.

15. b. Adhering to a regular, consistent daily schedule helps the patient to avoid confusion and anxiety and is important both during hospitalization and at home. Clocks and calendars may be useful in early AD but they have little meaning to a patient as the disease progresses. Questioning the patient about activities and events they cannot remember is threatening and may cause severe anxiety. Maintaining a safe environment for the patient is important but does not change the disturbed thought processes.

16. b. Family caregiver role strain is characterized by such symptoms of stress as the inability to sleep, make decisions, or concentrate. It is frequently seen in family members who are responsible for the care of the patient with AD. Assessment of the caregiver may reveal a need for assistance to increase coping skills, effectively use community resources, or maintain social relationships. Eventually the demands on a caregiver exceed the resources and the person with AD may be placed in an institutional setting.

17. a. Adult day care is an option to provide respite for caregivers and a protective environment for the patient during the early and middle stages of AD. There are also in-home respite care providers. The respite from the demands of care allows the caregiver to maintain social contacts, perform normal tasks of living, and be more responsive to the patient's needs. Visits by home health nurses involve the caregiver and cannot provide adequate respite. Institutional placement is not always an acceptable option at earlier stages of AD, nor is hospitalization available for respite care.

18. b, e. Dementia with Lewy bodies (DLB) is diagnosed with dementia plus two of the following symptoms: (1) extrapyramidal signs such as bradykinesia, rigidity, and postural instability but not always a tremor, (2) fluctuating cognitive ability, and (3) hallucinations. The extrapyramidal signs plus tremors would more likely indicate Parkinson's disease. Disturbed behavior, sleep, personality, and eventually memory are characteristics of frontotemporal lobe degeneration (FTLD).

19. a, b, d. All caregivers are responsible for the patient's safety. Basic care activities, such as those associated with personal hygiene and activities of daily living (ADLs) can be delegated to unlicensed assistive personnel (UAP). The RN will perform ongoing assessments and develop and revise the plan of care as needed. The RN will assess the patient's safety risk factors, provide education, and make referrals. The licensed practical nurse (LPN) could check the patient's environment for potential safety hazards.

20. a. Age; b. infection; c. hypoxemia (lung disease); d. intensive care unit (ICU) hospitalization (change in environment, sensory overload); e. preexisting dementia; f. dehydration. Also: hyperthermia and potentially medications to treat chronic obstructive pulmonary disease (COPD) and pneumonia.

21. d. Delirium is an acute problem that usually has a rapid onset in response to a precipitating event, especially when the patient has underlying health problems, such as heart disease and sensory limitations. In the absence of prior cognitive impairment, a sudden onset of confusion, disorientation, and agitation is usually delirium. Delirium may manifest with both hypoactive and hyperactive symptoms.

22. c. Care of the patient with delirium is focused on identifying and eliminating precipitating factors if possible. Treatment of underlying medical conditions, changing environmental conditions, and discontinuing medications that induce delirium are important. Drug therapy is reserved for those patients with severe agitation because the drugs themselves may worsen delirium.

23. d. In the severe stage of AD, the patient is at a developmental level of 15 months or less; therefore appropriate distractions would be infant toys. Watching

TV and playing games are more appropriate in the mild stage. Books to read would need to be at developmentally appropriate levels to be used as a diversion.

Case Study

1. The pathophysiology of AD includes cellular changes with neurofibrillary tangles with altered tau proteins and neuritic plaques containing β-amyloid protein in the cerebral cortex and hippocampus. There is also a loss of the connections between neurons.

2. AD is diagnosed by exclusion. When all other possible causes of mental impairment and persistence of dementia are ruled out, the diagnosis of AD remains. Brain atrophy and enlarged ventricles seen in some patients with AD are also seen in normal people and in other conditions. Positron emission tomography (PET) can be used to differentiate AD from other forms of dementia. Neuroimaging techniques detect changes earlier in the disease and can be used to monitor the response to therapy. Only on autopsy can AD be confirmed by the presence of amyloid plaques and neurofibrillary tangles in brain tissue.

3. All functions of mental capacity and ability to care for oneself are lost as the disease progresses. There will be deterioration of personal hygiene and all ADLs, progression of psychotic symptoms now evidenced by his hallucinations, loss of long-term memory and recognition of his family, and loss of communication.

4. The nurse should assess what the wife is doing now to manage his care, teach her about the expected progression of the disease, assist her in planning respite care or arranging for home health assistants, help her to identify problem areas, encourage her to keep G.D. awake and busy during the day so that he will sleep better at night and so will she, and refer her to community resources.

5. Community resources may include Alzheimer's support groups, adult day care, home health assistants and home nursing, and various forms of assisted living and long-term care facilities.

6. **Nursing diagnoses:**
   - Risk for injury *related to* impaired judgment (nighttime wandering) and sensory/perceptual alteration (hallucinations)
   - Risk for other-directed violence *related to* misinterpretation of environmental stimuli
   - Impaired memory *related to* effects of dementia
   - Wandering *related to* cognitive impairment
   - Disturbed sleep pattern *related to* circadian asynchrony
   - Self-neglect *related to* cognitive impairment

   Collaborative problems:
   Potential complication: depression, psychosis

7. **Nursing diagnoses:**
   - Anxiety *related to* erratic behavioral patterns and cognitive decline of husband
   - Ineffective health maintenance *related to* fatigue and chronic stress
   - Caregiver role strain *related to* grieving over the family member's illness
   - Risk for other-directed violence (patient abuse) *related to* ineffective coping

   Collaborative problems:
   Potential complication: depression, illness

CHAPTER 61

Answer Key

1. a, d, e, f. Bell's palsy affects the motor branches of the facial nerve. It is treated with corticosteroids, usually prednisone. Herpes simplex virus 1 may be a precipitating factor. Moist heat, gentle massage, electrical nerve stimulation, and exercises are prescribed. Care must be taken to protect the eye with sunglasses, artificial tears or gel, and possibly taping the eyelid closed at night. Oral hygiene is important but avoidance of hot foods is not needed.

2. a. The pain of trigeminal neuralgia is excruciating and it may occur in clusters that continue for hours. The condition is considered benign with no major effects except the pain. Corneal exposure is a problem in Bell's palsy or it may occur following surgery for the treatment of trigeminal neuralgia. Maintenance of nutrition is important but not urgent because chewing may trigger trigeminal neuralgia and patients then avoid eating. Except during an attack, there is no change in facial appearance in a patient with trigeminal neuralgia and body image is more disturbed in response to the paralysis typical of Bell's palsy.

3. a. Although percutaneous radiofrequency rhizotomy and microvascular decompression provide the greatest relief of pain, glycerol rhizotomy causes less sensory loss and fewer sensory aberrations with comparable pain relief and less danger. Gamma knife radiosurgery provides precise high doses of radiation useful for persistent pain after other surgery.

4. c. Because attacks of trigeminal neuralgia may be precipitated by hot or cold air movement on the face, jarring movements, or talking, the environment should be of moderate temperature and free of drafts and patients should not be expected to converse during the acute period. Patients often prefer to carry out their own care because they are afraid someone else may inadvertently injure them or precipitate an attack. The nurse should stress that oral hygiene be performed because patients often avoid it but residual food in the mouth after eating occurs more frequently with Bell's palsy.

5. a. The most serious complication of Guillain-Barré syndrome is respiratory failure and it is essential that respiratory rate and depth and vital capacity are monitored to detect involvement of the autonomic nerves that affect respiration. Corticosteroids may be used in treatment but do not appear to have an effect on the prognosis or duration of the disease. Rather, plasmapheresis or administration of high-dose immunoglobulin does result in shortening recovery time. The peripheral nerves of both the sympathetic and the parasympathetic nervous systems are involved in the disease and may lead to orthostatic hypotension, hypertension, and abnormal vagal responses affecting the heart. Guillain-Barré syndrome may affect the lower brainstem and cranial nerves (CNs) VII, VI, III, XII, V, and X, affecting facial, eye, and swallowing functions.

6. c. As nerve involvement ascends, it is very frightening for the patient but 85% to 95% of patients with Guillain-Barré syndrome recover completely with care, although 30% may have a residual weakness. Patients also recover if

ventilatory support is provided during respiratory failure. Guillain-Barré syndrome affects only peripheral nerves and does not affect the brain.

7. a. Tetanus is transmitted through wound contamination, causes painful tonic spasms or seizures, and can be prevented with immunization.

8. a, b, d. Neurosyphilis occurs 10 to 20 years after syphilis is contracted and is inadequately treated; it affects any part of the nervous system and causes degenerative changes in the spinal cord and brainstem in the later stages. The other options describe botulism.

9. d. Spinal cord injuries are highest in adolescent and young adult men between the ages of 16 and 30 and those who are impulsive or risk takers in daily living. Other risk factors include alcohol and drug abuse as well as participation in sports and occupational exposure to trauma or violence.

10. b. At the C7 level, spinal shock is manifested by tetraplegia and sensory loss. The neurologic loss may be temporary or permanent. Paraplegia with sensory loss would occur at the level of T1. A hemiplegia occurs with central (brain) lesions affecting motor neurons and spastic tetraplegia occurs when spinal shock resolves.

11. a. In central cord syndrome, motor weakness and sensory loss are present in both upper and lower extremities, with upper extremities affected more than lower extremities.

12. b. Brown-Séquard syndrome is characterized by ipsilateral loss of motor function and position and vibratory sense and vasomotor paralysis with contralateral loss of pain and temperature sensation below the level of the injury. Damage to the most distal cord and nerve roots with flaccid paralysis of the lower limbs and areflexic bowel and bladder is seen with cauda equine syndrome or conus medullaris syndrome. Posterior cord syndrome is rare, with cord damage resulting in loss of proprioception below the lesion level but retention of motor control and temperature and pain sensation. Anterior cord syndrome is often caused by flexion injury, with acute compression of the cord resulting in complete motor paralysis and loss of pain and temperature sensation below the level of injury but touch, position, vibration, and motion remaining intact.

13. c. The primary injury of the spinal cord rarely affects the entire cord but the pathophysiology of secondary injury may result in damage that is the same as mechanical severance of the cord. Complete cord dissolution occurs through autodestruction of the cord by hemorrhage, edema, and the presence of metabolites and norepinephrine, resulting in anoxia and infarction of the cord. Edema resulting from the inflammatory response may compress the spinal cord as well as increase the damage as it extends above and below the injury site.

14. c. Spinal shock occurs in about half of all people with acute spinal cord injury. In spinal shock, the entire cord below the level of the lesion fails to function, resulting in a flaccid paralysis and hypomotility of most processes without any reflex activity. Return of reflex activity, although hyperreflexive and spastic, signals the end of spinal shock. Rehabilitation activities are not contraindicated during spinal shock and should be instituted if the patient's cardiopulmonary status is stable. Neurogenic shock results from loss of vascular tone caused by the injury and is manifested by hypotension, peripheral vasodilation, and decreased cardiac output (CO). Sympathetic function is impaired below the level of the injury because sympathetic nerves leave the spinal cord at the thoracic and lumbar areas and cranial parasympathetic nerves predominate in control over respirations, heart, and all vessels and organs below the injury, which includes autonomic functions.

15. b. Until the edema and necrosis at the site of the injury are resolved in 72 hours to 1 week after the injury, it is not possible to determine how much cord damage is present from the initial injury, how much secondary injury occurred, or how much the cord was damaged by edema that extended above the level of the original injury. The return of reflexes signals only the end of spinal shock and the reflexes may be inappropriate and excessive, causing spasms that complicate rehabilitation.

16. a. Spinal injury below C4 will result in diaphragmatic breathing and usually hypoventilation from decreased vital capacity and tidal volume from intercostal muscle impairment. The nurse's priority actions will be to monitor rate, rhythm, depth, and effort of breathing to observe for changes from the baseline and identify the need for ventilation assistance. Loss of all respiratory muscle function occurs above C4 and the patient requires mechanical ventilation to survive. Although the decreased sympathetic nervous system response (from injuries above T6) and GI hypomotility (paralytic ileus and gastric distention) will occur (with injuries above T5), they are not the patient's initial priority needs.

17. b. Neurogenic shock associated with cord injuries above the level of T6 greatly decreases the effect of the sympathetic nervous system and bradycardia and hypotension occur. A heart rate of 42 bpm is not adequate to meet the oxygen needs of the body. While low, the blood pressure is not at a critical point. The oxygen saturation is satisfactory and the motor and sensory losses are expected.

18. c. With the injury at T4, the highest-level realistic goal for this patient is to be able to be independent in self-care and wheelchair use because arm function will not be affected. Indoor mobility in a manual wheelchair will be achievable but it is not the highest-level goal. Ambulating with crutches and leg braces can be achieved only by patients with injuries in T6–12 area. Independent ambulation with short leg braces and canes could occur for a patient with an L3–4 injury. (See Table 61-4.)

19. d. Although surgical treatment of spinal cord injuries often depends on the preference of the health care provider, surgery is usually indicated when there is continued compression of the cord by extrinsic forces or when there is evidence of cord compression. Other indications may include progressive neurologic deficit, compound fracture of the vertebra, bony fragments, and penetrating wounds of the cord.

20. a. The need for a patent airway is the first priority for any injured patient and a high cervical injury may decrease the gag reflex and the ability to maintain an airway as well as the ability to breathe. Maintaining cervical stability is then a consideration, along with assessing for other injuries and the patient's neurologic status.

21. c. The development of better surgical stabilization has made surgery the more frequent treatment of cervical injuries. However, when surgery cannot be done, skeletal traction with the use of Crutchfield, Vinke, or other types of skull tongs is required to immobilize the cervical vertebrae, even if a fracture has not occurred. Hard cervical collars or a sternal-occipital-mandibular immobilizer brace may be used after cervical stabilization surgery or for minor injuries or stabilization during emergency transport of the patient. Sandbags may also be used temporarily to stabilize the neck during insertion of tongs or during diagnostic testing immediately following the injury. Special turning or kinetic beds may be used to turn and mobilize patients who are in cervical traction.

22. c. Dopamine is a vasopressor that is used to maintain blood pressure during states of hypotension that occur during neurogenic shock associated with spinal cord injury. Atropine would be used to treat bradycardia. The temperature reflects some degree of poikilothermism but this is not treated with medications.

23. c. Because pneumonia and atelectasis are potential problems related to ineffective coughing and the loss of intercostal and abdominal muscle function, the nurse should assess the patient's breath sounds and respiratory function to determine whether secretions are being retained or whether there is progression of respiratory impairment. Suctioning is not indicated unless lung sounds indicate retained secretions. Position changes will help to mobilize secretions. Intubation and mechanical ventilation are used if the patient becomes exhausted from labored breathing or if arterial blood gases (ABGs) deteriorate.

24. d. During the first 2 to 3 days after a spinal cord injury, paralytic ileus may occur and nasogastric suction must be used to remove secretions and gas from the GI tract until peristalsis resumes. IV fluids are used to maintain fluid balance but do not specifically relate to paralytic ileus. Tube feedings would be used only for patients who have difficulty swallowing and not until peristalsis returns. Parenteral nutrition would be used only if the paralytic ileus was unusually prolonged.

25. a. During the acute phase of spinal cord injury, the bladder is hypotonic, causing urinary retention with the risk for reflux into the kidney or rupture of the bladder. An indwelling catheter is used to keep the bladder empty and to monitor urinary output. Intermittent catheterization or other urinary drainage methods may be used in long-term bladder management. Use of incontinent pads is inappropriate because they do not help the bladder to empty.

26. b. When spinal shock ends, reflex movement and spasms will occur, which may be mistaken for return of function; however, with the resolution of edema, some normal function may also occur. It is important when movement occurs to determine whether the movement is voluntary and can be consciously controlled, which would indicate some return of function.

27. a. 5; b. 2; c. 6; d. 3; e. 1; f. 4. The patient is experiencing autonomic dysreflexia. The initial response by the nurse should be to elevate the head of bed (HOB) to decrease blood pressure (BP) and then to remove noxious

stimulation. Frequently the trigger is bladder distention, which can be dealt with quickly. The physician needs to be notified as soon as possible and, depending on the communication system available to the nurse, he or she should have the call placed. Meanwhile, the nurse should stay with the patient and loosen any restrictive clothing. The physician may order an antihypertensive and documentation should be an accurate and thorough description of the entire episode.

28. b. Intermittent self-catheterization five to six times a day is the recommended method of bladder management for the patient with a spinal cord injury and reflexic neurogenic bladder because it more closely mimics normal emptying and has less potential for infection. The patient and family should be taught the procedure using clean technique and if the patient has use of the arms, self-catheterization should be performed. Indwelling catheterization is used during the acute phase to prevent overdistention of the bladder and surgical urinary diversions are used if urinary complications occur.

29. d. Most patients with a complete lower motor neuron lesion are unable to have either psychogenic or reflexogenic erections and alternative methods of obtaining sexual satisfaction may be suggested. Patients with incomplete lower motor neuron lesions have the highest possibility of successful psychogenic erections with ejaculation whereas patients with incomplete upper motor neuron lesions are more likely to experience reflexogenic erections with ejaculation. Patients with complete upper motor neuron lesions usually have only reflex sexual function with rare ejaculation.

30. a. Working through the grief process is a lifelong process that is triggered by new experiences, such as marriage, child rearing, employment, or illness, which the patient must adjust to throughout life within the context of his or her disability. The goal of recovery is related to adjustment rather than acceptance and many patients do not experience all components of the grief process. During the anger phase, patients should be allowed outbursts and the nurse may use humor to displace some of the patient's anger.

31. b. Most metastatic or secondary tumors are extradural lesions in which treatment, including surgery, is palliative. Primary spinal tumors may be removed with the goal of cure. Most tumors of the spinal cord are slow-growing, do not cause autodestruction, and, if removal is possible, can have complete function restored. Radiation is used to treat metastatic tumors that are sensitive to radiation and that have caused only minor neurologic deficits in the patient. Radiation is also used as adjuvant therapy to surgery for intramedullary tumors.

Case Study

1. S.M. is experiencing central cord syndrome of the cervical cord, which is an incomplete spinal cord injury with compression on anterior horn cells. It usually occurs as a result of hyperextension.

2. The cell bodies of lower motor neurons, which send axons to innervate the skeletal muscles of arms, trunk, and legs, are located in the anterior horn of the spinal cord. The cervical segments of the spinal cord contain the lower

motor neurons for the arms. A cervical injury that affects the anterior horn will affect the arms to a greater extent than it affects the legs.

3. Injury to the cord may occur without fracture of the vertebrae, with traumatic twisting or stretching of the cord. The response to the trauma includes secondary injury leading to edema, hemorrhage, and ischemia of the cord, impairing function.

4. High doses of methylprednisolone within 8 hours of injury have been found to significantly improve motor function and sensation in patients with incomplete as well as complete spinal cord injuries. It blocks lipid peroxidation by-products and is thought to improve blood flow and reduce edema in the spinal cord.

5. Shock and denial are common first reactions to the loss of function with spinal cord injuries, followed by anger and depression. During the acute phase, S.M. will probably have unrealistic expectations concerning her recovery, sleep a lot, and withdraw. It is best to explain the injury, provide honest information, and encourage the patient's recovery. As S.M. progresses, she will become angry and refuse to discuss her limitations. It is important for her to participate in self-care and the nurse should support family members and allow patient outbursts. Assist her through depression by encouraging family involvement and use of resources in planning graded rehabilitation steps to give S.M. success, avoid sympathy, and use kind firmness. Altered body image will be a big problem because she will see herself as different from her peers, an important developmental issue during adolescence.

6. Intensive rehabilitation that focuses on refined retraining physiologic function of her limbs should be planned and will involve much physical therapy over time. S.M. should be mobilized as quickly as appropriate to prevent hazards of immobility and to encourage her in her progress. Balance support systems to encourage independence, set goals with patient input, and emphasize potentials.

7. **Nursing diagnoses:**
   - Impaired physical mobility *related to* spinal cord injury and prescribed bed rest
   - Risk for disuse syndrome *related to* immobilization
   - Self-care deficit: feeding, bathing, and grooming *related* to upper extremity weakness
   - Risk for injury *related to* sensory deficit and lack of self-protective abilities
   - Ineffective coping *related to* loss of control over body
   Collaborative problems:
   Potential complications: progression of lesion, hypoventilation, spinal shock, skin lesions

CHAPTER 62

Answer Key

1. a. Epiphysis; b. diaphysis; c. articular cartilage; d. spongy bone; e. epiphyseal line; f. red marrow cavities; g. compact bone; h. medullary cavity; i. yellow marrow; j. periosteum
2. a. Periosteum; b. canaliculi; c. blood vessels; d. osteon

3. a. Joint cavity with synovial fluid; b. bursa; c. articular cartilage; d. tendon sheath; e. periosteum; f. bone; g. joint capsule; h. nerve; i. blood vessel; j. synovial membrane; k. bone
4. c. Osteoblasts form bone. Osteocytes are mature bone cells. Osteoclasts are responsible for the resorption of bone. A sarcomere is the contractile unit of myofibrils.
5. b. Atrophy is when the muscle size decreases. Hyaline is the most common type of cartilage tissue. Isometric is a muscle contraction that produces hypertrophy. Hypertrophy is the increase in the size of cells causing an increase in the organ.
6. d. A loss of elasticity in cartilage, ligaments, and tendons increases rigidity in the neck, shoulders, back, hips, and knees of older patients. Actin (thin) filaments and myosin (thick) filaments make up the contractile unit of the myofibrils, which decrease in strength with lack of use. Fascia is connective tissue that can withstand limited stretching.
7. d. Periosteum is the fibrous connective tissue covering bone. Synovium is the lining of a joint capsule. Striated is a characteristic of skeletal muscle. Hyaline is the most common type of cartilage.
8. a. The function of the tendon is to attach muscle to bone. The ligament attaches bone to bone at the joint. Fascia encloses individual muscles but does not connect cartilage to muscle in joints. The bursae are lined with a synovial membrane and are located in joints to relieve pressure and decrease friction between moving parts.
9. a, c, e, f. Abduction is moving the part away from the midline of the body and adduction is moving the part toward the midline of the body. These movements can be done with the hip, wrist, thumb, and shoulder. The knee and elbow move with flexion and extension.
10. d. Loss of water from discs between vertebrae, vertebral disc compression, and narrowing of intervertebral spaces all contribute to a loss of height in the older adult. Although bone density decreases and cartilage is lost from joints, these do not affect the long bones or the height of the person.
11. d. Loss of muscle mass and strength, decreased motor neurons, limited movement because of joint changes, and less flexible tendons and ligaments all contribute to the older adult's risk for falls. Although rest and nutrients are important, fatigue and a high risk for impaired skin integrity are not directly related to changes associated with aging in the musculoskeletal system. Being overweight will increase stress on joints. Providing all care only contributes to weakening of muscles and decreased independence.
12. a. Corticosteroids cause protein catabolism with skeletal muscle wasting and increased osteoclast activity with loss of bone mass, which can have a marked detrimental effect on mobility and activity. Potassium-depleting diuretics may cause hypokalemia, which is associated with muscle weakness and cramps. Oral hypoglycemic drugs and nonsteroidal antiinflammatory drugs (NSAIDs) are not known to affect the musculoskeletal system.

13.

Functional Health Pattern	Risk Factor for or Response to Musculoskeletal Problem
Health perception–health management	History of musculoskeletal injuries, poor use of body mechanics or excessive muscular or joint stress, family history of joint and bone disease; mechanism and circumstances of injury, methods of treatment, current status, need for assistive devices, interference with activities of daily living; safety practices
Nutritional-metabolic	Presence of obesity, inadequate calcium, vitamin D or C, or protein intake
Elimination	Inability to physically access toilet; constipation
Activity-exercise	Limitation or clumsiness of movement; pain, weakness, crepitus; extremes of occupational activity and recreational activities—sedentary or heavy use of body
Sleep-rest	Pain interfering with sleep; frequent position changes
Cognitive-perceptual	Musculoskeletal pain; pain management measures
Self-perception–self-concept	Loss of body image or self-worth caused by musculoskeletal deformity
Role-relationship	Change in work and family roles and responsibilities caused by immobility or pain
Sexuality-reproductive	Decreased sexual activity and satisfaction because of pain, deformity
Coping–stress tolerance	Decreased coping ability related to effect of musculoskeletal problems
Value-belief	Cultural or religious beliefs that influence the patient's acceptance of treatment related to diet, exercise, medication, or lifestyle modifications

14. c. Muscle strength is graded on a scale of 0 to 5, with 0 = no detection of muscle contraction and 5 = active movement against full resistance without evident fatigue (normal). Active movement against gravity and some resistance = 4.

15. b. There is no indication to measure the length of limbs during assessment unless a gait disturbance or limb length discrepancy is noted and then the limb should be measured between two bony prominences and compared with the measurement of the other extremity. Muscle mass measurement and joint movement may affect gait but differences in limb length will always affect gait. Palpating for crepitus will identify friction between bones, usually at joints.

16. c. A goniometer is a protractor device that measures the angle of joints and can be used to determine specific degrees of joint range of motion (ROM). It is used when a specific musculoskeletal problem that affects ROM has been identified.

17. b. Scoliosis is a lateral "S" curve of the thoracic and lumbar spine. Kyphosis is an exaggerated forward thoracic curvature. Lordosis is an exaggerated lumbar curvature or swayback. Ankylosis is fixation of a joint.

18. c. A contracture is shortening of a muscle or ligament that causes resistance of movement. A fluid-filled cyst is a ganglion cyst. Generalized muscle pain is myalgia. Crepitation is a grating sensation between bones with movement.

19. d. Torticollis is the neck twisted in an unusual position to one side, so the nurse should provide enough pillows to support the patient's head comfortably. An immobilizer to hold bones in place may be used with dislocation or for a joint with subluxation. Pillows to support the knees while sleeping may be done for valgum or varum deformities or for any patient's comfort. Exercises to increase or maintain muscle strength and maintain ROM are appropriate for most patients.

20. c. Plantar fasciitis presents as burning sharp pain at the sole of the foot that is worse in the morning. Pes planus is abnormal flatness of the sole and arch of the foot. Tenosynovitis is pain along a tendon sheath. Muscle atrophy presents as flabby-appearing muscle leading to decreased function and tone.

21. d. Steppage gait uses increased hip and knee flexion in order to clear the foot from the floor and then the foot slaps down on the walking surface. Ataxic gait is a staggering, uncoordinated gait, often with a sway. Spastic gait has short steps with dragging of the foot in a jerky cross-knee movement. Antalgic gait is a shorted stride with as little weight bearing as possible on the painful side.

22. c. A standard x-ray evaluates structural or functional changes of bones and joints and can determine density of bone. Myelogram is a sensitive test for nerve impingement and can detect very subtle lesions and injuries. Arthroscopy is used to visualize, diagnose, or repair joint problems. Magnetic resonance imaging (MRI) is used to view soft tissue.

23. d. Dual energy x-ray absorptiometry (DXA) measures bone mass of spine, femur, forearm, and total body and is used to diagnose and monitor changes in bone density with treatment. Bone scan is done with the injection of a radioisotope that is taken up by the bone to identify osteomyelitis, osteoporosis, and primary and metastatic malignant lesions. A diskogram is an x-ray with contrast media to evaluate intervertebral disc abnormalities. Quantitative ultrasound (QUS) evaluates density, elasticity, and strength of bone, which is commonly assessed at the calcaneus (heel).

24. c, d, e. Increases in rheumatoid factor (RF), antinuclear antibody (ANA), and erythrocyte sedimentation rate (ESR) as well as depletion of complement, total hemolytic, and

presence of human leukocyte antigen (HLA)-B27 may occur in rheumatoid arthritis. Uric acid may be elevated in gout. Anti-DNA antibody is the most specific test for systemic lupus erythematosus.

CHAPTER 63

Answer Key

1. d. Almost all older adults have some degree of decreased muscle strength, joint stiffness, and pain with motion. The use of mild antiinflammatory agents decreases inflammation and pain and can help the patient to maintain activity and prevent further deconditioning but other prescribed drugs and potential abdominal problems must be considered by the patient. Musculoskeletal problems in the older adult can be prevented with appropriate strategies, especially exercise. Stair walking can create enough stress on fragile bones to cause a hip fracture and use of ramps may help to prevent falls. Walkers and canes should be used as necessary to decrease stress on joints so that activity can be maintained.

2. c. Warm-up exercises "prelengthen" potentially strained tissues by avoiding the quick stretch often encountered in sports and also increase the temperature of muscle, resulting in increased speed of cell metabolism, increased speed of nerve impulses, and improved oxygenation of muscle fibers. Stretching is also thought to improve kinesthetic awareness, lessening the chance of uncoordinated movement. Muscle strength is not a key factor in soft tissue injuries and taping or wrapping joints may actually predispose a person to injury by weakening the joint, unless a previous injury is being treated.

3. b. An avulsion fracture occurs when a ligament pulls a bone fragment loose, with pain similar to a sprain. A fracture with two or more fragments is a comminuted fracture. It is a spiral fracture when it is twisted around a bone shaft. It is a transverse fracture when the line of fracture is at right angles to the longitudinal axis.

4. c. A pathologic fracture is a spontaneous fracture at the site of bone disease, such as osteoporosis. An open fracture is when there is communication with the external environment. The oblique fracture has a slanted fracture line. A greenstick fracture is splintered on one side and the other side is bent.

5. d. Carpal tunnel syndrome would be expected related to the continuous wrist movements. Injuries of the menisci, which are fibrocartilage in the knee, are common with athletes. Radial-ulnar fractures are seen with great force such as a car accident or a fall. Rotator cuff injuries occur with sudden adduction forces applied to the cuff while the arm is held in abduction. They are commonly seen with repetitive overhead motions.

6. c. Bursitis is inflammation of synovial membrane sac at friction sites. Tearing of a ligament is a sprain. Stretching of muscle and fascia sheath is a strain. Incomplete separation of articular surfaces of joints caused by ligament injury is subluxation.

7. b. Application of cold, compression, and elevation are indicated to prevent edema resulting from sprain and some strain injuries. Muscle spasms are usually treated with heat applications and massage and repetitive strain injuries require cessation of the precipitating activity and physical therapy. Dislocations or subluxations require immediate reduction and immobilization to prevent vascular impairment and bone cell death.

8. a, b, c, e. Consider the principle of RICE. Rest: movement should be restricted. Ice: cold should be used to promote vasoconstriction and to reduce edema. C: compression helps to decrease swelling. E: elevate the extremity above the level of the heart. Mild nonsteroidal antiinflammatory drugs (NSAIDs) may be needed to manage pain. Warm, moist compresses may be used after 48 hours for 20 to 30 minutes at a time to reduce swelling and provide comfort.

9. a. Ossification is the stage of fracture healing when there is clinical union and enough strength to prevent movement at the fracture site. Remodeling is the normal function of the bone. Consolidation is when the distance between bone fragments eventually closes and radiologic union first occurs. The callus formation stage appears by the end of the second week of injury when minerals and new bone matrix are deposited in the osteoid that is produced in the granulation tissue stage.

10. a, b, c, e. When the remodeling stage of healing occurs, radiologic union is present. Excess callus is reabsorbed, trabecular bone is laid, and the bone returns to its preinjury structure strength and shape. The osteoblasts and osteoclasts function normally in response to stress. The fracture hematoma stage is when the hematoma at the ends of the fragments becomes a semisolid blood clot. There is an unorganized network of bone composed of cartilage, osteoblasts, calcium, and phosphorus woven around fracture parts in the callus formation stage.

11. b. Deformity is the cardinal sign of fracture but may not be apparent in all fractures. Other supporting signs include edema and swelling, localized pain and tenderness, muscle spasm, ecchymosis, loss of function, crepitation, and an inability to bear weight.

12. a. A malunion occurs when the bone heals in the expected time but in an unsatisfactory position, possibly resulting in deformity or dysfunction. Nonunion occurs when the fracture fails to heal properly despite treatment and delayed union is healing of the fracture at a slower rate than expected. In posttraumatic osteoporosis, the loss of bone substances occurs as a result of immobilization.

13. a. Open reduction uses a surgical incision to correct bone alignment but infection is the main disadvantage, as well as anesthesia complications or the effect of preexisting medical conditions. Skin irritation and nerve impairment is most likely with skin traction. Prolonged immobility is possible with skeletal traction.

14. d. Complaints of abdominal pain or pressure, nausea, and vomiting are signs of cast syndrome that occur when hip spica casts or body jacket braces are applied too tightly, causing compression of the superior mesenteric artery against the duodenum. The cast may need to be split or removed and the health care provider should be notified. Elevation is not indicated for a spica cast and the patient with a spica cast should not be placed in the prone position during the initial drying stage because the cast is so large and heavy it may break. A cast should never be covered with a blanket because heat builds up in the cast and may increase edema.

15. b. Infection is the greatest risk with an open fracture and all open fractures are considered contaminated. Tetanus

prevention is always indicated if the patient has not been immunized or does not have current boosters. Prophylactic antibiotics are often used in management of open fractures but recent antibiotic therapy is not relevant, nor is previous injury to the site.

16. d. Pulses, sensation, and motor function distal to the injury should be checked before and after splinting to assess for nerve or vascular damage and documented to avoid doubts about whether a problem discovered later was missed during the original examination or was caused by the treatment. Elevation of the limb and application of ice should be instituted after the extremity is splinted.

17. b. Neurologic assessment includes evaluation of motor and sensory function and, in the upper extremity, includes abduction and adduction of the fingers, opposition of the fingers, and supination and pronation of the hands. It also includes sensory perception in the fingers. Evaluation of the feet would occur in lower extremity injuries. Assessment of color, temperature, capillary refill, peripheral pulses, and edema evaluates vascular status.

18. b. A patient with any type of cast should exercise the joints above and below the cast frequently and moving the fingers frequently will improve circulation and help to prevent edema. Unlike plaster casts, thermoplastic resin or fiberglass casts are relatively waterproof and, if they become wet, can be dried with a hair dryer on low setting. Tape petals are used on plaster casts to protect the edges from breaking and crumbling but are not necessary for synthetic casts. After the cast is applied, the extremity should be elevated at about the level of the heart to promote venous return and ice may be used to prevent edema.

19. c. Pain that is distal to the injury and is unrelieved by opioid analgesics is the earliest sign of compartment syndrome. Paralysis and absence of peripheral pulses will eventually occur if it is not treated but these are late signs that often appear after permanent damage has occurred. The overlying skin may appear normal because the surface vessels are not occluded.

20. a. Soft tissue edema in the area of the injury may cause an increase of pressure within the closed spaces of the tissue compartments formed by the nonelastic fascia, creating compartment syndrome. If symptoms occur, it may be necessary to incise the fascia surgically, a procedure known as a fasciotomy. Amputation is usually necessary only if the limb becomes septic because of untreated compartment syndrome.

21. c. The fractured humerus may cause radial nerve and brachial artery damage and it may be reduced nonsurgically with a hanging arm cast. A fractured tibia and femoral shaft are in the leg. The Colles' fracture is in the wrist and manifests with pronounced swelling and obvious deformity of the wrist; it is treated with closed manipulation and immobilization.

22. c. A Colles' fracture most often occurs in patients over 50 years of age with osteoporosis and frequently when the patient attempts to break a fall with an outstretched arm and hand. Dislocation is the complete separation of articular surfaces of the joint caused by a ligament injury. Open fracture is when there is communication with the external environment. A fracture is incomplete if only part of the bone shaft is fractured and the bone is still in one piece.

23. a, c. Airway patency and cervical spinal cord injury are the emergency considerations with facial fractures. Oral examination and cranial nerve assessment will be done after the patient is stabilized. Immobilization of the jaw is done surgically for a mandibular fracture.

24. b. The spine should be kept straight by turning the shoulders and hips together (logrolling). This keeps the spine in good alignment until union has been accomplished. Bed rest may be required for a short time but not until the pain is gone. Analgesics should be taken only as ordered. If they do not relieve the pain, the health care provider should be notified. Bone cement is used by the surgeon to stabilize vertebral compression fractures.

25. a. Initial manifestations of fat embolism usually occur 24 to 48 hours after injury and are associated with fractures of long bones and multiple fractures related to pelvic injuries, including fractures of the femur, tibia, ribs, and pelvis.

26. c. Patients with fractures are at risk for both fat embolism and pulmonary embolism from venous thromboembolism but there is a difference in the time of occurrence, with fat embolism occurring shortly after the injury and thrombotic embolism occurring several days after immobilization. They both may cause pulmonary symptoms of chest pain, tachypnea, dyspnea, apprehension, tachycardia, and cyanosis. However, fat embolism may cause petechiae located around the neck, anterior chest wall, axilla, buccal membrane of the mouth, and conjunctiva of the eye, which differentiates it from thrombotic embolism.

27. a. A hip prosthesis is usually used for intracapsular fractures. The other options are all extracapsular fractures.

28. d. The classic signs of a hip fracture are shortening of the leg and external rotation accompanied by severe pain at the fracture site and additional injury could be caused by weight bearing on the extremity. The patient may not be able to move the hip or the knee but movement in the ankle and toes is not affected.

29. c. Although surgical repair is the preferred method of managing intracapsular and extracapsular hip fractures, initially patients frequently may be treated with skin traction, such as Buck's traction or Russell's traction, to immobilize the limb temporarily and to relieve the painful muscle spasms before surgery is performed. Prolonged traction would be required to reduce the fracture or immobilize it for healing, creating a very high risk for complications of immobility.

30. a. Because the fracture site is internally fixed with pins or plates, the fracture site is stable and the patient is moved from the bed to the chair on the first postoperative day. Ambulation begins on the first or second postoperative day without weight bearing on the affected leg. Weight bearing on the affected extremity is usually restricted for 6 to 12 weeks until adequate healing is evident on x-ray. The patient may be positioned on the operative side following internal fixation and abductor pillows are used for patients who have total hip replacements.

31. d. Patients with hip prostheses with a posterior approach must avoid extreme flexion, adduction, or internal rotation for at least 6 weeks to prevent dislocation of the prosthesis. Gradual weight bearing on the limb is allowed and ambulation should be encouraged. The leg should be not be externally rotated.

32. c. The low-bulk, high-carbohydrate liquid diet and intake of air through a straw required during mandibular fixation often lead to constipation and flatus, which may be relieved

with bulk-forming laxatives, prune juice, or ambulation. Wires or rubber bands should be cut only in the case of cardiac or respiratory arrest and patients should be taught to clear their mouth of vomitus or secretions. The mouth should be thoroughly cleaned with water, saline, or alkaline mouthwashes or using a Water Pik as necessary to remove food debris. Hard candy should not be held in the mouth.

33. c. The compression dressing or bandage supports the soft tissues, reduces edema, hastens healing, minimizes pain, and promotes residual limb shrinkage. If the dressing is left off, edema will form quickly and may delay rehabilitation. Elevation and ice will not be as effective at preventing the edema that will form. Dressing the incision with dry gauze will not provide the benefits of a compression dressing.

34. b. Phantom sensation or phantom pain may occur following amputation, especially if pain was present in the affected limb preoperatively. The pain is a real sensation to the patient and will first be treated with analgesics and other pain interventions (i.e., tricyclic antidepressants, antiseizure drugs, transcutaneous electrical nerve stimulation [TENS], mirror therapy, acupuncture). As recovery and ambulation progress, phantom limb sensation usually subsides.

35. a. Because the device covers the residual limb, the surgical site cannot be directly seen and postoperative hemorrhage is not apparent on dressings, requiring vigilant assessment of vital signs for signs of bleeding. Elevation of the residual limb with an immediate prosthetic fitting is not necessary because the device itself prevents edema formation. Exercises to the leg are not performed in the immediate postoperative period to avoid disruption of ligatures and the suture line.

36. a. Flexion contractures, especially of the hip, may be debilitating and delay rehabilitation of the patient with a leg amputation. To prevent hip flexion, the patient should avoid sitting in a chair with the hips flexed or having pillows under the surgical extremity for prolonged periods and the patient should lie on the abdomen for 30 minutes three to four times a day to extend the hip.

37. a. Skin breakdown on the residual limb can prevent the use of a prosthesis so the limb should be inspected every day for signs of irritation or pressure areas. No substances except water and mild soap should be used on the residual limb and range-of-motion (ROM) exercises are not necessary when the patient is using a prosthesis. A residual limb shrinker is an elastic stocking that is used to mold the limb in preparation for prosthesis use but a cotton residual limb sock is worn with the prosthesis.

38. c. Debridement removes degenerative tissue from joints. Osteotomy corrects bone deformity by removal of a wedge or slice of bone. Arthrodesis surgically fuses a joint to relieve pain. Synovectomy removes tissue involved in joint destruction from rheumatoid arthritis (RA).

39. c. An arthroplasty is reconstruction or replacement of a joint to relieve pain and correct deformity, especially with osteoarthritis, RA, avascular necrosis, congenital deformities, or dislocations. Arthrodesis is the surgical fusion of a joint to relieve pain. An osteotomy removes a wedge of bone to correct a bone deformity. Synovectomy is used in RA to remove the tissue involved in joint destruction.

40. d. Physical therapy is initiated on the first postoperative day with ambulation and weight bearing using a walker for a patient with a cemented prosthesis and non–weight bearing on the operative side for an uncemented prosthesis. In addition, the patient sits in the chair at least twice a day and is turned to both sides and back with the operative leg supported.

41. b. Following a total hip arthroplasty with a posterior approach, during hospitalization an abduction pillow is placed between the legs to maintain abduction and the leg is extended. Extremes of internal rotation, adduction, and 90-degree flexion of the hip must be avoided for 4 to 6 weeks postoperatively to prevent dislocation of the prosthesis.

42. b. Continuous passive motion machines are frequently used following knee surgery to promote earlier joint mobility. Because joint dislocation is not a problem with knee replacements, early exercise with straight leg raises and gentle ROM is also encouraged postoperatively.

43. b. Neurovascular checks of the fingers following surgery of the hands are essential to detect compromised vascular and neurologic function caused by trauma or edema. Postoperatively, the hands are elevated with a bulky dressing in place and when the dressing is removed, a guided splinting program is started. Exercises are performed three to four times a day when the splints are removed and the patient is discharged. Before surgery, it must be made clear to the patient that the goal of the surgery is to restore function related to grasp, pinch, stability, and strength and the hands will not necessarily have good cosmetic appearance.

44. d. The patient with a tight cast may be at risk for neurovascular compromise (impaired circulation and peripheral nerve damage) and should be assessed first. The other patients should be seen as soon as possible. Providing analgesia for the patient with phantom pain would be the next priority. The patient in skeletal traction needs explanation of the purpose and functioning of the traction. She may need analgesia or muscle relaxants to help tolerate the traction.

Case Study

1. The knee and ankle should be immobilized with a splint. Unless the joints above and below the site are immobilized, the affected area is unstable.

2. The 6 Ps—pulses, paresthesias, pallor, pressure, paralysis, and pain—should be assessed, especially unrelieved pain, which may indicate compartment syndrome.

3. The wound should be cleaned with extensive irrigation using normal saline and if the wound is highly contaminated, surgical debridement may be necessary. Tetanus immunization is required if a dose of tetanus toxoid has not been given in the past 5 to 10 years. If the patient has had fewer than three doses of toxoid, then tetanus toxoid, reduced diphtheria toxoid, and acellular pertussis vaccine (Tdap) are recommended. Bleeding should be controlled with sterile dressings.

4. Measures to relieve pain include elevating the limb and applying ice to decrease swelling, administering analgesics, and keeping the limb immobilized.

5. It can take up to 1 year for complete healing of the fracture but ossification should take place in 3 weeks to 6 months. The limb can be casted and H.A. can be mobile with crutches with no weight bearing on the affected limb. Weight bearing will be restricted for 6 to 12 weeks, depending on the rate of healing. His return to work will depend on how he is able to perform on crutches.

6. The RN can delegate to unlicensed assistive personnel (UAP) positioning (position the casted leg above heart

level); applying ice as directed by the RN; maintaining body position; assisting the patient with passive and active ROM exercises; and notifying the RN about patient complaints of pain, tingling, or decreased sensation in the right leg.

7. H.A.'s wife should be called, informed of her husband's accident, and told that he is alert and oriented but has a fractured leg and will require hospitalization. Care should be taken not to panic her and to reassure her that his condition is stable.

8. **Nursing diagnoses:**
   - Acute pain *related to* edema and muscle spasms
   - Risk for peripheral neurovascular dysfunction *related to* vascular insufficiency and nerve compression secondary to edema
   - Risk for infection *related to* disruption of skin integrity and presence of environmental pathogens
   - Anxiety *related to* unknown outcome and restrictions
   - Readiness for enhanced self-health management *related to* questions about activity restrictions

   Collaborative problems:
   Potential complications: fat embolism, compartment syndrome, infection, malunion or nonunion

CHAPTER 64

Answer Key

1. b. Chronic infection of the bone leads to formation of scar tissue from the granulation tissue. This avascular scar tissue provides an ideal site for continued microorganism growth and is impenetrable to antibiotics. Surgical debridement is often necessary to remove the poorly vascularized tissue and dead bone and to instill antibiotics directly to the area. Involucrum is new bone laid down at the infection site, which seals off areas of sequestra. Antibiotics can be effective during acute osteomyelitis and prevention of chronic osteomyelitis requires early antibiotic treatment. Bone and skin grafting may be necessary following surgical removal of infection if destruction is extensive.

2. b. The patient with osteomyelitis is at risk for pathologic fractures at the site of the infection because of weakened, devitalized bone and careful handling of the extremity is necessary. Careful handling of dressings is necessary to prevent the spread of infection to others but is not related to preventing injury to this patient. Splints may be used to immobilize the limb, range-of-motion (ROM) exercises will be limited because of the possibility of spreading infection, and edema is not a common finding in osteomyelitis.

3. c. Because large doses of appropriate antibiotics are necessary in the treatment of acute osteomyelitis, it is important to identify the causative microorganism. The definitive way to determine the causative agent is by bone biopsy or biopsy of the soft tissue surrounding the site. The other tests may help to establish the diagnosis but do not identify the causative agent.

4. c. Activities such as exercise or heat application, which increase circulation and serve as stimuli for the spread of infection, should be avoided by patients with acute osteomyelitis. Oral or IV antibiotic therapy is continued at home for 4 to 6 weeks, weight bearing is contraindicated to prevent pathologic fractures, and notification of the health care provider if increased pain occurs is necessary.

5. b. One of the most common adverse effects of prolonged and high-dose antibiotic therapy is overgrowth of *Candida albicans* in the oral cavity and genitourinary tract. These infections are manifested by whitish-yellow, curdlike lesions of the mucosa. A dry, cracked, furrowed tongue is characteristic of severe dehydration and vesicles are characteristic of herpes simplex infections. Mouth and lip ulcers are characteristic of aphthous somatitis, or canker sores.

6. d. Osteochondroma is a benign overgrowth of bone and cartilage near the end of the bone at the growth plate, especially in long bones, pelvis, or scapula. It may transform to a malignant form. Osteoclastoma is a benign bone tumor with a high rate of recurrence, but does not become malignant. Endochroma is benign but is an intramedullary cartilage tumor found in a cavity of a single hand or foot bone. Ewing's sarcoma develops in the medullary cavity of long bones, especially the femur, humerus, pelvis, and tibia.

7. b. Osteosarcoma, the most common primary bone cancer, occurs in the metaphyseal region of long bones of the arms, legs, or pelvis. It is extremely malignant and metastasizes early and is often brought to attention by injury. A high rate of local recurrence occurs with osteoclastoma that arises in cancellous ends of long bones. Ewing's sarcoma develops in the medullary cavity of long bones as above.

8. b. Promotion of muscle activity is important in any patient with muscular dystrophy but when the disease has progressed to cardiomyopathy or respiratory failure, activity must be balanced with oxygen supply. At this stage of the disease, care should be taken to prevent skin or respiratory complications. The patient should be encouraged to perform as much self-care and exercise as energy allows but this will be limited.

9. d. Intervertebral disc herniation is generally indicated by radicular pain radiating down the buttock, below the knee, and along the distribution of the sciatic nerve. Cervical disc disease has pain radiating into the arms and hands. Acute lumbosacral strain causes acute low back pain. Degenerative disc disease is a structural degeneration of discs that is a normal process of aging and results in intervertebral discs losing their elasticity, flexibility, and shock-absorbing capabilities.

10. a. Proper daily exercise is an important part of the prevention of back injury, with the goal of maintaining mobility and strength in the back. Patients should sit with the knees higher than the hips and should sleep in a side-lying position, with knees and hips bent, or on the back, with a device to flex the hips and knees. Good body mechanics with proper transfer and turning techniques are necessary in all jobs and activities.

11. b. Urinary incontinence following spinal surgery may indicate nerve damage and should be reported to the health care provider. Paralytic ileus is common following surgery and is expected. Pain at the graft site, usually the iliac crest or the fibula, often is more severe than pain at the fused area. Although movement and sensation of the arms and legs should not be more impaired than before surgery, they often are not relieved immediately after surgery.

12. c. After spinal surgery, patients are logrolled to maintain straight alignment of the spine at all times, requiring the patient to be turned with a pillow between the legs and moving the body as a unit. The head of the bed is usually kept flat and the legs are extended.

13. a. A plantar wart is a papilloma growth on the sole of the foot. Thickened skin on the weight-bearing part of the foot is a callus. Local thickening of skin caused by pressure on bony prominences is a corn. A tumor on nerve tissue between the third and fourth metatarsal heads is a Morton's neuroma.

14. c. This patient has a hallux valgus (bunion) that will be treated surgically by removing the bursal sac and bony enlargement. Metatarsal arch support is conservative treatment for hammer toe. A corn is trimmed with a scalpel after softening. Intraarticular corticosteroids and passive manual stretching are conservative treatment for hallux rigidus from osteoarthritis.

15. c. Poorly fitted shoes selected for fashion rather than comfort are the primary factor in the development of foot problems. A few congenital problems predispose to foot problems. Poor hygiene in patients with peripheral vascular disease may lead to foot infections but these factors are in the minority compared with the effect of ill-fitting shoes.

16. c, f. Paget's disease is abnormal remodeling and resorption of bone with replacement of normal marrow with vascular connective tissue. Osteoporosis is loss of total bone mass and substance with abnormal remodeling and resorption of bone and is most common in bones of the spine, hips, and wrists. Osteomalacia results from vitamin D deficiency and causes generalized bone decalcification with bone deformity.

17. b, d, e. Risk factors for osteoporosis include age greater than 65, white or Asian ethnicity, cigarette smoking, inactive lifestyle, low body weight, and postmenopausal estrogen deficiency including premature menopause. Other factors include family history, excessive alcohol use, long-term use of medications such as corticosteroids, thyroid replacement, heparin, long-acting sedatives, or antiseizure drugs.

18. b, c. To specifically prevent osteoporosis in postmenopausal women, increased calcium and vitamin D intake and weight-bearing exercises (i.e., walking) are the best methods. Beef is not high in calcium or vitamin D. Although 20 minutes in the sun each day provides vitamin D for most women, it is recommended that postmenopausal women take supplemental vitamin D doses of 800 to 1000 IU per day. Although estrogen replacement will protect the woman against bone loss and fractures, it is no longer given specifically to prevent osteoporosis because of increased risk of heart disease and breast or uterine cancer.

19. a. The bisphosphonates, such as alendronate, must be taken at least 30 minutes before food or other medications to promote their absorption. As well, because they are very irritating to the stomach and esophagus, the patient must remain upright for at least 30 minutes after taking the medication to prevent reflux into the esophagus. These drugs will prevent further bone loss and increase bone density but calcium and vitamin D supplementation is still needed for bone formation.

Case Study

1. Risk factors for back pain in G.B. include excess body weight, cigarette smoking, and a job that requires heavy lifting and prolonged periods of sitting.

2. Preoperative preparation includes teaching about the restrictions on positioning and movement required following surgery, measures for pain control, and assessments that will be carried out postoperatively. The nurse should ensure that G.B. has received information about the procedure from the surgeon and understands the benefits and risks of the surgery.

3. G.B. will probably be restricted to flat bed rest for at least the first 24 hours to avoid straining the surgical area. Pillows may be used under the thigh of each leg to prevent strain on the back muscles and between the legs with turning to maintain alignment. When turning is allowed, he must be turned with the help of several personnel to avoid changing the alignment of the spine or he must be logrolled. Depending on the surgeon's preference, ambulation will usually begin by the second postoperative day, again keeping the spine in alignment.

4. The following postoperative assessments should be carried out by the nurse q2-4hr during the first 24 to 48 hours:
   - Sensation: In all extremities in all appropriate dermatomes
   - Circulation and vital signs
   - Movement: Of all extremities
   - Muscle strength: Note any new weakness of the extremities
   - Wound: Assess dressing for drainage and note amount, color, characteristics; clear or light yellow drainage should be tested for the presence of glucose, which would indicate spinal fluid leakage
   - Pain: Document location and intensity of pain; evaluate pain after administration of analgesia
   - Bowel activity: Assess bowel sounds, passage of flatus, and abdomen; paralytic ileus is common for several days
   - Urinary function: Incontinence or retention may indicate nerve damage and should be reported; intermittent catheterization may be required for bladder emptying, especially until G.B. is allowed to stand to void.

5. Discharge instructions include teaching G.B. to report any persistent limb weakness, abnormal sensations, or pain to the health care provider. He should be instructed to avoid standing or sitting for prolonged periods. Walking, lying down, and shifting weight from one foot to another should be encouraged. Twisting of the spine is harmful and he should be taught to think through any activity before bending, lifting, or stooping. A firm mattress or bed board should be used at home and sleeping on the side or back with knees and hips flexed should be encouraged. To prevent further back problems, weight loss and smoking cessation should be encouraged. He should be taught correct body mechanics and to do strengthening back exercises after recovery from the surgery.

6. **Nursing diagnoses:**
   - Acute pain *related to* nerve root compression, muscle spasms, and surgical incision
   - Impaired physical mobility *related to* pain
   - Ineffective self-health management *related to* lack of knowledge regarding posture, exercises, body mechanics, and weight reduction

   Collaborative problem:
   Potential complication: paralysis

CHAPTER 65

Answer Key

1. d. Cartilage destruction in the joints affects the majority of those affected by the age of 40 and when the destruction becomes symptomatic, osteoarthritis (OA) is said to be present. Degenerative changes cause symptoms after age 50 or 60 but more than half over age 65 have x-ray evidence

of OA. Joint pain and functional disability should not be considered a normal finding in aging persons. OA is not a systemic disease but is usually caused by a known event or condition that directly damages cartilage or causes joint instability.

2. a. 3; b. 5; c. 6; d. 1; e. 4; f. 2

3. d. The pain in later OA is caused by bone surfaces rubbing together after the articular cartilage has deteriorated. Crepitation occurs earlier in the disease with loose particles of cartilage in the joint cavity. Bouchard's nodes and Heberden's nodes are tender but occur as joint space decreases and as early as 40 years of age.

4. b. Principles of joint protection and energy conservation are critical in being able to maintain functional mobility in the patient with OA and patients should be helped to find ways to perform activities and tasks with less stress. Range-of-motion (ROM), isotonic, and isometric exercises of the affected joints should be balanced with joint rest and protection but during an acute flare of joint inflammation, the joints should be rested. If a joint is painful, it should be used only to the point of pain and masking the pain with analgesics may lead to greater joint injury.

5. a. Some relief for moderate to severe arthritic pain but not for mild arthritic pain has been observed with the use of over-the-counter glucosamine and chondroitin sulfate. These substances should be discontinued if there are no effects after consistent use over 90 to 120 days. They may decrease the effectiveness of antidiabetic drugs and increase the risk of bleeding.

6. a. Common side effects of nonsteroidal antiinflammatory drugs (NSAIDs) include gastrointestinal (GI) irritation and bleeding, dizziness, rash, headache, and tinnitus. Misoprostol (Cytotec) is used to prevent NSAID-induced gastric ulcers and gastritis and would increase the patient's tolerance of any of the NSAIDs. The use of naproxen would cause the same gastric effects as ibuprofen. The daily dose of acetaminophen should not exceed 4 g/day to prevent liver damage and antacids interfere with the absorption of NSAIDs.

7. a. OA is not systemic or symmetric. Morning joint stiffness resolves in about 30 minutes. Rheumatoid arthritis (RA) is rheumatoid factor (RF) positive and characterized by being systemic and affecting small joints symmetrically. Morning joint stiffness lasts 60 minutes to all day.

8. d. Pain and immobility of OA may be aggravated by falling barometric pressure. OA affects weight-bearing joints of knees and hips. Stiffness occurs on arising but usually subsides after 30 minutes. Pain during the day is relieved with rest. Fatigue, anorexia, and weight loss are nonspecific manifestations of the onset of RA.

9. c. In early disease, the fingers of the patient with moderate RA (1) may become spindle shaped from synovial hypertrophy and thickening of the joint capsule, (2) have no joint deformities but may have limited joint mobility, (3) have adjacent muscle atrophy, and (4) may be inflamed. Splenomegaly may be found with Felty syndrome in patients with severe nodule-forming RA. Heberden's nodes and crepitus on movement are associated with osteoarthritis.

10. d. The anti-citrullinated protein antibody (ACPA) is more specific than RF for RA and may allow for earlier and more accurate diagnosis. Other tests include C-reactive protein (CRP) that is elevated from inflammatory reactions of RA, a

finding that is useful in monitoring the response to therapy. The white blood cell (WBC) count may be increased in response to inflammation and is also elevated in synovial fluid. Anemia, rather than polycythemia, is common, and immunoglobulin G (IgG) levels are normal.

11. b. Rheumatoid nodules develop in 20% to 30% of patients with RA. Felty syndrome is most common in patients with severe, nodule-forming RA. It is characterized by splenomegaly and leukopenia. Sjögren's syndrome occurs as a disease by itself or with other arthritic disorders. Lyme disease is a spirochetal infection transmitted by an infected deer tick bite. Spondyloarthropathies are interrelated multisystem inflammatory disorders that affect the spine, peripheral joints, and periarticular structures but they do not have serum antibodies.

12. b. Entanercept binds to tumor necrosis factor (TNF) and blocks its interaction with the TNF cell surface receptors, which decreases the inflammatory response. Anakinra is an interleukin-1 receptor antagonist, thus decreasing the inflammatory response. Leflunomide is an antiinflammatory that inhibits proliferation of lymphocytes. Azathioprine is an immunosuppressant that inhibits DNA, RNA, and protein synthesis.

13. b. Certolizumab is a monoclonal antibody that is a TNF inhibitor and stays in the system longer and may show a more rapid reduction in RA symptoms. Parenteral gold alters immune responses that may suppress synovitis of active RA but it takes 3 to 6 months to be effective. Tocilizumab blocks the action of the proinflammatory cytokine interleukin-6 (IL-6). Hydroxychloroquine is an antimalaria drug used initially for mild RA and requires periodic eye examinations to assess for retinal damage.

14. c. Because older adults are more likely to take many drugs, the use of multidrug therapy in RA is particularly problematic because of the increased likelihood of adverse drug interactions and toxicity. Rheumatic disorders do occur in older adults but usually in milder form. Older adults are not less compliant with drug regimens but may need help with complex regimens. Interpretation of laboratory values in older adults is more difficult in diagnosing RA because of age-related serologic changes but the disease can be diagnosed.

15. b. Most patients with RA experience morning stiffness and morning activities should be scheduled later in the day after the stiffness subsides. A warm shower in the morning and time to become more mobile before activity are advised. Management of RA includes daily exercises for the affected joints and protection of joints with devices and movements that prevent joint stress. Splinting should be done during an acute flare to rest the joint and prevent further damage.

16. b. Pacing activities and alternating rest with activity are important in maintaining self-care and independence of the patient with RA, in addition to preventing deconditioning and a negative attitude. The nurse should not carry out activities for patients that they can do for themselves but instead should support and assist patients as necessary. A warm shower or sitting in a tub with warm water and towels over the shoulders may help to relieve some stiffness.

17. d. Cold therapy is indicated to relieve pain during an acute inflammation, can be applied with frozen packages of vegetables, and should last only 10 to 15 minutes at a time. Heat in the form of heating pads, moist warm packs,

paraffin baths, or warm baths or showers is indicated to relieve stiffness and muscle spasm. Heat should not be applied for more than 20 minutes at a time.

18. c. The best aerobic exercise is aquatic exercises in warm water to allow easier joint movement because of the buoyancy of the water. Water produces more resistance and can strengthen the muscles. Tai Chi is also a good form of gentle, stretching exercise that would be appropriate. Dancing and walking impact the joints of the feet and even low-impact aerobics could be damaging. Exercises for patients with RA should be gentle.

19. d. The diagnosis of gout is established by finding needle-like monosodium urate crystals in the synovial fluid of an inflamed joint or tophus. Hyperuricemia and elevated urine uric acid are not diagnostic for gout because they may be related to a variety of drugs or may exist as a totally asymptomatic abnormality in the general population. Although there is a familial predisposition to hyperuricemia, both environmental and genetic factors contribute to gout.

20. b. Colchicine has an antiinflammatory action specific for gout and is the treatment of choice during an acute attack, often producing dramatic pain relief when given within 12 to 24 hours. Allopurinol, a xanthine oxidase inhibitor, is used to control hyperuricemia by blocking production of uric acid. Probenecid is a uricosuric drug that is used to control hyperuricemia by increasing the excretion of uric acid through the kidney. Aspirin inactivates the effect of uricosuric drugs and should not be used when patients are taking probenecid and other uricosuric drugs.

21. b. During therapy with probenecid or allopurinol, the patient must have periodic determination of serum uric acid levels to evaluate the effectiveness of the therapy and to ensure that levels are kept low enough to prevent future attacks of gout. With the use of medications, strict dietary restrictions on alcohol and high-purine foods are usually not necessary. When the patient is taking probenecid, urine output should be maintained at 2 to 3 L per day to prevent urate from precipitating in the urinary tract and causing kidney stones. Patients should not alter their doses of medications without medical direction and the drugs used for control of gout are not useful in the treatment of an acute attack. Joint immobilization is used for an acute attack of gout.

22. d. An unusually high frequency of human leukocyte antigen (HLA)–B27 is found in patients with ankylosing spondylitis, psoriatic arthritis, and reactive arthritis and these diseases have a predilection for involvement of the spine, peripheral joints, and periarticular structures as well as an absence of rheumatoid factor and autoantibodies.

23. d. Kyphosis and involvement of costovertebral joints in ankylosing spondylitis lead to a bent-over posture and a decrease in chest expansion, manifestations that are managed with chest expansion and deep-breathing exercises. Postural training emphasizes avoiding forward flexion during any activities and the patient should sleep on the back without the use of pillows.

24. b, f. Reactive arthritis is self-limiting and follows GI or sexually transmitted infection, with symptoms including urethritis and conjunctivitis. Methotrexate is the treatment of choice for psoriatic arthritis. Hypersensitive tender points diagnose fibromyalgia. There is increased risk of septic arthritis in persons with decreased host resistance. Joint infection may be caused by the hematogenous route.

25. a. In systemic lupus erythematosus (SLE), autoantibodies are produced to nucleic acids, erythrocytes, coagulation proteins, lymphocytes, platelets, and many other self-proteins. This is a hypersensitive response, not immunodeficiency. Overproduction of collagen is characteristic of systemic sclerosis and abnormal IgG reactions with autoantibodies are characteristic of RA.

26. c. All body systems are affected by SLE. When the atrioventricular and sinus nodes are fibrosed and dysrhythmias occur, this is ominous. Although lupus nephritis can occur and lead to chronic kidney disease, treatment is available. Anemia, mild leukopenia, and thrombocytopenia are often present. Disordered thought processes, disorientation, memory deficits, and depression may occur.

27. b. Patients with SLE often find that one of the most difficult facets of the disease is its extreme variability in severity and progression. There is no characteristic pattern of progressive organ involvement, nor is it predictable as to which systems may become affected. SLE is now associated with a normal life span but patients must be helped to adjust to the unknown course of the disease.

28. a. Efficacy of treatment with corticosteroids or immunosuppressive drugs is best monitored by serial serum complement levels and anti-DNA titers, both of which will decrease as the drugs have an effect. A reduction in erythrocyte sedimentation rate (ESR) is not as specific and the patient with SLE often has a chronic anemia that is not affected by drug therapy.

29. a. Acute exacerbations of SLE may be precipitated by overexposure to ultraviolet light, physical and emotional stress, fatigue, and infection or surgery. Dietary recommendations include small, frequent meals and adequate iron intake. Although SLE has an identified genetic association with HLA-DR3, genetic counseling is not a usual recommendation. The major concern in planning a pregnancy is that there are increased risks for the mother and fetus during pregnancy and exacerbations are common following delivery. Although nonpharmacologic methods of pain control are encouraged, the use of NSAIDs is often necessary to help control inflammation and pain.

30. a. Scleroderma is a disorder of connective tissue that causes skin thickening and tightening, resulting in symmetric, painless swelling or thickening of the skin of the fingers and hands, expressionless facial features, puckering of the mouth, and a small oral orifice. It does not cause the swan neck or ulnar drift deformities seen in RA or SLE. Low back pain and spinal stiffness are associated with ankylosing spondylitis.

31. d. One of the most common and early manifestations of CREST syndrome (calcinosis, Raynaud's phenomenon, esophageal dysfunction, sclerodactyly, and telangiectasia) is Raynaud's phenomenon, which causes paroxysmal vasospasms of the digits with diminished blood flow to the fingers and toes on exposure to cold or stress, followed by cyanosis and then erythema on rewarming. The hands and feet must be protected from cold exposure and possible burns or cuts that might heal slowly and smoking is contraindicated. Sensitivity to ultraviolet light is not a factor in scleroderma, nor is fluid intake. Cardiovascular involvement may occur but it does not require patient monitoring.

32. b. Dermatomyositis produces symmetric weakness of striated muscle and weak neck and pharyngeal muscles may produce dysphagia. Weakened pharyngeal muscles lead to a poor cough, difficulty swallowing, and increased aspiration risk. Muscle tenderness or pain is uncommon, as is joint involvement. During an acute attack the patient is so weak that bed rest is needed and passive ROM is usually required.

33. b. People with fibromyalgia typically experience nonrestorative sleep, morning stiffness, irritable bowel syndrome, and anxiety in addition to the widespread, nonarticular musculoskeletal pain and fatigue. Fibromyalgia is nondegenerative, nonprogressive, and noninflammatory. Neither muscle weakness nor muscle spasms are associated with the disease, although there may be tics in the muscle at the tender points.

34. d. The American College of Rheumatology identifies two criteria for the diagnosis of fibromyalgia: (1) pain is experienced in 11 of the 18 tender points on palpation and (2) the patient has a history of widespread pain for at least 3 months. The other findings may also be present but are not diagnostic for fibromyalgia.

35. d. The pain and related symptoms of fibromyalgia cause significant stress and anxiety is a common finding. Stress management is an important part of the treatment and may include any of the commonly used relaxation strategies as well as psychologic counseling.

36. b, d, f, g. The Centers for Disease Control and Prevention, National Institutes of Health, and International Chronic Fatigue Syndrome Study Group identified the four major criteria for diagnosis of chronic fatigue syndrome: (1) fatigue not due to ongoing exertion; (2) fatigue not substantially alleviated by rest; (3) unexplained, persistent, or relapsing chronic fatigue of new and definite onset; and (4) a reduction in occupational, education, social, or personal activities from fatigue. The other options are some of the minor criteria; four or more minor criteria must be present with the major criteria for 6 months or more before the diagnosis can be made. (See Table 65-20.)

Case Study

1. N.M. needs to know that it is not known what causes RA but that in a genetically susceptible person autoantibodies, or RF, are formed that react with substances causing inflammation and damage to a variety of organs. Inflammation and fibrosis of the joint capsule and supporting structures may lead to complete immobilization of the joint and cause deformities similar to those she is developing in her hands. She should be told that RA is a disease that affects her whole body, even though her joints are primarily affected at this time. She should be told that the fatigue and low-grade fever she has are part of the disease and that with disease control these symptoms will improve.

2. Manifestations of RA include N.M.'s painful, stiff hands and feet; fatigue; low-grade fever; and ulnar drift deviation.

3. Although diagnosis of RA is often based on history and physical findings, positive RF occurs in approximately 80% of adult patients and titers rise during active disease. Testing for ACPA is a more specific test for RA than RF. Synovial fluid analysis in early disease will show an increase in the matrix metalloproteinase (MMP)-3 enzyme and WBC count. ESR and CRP are general indicators of active inflammation. An increase in antinuclear antibody (ANA) titers is also seen in some RA patients. X-rays are not specifically diagnostic of RA, although they may reveal soft tissue swelling and possible bone demineralization early in the disease. (See Table 65-7; a score of 6 or greater is definitive for RA.)

4. Methotrexate is a chemotherapeutic agent that is used as a disease-modifying antirheumatic drug (DMARD) because it has an antiinflammatory effect, reducing symptoms in days to weeks. However, it causes bone marrow suppression and hepatotoxicity, so frequent laboratory monitoring, including CBC and chemistry panel must be done. Its dosage in RA is much smaller than that used for cancer therapy and side effects are not as common. Teaching N.M. about methotrexate is an important nursing responsibility. Along with periodic laboratory monitoring, N.M could take a daily supplement of folic acid and should report signs of anemia or any infection. Methotrexate is teratogenic and N.M. should be informed that contraception must be used during and for 3 months after treatment.

5. Protection of N.M.'s joints will be enhanced if she can maintain a normal weight; avoid tasks that cause pain; use assistive devices to prevent joint stress; avoid forceful, repetitive movements; use good posture and proper body mechanics; seek assistance with tasks that cause pain; and modify home and work environments to create less stressful ways to perform tasks. To protect small joints N.M. should be taught to maintain joints in neutral position to minimize deformity, use the strongest joint available for any task, distribute weight over many joints instead of stressing a few, and change positions frequently (see Table 65-10). She should plan regularly scheduled rest periods alternated with activity throughout the day and should develop organizing and pacing techniques that spread tasks through the day or the week. Suggesting that she take a warm shower or bath in the morning to relieve her morning stiffness might be helpful. Exercise regimens will be prescribed and she should be encouraged to follow the regimens daily.

6. Because of the chronicity and disability associated with arthritis, patients are often vulnerable to claims of unproven remedies. The nurse should recognize that the copper bracelet will do no harm but may be a waste of money for N.M. It is important to encourage her to recognize that regular, proven methods of treatment used on a consistent basis are the best way to control her condition. The more she is taught about the disease and its management, the more compliant she will be with treatment regimens.

7. Additional sources of information and sharing are available from the Arthritis Foundation (www.arthritis.org) and should be suggested to N.M.

8. **Nursing diagnoses:**
   - Acute and chronic pain *related to* joint inflammation
   - Impaired physical mobility *related to* joint pain, stiffness, and deformity
   - Fatigue *related to* disease activity
   - Ineffective self-health management *related to* use of unproven remedies
   - Risk for infection *related to* altered immune function
   - Disturbed body image *related to* chronic disease activity, long-term treatment, deformities, stiffness, and inability to perform usual activities

   Collaborative problem:
   Potential complication: bone marrow suppression

CHAPTER 66

Answer Key

1. d. One of the primary characteristics of critical care nurses that is different from those of generalist medical-surgical nurses is the use of advanced technology to measure physiologic parameters accurately to manage life-threatening complications. All nursing addresses human responses to health problems and requires knowledge of physiology, pathophysiology, pharmacology, and psychologic support to the patient and family. Diagnosis and treatment of life-threatening diseases are roles of medicine.

2. a. 1; b. 2; c. 2; d. 3

3. b. Anxiety in the intensive care unit (ICU) patient is related to the environment, which has unfamiliar equipment, high noise and light levels, and an intense pace of activity that leads to sensory overload. The nurse should eliminate as much of this source of stress as possible by muting phones, limiting overhead paging, setting alarms appropriate to the patient's condition, and eliminating unnecessary alarms during care when possible. Offering flexible visiting schedules for family members and providing as much autonomy in decisions about care as possible are indicated when impaired communication and loss of control contribute to the anxiety. Use of sedation to reduce anxiety should be carefully evaluated and implemented when nursing measures are not effective.

4. b. The caregivers of the critically ill patient are very important in the recovery and well-being of the patient and the extent to which the family is involved and supported affects the patient's clinical course. Although the cost of planning and providing critical care is a concern to caregivers, it is not the major reason that caregivers are included in the patient's care. Caregivers may be responsible for making decisions about the patient's care only when the patient is unable to make personal decisions. Most caregivers have questions regarding the patient's quality of care because of anxiety and lack of information about the patient's condition.

5. b. Decreased heart rate (HR) causes decreased cardiac output (CO). The other options contribute to an increased CO.

6. d. Impedance cardiography (ICG) is noninvasive and transmits continuous or intermittent electric current through the chest that travels through the path of least resistance: the blood. Thoracic fluid status or impedance-based hemodynamic parameters (CO, stroke volume [SV], and systemic vascular resistance [SVR]) are calculated from the average impedance of fluid in the thorax. ICG measures the change in impedance in the ascending aorta and left ventricle over time. Generalized edema or third spacing interferes with accurate signals because of the excess volume.

7. c. Increased fluid administration increases preload, which will increase CO. Diuretics will decrease preload. Intropin (dopamine) does not affect preload but increases CO with increased cardiac contractility. Calcium channel blockers do not affect preload but decrease contractility.

8. c. CO is dependent on HR and SV. SV is determined by preload, afterload, and contractility. If CO is decreased and HR is unchanged, SV is the variable factor. If the preload (determined by pulmonary artery wedge pressure [PAWP]) and the afterload (determined by SVR) are unchanged, the factor that is changed is the contractility of the myocardium.

9. b. Referencing hemodynamic monitoring equipment means positioning the monitoring equipment so that the zero reference point is at the vertical level of the left atrium of the heart. The port of the stopcock nearest the transducer is placed at the phlebostatic axis, the external landmark of the left atrium. The phlebostatic axis is the intersection of two planes: a horizontal line midchest, halfway between the outermost anterior and posterior surfaces, transecting a vertical line through the fourth intercostal space at the sternum.

10. c. The pressure obtained when the balloon of the pulmonary artery catheter is inflated reflects the preload of the left ventricle. The pulmonary artery flow–directed catheter's balloon floats into the pulmonary artery. In the absence of mitral valve impairment, the left ventricular end-diastolic pressure or left ventricular preload is reflected by the PAWP. The low pressure alarm in the arterial catheter placed for arterial blood gas (ABG) sampling detects disconnection of the line, which is a medical emergency.

11. d. During insertion of a pulmonary artery catheter, it is necessary to monitor the electrocardiogram (ECG) continuously because of the risk for dysrhythmias, particularly when the catheter reaches the right ventricle. During the catheter insertion, the patient is placed supine with the head of the bed flat. It is the health care provider's responsibility to obtain informed consent regarding the catheter insertion. An Allen test to confirm adequate ulnar artery perfusion is performed before insertion of an arterial catheter in the radial artery for arterial pressure monitoring.

12. d. Although arterial pressure–based CO (APCO) monitoring is in use with patients on mechanical (control mode) ventilation with fixed respiratory rates and there is less risk of infection, more research is needed to determine the accuracy of the measures in comparison to pulmonary artery pressure monitoring. Pulmonary artery pressure monitoring is contraindicated for patients with coagulopathy and mechanical tricuspid or pulmonic valves.

13. c. The continuous CO (CCO) method of determining CO uses a heat exchange catheter that produces and detects the change in temperature. The bedside computer displays digital measurements every 30 to 60 seconds that reflect the average CO for the past 3 to 6 minutes. Fluid boluses are not needed, as with intermittent bolus thermodilution CO (TDCO). This makes the CCO method faster, easier, and safer for the patient. SVR can be calculated with either method.

14. a. Mean arterial pressure (MAP): 75 mm Hg = (90 mm Hg + 136 mm Hg)/3

    Pulmonary artery mean pressure (PAMP):

    26 mm Hg = (38 mm Hg + 40 mm Hg)/3

    SV: 25.8 mL/beat = (3.2 L/min × 1000 mL)/124 bpm

    SVR: 1525 dynes/sec/cm^{-5} = (75 mm Hg – 14 mm Hg × 80/3.2 L/min)

    b. All of the changes in the hemodynamic parameters are characteristic findings in the patient with heart failure: increased pulmonary congestion and pressures; increased pressure in the left atrium and ventricle; increased SVR; and decreased stroke volume, CO, and systemic blood pressure (BP).

15. b. The normal central venous oxygen saturation/mixed venous oxygen saturation (ScvO$_2$/SvO$_2$) of 60% to 80% becomes decreased with decreased arterial oxygenation, low

CO, low hemoglobin, or increased oxygen consumption. With normal CO, arterial oxygenation, and hemoglobin, the factor that is responsible for decreased $ScvO_2/SvO_2$ is increased oxygen consumption, which can result from increased metabolic rate, pain, movement, or fever.

16. d. When a pulmonary artery pressure tracing indicates a wedged waveform when the balloon is deflated, this indicates that the catheter has advanced and has become spontaneously wedged. If the catheter is not repositioned immediately, a pulmonary infarction or a rupture of a pulmonary artery may occur. If the catheter is becoming occluded, the pressure tracing becomes blunted and pulmonary edema and increased pulmonary congestion increase the pulmonary artery waveform. Balloon leaks found when injected air does not flow back into the syringe do not alter waveforms.

17. d. The counterpulsation of the intraaortic balloon pump (IABP) increases diastolic arterial pressure, forcing blood back into the coronary arteries and main branches of the aortic arch, increasing coronary artery perfusion pressure and blood flow to the myocardium. The IABP also causes a drop in aortic pressure just before systole, decreasing afterload and myocardial oxygen consumption. These effects make the IABP valuable in treating unstable angina, acute myocardial infarction with cardiogenic shock, and a variety of surgical heart situations. Its use is contraindicated in incompetent aortic valves, dissecting aortic and thoracic aneurysms, and generalized peripheral vascular disease.

18. d. During intraaortic counterpulsation, the balloon of the IABP is inflated during diastole and deflated during systole. This causes decreased HR, decreased peak systolic pressure, and decreased afterload. (See Table 66-6.)

19. c. Because the IABP is inserted into the femoral artery and advanced to the descending thoracic aorta, compromised distal extremity circulation is common and requires that the cannulated extremity be extended at all times. Repositioning the patient to prevent pneumonia is limited to side-lying or supine positions with the head of the bed elevated no more than 30 to 45 degrees. Assessment for bleeding is important because the IABP may cause platelet destruction and occlusive dressings are used to prevent site infection.

20. d. Weaning from the IABP involves reducing the pumping to every second or third heartbeat until the IABP catheter is removed. The pumping and infusion flow are continued to reduce the risk for thrombus formation around the catheter until it is removed.

21. b. Ventricular assist devices (VADs) are temporary devices that can partially or totally support circulation until the heart recovers and can be weaned from cardiopulmonary bypass or until a donor heart can be obtained. The devices currently available do not permanently support circulation.

22. c. A nasal endotracheal (ET) tube is longer and smaller in diameter than an oral ET tube, creating more airway resistance and increasing the work of breathing. Suctioning and secretion removal are also more difficult with nasal ET tubes and they are more subject to kinking than are oral tubes. Oral tubes require a bite block to stop the patient from biting the tube and may cause more laryngeal damage because of their larger size.

23. a. The patient is positioned with the mouth, pharynx, and trachea in direct alignment, with the head extended in the "sniffing position," but the head must not hang over the edge of the bed. The patient may be asked to extrude the tongue during nasal intubation. Speaking is not possible during intubation or while the oral ET tube is in place because the tube separates the vocal cords.

24. b. The first action of the nurse is to use an end tidal CO_2 detector. If no CO_2 is detected, the tube is in the esophagus. The second action by the nurse following ET intubation is to auscultate the chest to confirm bilateral breath sounds and observe to confirm bilateral chest expansion. If this evidence is present, the tube is secured and connected to an O_2 source. Then the placement is confirmed immediately with x-ray and the tube is marked where it exits the mouth. The patient should be suctioned as needed.

25. c. The minimal occluding volume (MOV) involves adding air to the ET tube cuff until no leak is heard at peak inspiratory pressure but ensures that minimal pressure is applied to the tracheal wall to prevent pressure necrosis of the trachea. The MOV should be between 20 and 25 cm H_2O of pressure to prevent tracheal injury. The cuff does not secure the tube in place but rather prevents escape of ventilating gases through the upper airway.

26. 100 to 120 mm Hg

27. c. Suctioning an ET tube is performed when adventitious sounds over the trachea or bronchi confirm the presence of secretions that can be removed by suctioning. Visible secretions in the ET tube, respiratory distress, suspected aspiration, increase in peak airway pressures, and changes in oxygen status are other indications. Peripheral wheezes or crackles are not an indication for suctioning. Suctioning as a means of inducing a cough is not recommended because of the complications associated with suctioning.

28. c. Nursing care for a patient with an ET tube includes (1) hyperoxygenation before and after suctioning, (2) keeping suctioning equipment and a self-inflating bag-valve-mask (BVM) at the bedside, and (3) using either one-time use sterile suction catheters for open suction technique or a suction catheter that is enclosed in a plastic sleeve connected directly to the patient ventilator circuit, which is changed per facility protocol for the closed suction technique. Used suction catheters are not left at the bedside.

29. d. If new dysrhythmias occur during suctioning, the suctioning should be stopped and the patient should be slowly ventilated via BVM with 100% oxygen until the dysrhythmia subsides. Patients with bradycardia should not be suctioned excessively. Ventilation of the patient with slow, small-volume breaths using the BVM is performed when severe coughing results from suctioning.

30. a, e. To prevent dislodgement of the oral ET tube during care, two nurses work together; one holds the tube while it is unsecured and the other performs care. After completion of care, confirm the presence of bilateral breath sounds to ensure that the position of the tube was not changed and reconfirm cuff pressure. Suction pressure less than 120 mm Hg will prevent tracheal mucosal damage. Although the use of water swabs prevents mucosal drying, humidified inspired gas helps to thin secretions. Secretions are moved to larger airways with turning, postural drainage, and percussion; these actions will not prevent or detect tube dislodgement.

31. b, c, e. Because the patient with an ET tube cannot protect the airway from aspiration and cannot swallow, the cuff should always be inflated and the head of the bed (HOB) elevated while the patient is receiving tube feedings or mouth care is being performed. The HOB elevated 30 to 45 degrees reduces risk of aspiration. The mouth and oropharynx should be suctioned with Yankauer or tonsil suction to remove accumulated secretions that cannot be swallowed. Clearing the ventilatory tubing of condensed water is important to prevent respiratory infection.

32. c. Sedation may be appropriate. As well, having someone the patient knows at the bedside talking to him and reassuring him may decrease his anxiety and calm him. Restraints have not been shown to be an absolute deterrent to self-extubation and the patient will need ongoing and frequent assessment of need. Reminding the patient of the need for the tube may help but it may not be enough to prevent him from pulling out the tube if he becomes extremely anxious. Moving the patient near the nurses' station will not be enough to prevent self-extubation since it can be done quickly.

33. b, e. Cystic fibrosis and acute respiratory distress syndrome (ARDS) are the most likely of these diagnoses to need mechanical ventilation related to severe hypoxia or respiratory muscle fatigue. Other indications for mechanical ventilation are apnea or impending inability to breathe and acute respiratory failure.

34. a, d. Positive pressure ventilators require an artificial airway and are most frequently used with acutely ill patients. The other options describe negative pressure ventilators.

35. a, c, e. Positive pressure ventilation has a predetermined peak inspiratory pressure, which increases the risk for hyperventilation and hypoventilation because the volume delivered varies based on the selected pressure and the patient's lung compliance. The other options describe volume ventilation.

36. d. Synchronized intermittent mandatory ventilation (SIMV) is described. Assist-control ventilation (ACV) has a preset tidal volume delivered at a set frequency and more frequently when the patient attempts to inhale. Pressure support ventilation (PSV) applies positive pressure only during inspiration that supplies a rapid flow of gas with spontaneous respirations. Pressure-controlled inverse ratio ventilation (PC-IRV) delivers prolonged inspiration and shortened expiration to promote alveolar expansion and prevent collapse.

37. a. Positive pressure ventilation, especially with end-expiratory pressure, increases intrathoracic pressure with compression of thoracic vessels, resulting in decreased venous return to the heart, decreased left ventricular end-diastolic volume (preload), decreased CO, and lowered BP. None of the other factors is related to increased intrathoracic pressure.

38. d. Decreased CO associated with positive pressure ventilation and positive end-expiratory pressure (PEEP) results in decreased renal perfusion, release of renin, and increased aldosterone secretion, which causes sodium and water retention. ADH may be released because of stress but ADH is responsible only for water retention. Increased intrathoracic pressure will decrease, not increase, the release of atrial natriuretic factor, causing sodium retention.

There is decreased, not increased, insensible water loss via the airway during mechanical ventilation.

39. a. LPN; b. RN; c. LPN; d. UAP; e. RN; f. LPN; g. RN; h. UAP; i. RN; j. UAP

40. c. Neuromuscular blocking agents produce a paralysis that facilitates ventilation but they do not sedate the patient. It is important for the nurse to remember that the patient can hear, see, think, and feel and should be addressed and given explanations accordingly. Communication with the patient is possible, especially from the nurse, but visitors for an anxious and agitated patient should provide a calming, restful effect on the patient.

41. c. The patient is experiencing effects of inadequate nutrition: anemia, delayed ventilator weaning with decreased respiratory strength, decreased resistance to infection, and prolonged recovery. Hypoxemia is related to anemia. Enteral feeding would provide needed nutrition. Decreased activity may be related to muscle weakness from lack of nutrition.

42. b. A leaking cuff can lower tidal volume or respiratory rates. An SIMV rate that is too low, the presence of lung secretions, or obstruction can decrease tidal volume. A decreased $PaCO_2$ and increased pH indicate a respiratory alkalosis from hyperventilation and cardiac dysrhythmias can occur with either hyperventilation or hypoventilation.

43. b. A variety of ventilator weaning methods is used but all should provide weaning trials with adequate rest between trials to prevent respiratory muscle fatigue. Weaning is usually carried out during the day, with the patient ventilated at night until there is sufficient spontaneous ventilation without excess fatigue. If the patient becomes hypoxemic, ventilator support is indicated.

44. a. Care of a ventilator-dependent patient in the home requires that the caregiver know how to manage the ventilator and take care of the patient on it. Before final decisions and arrangements are made, the nurse should ensure that caregivers understand the potential sacrifices they may have to make and the impact that home mechanical ventilation will have over time. Placement in long-term care facilities is not usually necessary unless the caregiver can no longer manage the care or the patient's condition deteriorates.

Case Study

1. The best indicators to use to monitor D.V.'s hemodynamic status are the values determined from the pulmonary artery catheter, the urinary output, and the BP because infectious processes are altering his level of consciousness (LOC), skin temperature, and other vital signs that may commonly be used to monitor hemodynamic status. Of the hemodynamic parameters, it is most important to monitor CO, SVR, and SvO_2 because these parameters are the most out of range and suggest septic shock.

2. PEEP is used for D.V. to increase his oxygenation because his PaO_2 is decreased. However, PEEP can increase intrathoracic pressure, suppressing venous return and increasing intracranial pressure (ICP). There may also be a risk of barotrauma with PEEP >5 cm H_2O.

3. D.V.'s MAP is 64 mm Hg ($100 + [46 \times 2]/3$). The MAP that is necessary to promote tissue and cerebral perfusion and not increase ICP would be one that maintains a cerebral perfusion pressure (CPP) of 70 mm Hg. With an ICP of 22

mm Hg, MAP needs to be 92 mm Hg to maintain cerebral perfusion and not increase ICP (CPP = MAP – ICP, or 70 = 92 – 22). D.V.'s current MAP results in a CPP of 42, which is inadequate to maintain cerebral perfusion.

4. Fluid therapy would include rapid administration of 0.9% sodium chloride, colloids, or both to expand vascular volume and maintain tissue perfusion, with monitoring of pulmonary artery pressure (PAP), PAWP, and CO to evaluate fluid replacement. Lactated Ringer's solution is contraindicated because of the patient's elevated lactate levels. Antibiotics specific for cryptococcal infections, such as fluconazole (Diflucan), should be initiated immediately and a broad-spectrum antibiotic, such as an aminoglycoside, is indicated for bacterial prophylaxis. Vasopressor agents, such as norepinephrine (Levophed), dopamine (Intropin), or phenylephrine (Neo-Synephrine), are indicated to promote vasoconstriction and increase SVR. After fluid therapy has been initiated, an osmotic diuretic, such as mannitol, may be used to pull water out of the brain tissue and decrease ICP. Aspirin or other antipyretics should be given to control D.V.'s temperature because increased temperature increases the metabolic rate and oxygen need. Sodium bicarbonate is not indicated to correct the patient's acidosis unless the pH is below 7.20.

5. Gastrointestinal ischemia may cause translocation of bowel bacteria into the systemic circulation, creating a source of further infection and sepsis. Early institution of enteral tube feedings may help to promote gastrointestinal function and prevent bacterial translocation.

6. **Assessment findings:**
   - Seizures reflect the cerebral irritation caused by the inflammation of the meninges and the increased ICP.
   - Increased ICP is responsible for the Glasgow Coma Scale (GCS) score of 6 and is reflected by the ICP of 22 mm Hg.
   - The infectious process of the meningitis is reflected by the increased body temperature and the WBC count of 18,500/μL.
   - The response of the sympathetic nervous system to the inflammation and sepsis is seen in the elevated blood glucose level.
   - Most of the other findings reflect the development of septic shock, systemic inflammatory response syndrome (SIRS), and possible development of multiple organ dysfunction syndrome (MODS).
   - Shock is evident from the lowered BP, metabolic acidosis, markedly reduced SVR, and decreased urinary output resulting from poor renal perfusion.
   - Septic shock is characterized by activation of mediators that cause widespread vasodilation and increased capillary permeability, resulting in decreased SVR and high CO because of the decreased peripheral resistance. The vasodilation causes the skin to be warm and dry. Septic shock also results in poor oxygen utilization, resulting in elevated mixed venous oxygen saturation (SvO_2). All of these processes are reflected in the assessment findings in this patient.
   - The ABGs and increased lactate indicate the metabolic acidosis resulting from anaerobic metabolism of cells.

The $PaCO_2$ and HCO_3^- are low and the respiratory rate is increased, indicating the body's attempt to compensate for the metabolic acidosis by using bicarbonate to buffer lactic acid and by hyperventilation to blow off extra carbon dioxide.
   - The decreased urinary output and decreased arterial oxygenation may reflect not only poor perfusion to the kidneys and lungs but also initial organ damage and development of MODS.

7. **Nursing diagnoses:**
   - Risk for ineffective cerebral tissue perfusion *related to* cerebral tissue swelling
   - Ineffective peripheral tissue perfusion *related to* deficit in capillary blood supply
   - Ineffective protection *related to* neurosensory alterations
   - Hyperthermia *related to* inflammatory process
   - Ineffective airway clearance *related to* unconsciousness and presence of artificial airway
   - Risk for injury *related to* endotracheal intubation, mechanical ventilation, seizure activity, and environmental hazards
   - Risk for aspiration *related to* presence of artificial airway
   - Imbalanced nutrition: less than body requirements *related to* increased caloric demands and inability to take nourishment orally
   - Risk for decreased CO *related to* impeded venous return by PEEP
   - Anxiety *related to* inability to communicate, fear of death/suffocation with being critically ill and ICU environment
   - Impaired physical mobility *related to* imposed movement restrictions

   Collaborative problems:
   Potential complications: ARDS; disseminated intravascular coagulation (DIC); organ ischemia—neurologic, renal, gastrointestinal, respiratory; pneumothorax or pneumomediastinum; MODS; delirium

CHAPTER 67

Answer Key

1. d. Although all of the factors may be present, regardless of the cause, the end result is inadequate supply of oxygen and nutrients to body cells from inadequate tissue perfusion.

2. b. Obstructive shock occurs when a physical obstruction impedes the filling or outflow of blood, resulting in reduced cardiac output (CO).

3. a, b, e, f. Hypovolemic shock occurs when there is a loss of intravascular fluid volume from fluid loss (as in hemorrhage or severe vomiting and diarrhea), fluid shift (as in burns or ascites), or internal bleeding (as with a ruptured spleen). Vaccines and insect bites would precipitate the anaphylactic type of distributive shock.

4. a. Older adults with chronic diseases and malnourished or debilitated patients are at risk of developing septic shock, especially when they have an infection (e.g., pneumonia, urinary tract infection) or indwelling lines or catheters.

5. b. Hemodynamic monitoring in cardiogenic shock will reveal increased pulmonary artery wedge pressure

(PAWP) and decreased CO. The characteristic signs of neurogenic shock are bradycardia and hypotension. Septic shock manifests with decreased systemic vascular resistance (SVR) and increased CO. Hypovolemic shock is characterized by increased SVR, decreased CO, and decreased PAWP.

6. a, d, e. After sympathetic nervous system activation of vasoconstriction, blood flow to nonvital organs, such as skin, kidneys, and the gastrointestinal (GI) tract is diverted or shunted to the most essential organs of the heart and the brain. The patient will feel cool and clammy, the renin-angiotensin-aldosterone system will be activated, and the patient may develop a paralytic ileus.

7. d. Angiotensin II vasoconstricts both arteries and veins, which increases blood pressure (BP). It stimulates aldosterone release from the adrenal cortex, which results in sodium and water reabsorption and potassium excretion by the kidneys. The increased sodium raises serum osmolality and stimulates the pituitary gland to release antidiuretic hormone (ADH), which increases water reabsorption, which further increases blood volume, leading to an increase in BP and CO.

8. a, c, f. In the compensatory stage of shock the patient's skin will be pale and cool (α-adrenergic stimulation). There may also be a change in level of consciousness but the person will be responsive, the BP will be lower than baseline, bowel sounds will be hypoactive (α-adrenergic stimulation), and tachypnea and tachycardia (β-adrenergic stimulation) will occur. Unresponsiveness and moist crackles in the lungs occur in the progressive stage of shock.

9. b. Thrombocytopenia can occur. When sepsis is the cause of shock, endotoxin stimulates a cascade of inflammatory responses that start with the release of tumor necrosis factor (TNF) and interleukin-1 (IL-1), which stimulate other inflammatory mediators. The release of platelet-activating factor causes formation of microthrombi and vessel obstruction. There is vasodilation, increased capillary permeability, and neutrophil and platelet aggregation and adhesion to the endothelium. The process does not occur in other types of shock until late stages of shock.

10. d. Decreased myocardial perfusion leads to dysrhythmias and myocardial ischemia, further decreasing CO and oxygen delivery to cells. The kidney's renin-angiotensin-aldosterone system activation causes arteriolar constriction that decreases perfusion. In the lung, vasoconstriction of arterioles decreases blood flow and a ventilation-perfusion mismatch occurs. Areas of the lung that are oxygenated are not perfused because of the decreased blood flow, resulting in hypoxemia and decreased oxygen for cells. Increased capillary permeability and vasoconstriction cause increased hydrostatic pressure that contributes to the fluid shifting to interstitial spaces.

11. b. During both the compensatory and the progressive stages of shock, the sympathetic nervous system is activated in an attempt to maintain CO and SVR. In the irreversible stage of shock, the sympathetic nervous system can no longer compensate to maintain homeostasis and a loss of vasomotor tone leading to profound hypotension affects perfusion to all vital organs, causing increasing cellular hypoxia, metabolic acidosis, and cellular death.

12. d. In every type of shock there is a deficiency of oxygen to the cells and high-flow oxygen therapy is indicated. Fluids would be started next, blood cultures would be done before any antibiotic therapy, and laboratory specimens then could be drawn.

13. b. In early compensatory shock, activation of the renin-angiotensin-aldosterone system stimulates the release of aldosterone, which causes sodium reabsorption and potassium excretion by the kidney, elevating serum sodium levels and decreasing serum potassium levels. Blood glucose levels are elevated during the compensatory stage of shock in response to catecholamine stimulation of the liver, which releases its glycogen stores in the form of glucose. Metabolic acidosis does not occur until the progressive stage of shock. At this stage compensatory mechanisms become ineffective and anaerobic cellular metabolism causes lactic acid production.

14. d. In late irreversible shock, progressive cellular destruction causes changes in laboratory findings that indicate organ damage. Increasing ammonia levels indicate impaired liver function. Metabolic acidosis is usually severe as cells continue anaerobic metabolism and the respiratory alkalosis that may occur in the compensatory stage has failed to compensate for the acidosis. Potassium levels increase and blood glucose decreases.

15. a. Lactated Ringer's solution may increase lactate levels, which a damaged liver cannot convert to bicarbonate. This may intensify the metabolic lactic acidosis that occurs in progressive shock, necessitating careful attention to the patient's acid-base balance. Sodium and potassium levels as well as hemoglobin (Hgb) and hematocrit (Hct) levels should be monitored in all patients receiving fluid replacement therapy.

16. b. The endpoint of fluid resuscitation in septic and hypovolemic shock is a central venous pressure (CVP) of 15 mm Hg or a PAWP of 10 to 12 mm Hg. The CO is too low and the heart rate is too high to indicate adequate fluid replacement.

17. a. A decreased mixed venous oxygen saturation (SvO_2) indicates that the patient has used the venous oxygen reserve and is at greater risk for anaerobic metabolism. The SvO_2 decreases when more oxygen is used by the cells, as in activity or hypermetabolism. All of the other values indicate an improvement in the patient's condition.

18. d. As a vasopressor, norepinephrine may cause severe vasoconstriction, which would further decrease tissue perfusion, especially if fluid replacement is inadequate. Vasopressors generally cause hypertension, reflex bradycardia, and decreased urine output because of decreased renal blood flow. They do not directly affect acid-base balance.

19. c. Vasoactive drugs are those that can either dilate or constrict blood vessels and are used in various stages of shock treatment. When using either vasodilators or vasoconstrictors, it is important to maintain a mean arterial pressure (MAP) of at least 60 mm Hg so that adequate perfusion is maintained. The other goals would be appropriate only with either vasodilators or vasoconstrictors, not with all vasoactive drugs.

20.

Type of Shock	Medical Therapies
Cardiogenic	Restore coronary artery blood flow with thrombolytic therapy, angioplasty, emergency revascularization; increase CO with inotropic agents; reduce workload by dilating coronary arteries, decreasing preload and afterload; use circulatory assist devices, such as an intraaortic balloon pump
Hypovolemic	Fluid and blood replacement, control of bleeding with pressure, surgery
Septic	Fluid resuscitation, antimicrobial agents, inotropic agents with vasopressors
Anaphylactic	Epinephrine, inhaled bronchodilators, colloidal fluid replacement, diphenhydramine, corticosteroids

21.

Drug	Action
Diuretics (e.g., furosemide [Lasix])	Decrease the workload of the heart by decreasing fluid volume and reducing preload.
Phosphodiesterase inhibitors (e.g., Milrinone [Primacor])	Increase cardiac contractility and output and decrease preload and afterload by directly relaxing vascular smooth muscles.
Nitroglycerin (Nitrol, Tridil)	Primarily dilates veins, reducing preload.
Nitroprusside (Nipride)	Acts as a potent vasodilator of veins and arteries and may increase or decrease CO, depending on the extent of preload and afterload reduction.

Others: Angiotensin-converting enzyme (ACE) inhibitors, β-adrenergic blockers

22. c. Prevention of shock necessitates identification of persons who are at risk and a thorough baseline nursing assessment with frequent ongoing assessments to monitor and detect changes in patients at risk. Frequent monitoring of all patients' vital signs is not necessary. Aseptic technique for all invasive procedures should always be implemented but will not prevent all types of shock. Health promotion activities that reduce the risk for precipitating conditions, such as coronary artery disease or anaphylaxis, may help to prevent shock in some cases.

23. a, b, c, e, f. Skin (color, temperature, moisture), urine output, level of consciousness, vital signs (including pulse oximetry), and peripheral pulses with capillary refill should be monitored to evaluate tissue perfusion.

24. c. If the metabolic acidosis is compensated, the pH will be within the normal range. If the patient is hyperventilating to blow off carbon dioxide to reduce the acid load of the blood, $PaCO_2$ will be decreased.

25. c, d, e. Antihistamines, oxygen supplementation, and colloid volume expansion are used to treat anaphylactic shock. Epinephrine, a vasopressor, is also frequently used. Only septic shock is treated with antibiotics. Vasodilators and inotropes are only used for cardiogenic shock. Volume expansion fluids vary with each type of shock.

26. d. Although some patients in shock may be treated with antianxiety and sedative drugs to control anxiety and apprehension, the nurse should always acknowledge the patient's feelings, explain procedures before they are carried out, and inform the patient of the plan of care and its rationale. Members of the clergy should be called only if the patient requests or agrees to a visit. Visits by family may have a therapeutic effect for some patients and may increase stress in others.

27. d. A common initial mediator that causes endothelial damage leading to systemic inflammatory response syndrome (SIRS) and/or multiple organ dysfunction syndrome (MODS) is endotoxin. MODS results from SIRS. Not all patients with septic shock develop MODS, although they do have SIRS. The respiratory system is frequently the first to show evidence of SIRS and MODS.

28. d. The ischemic or necrotic tissue mechanism triggers SIRS with myocardial infarction, pancreatitis, and vascular disease. Endotoxin release is seen with gram-negative and gram-positive bacteria. The abscess formation mechanism occurs with intraabdominal and extremitiy abscesses. Global perfusion deficits are seen post–cardiac resuscitation and in shock states.

29. a, d, e. Mechanical tissue trauma triggering of SIRS occurs with burns, surgical procedures, and crush injuries. Fungi, viruses, bacteria, and parasites cause microbial invasion.

30. a. Early enteral feedings in the patient in shock increase the blood supply to the GI tract and help to prevent translocation of GI bacteria and endotoxins into the blood, preventing initial or additional infection. Surgical removal of necrotic tissue, especially from burns, eliminates a source of infection in critically ill patients, as does the use of strict aseptic technique in all patient procedures. Known infections are treated with specific agents and broad-spectrum agents are used only until organisms are identified.

31. b. Generally, the first body system affected by mediator-induced injury in MODS is the respiratory system. Adventitious sounds and areas with absent breath sounds will be present. Other organ damage occurs but lungs are usually first.

32. b. The presence of MODS is confirmed when there is defined clinical evidence of failure of two or more organs. Elevated serum bilirubin indicates liver dysfunction, a

serum creatinine of 3.8 mg/dL indicates kidney injury, and a platelet count of 15,000/µL indicates hematologic failure. Other criteria include urine output less than 0.5 mL/kg/hr, blood urea nitrogen (BUN) ≥100 mg/dL, white blood cell (WBC) count >10000/µL, upper or lower GI bleeding, Glasgow Coma Scale (GCS) score ≤6, and Hct ≤20%. A respiratory rate of 45, $PaCO_2$ of 60 mm Hg, and chest x-ray with bilateral diffuse patchy infiltrates indicate respiratory failure but not other organ damage.

Case Study

1. A.M.'s risk factors were an indwelling catheter leading to urinary tract infection (UTI) and being a compromised patient: older; chronic illnesses of diabetes, heart failure, and history of prostate cancer and myocardial infarction.

2. The nursing home staff could have used aseptic technique in catheter placement, increased fluid intake to flush the catheter, consulted with the health care provider regarding prophylactic antimicrobials, and ensured early detection of changes in urine and body temperature.

3. Release of endotoxin by gram-negative bacteria that cause inflammatory responses is the initial insult. The endotoxin binds to monocytes and lymphocytes, stimulating the release of TNF and IL-1, which in turn causes release or activation of platelet-activating factor, prostaglandins, leukotrienes, thromboxane A_2, kinins, and complement. The result is widespread vasodilation and increased capillary permeability. Histamine is also released, which causes increased capillary permeability. The end result is decreased SVR and normal or increased CO as a result of the decreased SVR. Death is associated with persistent increase in heart rate and CO, with low SVR and refractory hypotension with progression to MODS. Respiratory failure is also common as the patient hyperventilates to compensate for metabolic acidosis, which results in fatigue and then respiratory acidosis. If acute respiratory distress syndrome (ARDS) develops, the patient will need intubation.

4. The widespread vasodilation caused by the inflammatory process and increased capillary permeability causing fluid loss to the interstitium cause hypotension.

5.

Assessment Finding	Physiologic Basis	Nursing Intervention
Decreased level of consciousness	Decreased tissue perfusion to the brain and hypoxia of brain cells	Reorientation and inform the patient of all care as given
Warm, dry, and flushed skin	Massive vasodilation and increased body temperature from gram-negative bacteria	Cover patient only with a sheet
Tachycardia	Activation of sympathetic nervous system with β-adrenergic stimulation, thus increasing heart rate	Monitor heart rate and other vital signs
Tachypnea	Compensation for tissue hypoxia and metabolic acidosis	Brush teeth every 12 hours and swab lips and oral mucosa every 2 to 4 hours
Fever	Bacterial infection	Provide antibiotics and antipyretics as ordered, monitor temperature, use aseptic technique to avoid further infections
Decreased SVR	Profound vasodilation	Administer vasopressors as ordered, encourage active range of motion (ROM) or provide passive ROM to decrease blood pooling in periphery
Increased CO	Occurs as a result of decreased vascular resistance	Monitor $SvO_2/ScvO_2$
Oliguria	Inadequate renal perfusion and possible renal failure	Administer fluids as ordered and monitor input and output
Hyperglycemia	Sympathetic nervous system stimulation causes glycogenolysis by the liver	Administer insulin as ordered

6. The overall goals for this patient on admission are (1) evidence of adequate tissue perfusion, (2) restoration of normal or baseline BP, (3) return or recovery of organ function, (4) avoidance of complications from prolonged states of hypoperfusion, and (5) prevention of health care–acquired complications of disease management and care.

7. A pulmonary artery catheter was needed to monitor fluid replacement and cardiac function because of multiple system involvement.

8. Arterial blood gases:
   - ↓pH: Indicates an acidosis, typical of the metabolic acidosis of anaerobic metabolism of shock

   - ↓PaO_2: Very low, indicating a marked hypoxemia
   - ↓$PaCO_2$: Low as a result of hyperventilation to compensate for the metabolic acidosis
   - ↓HCO_3: Bicarbonate is low because it is used to neutralize the acids of anaerobic metabolism.
   - ↓SaO_2: Very low oxygen saturation. Normal is 96% to 100% and the patient's level indicates severe hypoxemia.

9. Hemodynamic pressures:
   - Right atrial pressure (RAP): Normal is 2 to 8 mm Hg. Marked vasodilation would decrease venous return to the heart and it would be expected to be decreased.

- Pulmonary artery mean pressure (PAMP): Normal is 10 to 20 mm Hg and is an indicator of afterload or systemic vascular resistance. The patient's pulmonary artery pressure (PAP) would be expected to be decreased in septic shock, where there is profound vasodilation.
- PAWP: Normal is 6 to 12 mm Hg and is an indicator of afterload or systemic vascular resistance. The patient's PAWP would be expected to be low.
- CO: Normal is 4 to 8 L/min initially. The patient's CO would be expected to be elevated, illustrating the high CO typical of septic shock.
- SVR: Normal is 900 to 1400 dynes/sec/cm^{-5}. Vasodilation would produce a decreased SVR.

10. Fluid therapy is used to increase vascular volume and BP, which increases tissue perfusion. Intropin (dopamine) is used to increase vasoconstriction to elevate systemic vascular resistance and strengthen myocardial contractions to improve CO and BP.

11. **Nursing diagnoses:**
    - Ineffective peripheral tissue perfusion *related to* maldistribution of blood
    - Altered protection *related to* neurosensory alterations
    - Hyperthermia *related to* inflammatory process
    - Risk for disuse syndrome *related to* perceptual-cognitive impairment

    Collaborative problems:
    Potential complications: heart failure; ARDS; disseminated intravascular coagulopathy (DIC); organ ischemia—neurologic, renal, GI; MODS

CHAPTER 68

Answer Key

1. c. Respiratory failure results when the transfer of oxygen or carbon dioxide function of the respiratory system is impaired and, although the definition is determined by PaO_2 and $PaCO_2$ levels, the major factor in respiratory failure is inadequate gas exchange to meet tissue oxygen (O_2) needs. Absence of ventilation is respiratory arrest and partial airway obstruction may not necessarily cause respiratory failure. Acute hypoxemia may be caused by factors other than pulmonary dysfunction.

2. b, c, e, f. Hypoxemic respiratory failure is often caused by ventilation-perfusion (V/Q) mismatch and shunt. It is called oxygenation failure because the primary problem is inadequate oxygen transfer. There is a risk of inadequate oxygen saturation of hemoglobin and it exists when PaO_2 is 60 mm Hg or less, even when oxygen is administered at 60%. Ventilatory failure is hypercapnic respiratory failure. Hypercapnic respiratory failure results from an imbalance between ventilatory supply and ventilatory demand and the body is unable to compensate for the acidemia of increased $PaCO_2$.

3. c. Intrapulmonary shunt occurs when blood flows through the capillaries in the lungs without participating in gas exchange (e.g., acute respiratory distress syndrome [ARDS], pneumonia). Obstruction impairs the flow of blood to the ventilated areas of the lung in a V/Q mismatch ratio greater than 1 (e.g., pulmonary embolism). Blood passes through an anatomic channel in the heart and bypasses the lungs with anatomic shunt (e.g., ventricular septal defect). Gas exchange across the alveolar capillary interface is compromised by thickened or damaged alveolar membranes in diffusion limitation (e.g., pulmonary fibrosis, ARDS).

4. c. There will be more ventilation than perfusion (V/Q ratio greater than 1) with a pulmonary embolus. Pain and atelectasis will cause a V/Q ratio less than 1. A ventricular septal defect causes an anatomic shunt as the blood bypasses the lungs.

5. b. Diffusion limitation in pulmonary fibrosis is caused by thickened alveolar-capillary interface, which slows gas transport.

6. b. Hypercapnic respiratory failure is associated with alveolar hypoventilation with increases in alveolar and arterial carbon dioxide (CO_2) and often is caused by problems outside the lungs. A patient with slow, shallow respirations is not exchanging enough gas volume to eliminate CO_2. Deep, rapid respirations reflect hyperventilation and often accompany lung problems that cause hypoxemic respiratory failure. Pulmonary edema and large airway resistance cause obstruction of oxygenation and result in a V/Q mismatch or shunt typical of hypoxemic respiratory failure.

7. d. In a patient with normal lung function, respiratory failure is commonly defined as a PaO_2 ≤60 mm Hg or a $PaCO_2$ >45 mm Hg or both. However, because the patient with chronic pulmonary disease normally maintains low PaO_2 and high $PaCO_2$, acute respiratory failure in these patients can be defined as an acute decrease in PaO_2 or an increase in $PaCO_2$ from the patient's baseline parameters, accompanied by an acidic pH. The pH of 7.28 reflects an acidemia and a loss of compensation in the patient with chronic lung disease.

8. c, d, e, f. Morning headache, respiratory acidosis, the use of tripod position, and rapid, shallow respirations would be expected. The other manifestations are characteristic of hypoxemic respiratory failure.

9. a. Because the brain is very sensitive to a decrease in oxygen delivery, restlessness, agitation, disorientation, and confusion are early signs of hypoxemia, for which the nurse should be alert. Mild hypertension is also an early sign, accompanied by tachycardia. Central cyanosis is an unreliable, late sign of hypoxemia. Cardiac dysrhythmias also occur later.

10. a, d, e, f. Changes from aging that increase the older adult's risk for respiratory failure include alveolar dilation, increased risk for infection, decreased respiratory muscle strength, and diminished elastic recoil in the airways. Although delirium can complicate ventilator management, it does not increase the older patient's risk for respiratory failure. The older adult's blood pressure (BP) and heart rate (HR) increase but this does not affect the risk for respiratory failure. The ventilatory capacity is decreased and the larger air spaces decrease the surface area for gas exchange, which increases the risk.

11. d. The increase in respiratory rate required to blow off accumulated CO_2 predisposes to respiratory muscle fatigue. The slowing of a rapid rate in a patient in acute distress indicates tiring and the possibility of respiratory arrest unless ventilatory assistance is provided. A decreased inspiratory-expiratory (I/E) ratio, orthopnea, and accessory muscle use are common findings in respiratory distress but do not necessarily signal respiratory fatigue or arrest.

12. a. Patients with a shunt are usually more hypoxemic than patients with a V/Q mismatch because the alveoli are

filled with fluid, which prevents gas exchange. Hypoxemia resulting from an intrapulmonary shunt is usually not responsive to high O_2 concentrations and the patient will usually require positive pressure ventilation. Hypoxemia associated with a V/Q mismatch usually responds favorably to O_2 administration at 1 to 3 L/min by nasal cannula. Removal of secretions with coughing and suctioning is generally not effective in reversing an acute hypoxemia resulting from a shunt.

13. a. When there is impaired function of one lung, the patient should be positioned with the unaffected lung in the dependent position to promote perfusion to the functioning tissue. If the diseased lung is positioned dependently, more V/Q mismatch would occur. The head of the bed may be elevated or a reclining chair may be used, with the patient positioned on the unaffected side, to maximize thoracic expansion if the patient has increased work of breathing.

14. b. Augmented coughing is done by applying pressure on the abdominal muscles at the beginning of expiration. This type of coughing helps to increase abdominal pressure and expiratory flow to assist the cough to remove secretions in the patient who is exhausted. An oral airway is used only if there is a possibility that the tongue will obstruct the airway. Huff coughing prevents the glottis from closing during the cough and works well for patients with chronic obstructive pulmonary disease (COPD) to clear central airways. Slow pursed lip breathing allows more time for expiration and prevents small bronchioles from collapsing.

15. c. For the patient with a history of heart failure, current acute respiratory failure, and thick secretions, the best intervention is to liquefy the secretions with either aerosol mask or using normal saline administered by a nebulizer. Excess IV fluid may cause cardiovascular distress and the patient probably would not tolerate postural drainage with her history. Suctioning thick secretions without thinning them is difficult and increases the patient's difficulty in maintaining oxygenation. With copious secretions, this could be done after thinning the secretions.

16. a. It is most important to assess the patient for the cause of the restlessness and agitation (e.g., pain, hypoxemia, electrolyte imbalances) and treat the underlying cause before sedating the patient. Although sedation, analgesia, and neuromuscular blockade are often used to control agitation and pain, these treatments may contribute to prolonged ventilator support and hospital days.

17. d. Hemodynamic monitoring with a pulmonary artery catheter is instituted in severe respiratory failure to determine the amount of blood flow to tissues and the response of the lungs and heart to hypoxemia. Continuous BP monitoring may be performed but BP is a reflection of cardiac activity, which can be determined by the pulmonary artery catheter findings. Arterial blood gases (ABGs) are important to evaluate oxygenation and ventilation status and V/Q mismatches.

18. a, b, c. Morphine and nitroglycerin (e.g., Tridil) will decrease pulmonary congestion caused by heart failure; IV diuretics (e.g., furosemide [Lasix]) are also used. Inhaled albuterol (Ventolin) or metaproterenol (Alupent) will relieve bronchospasms. Ceftriaxone (Rocephin) and azithromycin (Zithromax) are used to treat pulmonary infections. Methylprednisolone (Solu-Medrol), an IV corticosteroid,

will reduce airway inflammation. Morphine is also used to decrease anxiety, agitation, and pain.

19. d. Noninvasive positive pressure ventilation (NIPPV) involves the application of a face mask and delivery of a volume of air under inspiratory pressure. Because the device is worn externally, the patient must be able to cooperate in its use and frequent access to the airway for suctioning or inhaled medications must not be necessary. It is not indicated when high levels of oxygen are needed or respirations are absent.

20. a. A sedation holiday is needed to assess the patient's condition and readiness to extubate. A hypermetabolic state occurs with critical illness. With malnourished patients, enteral or parenteral nutrition is started within 24 hours; with well-nourished patients it is started within 3 days. With these medications, the patient will be assessed for cardiopulmonary depression. Venous thromboembolism prophylaxis will be used but there is no reason to keep the legs still. Repositioning the patient every 2 hours may help to decrease discomfort and agitation.

21. a. Although ARDS may occur in the patient who has virtually any severe illness and may be both a cause and a result of systemic inflammatory response syndrome (SIRS), the most common precipitating insults of ARDS are sepsis, gastric aspiration, and severe massive trauma.

22. a, c, d. The injury or exudative phase is the early phase of ARDS when atelectasis and interstitial and alveoli edema occur and hyaline membranes composed of necrotic cells, protein, and fibrin line the alveoli. Together, these decrease gas exchange capability and lung compliance. Shortness of breath occurs but it is not a physiologic change. The increased inflammation and proliferation of fibroblasts occurs in the reparative or proliferative phase of ARDS, which occurs 1 to 2 weeks after the initial lung injury.

23. c. In the fibrotic phase of ARDS, diffuse scarring and fibrosis of the lungs occur, resulting in decreased surface area for gas exchange and continued hypoxemia caused by diffusion limitation. Although edema is resolved, lung compliance is decreased because of interstitial fibrosis. Long-term mechanical ventilation is required. The patient has a poor prognosis for survival.

24. a. Refractory hypoxemia, hypoxemia that does not respond to increasing concentrations of oxygenation by any route, is a hallmark of ARDS and is always present. Bronchial breath sounds may be associated with the progression of ARDS. $PaCO_2$ levels may be normal until the patient is no longer able to compensate in response to the hypoxemia. Pulmonary artery wedge pressure (PAWP) that is normally elevated in cardiogenic pulmonary edema is normal in the pulmonary edema of ARDS.

25. c. Early signs of ARDS are insidious and difficult to detect but the nurse should be alert for any early signs of hypoxemia, such as dyspnea, restlessness, tachypnea, cough, and decreased mentation, in patients at risk for ARDS. Abnormal findings on physical examination or diagnostic studies, such as adventitious lung sounds, signs of respiratory distress, respiratory alkalosis, or decreasing PaO_2, are usually indications that ARDS has progressed beyond the initial stages.

26. b. Ventilator-associated pneumonia (VAP) is one of the most common complications of ARDS. Early detection requires frequent monitoring of sputum smears and cultures

and assessment of the quality, quantity, and consistency of sputum. Prevention of VAP is done with strict infection control measures, ventilator bundle protocol, and subglottal secretion drainage. Blood in gastric aspirate may indicate a stress ulcer and subcutaneous emphysema of the face, neck, and chest occurs with barotrauma during mechanical ventilation. Oral infections may result from prophylactic antibiotics and impaired host defenses but are not common.

27. a. Because ARDS is precipitated by a physiologic insult, a critical factor in its prevention and early management is treatment of the underlying condition. Prophylactic antibiotics, treatment with diuretics and fluid restriction, and mechanical ventilation are also used as ARDS progresses.

28. a. Positive end-expiratory pressure (PEEP) used with mechanical ventilation applies positive pressure to the airway and lungs at the end of exhalation, keeping the lung partially expanded and preventing collapse of the alveoli and helping to open up collapsed alveoli. Permissive hypercapnia is allowed when the patient with ARDS is ventilated with smaller tidal volumes to prevent barotrauma. Extracorporeal membrane oxygenation and extracorporeal CO_2 removal involve passing blood across a gas-exchanging membrane outside the body and then returning oxygenated blood to the body.

29. b. PEEP increases intrathoracic and intrapulmonic pressures, compresses the pulmonary capillary bed, and reduces blood return to both the right and left sides of the heart. Increased PaO_2 is an expected effect of PEEP. Preload (CVP) and cardiac output (CO) are decreased, often with a dramatic decrease in BP.

30. d. When a patient with ARDS is supine, alveoli in the posterior areas of the lung are dependent and fluid-filled and the heart and mediastinal contents place more pressure on the lungs, predisposing to atelectasis. If the patient is turned prone, air-filled nonatelectatic alveoli in the anterior portion of the lung receive more blood and perfusion may be better matched to ventilation, causing less V/Q mismatch. Lateral rotation therapy is used to stimulate postural drainage and help mobilize pulmonary secretions.

Case Study

1. The patient is experiencing hypercapnic respiratory failure, reflected by the elevated $PaCO_2$ and pH of 7.3. In this case, severe COPD, with destruction of alveoli and terminal respiratory units, has led to hypoventilation, with less removal of CO_2 and less space for O_2 in the alveoli. The patient with severe COPD always has some degree of decompensation resulting in chronic respiratory failure but an acute exacerbation or infection may cause an acute decompensation, thus producing an acute chronic respiratory failure.

2. The primary contributing factor to the onset of the acute respiratory failure is the pneumonia, with inflammation, edema, and hypersecretion of exudates in the bronchioles and obstructed airways (V/Q mismatch). Other factors include the presence of chronic lung disease, her age, and immunosuppression with corticosteroids. An episode of respiratory failure may represent an acute decompensation in a patient whose underlying lung function has deteriorated to the point that some degree of decompensation is always present (chronic respiratory insufficiency).

3. The primary pathophysiologic effects of hypercapnia are a respiratory acidosis resulting from retained CO_2 and hypoxemia resulting from alveolar retention of CO_2. In addition to the patient's ABG values, clinical manifestations of hypercapnic respiratory failure that she is experiencing include the dyspnea, shortness of breath, sitting in a tripod position, and using pursed lip breathing. Other manifestations of hypercapnia that the nurse should assess the patient for include morning headache, somnolence, confusion, dysrhythmias, and muscle weakness. Because the patient is also hypoxemic, she should be assessed for mild hypertension, tachycardia, prolonged expiration, and accessory respiratory muscle use.

4. The tripod position helps to decrease the work of breathing (WOB) because propping the arms up increases the anterior-posterior diameter of the chest and changes pressures in the thorax. Pursed lip breathing causes an increase in SaO_2 because it slows respiration, allows more time for expiration, and prevents the small bronchioles from collapsing.

5. NIPPV is delivered by placing a mask over the patient's nose or nose and mouth; the patient breathes spontaneously while positive pressure is delivered. It may be used as a treatment for patients with acute or chronic respiratory failure and helps to decrease the WOB, without the need for endotracheal intubation. It is not appropriate for the patient who has absent respirations, excessive secretions, a decreased level of consciousness, high O_2 requirements, facial trauma, or hemodynamic instability.

6. The nurse should monitor the patient for change in mental status, anxiety, agitation, increased pulmonary congestion, decreased I/E ratio, retraction or use of accessory muscles, pain, oxygen saturation, fatigue with breathing, dysrhythmias, decreased CO, and adequate hemoglobin concentration (should be $\geqslant$9g/dL to ensure adequate O_2 saturation). Maintaining protein and energy stores with enteral or parenteral nutrition will also help.

7. Treatment of acute respiratory failure is directed toward reversing the disease process that resulted in the failure. This patient's COPD is chronic and irreversible but the IV antibiotics are critical in treating the pneumonia that precipitated the acute respiratory failure. The bronchodilators and corticosteroids will help with airway inflammation and spasm but it cannot be expected that this patient will recover without treatment of the infection.

8. Because the patient will be at increased risk for respiratory failure, her discharge teaching should include a focus on preventing pneumonia with deep breathing and coughing, use of incentive spirometry to keep airways open, and ambulation. Optimizing hydration (2 to 3 L/day if cardiac and renal status can tolerate it) and nutrition are also important to decrease her risk by making secretions easier to expel. Because she already uses O_2 therapy at home, she should use the appropriate amount and delivery device to prevent blunting of her respiratory drive. She will also need to be taught about the medications she is receiving while in the hospital and before she goes home, especially if medications have changed from those she was previously taking at home.

9. **Nursing diagnoses:**
   - Impaired gas exchange *related to* alveolar hypoventilation
   - Ineffective airway clearance *related to* increased airway resistance and secretions
   - Ineffective breathing pattern *related to* expiratory obstruction to airflow
   - Risk for imbalanced nutrition: less than body requirements *related to* shortness of breath and decreased energy level
   - Risk for impaired skin integrity *related to* NIPPV mask

   Collaborative problems:
   Potential complications: hypoxia, hypercapnia, respiratory and metabolic acidosis, dysrhythmias, malnutrition, muscle mass atrophy

CHAPTER 69

Answer Key

1. a. 2; b. 1; c. 2; d. 4; e. 1; f. 5; g. 2; h. 3 (See Table 69-2.)
2. d. During the primary survey of emergency care, assessment and immediate interventions are made for life-threatening problems affecting airway, breathing, circulation, disability, and exposure/environmental control. The triage system is used initially to determine the priority of care for patients and history of the illness or accident is part of the secondary survey. Any emergency department should be able to stabilize and initially treat a patient who requires specialized care before transferring to another facility if needed.
3. d. Asymmetric chest wall movement may indicate a flail chest, which requires bag-mask ventilation with 100% oxygen and may require intubation. A central pulse is checked and pressure is applied to a wound when there is profuse bleeding. The cervical spine is stabilized if there is any suspicion of a head or neck injury.
4. a. Specific injuries are associated with specific types of accidents and events surrounding an incident and details of the incident and the trajectory of penetrating injuries are important in identifying and treating injury. Alcohol use is assessed with blood testing and although information may be used for regulatory agencies, the primary use of the information is for treatment of the patient.
5. b. During the "E" step (exposure/environmental control), the nurse will remove the patient's clothing and perform a thorough physical assessment. A full set of vital signs are obtained in the "F" step (full set of vital signs/focused adjuncts/facilitate family presence). The "H" step involves eliciting history and head-to-toe assessment. The "C" step (circulation) includes assessing mental status and capillary refill for signs of shock.
6. b. A nasally placed tube is contraindicated if the patient has facial fractures or a possible basilar skull fracture because the tube could enter the brain. It would not be contraindicated in the other conditions.
7. c. The mnemonic AMPLE stands for allergies, medications, past health history, last meal, and events/environment leading to the illness or injury. These things will provide information to deal with the emergency situation. The other options will be assessed if pertinent but not all of them relate to health history; many are physical assessments.
8. c. Tetanus immunoglobulin provides passive immunity for tetanus and is used in treatment of a tetanus-prone wound if the patient has not had at least three doses of active tetanus toxoid. The patient would also receive tetanus toxoid to initiate active immunity in the case of tetanus-prone wounds. If the patient has fewer than three doses of tetanus toxoid and a non–tetanus-prone wound, only tetanus and diphtheria toxoid (Td) would be administered to initiate active immunity. In the actively immunized patient, Td is administered for tetanus-prone wounds if it has been more than 5 years since the last dose and is administered for non–tetanus-prone wounds if it has been more than 10 years since the last dose.

9. b. Therapeutic hypothermia post–cardiac arrest for 24 hours after the return of spontaneous circulation (post defibrillation) improves mortality and neurologic outcomes. Patient "b" might benefit from this therapy. Patient "a" will need airway maintenance and evaluation of the cause of unconsciousness. Patient "c" should have ABCs monitored and begin the cooling process. Watch for dysrhythmias and provide fluid and electrolyte replacement. Patient "d" will need mechanical ventilation and diuretics.
10. b. Organ procurement organizations are now called to talk with families, as they are trained to screen and counsel families, obtain informed consent, and harvest organs.
11. c. Heat cramps are related to physical exertion during hot weather without adequate fluid replacement. Heatstroke is from failure of hypothalamic thermoregulatory processes. Heat exhaustion is from prolonged exposure to heat over hours or days.
12. a, d, e. In heat exhaustion, volume and electrolyte depletion, elevated rectal temperature, profuse diaphoresis, mild confusion, headache, and pupil dilation occur. Heatstroke is characterized by an elevated core temperature (above 104°F [40°C] without sweating), the need for oxygen administration and treatment with cooling methods, and a high risk of mortality and morbidity.
13. c. Rewarming of frostbitten tissue is extremely painful and analgesia should be administered during the process. The affected part is submerged in a warm water bath at approximately 98.6°F to 104°F (37°C to 40°C). Massage or scrubbing of the tissue should be avoided because of the potential for tissue damage. Blisters form in hours to days following the injury and are not an immediate concern.
14. c. Rigidness, bradycardia, and slowed respiratory rate are signs of moderate hypothermia. The ABCs are the initial priority. Active core rewarming is indicated for moderate to severe hypothermia. Axillary temperatures are inadequate to monitor core temperature, so esophageal, rectal, or indwelling urinary catheter thermometers are used. The patient should be assessed for other injuries but should not be exposed, to prevent further loss of heat.
15. b. Patients with profound hypothermia appear dead on presentation and exhibit fixed, dilated pupils; difficult-to-detect vital signs; unconsciousness; and apnea. Shivering is seen in mild hypothermia. Moderate hypothermia is characterized by slowed respirations, blood pressure (BP) obtainable only by Doppler, and rigidity.
16. d. With saltwater near-drowning fluid is drawn from the vascular space into the alveoli, impairing alveolar ventilation and resulting in hypoxia. Surfactant destruction and noncardiogenic pulmonary edema occur with both saltwater near-drowning and freshwater near-drowning. Water leaks from the alveoli to the circulation with freshwater near-drowning.
17. a. Airway and oxygenation are the first priorities. A life-threatening consequence of near-drowning of any type is

hypoxia from fluid-filled and poorly ventilated alveoli. Correction of metabolic acidosis occurs with effective ventilation and oxygenation. Lactated Ringer's solution or normal saline solution is started to manage fluid balance and mannitol or furosemide may be used to treat free water and cerebral edema.

18. a. Wood ticks or dog ticks release a neurotoxin as long as the tick head is attached to the body. Tick removal is essential for effective treatment. Tick removal leads to return of muscle movement, usually within 48 to 72 hours. There is no antidote and hemodialysis is not known to remove the neurotoxin. Antibiotics are used to treat Lyme disease and Rocky Mountain spotted fever, which are infections spread by tick bites.

19. c. The priority care for a patient with an animal bite is to clean it with copious irrigation and debridement (if necessary). Antibiotics will be prescribed prophylactically because this patient is at greater risk for infection because of his age and because the bite occurred 8 hours ago. Caring for the patient should be done before reporting the bite to authorities, if required. Rabies prophylaxis would be needed only if the neighbor's dog had not been vaccinated. The neurotoxin virus that mammals carry is rabies and the dressing will not prevent this exposure.

20. c. Hemodialysis is reserved for patients who develop severe acidosis from ingestion of toxic substances. Milk or water may be used for immediate dilution of acids such as toilet bowl cleaners. Cathartics are given with activated charcoal. Whole bowel irrigation is controversial and can cause electrolyte imbalance.

21. a, b, d, e. Gastric lavage is used for patients who ingest bleach, aspirin, iron supplements, and tricyclic antidepressants (e.g., amitriptyline). Patients who ingest caustic agents, co-ingest sharp objects, or ingest nontoxic substances should not receive lavage.

22. d. Activated charcoal will absorb any of the medication left in the stomach. Cathartics are usually given with activated charcoal to increase elimination of the toxins absorbed by the charcoal. *N*-acetylcysteine (Mucomyst) will be administered for acetaminophen toxicity. Vomiting should never be induced in a patient who is unconscious.

23. b. Botulism caused by *Clostridium botulinum* is a lethal neurotoxin that is treated by inducing vomiting, enemas, antitoxin, and mechanical ventilation. Sarin is a colorless, odorless chemical agent of terrorism that affects the nervous system. Smallpox is from a virus and causes skin lesions. Tularemia is a bacterium that primarily infects rabbits and causes influenza-like symptoms in humans.

24. d. There is no established treatment for most viruses that cause hemorrhagic fever. Plague, anthrax, and tularemia are effectively treated with antibiotics if there is a sufficient supply of the antibiotics and the organisms are not resistant to them.

25. b, c, d. There are vaccines available to protect patients against anthrax, botulism, and smallpox. There are currently vaccines in development for plague and tularemia, as well as a new one for botulism. There are no vaccines for the viruses that cause hemorrhagic fever.

26. b. Because hemorrhagic fever (e.g., Marburg virus, Ebola virus) causes hemorrhage of tissues and organs, care is primarily supportive. Intramuscular injections and anticoagulants are avoided. Care of the rodent or mosquito bite, if needed, is included in supportive treatment.

27. d. Disaster medical assistance teams (DMATs) are composed of members with health or medical skills and directly provide medical care in disaster situations. Triage is performed by first responders such as police and designated emergency medical personnel. The hospital's emergency response plan is a specific plan that addresses how personnel and resources will be used at that facility in case of a disaster and community emergency response teams provide training to communities in general to respond to disasters.

Case Study

1. Advanced age and prolonged exposure to heat over several days are risk factors for M.M.'s development of heatstroke.

2. The nurse would expect the following laboratory tests and alterations:
   - Arterial blood gases (ABGs): decreased PaO_2
   - Electrolytes: decreased serum sodium, chloride, potassium
   - Complete blood count (CBC): hemoconcentration with elevated hemoglobin and hematocrit
   - Blood urea nitrogen (BUN) and creatinine: elevated
   - Serum glucose: decreased
   - Coagulation studies: decreased prothrombin time, decreased bleeding times
   - Liver function tests: elevated enzymes
   - Urinalysis: elevated specific gravity, protein; possible microscopic hematuria; myoglobinuria

3. To cool M.M., clothing would be removed and he would be covered with wet sheets and placed in front of a fan. Consider immersion in a cool water bath. If the temperature is not reduced by these methods, administer cool fluids IV or lavage with cool fluids. Closely monitor the patient's temperature and prevent shivering, which increases core temperature.

4. The following treatment is indicated: 100% oxygen to compensate for the hypermetabolic state, with intubation and mechanical ventilation if necessary; IV crystalloid salt solution with central venous pressure (CVP) or pulmonary artery pressure (PAP) monitoring to evaluate fluid status; continuous cardiac monitoring for dysrhythmias; cooling methods with monitoring of core temperature and prevention of shivering; administration of chlorpromazine (Thorazine) if needed to control shivering during cooling process; and indwelling catheter and monitoring on intake and output.

5. M.M.'s wife should be told that M.M. is seriously ill and that there is a chance he might not recover, because heatstroke has a very high morbidity and mortality rate. She should be kept informed of the treatment he is receiving and his response to treatment and she should be provided with emotional support and an opportunity to be at her husband's bedside.

6. **Nursing diagnoses:**
   - Hyperthermia *related to* environmental exposure
   - Decreased cardiac output *related to* hypermetabolic process
   - Deficient fluid volume *related to* fluid loss greater than intake
   - Altered protection *related to* altered mental state
   - Risk for impaired skin integrity *related to* immobility

   Collaborative problems:
   Potential complications: hypovolemic shock, cerebral edema, seizures, hypoxia, electrolyte imbalance, acute kidney injury, disseminated intravascular coagulation (DIC)